NUTRITION

Second Edition

NUTRITION

Second Edition

Eva May Nunnelly Hamilton • Eleanor Noss Whitney

Second Edition
Prepared by
Eleanor Noss Whitney

WEST PUBLISHING COMPANY

St. Paul New York Los Angeles San Francisco

50 West Kellogg Boulevard
P.O. Box 3526
St. Paul, Minnesota 55165

Printed in the United States of America

Library of Congress Cataloging in Publication Data

Hamilton, Eva May Nunnelley.
Nutrition.

Slightly modified version of the 2nd ed.
Includes bibliographical references and index.
1. Nutrition. 2. Food. I. Whitney, Eleanor Noss. II. Title.
QP141.H343 641.1 82-4886
ISBN 0-314-66862-4 AACR2

Photo Credits

Cover Photo: Country Wedding by P. Bruegel. Reprinted with the permission of the Kunsthistorisches Museum, Vienna. Photo © by Meyer Wien Vl. **13** Photo © Robert Gaylord. **363** Photo courtesy of INFACT, 1701 University Avenue, S.E., Minneapolis, MN 55415.

Dedication

To my dear friend May Hamilton. You dared to embark on the writing of our books with me, and together we navigated the smooth and the rough waters. I shall always treasure our many hours together: the laughter, the excitement, the arguments, the shared sense of mission. Your spirit is still on every page and always will be.

Ellie Whitney

Acknowledgments

Annette Franklin, I thank you for your cheerful, consistent, and careful work in typing your way through all of this how many times? You've been a good sport, a willing learner, and a competent director of the efforts of Hal, Peggy, and Daisy.

Russell, I appreciate your speedy and skillful help on the computer and your honest reactions to the contents of these pages.

Thank you, too, to reviewers Sally McGill, Anne Popma, Agnes Hartnell, Mae Cleveland, and Wendy Schiff, and a special thank you to Sam Smith whose efforts far exceeded his duties. I am also grateful to Natholyn Harris, who provided the material for the Chapter 11 Food Feature, to Debbie Cleneay and Chris Kelchner for their cheerful and efficient assistance, to my colleagues, students, and friends, and to my family for your criticism, suggestions, and support.

About the Authors

Eva May Nunnelley Hamilton is an adjunct faculty with The Florida State University. She received her B.A. from the University of Kentucky and her M.S. from The Florida State University. She has been associated with science and nutrition education for over thirty-five years.

Eleanor Noss Whitney is an Associate Professor of Nutrition at The Florida State University. She received her B.A. from Radcliffe/Harvard College and her Ph.D. from Washington University in St. Louis. She has done research in nutrition as it relates to growth and development, alcoholism, and cancer, and has published articles in *Science, Journal of Nutrition, Genetics,* and *American Journal of Clinical Nutrition,* among others.

The authors have also written the college textbooks *Understanding Nutrition* (2nd ed., West, 1981) and *Nutrition: Concepts and Controversies* (2nd ed., West, 1982). This book is a slightly modified version of the latter.

Contents

Controversy List

Preface

This book is written for the reader who wants to understand nutrition as it really is, with all of its complexity, uncertainty, and controversy. If you are interested in nutrition, then you have probably already read one or many other books and have begun to be troubled by what you suspect is oversimplification, exaggeration, or inaccuracy. This book avoids those misdeeds; it is a scholarly book based on research, and it cites its many references. It tells you honestly when the answers are not known, even when it is tempting to offer answers. But it is not a dull book, nor does it require you to have a college degree in chemistry before approaching it. Nutrition is a fascinating subject, and today more than ever it is important for each person to learn and apply its principles.

In *Nutrition* we are trying to do two things. We are using the chapters mostly for solid information, on which the experts in our field largely agree. Then, to meet your interest in current "hot topics" in nutrition, we are presenting the available evidence for and against some of the most newsworthy claims in the Controversies, which are set aside on pages of a different color.

In presenting the Controversies, we have made every effort to make the issues clear and our treatment brief. But we have not watered them down. Some of today's nutrition issues are truly complex. One of the most important things we can do for you as a consumer is to help you see through oversimplifications so that you will not be misled by them. If you choose to put the effort into studying the issues, you deserve to see them presented fully and fairly, with documentation so that you can pursue them further if you wish. As a result, some of the Controversies are not light reading, but perhaps you will see between the lines the intense interest and excitement with which investigators are pursuing the questions.

In each Controversy, we have felt compelled to remain tentative in presenting conclusions. This may be frustrating for the person who wants yes or no answers, but for the questions being asked in science today, there are no firm answers yet. We would like to take credit for a certain amount of courage in presenting conclusions at all. As the editor of *Nutrition Today* points out, "These days in nutrition only one thing is certain. Neutral territory is the only place where one is sure to be shot at from both sides."*

If you find the information presented here to be useful and important, you will want to apply it in your shopping, eating out, and cooking. In anticipation of your questions, each chapter includes a Food Feature, which translates the chapter concepts into practical suggestions.

You probably agree with us that nutrition has some relation to your health. You may be motivated—if only you can get it all straight—to adopt a diet for yourself that will help you maintain your health. No doubt you are also aware of the many links between "poor" nutrition (whatever that is) and disease and would like to learn to avoid food habits that will get you into medical trouble. That is, you would like to exercise preventive nutrition. In response to that need, this book offers more information on the relationship between nutrition and disease than most others do.

But right away, you may react defensively: "Yes, but not if that means I have to give up my favorite foods." This reaction is universal, natural, and entirely understandable. In voicing it you are showing your awareness that your food preferences are deep and possibly unchangeable. You are saying (and you are right), "I don't eat what my parents and teachers tell me to eat; I eat what I like." It is a known fact that people do choose foods mostly for pleasure; you are not alone in this.

You should know right away that this book will not tell you that you must eat certain foods. Its message is not "Drink orange juice every morning" or "Eat a carrot every other day." Neither of these habits is necessary to good health. This book presents foods unemotionally as bearers of nutrients and calories, and leaves you free, if you choose, to make enlightened choices. Suppose you like chocolate bars and chocolate chip cookies equally well and must decide which to take along on an outing. Because they are equally inviting, your knowledge of what nutrients they contain may tip the balance in favor of the choice that better squares with your nutritional good judgment.

Eating is, or can be, one of life's greatest pleasures. For most people (at least in the developed countries), this pleasure is available several times a day. Yet for many, it is associated with strong mixed feelings: guilty pleasure, enjoyment mingled with anxiety. If we have a mission on your behalf, it is to relieve the guilt and anxiety and free you to choose with pleasure those foods you already like and enjoy. Many a student, after taking a nutrition course and reviewing his or her own diet, has reported, "I was surprised to find that my diet was so well-balanced and adequate"—and with a sigh of relief has continued to choose as before, only this time knowing the choices are sound. Many another has said, "I see, now, what is wrong with my diet, and I see that it's easy to change"—and then has made the change and continued to enjoy good eating, improved health, and well-being as a result. We expect this will be your experience as well.

The sequence of chapters seems logical to us, but there is no law that says you may not pass Go, that you must begin on page 1 and step on every space until you reach Stop. We encourage you to explore the entire book before you begin, especially the appendixes and index.

Appendix A, The Human Body, presents the background anatomy and physiology for those who need to review the body systems, and it may make enjoyable reading before you begin your reading of the chapters. Appendix B is a master glossary of nutrition terminology; all terms you'll see in boldface type on the pages to come are included there, as well as others you may want to look up. The composition of standard foods is presented in Appendix H (calories, protein, fat, carbohydrate, five vitamins, and two minerals). The composition of the more modern "fast foods" is prescribed in Appendix G. Other constituents of foods you might want to look up are fiber, cholesterol, and fats, sodium, potassium, and sugar; see the outside back cover to find these easily. The Recommended Dietary Allowances (RDA) for the various age-sex groups, and the U.S. RDA, used on food labels, are on the inside covers, front and back. For Canadian readers, the Canadian Dietary Standard, Exchange System, and Food Groups also appear in the Appendixes.

Sometimes people want to accumulate nutrition materials of their own. Appendix J provides a list of recommended references with the addresses from which they can be obtained. References that you might find interesting, relating to the individual chapter topics, are listed at the end of each chapter.

When I set out to prepare the index for the second edition, I tried to make it as complete as possible. The book cautions you repeatedly not to self-diagnose or self-prescribe but to seek medical advice whenever you have a condition that suggests something may be amiss. However, some of the symptoms you may encounter may indicate a nutritional problem, and if the information to help you solve that problem is in this book or its many references, then I want to be sure you find it. I have therefore collected together in the index all the behavioral and physical symptoms described here under the terms *Behavior* and *Symptoms* respectively, so that you can look them up. A moment's scrutiny of those entries shows the tremendous impact nutritional deficiencies, excesses, and imbalances can have on both mental and physical health, and should provide you with still further motivation to study the subject. But the caution should be repeated here: finding a symptom that happens to match a particular nutritional problem is *not* evidence that you have that problem, for many different kinds of medical and emotional as well as nutritional problems can give rise to the same symptoms. Please use what you find here with judgment and care.

With this caution, I invite you to enjoy reading and using this book as much as I have enjoyed writing it. And I earnestly hope it will enhance your health and your life.

Eleanor N. Whitney, January 1982

*C. F. Enloe, Jr., The dangers of being neutral (editorial), *Nutrition Today*, May/June 1977, p. 12.

NUTRITION

Second Edition

PART ONE

INTRODUCTION

Chapter 1 describes the body's basic needs and shows how newly available food choices complicate the problem of designing and consuming an adequate and balanced diet.

Chapter 2 provides the background for the study of foods and diets. To help you begin to become acquainted with foods, the most commonly used food-grouping systems are described, together with some guidelines for designing diets.

Chapter 3 provides the background for the study of the nutrients and human nutrient needs. The Recommended Dietary Allowances (RDA) and other such recommendations are introduced, and their use as a standard for assessing the nutritional status of groups of people is demonstrated. A brief overview of our most recent nutritional status surveys highlights the nutrients of greatest concern.

CHAPTER 1

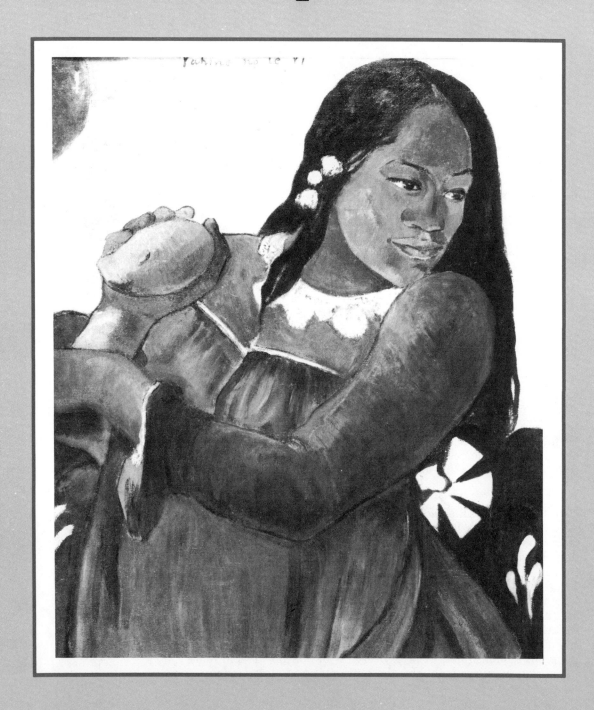

The Problem of Food Choices

You may be clothed in the latest fashions, and your car may be the latest model out of Detroit, but the body you live in is that of a caveman or cavewoman. You have come a long way from the cave dwellers in many ways: in language skills, in the arts, in medicine, and especially in the use of machinery. But in the ways your body handles food, bacteria, toxins, and air pollutants, there have been few, if any, changes. You now have essentially the same body and brain your ancestors had 12,000 years ago.

Although the body has remained the same, the world has greatly changed, especially in the last hundred years. The technological era has brought great advantages to the developed countries: an abundant, relatively low-cost food supply, massive transportation and communication networks to distribute it, the luxuries of convenience foods and high-speed cooking equipment, and many others. But with these advantages have come the attendant ills of smog, water pollution, and the necessity of mixing additives into the food supply to preserve it on its way around the world. Your cave-dweller body has no way of contending with these new problems.

Thanks to modern technology, you have far greater freedom to choose foods from a far greater variety in the local stores than people ever have had before. But with freedom comes both risk and responsibility: You have to make choices.

Opposite: A detail from Girl with Mango *by Paul Gaugin. The Baltimore Museum of Art. The Cone Collection, formed by Dr. Claribel Cone and Miss Etta Cone of Baltimore, Maryland.*

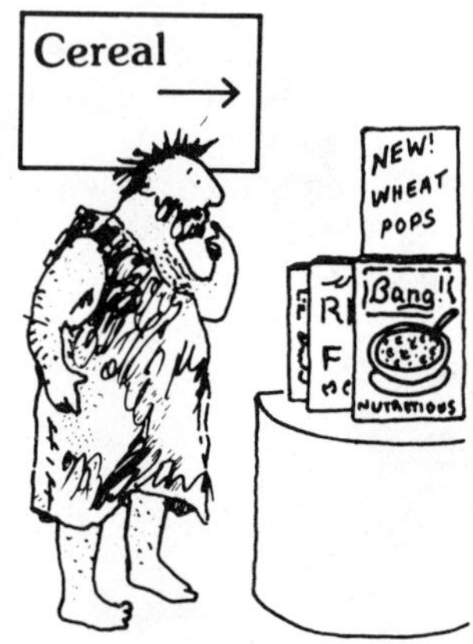

What foods best meet the needs of your cave-dweller body?

This chapter begins by describing the human body and showing the twentieth-century problems it has to deal with. Then it explains the factors affecting food choices to help you deal with them successfully.

The Ancient Body in the Modern World

At the moment of conception, you received from your mother and father the genes that determine how your body works. Many of these genes are thousands of centuries old and have not changed since your ancestors walked the earth coated with fur and carrying clubs. To know, then, what your body is equipped to do, it helps to understand the life early humans led.

For a complete description of the human body systems relevant to the study of nutrition, see Appendix A.

Hunger and food. Food was not always available. Times of famine alternated with times of feast. But with its flexible and sensitively regulated equipment the cave-dweller's body worked well. It had evolved to be able to digest food and to use the nutrients from both plants and animals. This made wide food choices possible and presented the least likelihood of starvation. The body could store excess energy nutrients when food was plentiful; then, when threatened by starvation, it could burn these energy nutrients and so stay alive. Some of the extra energy was stored in the liver, where it could quickly be retrieved to keep the body going on a minute-to-minute basis between meals. Thus the cave-dweller was relieved of the burden of eating throughout the waking hours, as many other animals still must do. The body stored the remainder of the excess energy in its fat cells to help it survive long famines and debilitating illnesses. In addition, the body had acquired a system whereby the fuel from the liver and fat cells could be called on for an immediate surge of energy in case of emergency. The extra energy helped in overcoming or outrunning enemies and was frequently needed for these purposes.

The cave-dwellers were equipped with a number of drives that helped them survive. One of these, the hunger drive, pushed them to walk long distances or work long hours to provide themselves with food. Hunger—felt frequently—drove the cave-dweller to replenish his body's fuel from the available food even when he had sufficient fuel in his own fat stores to meet temporary needs. Thus he was never likely to dip into those stores until and unless no food was forthcoming from his environment. Then he would go through an uncomfortable transition period. First, his hunger pangs would become keen and devastating, driving him to put forth his utmost effort to find food to eat. If all else failed, his body would shift to an alternative fuel source, its own fat. After this shift had occurred, the hunger pangs would be suppressed; and they would not be felt again so keenly until after he had found food and started to eat again.

Ketosis is explained in Chapters 4 and 7.

In today's world, these adaptations of the body do not provide such a great advantage because—at least in the developed countries—the food supply is no longer unreliable. In fact, many of the very characteristics that served the cave-dweller so well are now producing conditions that shorten life. The storage of excess energy, so much needed when the food supply was unreliable, is now producing obesity. Obesity is responsible for many of today's ills: It precipitates diabetes in susceptible people, it aggravates high blood pressure, it worsens arthritis, and it harms health in many other ways. We store fat in case we should need energy during famine; then, the trouble is, the famine never comes. We stay fat.

Thus today, although you have the same body and the same drives the cave-dweller had, your needs are not the same. Cave-dwellers used their brains to discover ways to obtain food—because tomorrow might bring famine or violent physical exertion. You must use yours, sometimes, to refuse delicious food and battle the ancient instincts which cry out for you to eat.

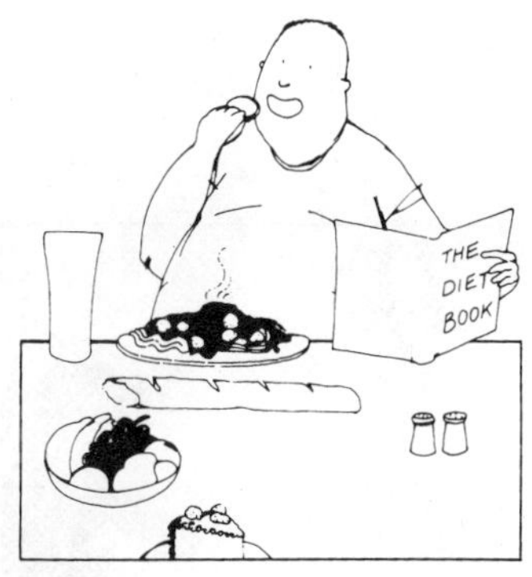

The dieter's dilemma: Help is offered in Chapters 7 and 8.

The taste for sugar and salt. Another way in which your body is like the cave-dweller's is in the taste buds on your tongue and in other parts of your mouth. The taste sensors probably helped early humans to distinguish between edible and toxic substances. Also, their enjoyment of the taste of food enhanced the hunger drive, so that they would eat large enough amounts to keep them alive until they found more food. The generally held belief is that there are four basic kinds of taste buds, each sensitive to a single taste sensation: sweet, sour, bitter, or salty.[1] Sweet and salty tastes seem to be universally desirable, but generally there is an aversion to bitter and sour tastes. The enjoyment of sweetness ensured that the cave-dwellers would consume ample energy, especially from foods containing natural sugars, the energy fuel for the brain. The pleasure of a salty taste prompted them to consume sufficient amounts of two very important minerals—sodium and chloride.

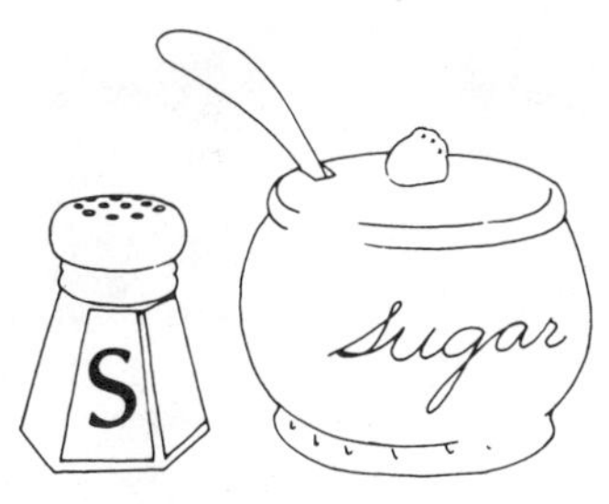

Two substances new to the body.

In modern humans, the instinctive liking for sugar and salt can lead to drastic overeating of these substances. Sugar has become available in pure form only in the last hundred years, so for the first time we can really overconsume it. And it can be added to all kinds of foods to capitalize on our sweet tooth—a problem the cave-dweller never had to deal with. As for salt, in pure form, it too is relatively newly available, and food sellers add it liberally to their products to tempt us. North Americans and Japanese are thought to eat too much salt and so to worsen their blood pressure problems.

Stress and activity. In ancient times, stress was usually physical danger, and the response to it was violent physical exertion. The body has a magnificent adaptation to the needs for emergency action. The moment danger is detected, nerves and glands pour forth the stress hormones and every organ of the body responds. The pupils of the eyes widen so that you can see better; the muscles tense up so that you can jump, run, or struggle with maximum strength; breathing quickens to bring more oxygen into the lungs; and the heart races to rush this oxygen to the muscles and enable them to burn the fuel they need for energy. The liver pours forth the needed fuel—glucose—from its stored supply, while the fat cells release fat as an alternative fuel. With all its action systems at peak efficiency, the body can respond with amazing speed and strength to whatever threatens it. This is the famous **fight-or-flight reaction**.

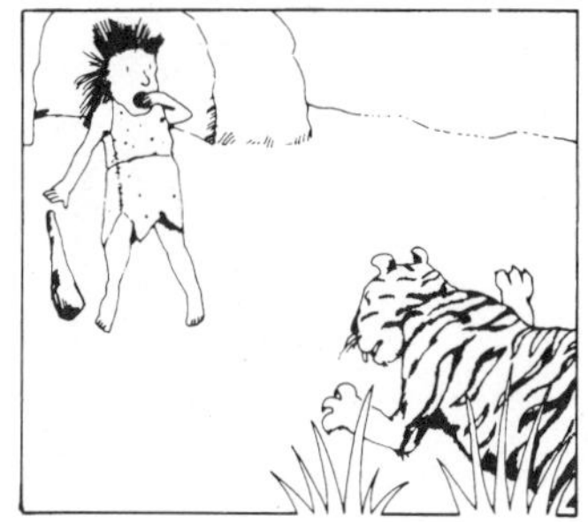
The fight-or-flight reaction, the cave-dweller's response to physical danger.

In the modern world, stress is seldom physical, but the body's reaction to it is still the same. What frightens you today may be a boss who threatens to fire you or a teacher who gives you an undeserved low grade. Under these stresses, you are not supposed to fight or run as the cave-dweller did. You smile at the enemy and suppress your fear. But your heart races, you feel it pounding, and hormones still flood your bloodstream with glucose and fat. Then the fat isn't used for fuel by your muscles but instead ends up clinging to the walls of your arteries, which harden and bring on cardiovascular disease. Your number one enemy today is not a man-eating tiger who prowls around your cave, but a disease of modern civilization: atherosclerosis. Years of fat accumulation in the arteries incur a strain on the heart that leads to heart attacks—not from overexertion but from underexertion paired with high blood pressure. It would be better, whenever you feel threatened or upset, to run, scream, or punch a pillow: to use up the fuel and exercise the heart and muscles that have been geared up for action.

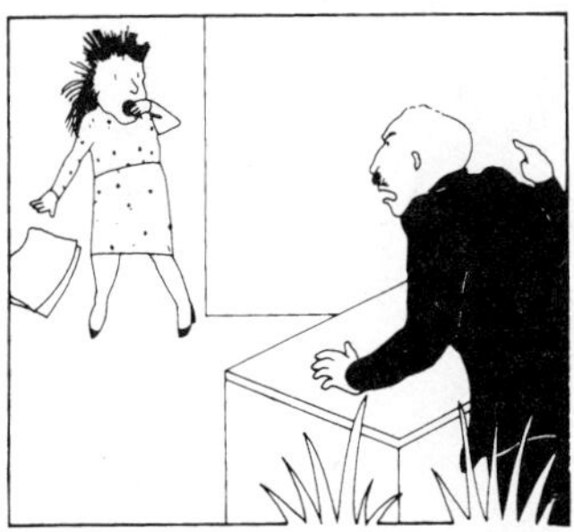

The stress reaction of today affects the body the same way as it did 12,000 years ago.

Not only our experience of stress/threat but also our experience of the "good" stress—exercise—is different from earlier times. The amount of heavy physical activity built into our lives is far less than in the past. In the last fifty years in the industrialized countries, the automobile has become an extension of the legs. Instead of walking to school or work, you probably ride; when you arrive you sit at a desk or stand at an assembly line. You probably spend several hours in the evening studying or watching television. Even a generation ago children still played games outdoors for hours every day with other neighborhood children, but now they sit passively in front of the television set watching others perform. People spend as many hours now as formerly performing the work of house and child care, but many of those hours are spent at sitting-down jobs.

The sedentary life that many people lead has serious implications for their health. Heredity gave humans a body that needs exercise. The muscles, heart muscles included, need to be used to be in the best possible condition. You should be fighting your enemies, plowing the north forty acres, or scrubbing clothes on a rock by a stream. Instead, you may get hardening of the arteries and heart attacks. People today have to make special efforts to plan exercise into their daily routines.

Protection from poisons. The body has always had to defend itself against harmful substances ingested by mistake. The sense of taste is the front line of this defense; you refuse foods that don't taste right. The second line of defense is the stomach's rejection response; you vomit up or wash out via diarrhea whatever "disagrees" with the digestive system. The third line is the liver's filtering and detoxifying systems: Toxins that get into the bloodstream are removed from it by the liver cells, which then render them harmless and put them away in permanent storage or release them for excretion in the urine.

For example, protection against the harmful effects of one ancient and familiar substance—alcohol—is built into your genes. One of those genes, expressed in your liver, codes for an enzyme that converts alcohol into substances the body can use or excrete. So long as the liver is not overwhelmed with alcohol, the system works efficiently. But alcohol has been around ever since the first fruit ripened and fermented, so there have been millions of years for natural selection to mold a detoxifying system for it.

On the other hand, most of the additives intentionally put into foods and the pollutants and toxins that get in by mistake are new to the body. If it can't excrete them, it may accumulate harmful quantities or convert them to odd, unfamiliar substances that can interfere with metabolism or cause cancer or birth defects. An important new area of study in nutrition is the study of the body's handling of these substances.

All of these differences add together into a set of circumstances that challenge your body and mind to maintain health against many odds. You are living with the food, the luxuries, the smog, the additives, and all the other problems and pleasures of the twentieth century. However, you are housed in a body designed for another era, when the weak died before they could procreate and strong men and women survived on simple foods obtained through hard physical labor. You have the freedom to choose many different kinds of foods, to eat often or seldom, to eat a lot or a little. But you have not inherited any instincts for choosing correctly. And in this country's melting pot of cultures and traditions, you may not have learned any time-tested and proven way of patterning your food intake. There is no guarantee that your diet, haphazardly chosen, will meet the needs of your cave-dweller body. Unlike your ancestors, you have to learn how your body works and what it needs from food in order to serve it best. You have to make your food choices consciously, bringing your mind into the act of nourishing your body. You have to learn how to eat—hence this book. But there is something else to be aware of as you assign to your conscious mind the task of making your food choices; it has to do with the economy of the modern world.

Food and Money

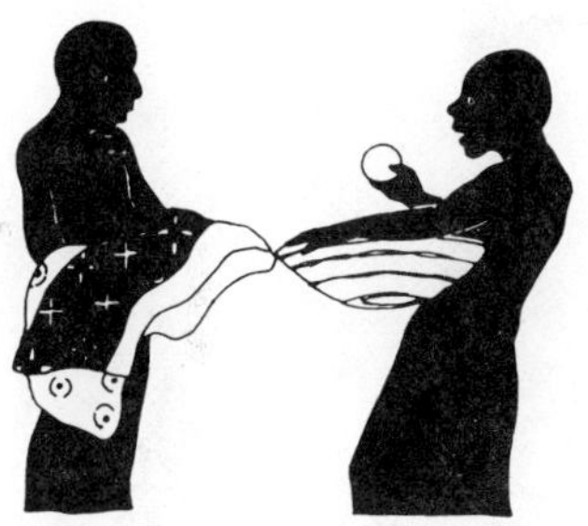

Food itself used to be the medium of exchange.

Food itself—in the form of cattle, sacks of grain, and the like—used to be the medium of exchange, because it was the most important means of survival. Now money has replaced food, and the motivation to make money has become as strong a "greed" as that for food has ever been.

Those who make money from the sale of food now bombard you with advertisements to persuade you to buy their products. The advertising and food industries have combined forces to make money from your appetite for food.

In selling their products the people of the food industry use every technique they know of. They make their food as attractive to the senses of taste, smell, and sight as they can. If this means adding sugar and salt, they do so. They process their foods so that they will remain attractive even after being on the shelf for a while.

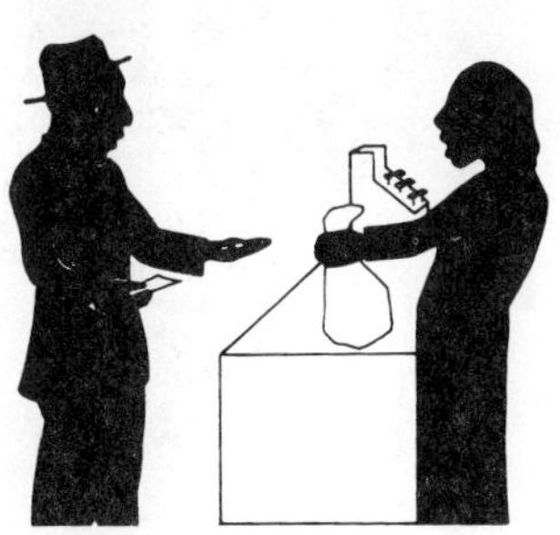

Now money has replaced food and people are "greedy" for money.

As consumers have become sophisticated enough to begin selecting foods not only on the basis of their taste appeal but also for their nutritional value, the food industry has responded by advertising its products as "nutritious." This puts you, the consumer, in the position of being bombarded from all directions with claims that "our" foods are good for you, and that "their" foods are bad for you.

You thus have a new problem deciding whom to believe in the realm of nutrition information. Some well-established food companies that formerly provided a quality-controlled, healthful product now

The primary interest of the agricultural enterprise is the financial well-being of the food producers—not the well-being of the consumers. The nutritional message of the future will be increasingly directed toward a limitation of consumption of many products. Thus the primary interests of the nutrition community and of the [food producers] will become increasingly difficult to reconcile.

—D. M. Hegsted

have gone into the business of enticing children to eat something akin to candy bars for breakfast. The advertised claim is that the bars are equivalent to a breakfast of ham and eggs. Some companies are putting out what they call cereal products that are, in reality, sugar with some added cereal. They conduct massive campaigns via children's television programs. Others offer snack foods "for energy" that are little more than fat and salt with a little flavoring. The list of food companies now producing inferior foods is endless, and the advertising for their products is convincing.

The person who wants to learn what is needed in order to achieve the best nutritional state has at least a twofold task:

> To learn what nutrients the body needs and what kinds and combinations of foods supply them.
>
> To learn what kinds of claims are made by people who sell or write about foods and nutrients and how to tell whether the claims are valid.

Basic needs of cells supplied by nutrition:
Energy fuel.
Water.
Essential nutrients.
More about essential nutrients—Chapter 2.

To help with the first task: The most basic need of the body's cells, always, is for energy fuel and the oxygen with which to burn it. Next, the cells need water, the environment in which they live. Then they need building blocks to maintain themselves—especially the ones they can't make for themselves. These building blocks—the essential nutrients—must be supplied preformed from food. These needs are among the limitations of our heredity from which there is no appeal, and they underlie the first principle of diet planning: Whatever foods we choose must provide energy, water, and the essential nutrients. The chapters of Part II are devoted to studying these needs in detail.

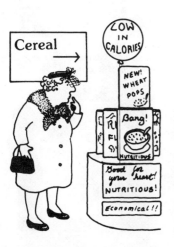

Today's buyer faces many bewildering nutrition claims.

As for the second task: Help with consumer problems will be offered throughout this book in the form of digressions like this one. Becoming skillful at recognizing false, misleading, or unproven nutrition information means learning the kinds of tricks that are used to mislead the unwary reader, viewer, or listener. One way to do this is to have a collection of "tags" to identify these tricks, like the following:

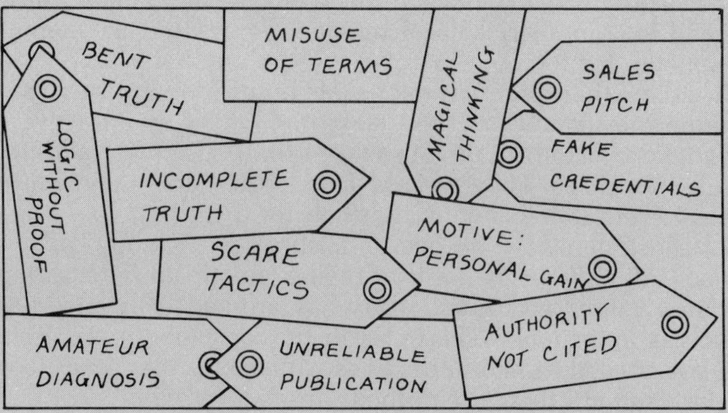

The more of these tags you can tie on a package of nutrition information, the less likely it is to be valid.

If you want not only to learn about nutrition but also to apply that knowledge, you have a third task:

> To learn what foods contain the nutrients to meet your body's needs and how to design your diet.

Part III helps with this task, while Part IV applies all these learnings to people at all stages of life, from birth to old age.[1]

For Further Information

The reader who wants to pursue this chapter's topics or any other nutrition topics further will find many references of interest described in Appendix J. In addition, we especially recommend the following.

The *Journal of Nutrition Education*, in an issue entitled "Food—Custom and Nurture," presented an annotated bibliography including several hundred references:

- *Journal of Nutrition Education* 11: Supplement 1, 1979.

An insightful paper, written long ago by the famous anthropologist Margaret Mead, shows how an understanding of puritanical feelings about food is a prerequisite to changing food habits, and how deeply they are imbedded in human nature:

- Mead, M. The problem of changing food habits. *Bulletin of the National Research Council* 108 (1943): 20-31.

According to an archaeological study on our hominid ancestors, one of the most significant steps in our evolution into human beings was our learning to share food to help each other survive:

- Isaac, G. The food-sharing behavior of protohuman hominids. *Scientific American* 200 (1978): 90-106.

A delightful paper about people's food choices is:

- Star, J. The psychology and physiology of eating. *Today's Health*, February 1973, pp. 32-37.

Star describes how he loves eating red hot peppers and explains, "Some people apparently derive pleasure from a certain degree of pain." He also describes with loving detail the modern American way of eating on the run. Star's article is reprinted in L. Hofmann's book of readings, *The Great American Nutrition Hassle*, pp. 11-21 (complete reference in Appendix J).

On human societies and their relation to food:

- Graubard, M. *Man's Food, Its Rhyme or Reason*

[1]*Chapter Notes can be found at the end of the Appendixes.*

Five short papers revealing the deep connections between primates' and people's customs and traditions and their food behavior are:

- Babcock, C. G. Food and its emotional significance. *Journal of the American Dietetic Association* 24 (1948): 390-393.
- Knutson, A. L., and Newton, M. E. Behavioral factors in nutrition education. *Journal of the American Dietetic Association* 37 (1960): 222-225.
- Mead, M. Dietary patterns and food habits. *Journal of the American Dietetic Association* 19 (1943): 1-5.
- Mead, M. Cultural patterning of nutritionally relevant behavior. *Journal of the American Dietetic Association* 25 (1949): 67-68.
- Wenkaw, N. S. Cultural determinants of nutritional behavior. *Nutrition Program News*, July/August 1969.

Controversy 1

Natural Foods

Are they better for you?

This is the first of the many controversies discussed in this book, and it deals with a subject close to many people's hearts—the foods we choose to buy and eat. No one will be completely in agreement with all that is said here. If your own view is not the first to be presented, please be aware that it will probably receive fair treatment later on. If you love whole-grain bread, for example, be assured that some very favorable statements are made about it in the chapters to come. First the cons, then the pros, of "natural" foods are given, before a balanced view is reached.

Long ago, an experiment was performed in which six rats were fed a diet of white bread and water. Within thirteen weeks, all of them were sick and their hair was falling out.[1] This experiment has been widely reported, and some people have taken it as "proof" that white bread is not nutritious, and in fact is even bad for health. Actually, however, the experiment only proved that white bread by itself does not provide all the nutrients animals need to grow and stay healthy. No other single food—not even hamburger—supports life much better. In fact, in that same experiment, six animals were fed

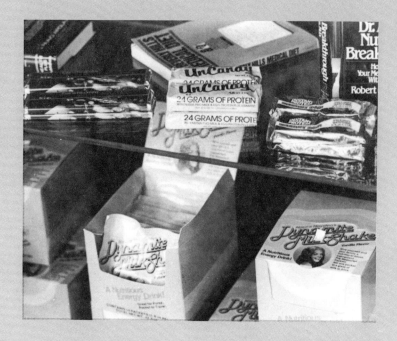

hamburger and all developed paralysis; all but one were dead by the thirteenth week. Dr. D. M. Hegsted, professor of nutrition, Harvard School of Public Health, in reporting the experiment, called these feeding routines "sole foods" and cautioned that any single food consumed in excess and in the absence of other foods may appear to be toxic.[2]

Rather than feeding them single foods, it is possible to offer rats—or human beings, for that matter—a mixed diet that includes members of all four food groups; they will then stay healthy and active and suffer no apparent ill effects. In such a diet, the bread group could be represented by the same white bread fed previously, and the meat group by hamburger as before, but two other food groups would also be represented: fruits/vegetables and milk/milk products. In this diet, the nutrient deficits of each food would be compensated for by the other foods.

Miniglossary

botulism (BOTT-you-lizm): Poisoning by the toxin produced by a certain species of bacteria (*Clostridium botulinum*); this toxin is the most potent biological poison known.

chamomile (CAM-oh-meel): One of a number of plants whose leaves, flowers, or other parts are popularly used for the making of herbal teas. Hazards are associated with the overuse of this and many others.

ginseng (JINN-seng): See *chamomile*.

health food: A misleading term used on labels, usually of organic or natural foods, to imply unusual power to promote health. This term has no legal definition as of 1981.

natural food: A food that has been altered as little as possible from the original farm-grown state. As used on labels, this term may misleadingly imply unusual power to promote health. Not legally defined as of 1981.

organic (chemist's definition): Containing carbon atoms or, more precisely, containing carbon-carbon or carbon-hydrogen bonds.

organic (popular definition): Referring to foods and nutrients, produced without the use of chemical fertilizers, pesticides, or additives. As used on labels, this term may misleadingly imply unusual power to promote health. Not legally defined as of 1981.

sassafras: See *chamomile*.

shock: An emergency reaction of the body in which the blood pressure drops suddenly; a dangerous condition.

staple: With respect to food, one which is used frequently or daily in the diet; for example, potatoes (in Ireland) or rice (in the Far East).

Would this diet of white bread, hamburger, fruit/vegetable, and milk be a healthy diet? There are two schools of thought on the merits of ordinary foods bought in ordinary grocery stores.

An article in *The Miami Herald* is typical of the "No!" answer to this question. Its headline states "OUR FOOD IS KILLING US," and it refers to grocery-store foods as "denutrified, contaminated and deeply embalmed garbage."[3] The quoted writer subscribes to the view that our food has been subjected to all kinds of violence:

- It has been processed to the point where it no longer contains any nutrients worth mention ("denutrified").
- It has been sprayed or otherwise treated with poisons that can do us harm when we eat it ("contaminated").
- It has been pumped full of additives to change its texture, color, and flavor (more "contaminated"); and it has preservatives added to make it imperishable ("embalmed").
- Furthermore, it was grown on such poor soil that it had virtually no nutritive value to begin with ("garbage").

It is dangerous, in this view, to eat such unnatural food.

People who hold this view, and there are many of them, urge consumers to abandon the grocery store and shop instead at stores that sell foods described as "organic," "natural," or "health" foods.

There are actually several issues here, and none of them is simple. All of the above accusations have to be translated into more objective language before they can be dealt with at all, and discussion of some will be postponed to later places in the book. Regarding the "denutrification" of foods, an objective wording of the question might be "Does food processing cause such great nutrient losses that consumers should seek out unprocessed foods?" A first attempt at answering this question is the discussion of refined, enriched, and whole-grain bread in the Chapter 4 Food Feature. Regarding "contamination" and "embalming" (incidental and intentional additives), a whole chapter (Chapter 11) addresses these issues. Here, let us begin to deal with the merits of "natural" foods. It is necessary to start with some definitions.

Organic, natural, and health foods. The term *organic* has two meanings. One meaning was made popular by R. Rodale, a Pennsylvania editor whose magazine *Prevention* has enjoyed a wide readership for several decades among people interested in health. According to Rodale, an organic food is a food "fertilized with manure rather than chemical fertilizers, grown without application of pesticides, and processed without the use of food additives." However, as used by chemists, the term *organic* has an entirely different meaning: it means containing organic compounds, or molecules with carbon atoms in them.[4] By this definition, all foods are organic.[5]

Anyway, when you read the word *organic* on a food label it usually conveys the Rodale meaning: free of chemical fertilizers, pesticides, and additives. The word *natural* has similar connotations but means more generally foods altered as little as possible from their original farm-grown state. *Health foods* encompass both organic and natural foods. They include "conventional foods which have been subjected to less processing than usual (such as unhydrogenated nut butters and whole-grain flours) and less conventional foods such as brewer's yeast, pumpkin seeds, wheat germ, and herb teas."[6] The latter items are supposed to have special power to promote health. None of these words has any legal meaning so they may express different intents when used on different labels.

Cons of health foods. Does the consumer buy any advantage in buying health foods? When the foods themselves have been studied, no evidence has ever been collected to show that they confer any special health benefit to the users, at least physically. But when the *users* are observed it is found that what they are trying to buy is "peace of mind." They are described as people who long for purity, who distrust technology and especially "chemicals," and who are anxious about their health.[7] Health food store operators have been seen to play the role of doctors. They "diagnose" the ailments their customers complain of and "prescribe" foods or pills or powders to relieve the symptoms. For this service, customers may pay prices inflated 50 percent or more above the prices of comparable grocery-store items.

Mail-order houses also cater, often dishonestly, to people's anxiety and needs for reassurance. Herbal products available for order by mail are required by law to carry the label:

> *The following information should not be used for the diagnosis, treatment or prevention of diseases. . . [and] should not be used to. . . replace the services of a physician. . . .*

But the people selling these products correctly anticipate that the buyers will overlook the label. Right below the disclaimer are promises that these products will help "impotence, memory, kidney and bladder complaints, arthritis, cancer . . ." (the list goes on and on). They will correct "miscarriage even after hemorrhaging and pain have begun."[8] (Imagine a woman beginning to bleed, with an impending miscarriage, delaying her trip to the doctor or hospital in order to take an herbal preparation! And yet it is easy to see why a young woman fearful of doctors and hospitals and trusting "nature" would make such a choice, even against all reason and evidence.) Almost $100 million a year are spent on herbal products, much of it by mail.[9]

Taking herbal products is risky for several reasons. They cannot be monitored or held to defined standards by government agencies, as packaged, labeled foods can be. Many contain natural toxins and should be used with great moderation, if at all. Sassafras, for example, contains the liver toxin safrole.[10] The overuse of ginseng produces a cluster of symptoms including high or low blood pressure, nervousness, sleeplessness, diarrhea, depression, confusion, and many others.[11] The popular herb chamomile can cause shock.[12] *The Journal of the American Medical Association* warns its physician readers that when they see food poisoning symptoms they should keep in mind the possibility that herbal teas from natural food stores may be involved:

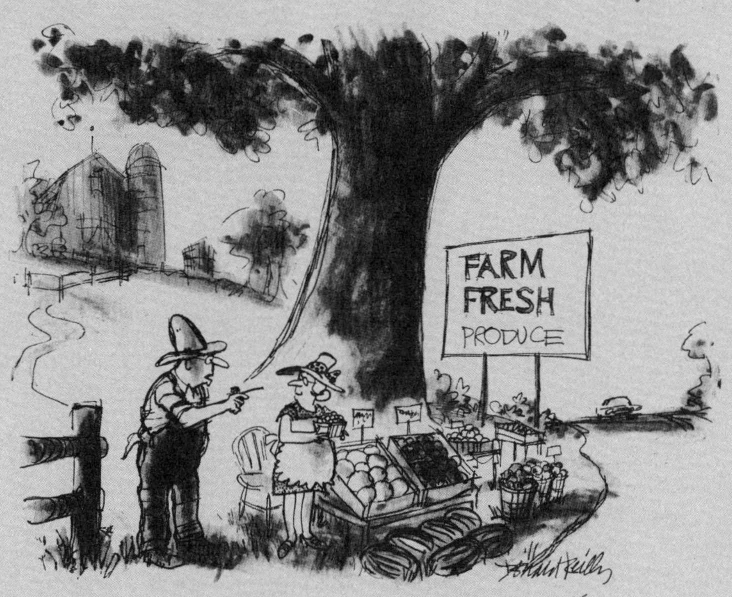

"Remember, now, the stuff is organic for those that want organic."

Drawing by Donald Reilly; © 1971 The New Yorker Magazine, Inc.

The American public is unaware of the potential dangers of certain of these products; they assume and are accustomed to the fact that foods purchased from retail stores generally have been tested and approved for human use. However, many . . . plant products have not been tested; their effects on the body are not fully understood, or their effects simply are unknown to the majority of casual purchasers. . . Unfortunately the Food and Drug Administration [FDA] does not have the authority to require such labels except via a cumbersome product-by-product procedure.[13]

As of the fall of 1979, 700 different plants had been reported to cause deaths or serious illnesses in the Western hemisphere.[14] (At the same time, there had been—apparently—no cases of food-borne illness attributed to the consumption of legally-permitted levels of artificial additives in processed foods.[15])

Among other health foods, none is innocent of all charges, even honey. Honey is susceptible to the growth of bacterial spores which produce the deadly botulism toxin. The small amounts normally involved may constitute no risk for most people, but infants under one year of age should probably never be fed honey.[16] It can also be contaminated with environmental pollutants picked up by the producer bees and is believed to be implicated in several cases of sudden infant death.[17]

More dangerous by far than either herbals or foods like honey are pills and supplements, especially of minerals. Controversy 2 deals with some of these.

From all of this information it is apparent that products sold under the label "health" may not be so healthy after all. In fact, the term is considered so misleading that the Federal Trade Commission has proposed a law that the terms *health food*, *natural*, and *organic* be prohibited from use on labels.[18] The term *organic* may also sometimes be an outright lie. Many foods sold as organic contain pesticide residues at the same levels as conventional foods, in some cases because the farmers secretly spray them and in others because pesticide residues remain in the environment from previous uses. Moreover, organic foods in several experiments have been found not to differ chemically from conventional foods.[19] And it is not surprising—even if it is disappointing—that some sellers will label their products organic just to be able to sell them at twice the price they would get for the same foods without the label. Even though this is unethical, it is not illegal; nor is it false advertising, since *organic* is not legally defined.

All of this is not to say that all health food operators are dishonest. Many are utterly sincere and are trying to sell their customers the purest and finest products. But on the whole, as you might expect, most people turning to health foods sooner or later become disillusioned. One health food store owner gave up the business because she couldn't square it with her conscience. "I just didn't believe it any more. It got to the point where I was almost hiding from my customers. I couldn't look them in the eye. After I stopped believing I just couldn't sell it any more."[20]

If health food store products often are not what they appear to be and will not do for the consumer what he hopes they will do, some questions still remain about their merits. One question of great concern in this shrinking, pollution-threatened, energy-starved world relates to the methods of organic farming. Even if organic foods do not differ chemically from conventional foods, they are produced differently. Does the method of production make any difference—to anybody?

Pros of organic farming. Organic foods are grown in soil that is fertilized only with natural waste materials such as manure and compost (rotted vegetable matter and garbage). Like "chemical" fertilizers, these materials are composed of chemicals, and they support the growth and health of plants only to the extent that they provide the chemicals the plants need: potassium, nitrogen, phosphate, and others. There is nothing superior about organic fertilizer from that standpoint. Both organic and "chemical" fertilizers can be excellent for a plant if they provide it with a "balanced diet" of nutrients, and both types of fertilizer can be poor if they provide an imbalance of nutrients or are missing one or more.[21] The ultimate chemical composition achieved by a plant depends on the genetic program it has received from its seed. It makes protein, or vitamins, or fiber according to those inherited instructions and is not at the mercy of the quality of the soil—as long as the needed raw materials are there in a usable form. Plants grow normally if they grow at all. If the fertilizer is inadequate, then the crop yield will be less—but what plants there are will be of the usual composition. The only exception to this relates to minerals. Plants grown in soil lacking iodine will produce iodine-poor fruits and vegetables, for example. But crop rotation, soil testing, soil enrichment, and crop analysis ensure that plants don't lack minerals.[22]

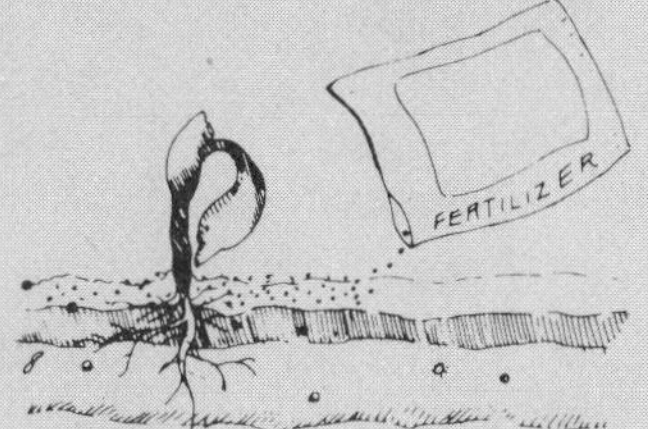

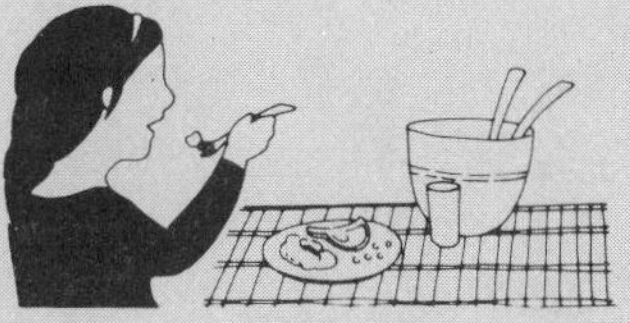

There may, however, be fringe benefits to the use of natural fertilizers like compost. For example, such fertilizers affect the structure (tilth) of the soil to give a mechanical advantage to the plant. Moreover, organic material returned to the soil is recycled in the natural way. It might otherwise be burned (polluting the air) or dumped to wash into the rivers, lakes, and oceans (polluting the water).

The recycling aspect may be one of the most significant differences between organic and conventional farming, and its chief advantage may be not to the nutrition of the individual consumer but to the ecology. J. D. Gussow, professor of nutrition, Columbia University, points out that organic farming conserves energy and doesn't pollute. In contrast, conventional agriculture consumes vast amounts of energy and produces fully *half* of the more than four billion tons of solid waste the United States generates each year. Organic farming attempts to make use of its own waste: It is "ecologically sound agriculture." Besides, it breaks no laws, and it can produce foods as safe and as nutritious as conventional foods.[23]

To sum up what has been said so far, foods carrying the labels *organic*, *health*, and *natural* have no proven nutritional advantage over conventional, comparable grocery-store foods. They are often considerably more expensive; they are often fraudulently advertised; and their use—especially that of herbal preparations—may be risky because they are not well regulated or inspected. When substituted for competent medical advice and treatment they may be tragically ill-chosen. Organic foods are often not pesticide-free, as they are claimed to be, and are not different chemically from their conventional counterparts. If any reason exists to recommend organic over conventional agriculture, it relates to the ecology, not to the food produced.

Personal strategy: What about natural foods? Does all of this mean there is *no* advantage to natural foods? The questions of food processing and additives have been postponed to later parts of the book and they need to be considered before a full answer can be given, but for the moment it might be fair to conclude with some personal recommendations. Generally speaking, the more a food resembles the original, farm-grown product, the more nutritious it is likely to be. Nutrients are lost, and often nutrient-empty additions like sugar, salt, and fat are made, during processing. A potato contains 20 milligrams of vitamin C; the same number of calories in french fries contains only about 7 milligrams of vitamin C. (By this standard, it isn't really fair to call potato chips "natural" even if they are organically grown!) An apple contains 50 international units of vitamin A, the same number of calories of applesauce contains about 30, and apple jelly contains less than 1. And so forth. Regardless of where these products were purchased—whether at the health food store or at the grocery store—there is something to be said for buying the potato and the apple. They don't have to be *labeled* natural, they only have to *be* natural, to win points in this scoring system.

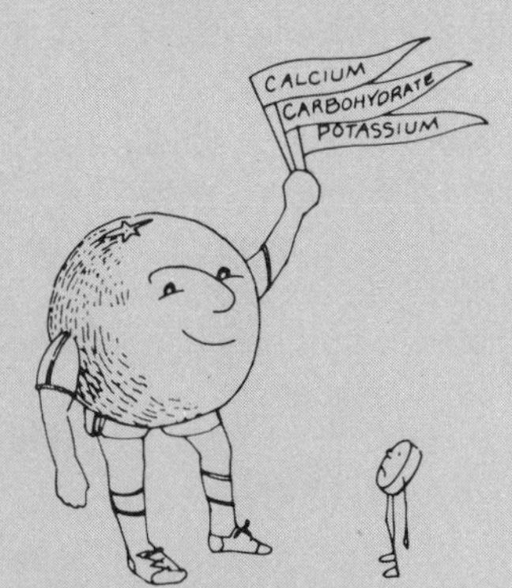

(Incidentally, something funny about health food stores is that they ignore the nutrient density principle being used here. Among their most popular items are candy bars loaded with sugar and fat which—because they are made from sources labeled "natural" like fruit sugar, honey, and carob beans rather than from cane sugar and chocolate—are advertised as superior sources of nutrients.)

When you want to choose nutritious foods, then, a useful

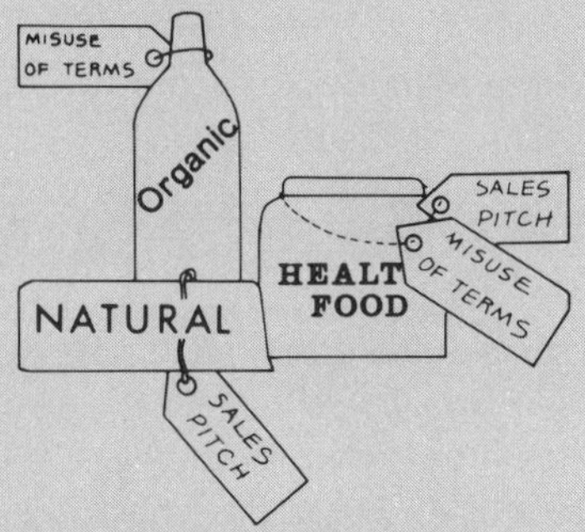

guideline is to choose whole, natural foods. But you don't have to do this all the time. Not every potato product you use must be recognizably potato. A principle that helps a great deal with making food choices is to ask, "What am I using this food for?" or "How much of a contribution does this food make to my diet?" The more you depend on a food as a staple item, the more important is its wholesomeness. In the same way, the less often or heavily you use a food, the less its quality matters. An example is the use of candy bars. If you eat them only on picnics and you picnic only once a year, fine. They'll hardly detract from your nutrition on a year-round basis. But if you are eating nothing but candy bars for breakfast and lunch every day, then they are a staple item in your diet and a very poor choice indeed. You can no doubt think of many similar examples of harmless versus harmful food practices.

Something else to keep in mind is that not all choices are necessarily positive or negative; some are simply neutral. If you happen to know an organic farmer locally and want to buy his produce, there is certainly no reason not to. His products may be more attractive, more flavorsome, more desirable to you as consumer than the same kind of foods available elsewhere. You may want to encourage him and support his "ecologically sound agriculture" even if it means paying a higher price to do so. And if you have taken a fancy to a particular product sold at the local health food store, whatever it may be, there is no reason why you should not buy it and use it in moderation. Some products sold as natural (such as the local baker's whole-grain bread, for example) are truly delicious, nourishing, and worth the extra price to consumers who have the money to spend.

But if you don't have the money, or don't have a personal preference for specific products in these special categories, there is no reason why you should make any effort in that direction. It is perfectly possible to obtain all the wholesome, nutritious foods you need for a balanced and adequate diet by making educated choices in the grocery store.

The Controversy Notes and For Further Information follow the Appendixes.

CHAPTER 2

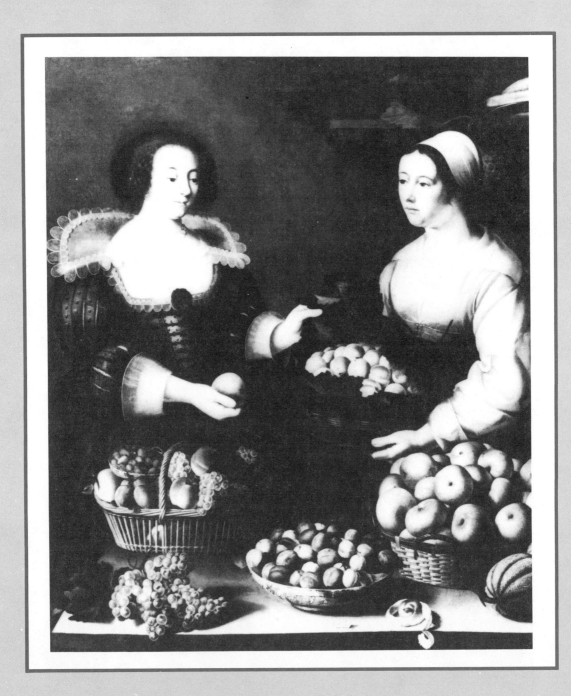

First Facts: Foods

Eating well is not difficult, in principle. All that is needed is to eat a selection of foods that supplies appropriate amounts of the essential nutrients and energy. Yet to master that principle and put it into practice may seem to be extraordinarily difficult. Consider all the people who are overweight or the tens of thousands of women and children in the United States who have iron deficiency.

Supposing that mastery is the objective, there are several questions to be answered. What are the essential nutrients? Which foods supply these nutrients? How can we eat all these foods without getting fat? This chapter answers these questions.

The Nutrients

The **nutrients** fall into six classes, and all six are found in most **foods**. Usually water predominates; the three energy nutrients—carbohydrate, fat, and protein—are next in abundance. Last come the vitamins and minerals in smaller yet significant amounts.

The six classes of nutrients:
Carbohydrate.
Fat.
Protein.
Vitamins.
Minerals.
Water.

The human body is made of similar materials, in roughly the same order of predominance. If you weigh 150 pounds, your body contains about 90 pounds of water and (if 150 pounds is the proper weight for you) about 30 pounds of fat. The other 30 pounds are mostly protein, carbohydrates (and related organic compounds made from them), and the major minerals of your bones—calcium and phosphorus. Vitamins, other minerals, and incidental extras constitute a fraction of a pound.

Opposite: A detail from At the Greengrocer *by Louise Moillon, at the Musées Nationaux de Louvre, Paris. Used with permission.*

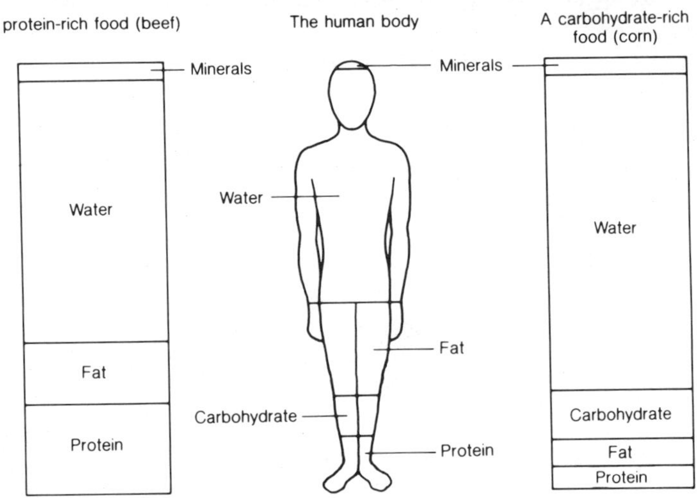

Composition of foods and of the human body. Vitamins are not shown because the quantities are too small to be seen on a graph of this size.

The next seven chapters are devoted to these nutrients. (As you are aware, however, other constituents are found in foods and in your body —organic additives, both intentional and incidental, and trace minerals, which are of no recognized positive value to humans. Some may even be harmful. Additives and pollutants are discussed in later sections of the book.)

All of the nutrients are composed of elements, or atoms, bonded together by energy. Of the six classes of nutrients, four contain atoms of carbon and are therefore **organic** (carbon-containing)—carbohydrate, fat, protein, and vitamins. This means that they can be oxidized or burned (to carbon dioxide and water) and that, when they are, energy will be released. But only three of these four—carbohydrate, fat, and protein—are oxidized in the body in such a way as to yield energy the body can use. One of the most common misconceptions prevalent among the general public is that the vitamins in some way yield energy for human use. They do not. The only significance to us of their being organic is that they are easily destroyed by chemical and physical agents such as heat and light. Therefore, we have to be somewhat careful in cooking foods that contain them.

The organic nutrients:
Carbohydrate.
Fat.
Protein.
Vitamins.
More about cooking to preserve vitamins—Chapter 9.

The energy nutrients. Only three nutrient classes—carbohydrate, fat, and protein—are **energy nutrients**. The energy they contain is measured in **calories**, familiar to everyone as the constituent in foods that makes them fattening. (Properly speaking, however, in nutrition they are kilocalories, and you will often see them referred to as ***k*calories** or ***k*cal**.) The energy they contain may be used by the body in several ways: to heat the body, to build its structures, to move its parts, or to be stored in body fat and other compounds for later use. The energy values of these nutrients appear in the margin.

The energy nutrients:
Carbohydrate.
Fat.
Protein.

1 g carbohydrate = 4 cal.
1 g fat = 9 cal.
1 g protein = 4 cal.

Not many people realize that protein can be fattening. Carbohydrate and fat are well known as calorie-laden villains against which the overweight wage constant war, but protein is not innocent in this respect. Protein does much more for the body than simply contribute calories, but an excess of any of the three energy nutrients can pad the body with an unwanted blanket of fat.

It is important not to forget one other organic compound—the alcohol found in beverages people consume. Alcohol isn't a nutrient, because it can't be used in the body to promote growth, maintenance, or repair. But it does serve as an energy (calorie) source and can be converted to fat. When alcohol contributes a substantial portion of the energy in a person's diet, its effects are damaging.

1 g alcohol = 7 cal.
More about alcohol—Chapter 14.

Practically all foods contain mixtures of the three energy nutrients, although they are sometimes classed by the predominant nutrient. A protein-rich food like beef actually contains a lot of fat as well as protein. A carbohydrate-rich food like corn also contains fat (corn oil) and protein. Thus it is incorrect to say that you are eating a protein when you eat meat; you are eating a protein-rich food. Only a few foods are exceptions to this rule, the common ones being sugar (which is almost pure carbohydrate) and oil (which is almost pure fat).

The essential nutrients. The body can make some nutrients from others. For example, it can convert some of the amino acids (parts of protein) into carbohydrate, if need be. It can manufacture one of the vitamins—niacin—from a certain amino acid. It can make most of its fats and oils from any of several different raw materials. But there are certain compounds absolutely indispensable to body function that the body cannot make for itself, and these are termed the **essential nutrients**. When used this way, the word *essential* doesn't mean just necessary. Many compounds the body makes for itself are necessary for good health. But *essential nutrient* means a nutrient that is needed in the diet because the body cannot make it for itself.

The essential nutrients:
- *Carbohydrate.*
- *Fat (linoleic acid).*
- *Protein (eight amino acids plus one for infants).*
- *Vitamins (thirteen now known).*
- *Minerals (fifteen now known).*
- *Water.*

The nutrients now known to be essential for human beings are listed in the margin. The list shows that there are about forty nutrients to be concerned about. Each nutrient also has an amount tied to it—how much you need. It may be a relief to discover, after a little more reading and thought, that diet planning can be reduced to a few simple principles to ensure that you take in all the nutrients in appropriate amounts without having to count and weigh each one. After all, you don't buy and cook nutrients; you usually think in terms of foods. The use of a food group plan makes it possible to design a diet that meets all your nutrient needs. (If you choose to think in terms of nutrients, however, you use a standard such as the Recommended Dietary Allowances of the United States, the Dietary Standard for Canada, or the standards of the World Health Organization. These standards are presented in the next chapter.)

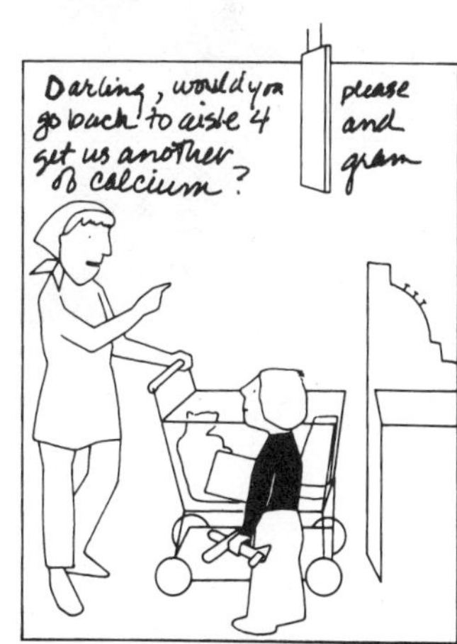
Darling, would you go back to aisle 4 get us another ℔ calcium?
please and gram
When you shop for food, you're really buying nutrients.

Food Group Plans

The individual nutrients are treated in later chapters, but two of them —iron and calcium—are used here to show why dietary balance is

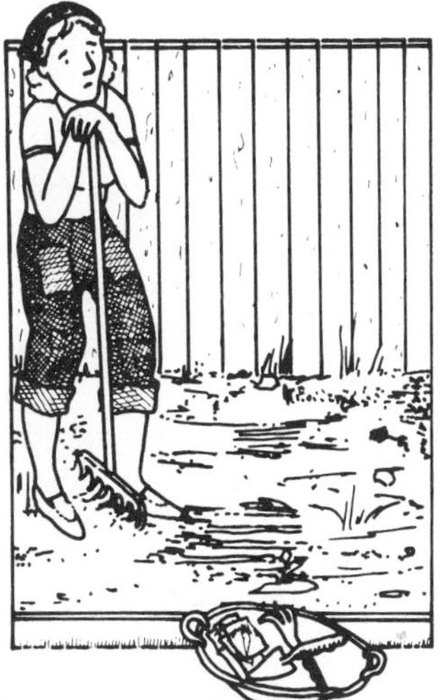
An iron deficiency makes a person tired.

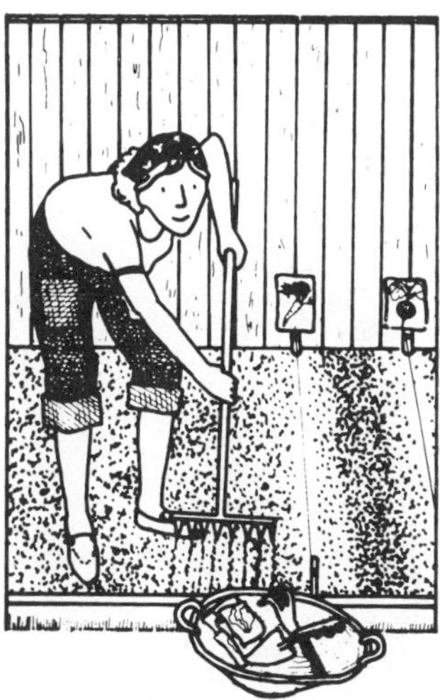
When iron is replenished, energy returns.

important. Iron is one of the essential nutrients: You can only get it into your body by eating foods that contain it. If you miss out on these foods you can develop iron-deficiency anemia: You feel weak, tired, and unenthusiastic, may have frequent headaches, and can do very little muscular work without disabling fatigue. If you make the needed correction and add iron-rich foods to your diet, you soon feel more energetic.

Some foods are rich in iron; others are notoriously poor. Meats, fish, poultry, and legumes are in the iron-rich category, and an easy way to obtain the needed iron is to include these foods in your diet regularly. Most food group plans recommend two or more servings a day.

Calcium is another essential nutrient. A diet lacking calcium causes poor bone development during the growing years and a gradual bone loss in adults that can totally cripple a person in later life. The foods just named (meats and meat substitutes) are poor sources of calcium; you can get enough of this nutrient only by making frequent use of milk and milk products or carefully selected milk substitutes. Most food group plans recommend two or more cups of milk or the equivalent every day for adults and more for growing children, teenagers, and women who are either pregnant or breastfeeding their babies.

Foods that are rich in iron are poor in calcium and vice versa. In fact, milk (except breast milk) and milk products are so poor in iron that the overuse of these foods can actually cause iron-deficiency anemia by displacing iron in the diet. The anemia even has a special name: milk anemia. And yet no one could accuse milk of being a nonnutritious food: It is the single most nutritious food for children and is important in the diet of people of all ages.

The concept being developed here is that of dietary **balance**. Use enough—but not too much—meat/meat substitutes for iron; use enough—but not too much—milk/milk products for calcium. Save some space in the diet for other foods needed for other nutrients.

Iron and calcium are only two of the nearly forty essential nutrients. What foods provide the others? One of the most familiar systems of grouping foods fits them all into four groups, as shown in Table 1. Each of the four groups contains foods that are similar in origin and nutrient content. The nutrients named in the table are representative of all the nutrients, and the assumption is that once you've got adequate amounts of these you'll probably have enough of the other two dozen or so essential nutrients as well, because they occur in the same groups of foods.

The Four Food Group Plan specifies that a certain quantity of food must be consumed from each group. For the adult, the number of servings recommended is two, two, four, and four (see Table 2).

Many foods that we eat don't fit into any of the four food groups. Consider butter, margarine, cream, sour cream, salad dressing, mayonnaise, jam, jelly, broth, coffee, tea, alcoholic beverages, synthetic products, and others. These items are grouped together into a miscellaneous category. Some of them do contribute some nutrients to the day's intake. However, either they are not foods, their nutrient content is not significant in enough of the nutrients characteristic of a

Table 1. The Four Food Groups[a]

Food Group	Sample Foods	Main Nutrient Contributions
Meat and meat substitutes	Beef, pork, lamb, fish, poultry, eggs, nuts, legumes	Protein, iron, riboflavin, niacin, zinc, vitamin B_{12}[b]
Milk and milk products	Milk, buttermilk, yogurt, cheese, cottage cheese, soy milk, ice cream	Calcium, protein, riboflavin, zinc, vitamin B_{12}[b]
Fruits and vegetables	All	Vitamin A, vitamin C[c]
Grains (bread and cereal products)	All whole-grain[d] and enriched flours and products	Additional amounts of niacin, iron, thiamin[e]

[a] This is a U.S. plan. A similar plan developed for Canada is presented in Appendix M.

[b] Vitamin B_{12} is contributed only by the animal food members of this group.

[c] Dark green and deep orange vegetables are especially reliable vitamin A sources; other fruits and vegetables are not. For vitamin C, citrus fruits, green leafy vegetables, and selected other fruits and vegetables are superior sources. See Chapter 9 for more details.

[d] Whole grains include wheat, oats, rice, barley, millet, rye, bulgar.

[e] One serving is not a significant source of any of these nutrients but if the recommended four or more servings are eaten, they contribute significant quantities to the diet. This group also contributes most of the complex carbohydrate of the diet. Whole-grain products are highly recommended in place of refined enriched products. For more details, see Chapter 4.

food group, or their nutrient content has been greatly diluted by fat, sugar, or water.

The Four Food Group Plan appears quite rigid, but it can be used with great flexibility once its intent is understood. For example, cheese can be substituted for milk because it supplies protein, calcium, and riboflavin in about the same amounts. Legumes and nuts are alternative choices for meats. The plan can be adapted to casseroles and other mixed dishes and to different national and cultural cuisines.

The Modified Four Food Group Plan

Since the Four Food Group Plan was originally devised, many more nutrients have been discovered and studied. A test of the plan as real people apply it shows that a person can follow all its guidelines and still fail to meet the day's needs for some of these nutrients—especially

Table 2. Servings in the Four Food Group Plan

Food Group	Servings (adult)	Serving Size
Meat and meat substitutes	2	2–3 oz cooked meat, fish, or chicken; ¼ cup tuna; 2 eggs; 4 tbsp peanut butter; 1 cup cooked legumes; ½ cup nuts
Milk and milk products	2[a]	1 cup (8 oz) milk; 1 cup yogurt; 1 ½ cup cottage cheese; 2 cups ice cream; 5 tbsp milk pudding; 1–2 oz cheese
Fruits and vegetables	4[b]	½ cup fruit, vegetable, or juice; 1 medium apple, orange, banana, or peach
Grains (bread and cereal products)	4[c]	1 slice bread; ½ cup cooked cereal, 1 cup (1 oz) ready-to-eat cereal; ½ hamburger or hot dog bun or English muffin; ½ cup cooked rice, grits, macaroni, or spaghetti; 2 tbsp flour; 6 saltines; 1 6-inch tortilla

[a] For children up to 9, 2–3 cups; for children 9 to 12, 3–4 cups; for teenagers and pregnant women, 3–4 cups; for nursing mothers, 4 cups or more.

[b] One should be rich in vitamin C; at least one every other day should be rich in vitamin A.

[c] Enriched or whole-grain products only.

vitamin B_6, magnesium, zinc, and vitamin E. Iron is also a problem, as it has been from the beginning.

A modification of the Four Food Group Plan devised to solve these problems was published in 1978. It recommends:

Two servings milk/milk products (as before).

Two servings meat, fish, or poultry (serving size 3 ounces, not 2 to 3 ounces).

Two servings legumes and/or nuts (portion size ¾ cup), to provide more of the five nutrients just mentioned.

Four servings fruits and vegetables (as before).

Four servings whole-grain (not enriched) products, for more of those same nutrients.

One serving fat or oil (for vitamin E).

Most selections of food based on this plan would supply 100 percent of the recommended amounts of all nutrients for men and all except iron for women and would miss providing a woman's full recommended amount of iron by only 10 percent. The average energy content of a diet selected according to this plan, however, is high—2200 calories—and the authors of the plan acknowledge that this is a disadvantage. It restricts the freedom of food choices for a person who may have a calorie allowance no higher than 2200 calories. But they feel that this disadvantage is outweighed by the advantage of a virtual guarantee of diet adequacy.[1]

Food Groups for Vegetarians

The vegetarian faces a special problem in diet planning—that of obtaining the needed nutrients from fewer food groups. There are two major classes of vegetarians (with many variations): The **lacto-ovo-vegetarian** uses milk and eggs (animal products) but excludes meat, fish, and poultry (animal flesh) from the diet, while the **pure vegetarian**, or **vegan**, excludes all of these foods and uses only plant foods. For both lifestyles it is necessary to know how to combine foods to obtain the nutrients nonvegetarians get from the meat and milk groups.

For the lacto-ovo-vegetarian, the Four Food Group Plan can be adapted by making a change in the meat group (see margin). The strict vegetarian, who doesn't use dairy products, should take a vitamin B_{12} supplement or use vitamin B_{12}-fortified soy milk. There is much more the vegetarian needs to learn, and additional pointers are offered in later chapters.

Four Food Group Plan for the Vegetarian

2 servings milk or milk products (or soy milk fortified with vitamin B_{12})

2 servings protein-rich foods (include 2 cups legumes daily to help meet iron requirements for women; count 4 tbsp peanut butter as 1 serving)

4 servings whole-grain foods

4 servings fruits and vegetables (include 1 cup dark greens to help meet iron requirements for women)

Adapted from a pamphlet, Vegetarian Food Choices, *The Shands Teaching Hospital and Clinics, Food and Nutrition Service, University of Florida, Gainesville, 1976*

Calorie Control and Nutrient Density

The preceding discussion has highlighted a problem that concerns many people today: Eating well seems to necessitate eating a lot. Some people don't even spend 2200 calories in their daily activities. If they were to eat this many calories, they would get fat.

How can a person get all the essential nutrients without overeating? The answer lies in selecting the foods within each group that deliver the most nutrients at the lowest calorie cost: foods with high **nutrient density**. Taking iron, for example: a 3-ounce serving of sirloin steak or of sardines provides 25 milligrams of iron; but the beef supplies 330 calories, the sardines 175.[2] The sardines, then, are more iron-dense (they have more iron for the same number of calories). If you asked a nutritionist whether beef or sardines were more nutritious, he or she would have to say both were nutritious, in the sense that both provide nutrients and not just calories. But using the new concept of

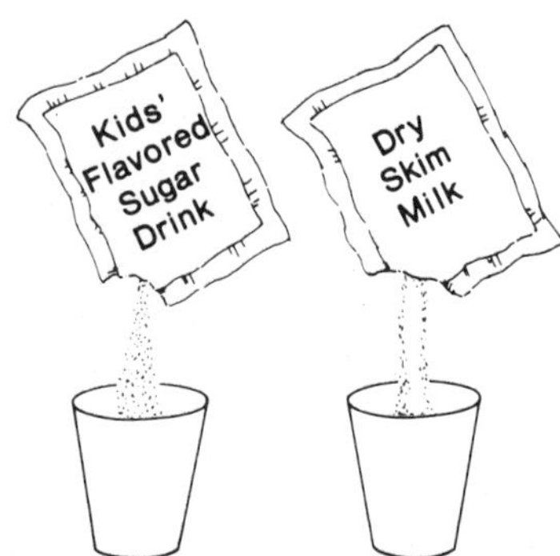

84 cal from sucrose.

36 cal from protein; 48 cal from lactose; 296 mg calcium; 10 IU vitamin A; 0.44 mg riboflavin; and more.

Another example of nutrient density. Both items are 84 calories, but there are many more nutrients in the milk.

nutrient density the nutritionist could tell you that the sardines were more nutritious than the beef, at least with respect to iron. (Remember, both provide the *same* amount of iron in a serving, but the sardines provide it at a lower calorie cost). The concept of nutrient density may someday become the basis for a new kind of nutritional labeling of foods in the market: Foods that provide more nutrients than calories, relative to a person's need, will qualify to be labeled **nutritious foods**.

The concept of a nutritious food as one which delivers nutrients at a low calorie cost can help the weight-conscious consumer to make informed choices. The food industry has enthusiastically endorsed the selling of the nutritional **adequacy** concept. The dairy people proclaim, "Drink milk—it's good for you." The meat people boast that meat is rich in protein and iron, as indeed it is. Every food can be advertised on the claim that it is loaded with nutrients, bursting with vitamins, high in health value. But the aware consumer realizes that milk and meat can also contribute many fat calories. Thus the advertisement of these and other products may benefit the milk and meat industries more than it benefits our bodies. This doesn't mean we should avoid them, but that we should use them with moderation.

Another case in point is honey, a much-beloved and much-advertised health-food product. Honey does provide a few B vitamins and trace minerals in very small amounts in contrast to white sugar, which does not supply them at all. But to say that honey is actually nutritious is to mislead the consumer. On the other hand, wheat germ, another favorite item in health-food stores, provides abundant B vitamins, iron, and other nutrients relative to its calorie amount. If the two should enter a contest for the title of "nutritious food," the wheat germ would win, hands down.

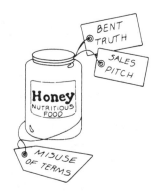

When honey claims to be nutritious, it's bending the truth. There's more on honey in Chapter 4.

No list of nutritious foods (by this definition) has been published as yet, but systems already exist that are useful to the consumer who wants to eat well and control calories at the same time. These are known as exchange systems.

Exchange Systems

Unlike a food group system, which sorts foods by their nutrient contents only, an **exchange** system pays special attention to calories and serving sizes. All the food servings on one list have the same number of calories and the same amount of energy nutrients (protein, fat, and carbohydrate). The U.S. exchange system will be presented here as an example. There are six, not four, groups of foods in the exchange system, and each has a typical member you can remember it by. The groups, and their typical representatives, are:

MILK—1 cup skim milk—80 calories.

VEGETABLE—½ cup green beans—25 calories.

FRUIT—½ small banana—40 calories.

BREAD—1 slice bread—70 calories.

MEAT—1 ounce lean meat or cheese—55 calories.

FAT—1 teaspoon butter—45 calories.

Table 3. The Six Exchange Groups[a]

Group	Serving Size	Carbohydrate (g)	Protein (g)	Fat (g)	Energy (cal)
Milk (skim)[b]	1 cup	12	8	0	80
Vegetable[c]	½ cup	5	2	0	25
Fruit (see fruit list)	1 serving	10	0	0	40
Bread[d]	1 slice	15	2	0	70
Meat (lean)[e]	1 oz	0	7	3	55
Fat	1 tsp	0	0	5	45

[a] This is the U.S. exchange system. The complete details, and those of the Canadian system, are shown in Appendix L.

[b] 1 cup low-fat milk = 1 skim milk + 1 fat. 1 cup whole milk = 1 skim milk + 2 fat.

[c] This group includes low-calorie vegetables only. See the vegetable list.

[d] This group includes starchy vegetables such as lima beans and corn, as well as cereal, bread, pasta, and other grain products. For serving sizes see Appendix L.

[e] This group includes cheese and peanut butter as well as meat.

The complete details of the U.S. and Canadian systems are in Appendix L.

Table 3 shows the protein, fat, and carbohydrate values that belong to each group, and Figure 1 shows the foods that belong together in this system. Notice that cheese is classed as a "meat" in this system because its protein and fat contents are similar to those of meat.

Keeping calorie-consciousness very much in mind, the user of this system is encouraged to think of skim milk as milk and of whole milk as milk with added fat: A glass of whole milk is described, in fact, as "one milk plus two fats," and a glass of low-fat milk as "one milk plus one fat." The vegetable list includes only low-calorie vegetables, so that ½ cup of any of them will provide about 25 calories. The fruit list specifies "no added sugar or sugar syrup"—not to forbid the user from eating fruits with sugar but to make you aware when you do and to help you keep track of sugar consumption. Serving sizes are adjusted so that fruit helpings are equal in calories. One small banana counts as "two fruits." But a piece of cherry pie is not a fruit. It includes a fruit if it contains ten large cherries, but it also includes bread exchanges, fat exchanges, and sugar. The bread list also clearly specifies serving sizes and makes clear which grain products contain added fat. Corn, lima beans, and other starchy vegetables are grouped with the breads because they are similar to them in calorie and carbohydrate content.

The well fed person is not necessarily well nourished.
—R. Fremes and Z. Sabry

Perhaps most important of all, meats and cheeses are separated into three categories—lean, medium-fat, and high-fat—and the fat list, by including items like bacon and olives, alerts the user to foods that

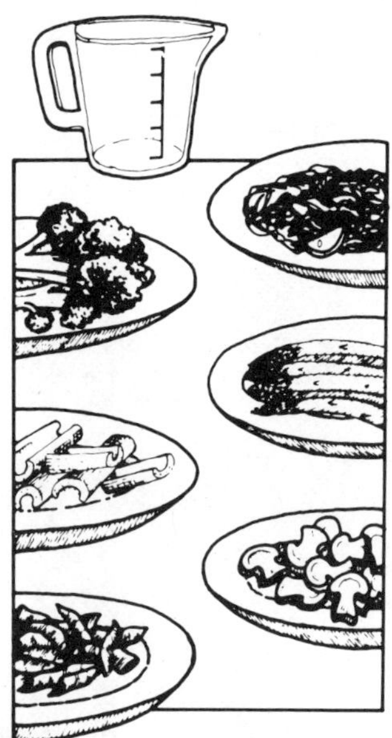

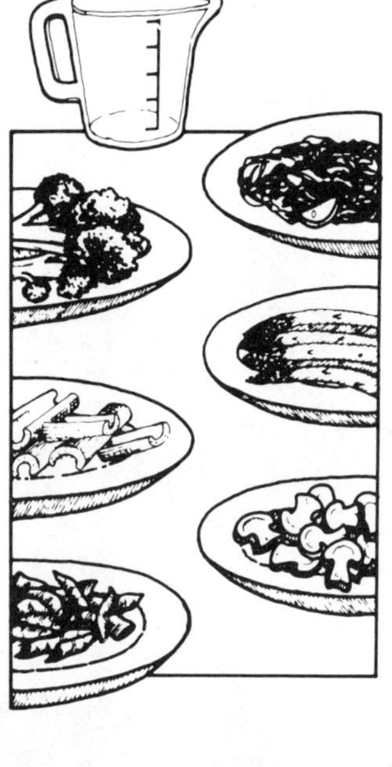

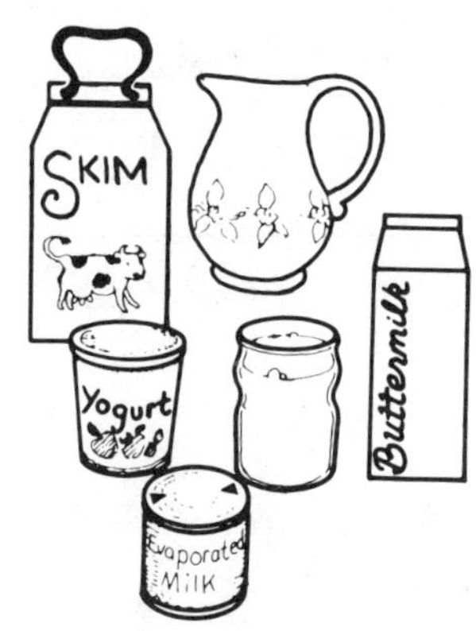

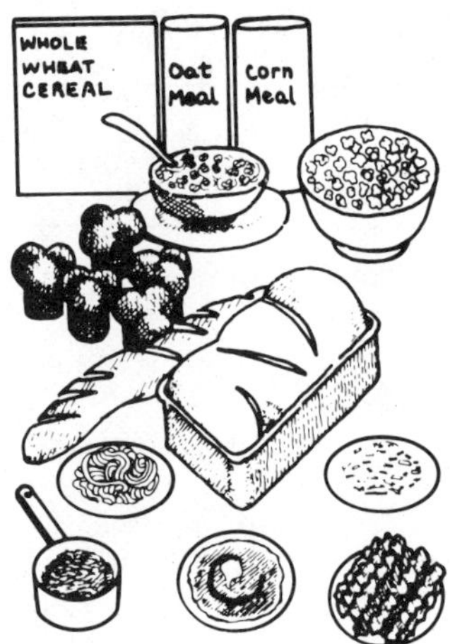

Figure 1. Groups of similar foods: exchange system (by calorie, carbohydrate, protein, and fat content).

Breads

1 slice bread is like:

¾ cup ready-to-eat cereal
½ cup cooked beans
⅓ cup corn
1 small potato

(1 bread = 15 g carbohydrate, 2 g protein, and 70 cal)

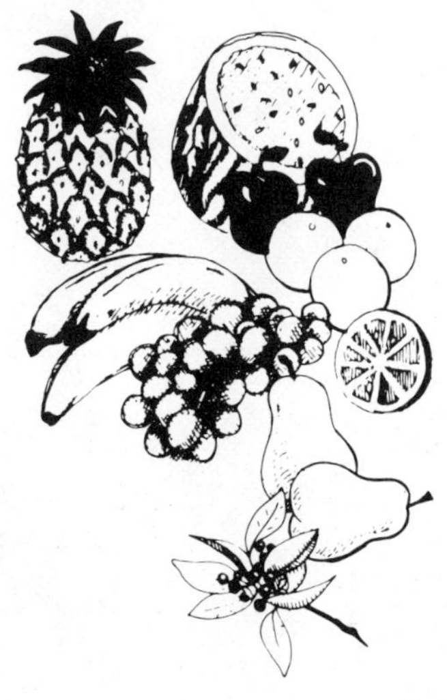

Milks

1 cup skim milk is like:

1 cup skim milk yogurt

(1 milk = 12 g carbohydrate, 8 g protein, and 80 cal)

Vegetables

½ cup green beans is like:

½ cup greens
½ cup carrots
½ cup beets

(1 vegetable = 5 g carbohydrate, 2 g protein, and 25 cal)

Fruits

½ small banana is like:

1 small apple
½ grapefruit
½ cup orange juice

(1 fruit = 10 g carbohydrate and 40 cal)

(continued on next page)

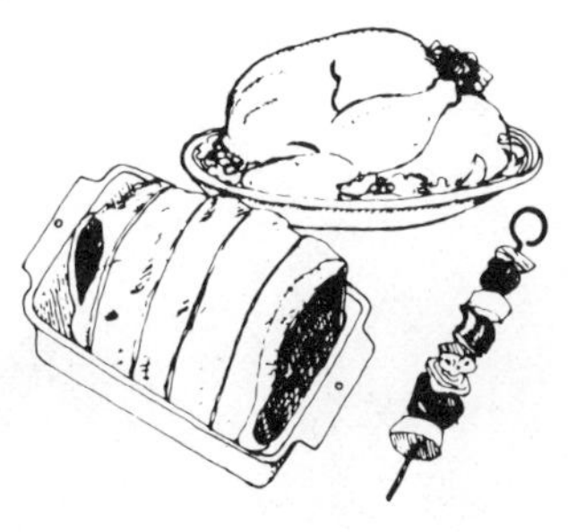

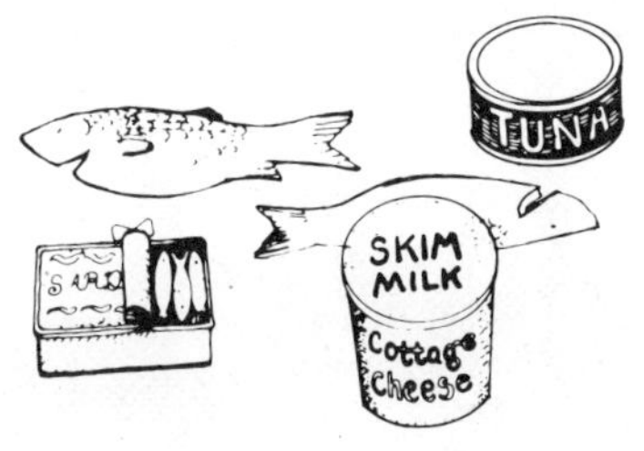

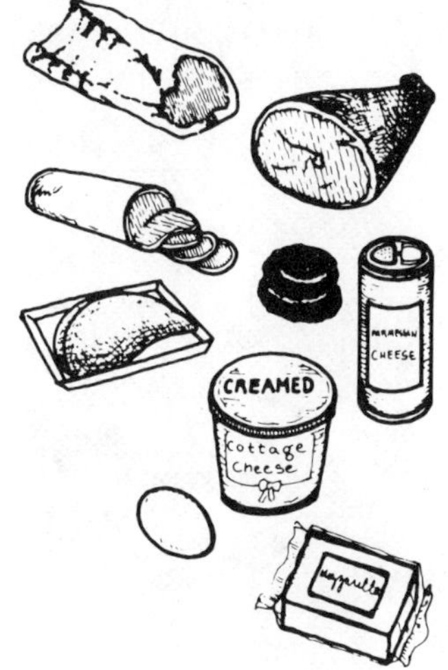

Meats (lean)

1 oz lean meat is like:

1 oz chicken meat without the skin
1 oz any fish
¼ cup canned tuna
1 oz low-fat cheese

(1 low-fat meat = 7 g protein, 3 g fat, and 55 cal)

Meats (medium-fat)

1 oz medium-fat meat is like 1 oz lean meat in protein content but is estimated to have an extra "½ fat"— that is, to have the 3 g fat of a lean meat and 2½ g additional fat. Examples:

1 oz pork loin
1 egg
¼ cup creamed cottage cheese

(1 medium-fat meat = 7 g protein, 5½ g fat, and about 80 cal)

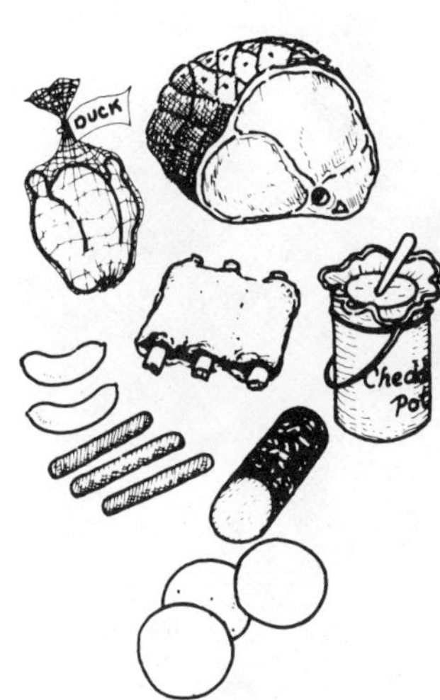

Meats (high-fat)

1 oz high-fat meat is like 1 oz lean meat in protein content but is estimated to have an extra "1 fat"— that is, to have the 3 g fat of a lean meat and 5 g additional fat. Examples:

1 oz country-style ham
1 oz cheddar cheese
1 small hot dog

(1 high-fat meat = 7 g protein, 8 g fat, and 100 cal)

Peanut Butter

Peanut butter is like a meat in terms of its protein content but stands alone in being very high in fat. It is estimated as:

2 tbsp peanut butter = 1 lean meat + 2½ fat

(2 tbsp peanut butter = 7 g protein, 15½ g fat, and 70 cal)

(Don't stop reading now, and don't swear off peanut butter, necessarily. You'll need to read about the polyunsaturated character of its fat in Chapter 5, and the B-vitamin contributions it makes in Chapter 9, before deciding how much of a place it should have in your diet.)

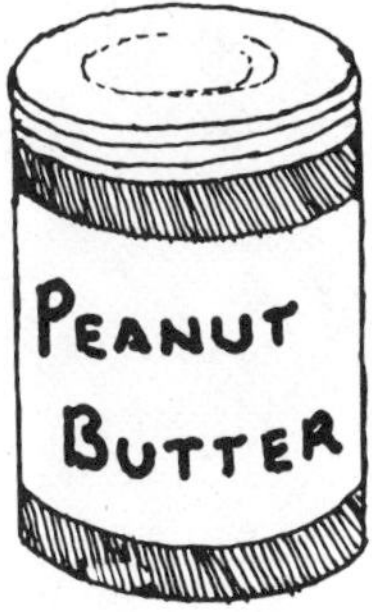

Note: Cheeses are grouped with milk in food group plans because of their calcium content but with meats in this system because, like meat, they contribute calories from protein and fat and have negligible carbohydrate content.

(continued on next page)

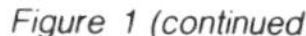

Figure 1 (continued)

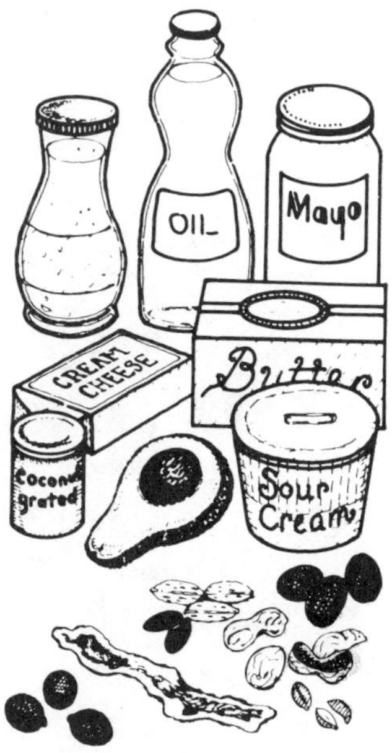

Fats

1 tsp butter is like:

1 tsp margarine
1 tsp any oil
1 tbsp salad dressing
1 strip crisp bacon
5 small olives
10 whole Virginia peanuts

(1 fat = 9 g fat and 45 cal)

Legumes

Legumes are an odd kind of plant food, odd in the sense that food grouping systems have a hard time fitting them into any group. They are like meats in a sense because they are rich in protein and iron and many are low in fat. But they contain a lot of starch—so they can be treated as:

½ cup legumes = 1 lean meat + 1 bread

(1 serving legumes = 15 g carbohydrate, 9 g protein, 3 g fat, and 125 cal)

(Or they can be considered similar to breads in being rich in complex carbohydrate, and the additional protein can be ignored; but this treatment underestimates their calorie value, especially that of the higher-fat legumes such as peanuts.) Whatever you do with them on paper, however, use them often in cooking. You will learn many more reasons why they are an inexpensive, nutritious, high-quality, and health-promoting food as you read on. Note: The Modified Four Food Group Plan recommends the use of two ¾-cup servings of legumes a day. For calculating, this would amount to *three* ½-cup servings.

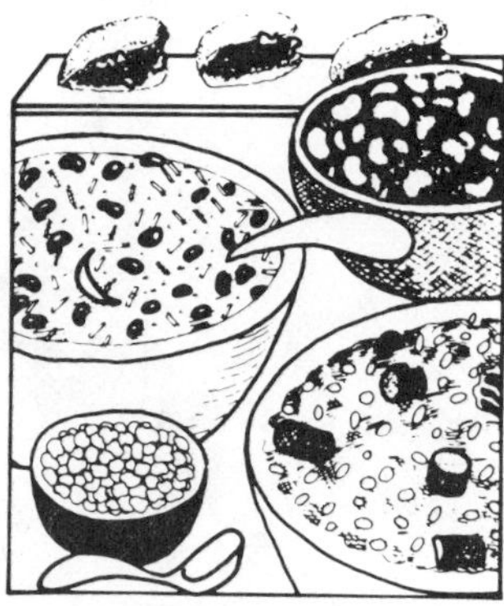

are unexpectedly high in fat calories. More details of the exchange system will appear in later chapters.

If you are a diet planner who wants to ingest all the nutrients you need, you are well advised to follow a food group plan, because it promotes adequacy and provides balance among the different kinds of foods that will help you avoid overemphasis on any one. But if you want to control calories as well, you will find it convenient to use the exchange lists as lists of nutritious foods from which to make your selections. You need to be aware of only one additional principle of diet planning to do very well for yourself: variety. It is generally agreed that people should not eat the same foods day after day, for two reasons. One reason is that there may still be undiscovered nutrients, and some foods may be better sources of these than others. The second reason is that a monotonous diet may deliver unwanted amounts of undesirable food constituents, such as incidental additives and pollutants. Each additive is diluted by all the other foods eaten with it and even further diluted if several days are skipped before it is eaten again.

Diet principles:
Adequacy.
Balance.
Calorie control.
Variety.

Thoughtful diet planning is simplified by grasping the concepts of adequacy, balance, calorie control (nutrient density), and variety. But even if these concepts are clearly understood, diet planning may seem a sizable job to undertake. This chapter's Food Feature acknowledges that and puts together some practical pointers to help.

Food Feature: How to Manage It All?

An important person in the delivery of good nutrition is often overlooked by the professional personnel (nutritionist, doctor, dietitian). That person is the one who invests time, skill, and personal energy in delivering the needed nutrients. If three fruit servings a day are required, someone must travel to the market—select fruit from the fresh, canned, frozen, or dried fruits—pay for it—carry it home—store it in the refrigerator or freezer or on the shelf—decide which fruit will be served next—wash, pare, and serve the fresh—unwrap, thaw, and serve the frozen—open the canned and serve the contents. If any of the fruit is to be cooked, the person must find a pan for it, have a stove to cook it on, and know how to prepare it. After the food is eaten, he or she must wash, dry, and put away the dishes, utensils, and pans; wrap and store the leftovers; wipe the kitchen counters and sink; and carry out of the house the wrappings, cans, parings, and table scraps.

All this activity must be performed by oneself or by a parent, caretaker, or "wife." Many people are unable to perform these tasks for themselves. Children, the handicapped, the poor, and the elderly must depend on others for some or all of these services. Moreover, some able-bodied and intelligent people can't perform these services because they haven't acquired the marketing and food preparation skills needed. For example, a boy may not receive instruction in food-related skills, although his sister may be encouraged to develop a lot of expertise. Yet at an early age, when he leaves home to work or to go to college, the boy may find himself responsible for his own food. Prior to a divorce or the death of a spouse, a man may have given no thought to this important aspect of his body's health and then be plunged suddenly into the world of marketing, cooking, and garbage.

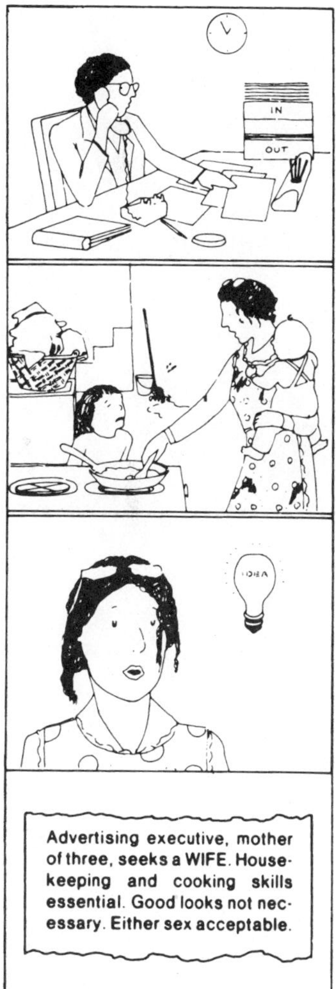
IN
OUT
Advertising executive, mother of three, seeks a WIFE. Housekeeping and cooking skills essential. Good looks not necessary. Either sex acceptable.
Managing the food is a hassle.

The story is told of a man in his mid-fifties who, on the death of his wife, was forced for the first time to make decisions about his own food. During the year following his wife's death, his doctors treated him for numerous ailments. Finally, he was seen by a dietitian who made the correct diagnosis: scurvy, the vitamin C-deficiency disease. He had been subsisting on a diet of black coffee, hamburgers, martinis, and steak. Even an occasional baked potato with his steak would have saved him, but baking it was beyond his skill or interest.

People living alone, like this widower, are apt to have great difficulty obtaining a good diet. Vegetables, meat, and fruits are prepackaged in the market in a size suitable for families. They spoil before a single person can eat them. A quart of milk sours before it can be used, and cereals and bread become stale. Cleaning up the mess in the kitchen after the preparation of a meal for one is as big a chore as if several had been fed. Small wonder that a solitary person often gives up trying to have fruits and vegetables and resorts to eating a hamburger at a fast-food restaurant. Food Features in all of the chapters to come will provide pointers to promote diet adequacy and ease of food preparation. For the moment, let's concentrate on the planning part.

Suppose you want to plan menus that are adequate but not excessive in calories. The Four Food Group Plan promotes adequacy, but most people (notably young college women) say, "I couldn't possibly eat all that food without getting fat!" The following demonstration shows that it can be done; it may come as a surprise that it can be done extremely well.

A person who wants to include all the nutrients but limit consumption of excess calories at the same time can use a food group plan as a guide for selecting the foundation foods and an exchange system to choose the actual items, as shown in Table 4. This shows that for a total of 900 calories, adequacy for most of the major nutrients can probably be achieved. An average adult woman would still have more than 1000 calories to spend. A wise choice would be to invest many of these calories in additional fruits, vegetables, and whole-grain foods, or in the two large servings of legumes/nuts and the one serving of fat recommended by the Modified Four Food Group Plan. (Two ¾-cup servings of legumes at about 180 calories each and 1 teaspoon of margarine at 45 calories would add only about 400 calories to the total and still leave some room to spare.) Some of the extra calories could be spent adding more starch-containing foods like

Table 4. How to Use a Food Group Plan and an Exchange System to Plan Diets

Four Food Group Plan	Using the Exchange System	Example	Energy Cost (cal)
Milk—2 cups	Milk list—select 2 exchanges	2 cups skim milk	160
Meat—2 servings (2–3 oz each)	Meat list—select 6 exchanges[a]	6 oz lean meat	330
Fruits and vegetables—4 servings	Fruit and vegetable lists—select 4 exchanges	2 vegetable exchanges;	50
		2 fruit exchanges	80
Grains (breads and cereals)—4 servings	Bread list—select 4 exchanges	4 bread exchanges	280
Total			900

[a] In the Four Food Group Plan, 1 serving is 2–3 oz. In the exchange system, 1 exchange is 1 oz.

additional whole-grain bread or snacks like popcorn. Others could be invested in occasional sweet desserts, even alcohol. If these additions were made, they would be made by choice rather than through the unintentional use of high-calorie foods to begin with. The goal is adequacy and balance, not necessarily at each meal, but within each day.

With judicious selections, the diet can meet the need for all the nutrients and provide some luxury, fun items as well. The final plan might be like that outlined in the margin (one of many possible examples). The planner then could achieve variety by selecting different foods each day from the exchange lists.

A last refinement that is useful to the conscientious diet planner is to learn to use different patterns of exchanges for different calorie levels. A person eating 3000 calories a day could use considerably more bread exchanges, for example, than a person eating only 1500 calories a day. Table 5 shows diet plans for different calorie intakes.

A Sample Diet Plan

Exchanges	Energy (cal)
2 skim milk	160
2 vegetable	50
3 fruit	120
7 bread	490
6 medium-fat meat	465
4 fat	180
	1465

This diet derives about 20 percent of its calories from protein, about 30 percent from fat, and nearly 50 percent from carbohydrate.

Table 5. Diet Plans for Different Calorie Intakes

	Energy Level (cal)						
Number of Exchanges	1000	1200	1500	1800	2100	2600	3000
Milk	2	2	2	2	2	2	2
Vegetable	1	2	2	3	3	4	4
Fruit	3	3	3	3	4	4	5
Bread	4	5	7	8	10	12	15
Meat (Medium-fat)	5	5	6	8	8	10	10
Fat	1	3	4	5	8	12	15

In summary, you eat foods, but what you obtain from them is nutrients. These fall into six classes—carbohydrate, fat, protein, vitamins, minerals, and water. The first four are organic (carbon-containing), but only the first three provide energy the human body can use.

This energy and that of alcohol (a nonnutrient) can power body activities or be stored as fat or other body compounds. Food energy is measured in calories.

The objective of thoughtful diet planning is to provide adequate intakes of the essential nutrients for a reasonable calorie cost. To manage this it helps to think in terms of food groups, following a plan that specifies a certain number of servings from each group daily. The members of each food group and the amounts considered to constitute a serving are itemized in any exchange system.

An additional aid in diet planning is a set of standards or recommendations specifying how much of each nutrient to aim for. Examples of such recommendations, including the RDA (Recommended Dietary Allowances) are presented in the next chapter.[1]

For Further Information

The Modified Four Food Group Plan was published in the *Journal of Nutrition Education* in 1978. See this chapter's note 1.

The exchange system referred to here is printed in its entirety in Appendix L and is available for about $1 from the American Dietetic Association (address in Appendix J).

The evolving concept of nutrient density has been elucidated by many sources, including:

- Wittwer, A. J.; Sorenson, A. W.; Wyse, B. W.; and Hansen, R. G. Nutrient density—evaluation of nutritional attributes of foods. *Journal of Nutrition Education* 9 (January-March 1977): 26-30.

[1] *Chapter Notes can be found at the end of the Appendixes.*

Controversy 2

Vitamin Supplements

Do you need to take them?

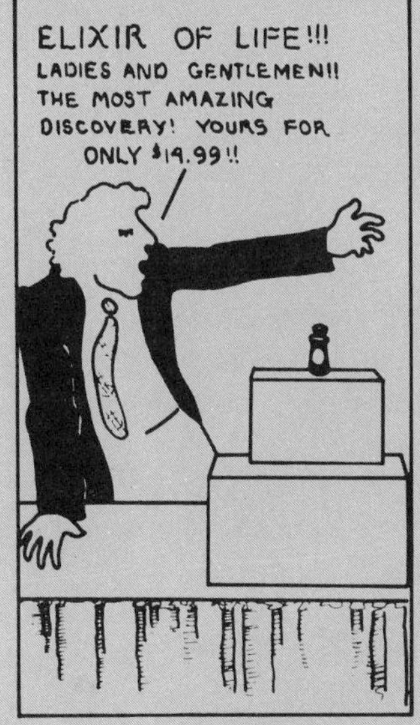
ELIXIR OF LIFE!!!
LADIES AND GENTLEMEN!!
THE MOST AMAZING DISCOVERY! YOURS FOR ONLY $19.99!!

Of the billions of dollars spent on drugs in the United States each year, hundreds of millions are spent on vitamin pills. They find their way into 75 percent of U.S. households.[1] Some people buy them because their doctors have told them to, but most people decide independently that they need them. One person takes a single pill every morning, expecting it to deliver all the vitamins she needs. Another puts together a veritable arsenal of pills and powders in a pattern tailored to what he sees as his own personal needs.

Who's right? Or is it necessary to take vitamin pills at all? The vitamins are not dealt with individually until Chapter 9, but it seems only fair to introduce the issue early because it is of such general concern.

Many takers of the single, daily pill seem to view it as a kind of nutritional insurance. This attitude (to anticipate the conclusion of this discussion) is not an extreme practice and, even if unnecessary, does little harm even to the pocketbook. If you engage in this practice, however, you will probably find as you read on that you can, if you wish, learn to adjust your diet to meet your vitamin needs from foods. All you need in order to feel secure in doing this is an understanding of a plan like the Four Food Group Plan (Chapter 2), and an understanding of the RDA (Chapter 3), and an acquaintanceship with the vitamins (Chapter 9).

The supplement-taker of concern here is the one with the arsenal, the one who takes before breakfast, say, 500 milligrams of vitamin C, 1000 units of vitamin E, several tablespoons of "nutritional yeast," some kelp tablets, a capsule of vitamins A and D, and assorted pills containing trace minerals and who sprinkles dessicated liver, powdered bone, and wheat germ on his granola, followed by powdered skim milk. This person is asking pills and powders to play a role that is better delegated to food. (Not all the choices just listed are equally questionable, however. The wheat germ, granola, and milk are nutritious foods.)

What such a person is trying to do is to obtain all the nutrients he needs. He is persuaded that he can't do this using ordinary foods. Controversy 1 dealt with one aspect of this belief—the "magic" associated with health foods—but even if this person agreed with the conclusion reached there, he would still use his pills and powders. "I need them," he would say, "because I may have unusually high needs for vitamins and minerals, and besides, it can't hurt to take a little extra."

These beliefs are typical of nutritional faddism, which has been aptly said to have its roots in "interest, accompanied by inadequate knowledge."[2] Our supplement-taker, then, is a faddist because he sincerely wants to care for his nutritional health. Let us take a close look at the first of his reasons: "I may have unusually high needs."

Nutritional individuality. Biologically speaking, no two people are exactly alike except identical twins, and no two people have exactly the same nutritional needs. I may need a bit more vitamin C than you, and you a bit more protein than I, to maintain peak health. Not only are we different biologically, but our different lifestyles affect our nutritional needs. Even identical twins, if they live differently, may not have identical nutritional needs. If one of them has a highly stressful job, for example, she may need slightly more of certain B vitamins than the other. These differences between individuals—which are called normal variation—may make our nutrient requirements differ as much as two- or three-fold, one from another; that is, you may need up to twice or three times as much vitamin C as I do, assuming my needs are average.[3]

In some instances, very large differences in nutritional needs are seen. Some people are born with rare genetic defects so that they cannot use certain nutrients in the normal way. These people may have extraordinarily high or low nutrient requirements, differing ten- or a hundred-fold from the average. But these are special cases. Only one may arise among 10,000 people.

Illness also imposes differences in nutrient requirements. Under the stress of surgery or high fever or after suffering extensive burns, for example, a hospital patient's needs for protein are much greater than usual, up to perhaps five times the normal needs, and the needs for vitamins and minerals may be increased even more. Some prescription and over-the-counter medicines also increase specific vitamin and mineral needs. These special needs have been intensively studied and are the subject of large volumes of diet therapy studied by dietitians in training for hospital work.

Miniglossary

cell salts: A mineral preparation sold in health food stores supposed to have been prepared from living, healthy cells. It is not necessary to take such preparations and it may be dangerous.

dessicated liver: Dehydrated liver, a powder sold in health food stores and supposed to contain in concentrated form all the nutrients found in liver. Possibly not dangerous, this supplement has no particular nutritional merit, and grocery-store liver is considerably less expensive.

granola: A cereal made from mixed oats and other grains.

homeopathy (home-ee-OPP-path-ee): A branch of medicine (supposedly) that focuses on prevention of disease, promotion of health, and restoration of disturbed body balances by feeding needed nutrients. Homeopathic "physicians" may or may not have M.D. degrees.

kelp: A kind of seaweed used by the Japanese as a foodstuff. Kelp tablets are made from dehydrated kelp.

subclinical deficiency: A nutrient deficiency that has no visible or otherwise detectable (clinical) symptoms. It is possible for such a deficiency to develop (see the discussion of loss of iron from body stores in Chapter 3), but the term is often used as a scare tactic to persuade consumers to buy nutrient supplements they don't need.

supplement: A preparation (such as a pill, powder, or liquid) containing nutrients that can be used to supplement the diet. Breakfast cereals that contain "100 percent of the U.S. RDA" for certain nutrients are also considered dietary supplements.

trace minerals: See Chapter 10.

What we are concerned with here, however, are normal variations, and these don't justify the taking of large quantities of vitamins in concentrated form by the normal, healthy person. Foods contain enough vitamins so that a reasonably careful selection of them will supply all the vitamins most people need. The food group plan described in the last chapter provides a healthful balance of nutrients, and the modified plan takes care of the nutrients that might otherwise be lacking. The amounts of nutrients supplied by such a plan are enough to meet the needs of people at the top of the range of normal variation.

"But," the supplement-taker may say, "that argument is based on too many assumptions for my comfort. You assume that the foods you speak of have the nutrients in them—whereas they may be poor in nutrients. You assume that they haven't lost those nutrients in cooking—when in fact they could be cooked to pieces and have no nutritional value." The nutrient contents of ordinary grocery-store foods were the subject of Controversy 1 and will come up again. Losses in cooking are moderate if you are careful (see Chapter 9). But the debate between the self-doser and the ordinary-food user goes on and on, and will pop up again often in the chapters to come.

One other aspect of the self-dosing practice should at least be mentioned here: the risks. It is a myth that the vitamins are nontoxic. All of them, including the water-soluble vitamins B and C, have been shown to have toxic effects when taken in large doses, at least in some people.

How vitamins are promoted. "Three-fourths of the public believe that extra vitamins provide more pep and energy. Twenty-six percent [use] nutritional supplements expecting observable benefits—without a physician's advice," reports Dr. P. L. White, director of the Department of Foods and Nutrition of the American Medical Association.[4] If it isn't necessary to do this, why have so many people been bamboozled into believing that it is? Dr. White has identified one of the kinds of claims made by pill-pushers: "The idea of nutritional individuality promotes the notion that you should try it [a fad] even though it didn't work for me."[5] Dr. V. Herbert, professor of medicine and pathology at Columbia College of Physicians and Surgeons, has noted many of the earmarks of faddism. You can tell it may be a quack talking if he tries to persuade you:

- That you should buy something you wouldn't otherwise buy.
- That your disease condition is due to a faulty diet.
- That you have a "subclinical" deficiency.
- That, in fact, you should take supplements of any kind.
- That you should take "natural" vitamins.[6]

The last of these notions, that "natural" vitamins are of more virtue than synthetic vitamins, resembles the now-familiar argument about fertilizers. The body cannot tell whether a vitamin it finds in its bloodstream came from an organically grown cantaloupe melon or from a chemist's laboratory. Pills made either from the melon or from some chemical in the lab may differ from one another in their *other* ingredients, but insofar as they contain a certain vitamin, they are identical. If either kind of pill has an advantage of any kind, it is as often the synthetic as the "natural" pill. In one instance, vitamin C from *synthetic* pills has been found to be absorbed better into the body than that from "natural" pills;[7] in another, the "natural" pills have been found to be so weak that synthetic vitamin C has had to be added to them to bring the concentration up to acceptable levels.[8]

In any case, there is nothing natural about a pill, no matter what its source. If we define *natural* more carefully and insist that the word be used only to refer to foods, not pills, and only to foods in their original, farm-grown state, then we can make a statement that will hold up to critical inspection. The natural food (like a cantaloupe melon) may be better for you than any pill—not because it has better vitamin C in it but because it conveys "fringe benefits" along with the vitamin C: carbohydrate, fiber, and fluid with dissolved calcium, potassium, and many other nutrients:

There is no advantage to eating a nutrient from one source as opposed to another, but there may be fringe benefits to eating that nutrient in a natural food as opposed to a purified nutrient preparation.[9]

Minerals are even more dangerous. Takers of self-prescribed pills need a warning about the risks of overdosing with vitamins, but if they also take minerals they need a more urgent warning. Minerals are often "prescribed" by people calling themselves *homeopathic physicians.* "Homeopathy is a therapeutic system based on minute doses of various remedies, many of which are mineral salts. . . . These 'cell salts' are alleged to have therapeutic value in a wide range of diseases."[10] The reasons why ill-informed dosing with minerals is especially dangerous will become fully apparent in Chapter 10; Dr. White expresses his concern this way:

The newer research on the trace minerals has been exploited by the health food set; one sees glowing claims for zinc, selenium and chromium, the last being promoted as GTF, or glucose tolerance factor. Laboratories that "evaluate" nutritional status by hair analysis flourish, as does their business in food supplements to "correct" the "metabolic imbalances" uncovered by such analysis. Admittedly useful for certain determinations, hair analysis has not yet been found appropriate for general nutritional evaluation.

A most disturbing aspect is that some physicians and dentists are utilizing the "services" of hair analysis laboratories.[11]

Personal strategy. With all there is to be said against the use of vitamin pills, is there anything to be said *for* them? Yes, when a doctor prescribes them, and yes, in at least two other instances:

- When your calorie intake is below about the 1500 level, so that you can't eat enough total food to be sure of meeting your vitamin needs.
- When you know that—for whatever reason—you are going to be eating irregularly for a limited time.

On these occasions, a one-a-day type vitamin pill should suffice. It is then important to remember that, if vitamins are needed, minerals will be needed too and a vitamin-mineral supplement is called for.

A problem that remains for the reader who is persuaded of the view presented here is "How do I tell my friends?" Trying to convince a pill-popping friend not to take pills and powders can easily turn into the unfortunate experience of losing the friend. As Dr. A. E. Harper, professor of nutritional sciences, University of Wisconsin, has put it, "Isn't it amazing how when you explain to someone that what they have accepted as fact is not so, they become angry with you rather than with the person who gave them the inaccurate information in the first place?"[12] Yes, it is amazing and painful. But the response is not surprising when you recall that the person who has paid his or her own money as the price for believing a bogus fact has a personal stake in having the fact be true.

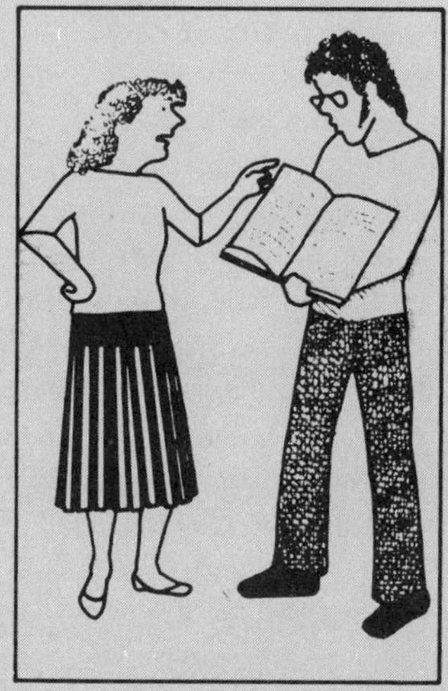

To avoid alienating the people we try to reach with valid information we can adopt several strategies. For one thing, we can always acknowledge the validity of the feelings and values that underlie the faddist's practices. Then, we can distinguish between practices that are dangerous and those that are merely neutral. We can ignore the neutral ones and confront only the dangerous ones. Finally, we can make ourselves responsible for learning the facts of the matter as thoroughly as we can, getting them all in perspective, and communicating them clearly.

In closing, it may be of interest to demonstrate how nutritional good judgment would rank the items selected by the pill and powder breakfaster described at the start. They can be sorted into groups as follows:

- Most risky: The A and D capsules and the minerals, because overdoses are a real possibility and have serious ill effects. Potassium chloride, for example, is sold in health food stores, carries no warning label, and is known to have caused deaths of otherwise healthy individuals. One case was that of a baby whose mother had read the book *Let's Have Healthy Children* by Adelle Davis and had given the supplement to the infant, as the book suggested, for colic.[13]

- Next: The nutritional yeast, which is not needed (and live yeast actually consumes nutrients[14])—the powdered bone (the calcium from such a source is very poorly absorbed, and some bonemeal has been found to contain high levels of lead[15])—and the kelp tablets (the urine of people who use kelp tablets has been found to contain raised concentrations of arsenic, a poison and a possible cancer-causing agent.[16])

- Next: The vitamin C and the vitamin E. These are not the highest doses people take and get away with, but they are high enough to be toxic in some individuals. (See Chapter 9 and Controversy 20 for more about vitamin C and E toxicity.)

- Next: The dessicated liver. This is probably a neutral practice (although some risks could still come to light); it is easy to get the nutrients delivered in ordinary foods, but there may be no harm in this practice other than to the pocketbook.

- Last: The wheat germ, the granola, and the powdered skim milk. These are nutritious foods, they can be bought in the grocery store, and the skim milk in particular is a very economical source of valuable nutrients.

In counseling the user, you might praise the value system that puts such a high premium on health and express support of the desire to take such good care of the body. Then, you might reinforce the use of the last three items, agreeing that they are nutritious, reasonable in cost, and delicious. If you are sure of your listener's openness to whatever else you might have to say, you might offer a caution about the use of the potent supplements listed first and keep your own counsel about the remaining ones unless you are asked. Hopefully this way you won't lose a friend, and you may provide a substantial boost to exactly what he treasures most —his good health.

The Controversy Notes and For Further Information follow the Appendixes.

CHAPTER 3

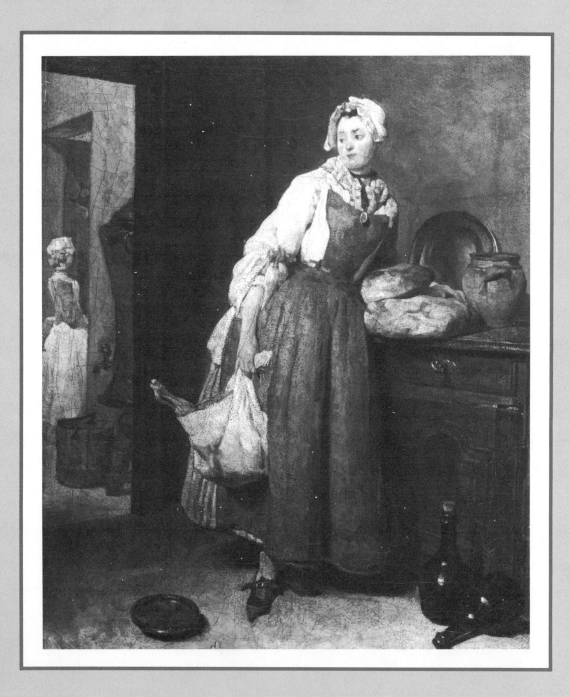

First Facts: Nutrient Needs and Nutritional Surveys

The last chapter showed that it is not necessary to think always in terms of nutrients. Diet adequacy can be achieved through the use of a food group plan aided by the principles of nutrient density and calorie control. However, the science of nutrition is actually based on the study of how the body uses nutrients, and one of the most important aspects of that study is to ask how much of each nutrient the body needs and how we can tell if it is getting enough. This chapter shows how nutrition scientists arrive at recommended nutrient intakes, how the adequacy of people's nutrition intakes is assessed, and how well the people of the United States and Canada are doing, nutritionally, as judged by these standards.

The following section introduces the RDA as an example of recommended intakes. (The U.S. RDA used on food labels is different from the RDA and is described later in this chapter.)

Recommended Nutrient Intakes

The RDA. The United States government publishes recommendations concerning appropriate nutrient intakes for the people in this country.

Opposite: Back from the Market *by Jean Baptiste Siméon Chardin. Reprinted with the permission of the National Gallery of Canada, Ottawa.*

RDA are set for:
Energy (cal)—a range.
Protein (g).
Vitamins:
A, D,E, C, folacin, niacin, riboflavin, thiamin, B_6, B_{12}.
Minerals:
Calcium, phosphorus, iodine, iron, magnesium, zinc.

"Estimated safe and adequate intakes" as of 1980 are set (in ranges) for:
Vitamins:
K, biotin, pantothenic acid.
Minerals (trace elements):
Copper, manganese, fluoride, chromium, selenium, molybdenum.
Minerals (salts):
Sodium, potassium, chloride.
See inside front cover and Appendix I.

These are the **Recommended Dietary Allowances (RDA)**, and they are used and referred to so often that they are presented on the inside front cover of this book. As you can see, the main RDA table includes recommendations for protein, ten vitamins, and six minerals, while the additional tables (Appendix I) include three more vitamins and nine more minerals, as well as energy (calories). About every five years, the Committee on RDA[1] meets to re-examine and revise these recommendations on the basis of new evidence regarding people's nutrient needs. It then publishes an updated set of RDA.[2]

The RDA have been much misunderstood. One young woman, on first learning of their existence, was outraged: "You mean Uncle Sam tells me that I must eat exactly forty-five grams of protein every day?" This is not the government's intention, and the RDA are not commandments. The following facts will help put the RDA in perspective:

They are published by the government, but the study group that recommends them is composed of nutritionists and other scientists.

They are based on available scientific evidence to the greatest extent possible and are revised about every five years for this reason.

They are recommendations, not requirements, and certainly not minimum requirements. They include a margin of safety so substantial that two-thirds of the RDA is often deemed adequate, except for energy.

They recommend a range within which most healthy persons' intakes of nutrients probably should fall. Individual needs differ.

They are for healthy persons only. Medical problems alter nutrient needs.

Separate recommendations are made for different groupings of people. Children aged four to six are distinguished from men aged nineteen to twenty-two, for example. Each individual can look up the recommendations for his or her own age and sex group. No RDA is set for carbohydrate or fat. The assumption is that you will use a certain number of calories meeting your protein RDA and then will distribute the remaining calories among carbohydrate and fat and possibly alcohol, according to your personal preference, to meet your energy RDA.

The setting of recommended allowances. It is important to understand the way the RDA and other such recommendations are set. Especially if you use them to guess at the adequacy of your own diet, you need to be aware that individuals' nutrient needs may vary widely, that the allowances have to be chosen so that they will be practical for use for whole groups of people, and that you must keep these limitations and qualifications in mind when you use them. A theoretical discussion based on the way the Committee on RDA made its recommendation for protein will illustrate these points.

Suppose we were the Committee on RDA and we had the task of setting an RDA for nutrient X (any nutrient). Ideally, our first step would be to try to find out how much of that nutrient individual persons need. We would review and select the most valid studies of deficiency states, of nutrient stores and their depletion, and of the factors infuencing them. We could also measure the body's intake and excretion (in the case of nutrients that aren't changed before they are excreted) and find out how much of an intake is required for a balance (this is called a **balance study**). For each individual subject, we could determine a **requirement** for nutrient X. Below the requirement, that person would slip into negative balance or experience declining stores.

We would find that different individuals have different requirements. Mr. A might need forty units of the nutrient each day to maintain balance; Ms. B might need thirty-five; Mr. C, sixty-five. If we looked at enough individuals, we might find that their requirements fell into an even distribution, that most were near the midpoint, and only a few were at the extremes. Figure 1 depicts this situation.

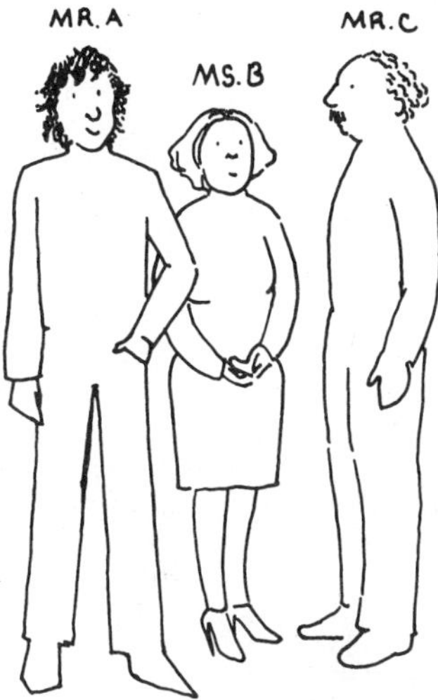

Different individuals have different requirements.

Then we would have to decide what intake to recommend for everybody: We would have to set the RDA. Should we set it at the mean (shown in Figure 1 at forty-five units)? This is the average requirement for nutrient X; it is the closest to everyone's need. But if people took us literally and consumed exactly this amount of nutrient X each day, half of the population would develop deficiencies, Mr. C among them.

Perhaps we should set the RDA for nutrient X at or above the extreme—say, at seventy units a day—so that everyone would be covered. (Actually, we didn't study everyone, so we would have to worry that some individual we didn't happen to test would have a still higher requirement.) This might be a good idea in theory, but what if nutrient X is expensive or scarce? A person like Ms. B, who needs only thirty-

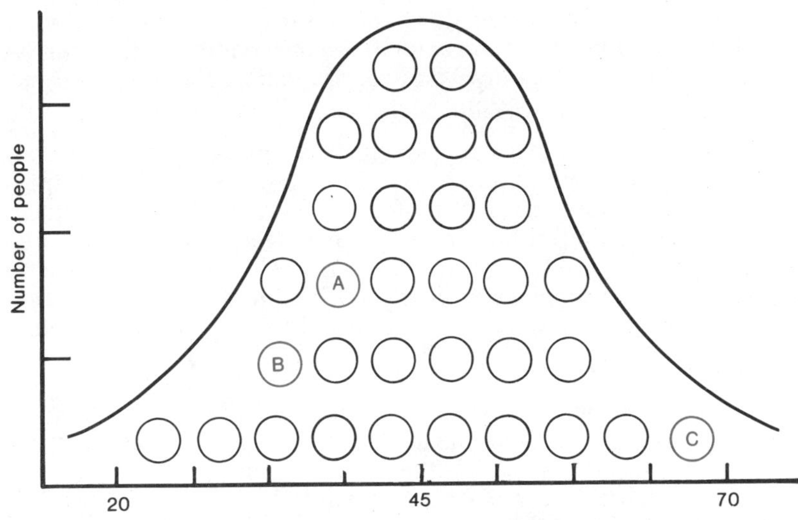

Figure 1. *Each dot represents a person. A, B, and C are Mr. A, Ms. B, and Mr. C.*

five units a day, would then try to consume twice that, an unnecessary strain on her pocketbook. Or she might overeat as a consequence or overemphasize foods containing nutrient X to the exclusion of foods containing other valuable nutrients.

The choice we would finally make, with some reservations, would be to set the RDA at a reasonably high point so that the bulk of the population would be covered. In this example, a reasonable choice might be to set it at sixty-three units a day. By moving the RDA further toward the extreme we would pick up very few additional people but inflate the recommendation as it applies to most people (including Mr. A and Ms. B).

It is this kind of choice that the committee makes in setting the RDA for nutrients. They set it well above the mean requirement as best they can determine it from the available information. (Actually, they don't usually have enough data to be sure that the population's requirements are evenly distributed.) Relatively few people's requirements, then, are not covered by the RDA.

If you have followed this line of reasoning, you will see why the RDA cannot be taken literally by any individual. Remember, you can't know exactly what your own personal requirement may be. Remember, too, that the Committee on RDA makes several assumptions that do not apply to all real situations. They assume, among other things, that you are eating a generally adequate diet including protein of good quality and that you are consuming adequate calories and nutrients. They assume that you cook your foods with reasonable care and that nutrients aren't lost in preparation. When you use the RDA for yourself and compare your nutrient intakes with them, you should keep two principles in mind:

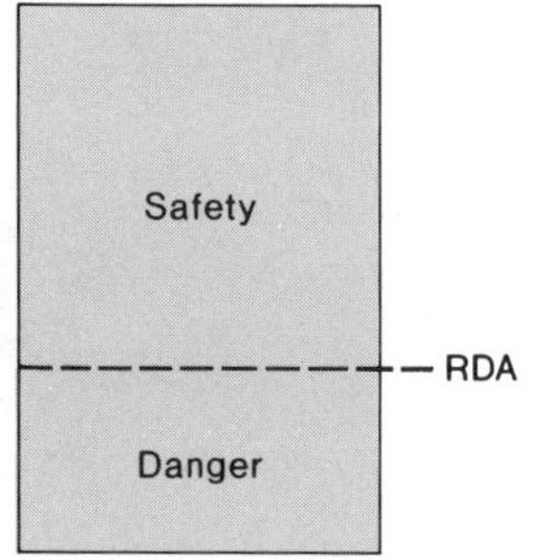

The naive view of the RDA: that all intakes above the line are safe.

> They are not minimum requirements. "R" stands for "recommended," not for "required." They are allowances, and they are generous. Even so, they do not necessarily cover every individual for every nutrient. If you want to be conservative in planning your own diet, it is probably wise to aim at getting 100 percent or more of the RDA for every nutrient.
>
> Beyond a certain point, though, it is unwise to consume large amounts of any nutrient. It is naive to think of the RDA simply as minimum amounts. A more accurate view is to see your nutrient needs as falling within a range, with danger zones both below and above it. Figure 2 illustrates this point. The 1980 RDA reflect this consideration especially clearly in the tables for the trace minerals (Appendix I) which are stated in terms of "safe and adequate" ranges of intakes.

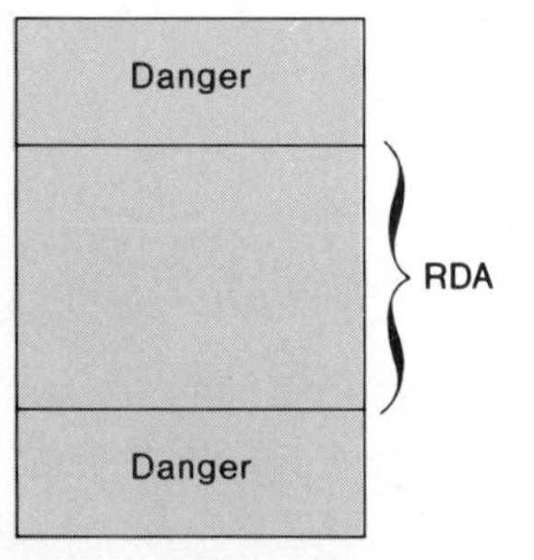

The accurate view of the RDA is that they represent a range. Intakes above or below certain limits are dangerous.

Figure 2.

It is also important to remember that the RDA and other such recommendations are for the maintenance, not the restoration, of health. Under the stress of illness or malnutrition, a person may require a much higher intake of certain nutrients. Separate recommendations are made for therapeutic diets; for use after surgery, burns, or fractures; or in the treatment of illness.

With the understanding that they are approximate, flexible, and generous, we can use the RDA as a yardstick to measure the adequacy of diets in whole populations, like that of the United States. For example, a diet providing at least two-thirds of the RDA for seven indicator nutrients is deemed good by the USDA; one providing less than two-thirds for one or more is poor.[3] These and other standards have been applied in a number of surveys of the U.S. population to determine the people's nutritional status.

The RDA for energy (calories). In setting allowances for calorie intakes, the Committee on RDA took a different tack than for the nutrients. It had reasoned that it would be sensible to set generous allowances for protein, vitamins, and minerals. It felt that small amounts of a *nutrient* in excess of the minimum required to maintain freedom from deficiency symptoms would be less harmful than small deficits. However, *energy* intakes either above or below need are harmful: Obesity is as much to be avoided as undernutrition. The Committee on RDA therefore set the energy RDA at the mean—halfway between the lowest and highest needs of the individuals it studied. This choice minimizes the risk of encouraging excessive energy intakes. Figure 3 illustrates the difference between the nutrient and calorie RDA set by the committee.

The energy RDA is thus a recommendation for the "average" person. The average U.S. female aged twenty-three to fifty, is 5 feet 5 inches tall and weighs 128 pounds (58 kilograms). This **reference woman** requires (on the average) 2000 calories a day to maintain her weight. The **reference man**, who is 5 feet 9 inches tall and weighs 154 pounds (70 kilograms), requires about 2700 calories. Both sleep or lie down for eight hours a day, sit for seven hours, stand for five, walk for two, and spend two hours a day in light physical activity. Very few people fit these descriptions exactly; but as Figure 3 shows, most people fall close to the mean. The best way to ensure that your calorie intake actually fits your own particular requirements is to monitor your weight over a period of time.

As mentioned previously, no RDA is set for carbohydrate and fat. The committee expects that you will use these nutrients as you choose to meet the energy RDA.

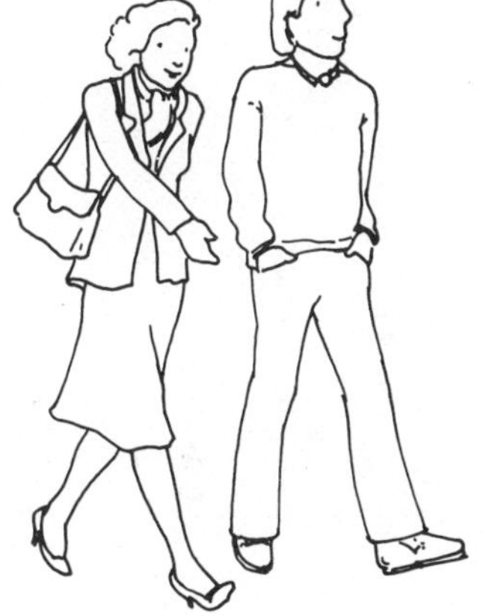

The reference man and woman are average figures used as standards.

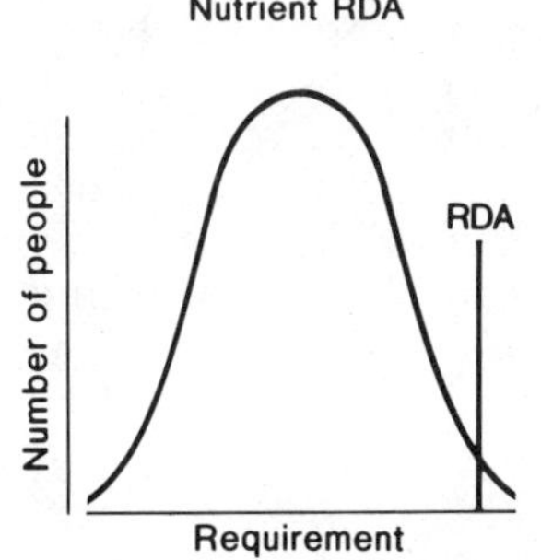

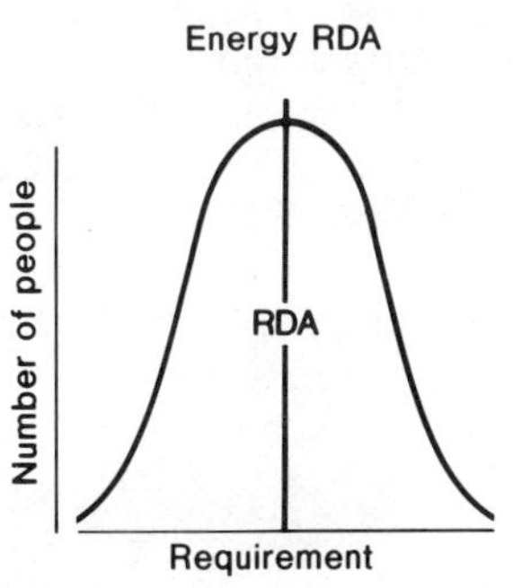

Figure 3. The difference between the nutrient RDA and the energy RDA.

The U.S. RDA. The term "U.S. RDA" appears on food labels and so deserves a paragraph of explanation. When you read a food label, you may want to have its nutrient contents expressed as a percentage of your need. For example, it would be useful to see on the label of a cereal box that one serving of the cereal provides you with 25 percent of your needed iron for the day. Your RDA could be used to give you this information; but the trouble is, the makers of the label don't know who you are: a ten-year-old boy, a seventy-year-woman, or a pregnant teen-age girl. The idea behind the U.S. RDA was to develop a single set of standards for a sort of generalized adult human being whose nutrient needs are high—as high as people's needs generally go. So if you read on a label that a serving of cereal provides 25 percent of the U.S. RDA of iron, you can be sure that it will also provide at least 25 percent of *your* iron RDA. Your need, if it is different from the U.S. RDA, is sure to be lower.

The **U.S. RDA**, then, are a set of figures chosen by the Food and Drug Administration (the FDA, which is responsible for nutrition labeling) out of the 1968 RDA tables. In most cases, the U.S. RDA is the same as the RDA for an adult man. But for iron—because a woman's need is greater than a man's—the woman's RDA is used for U.S. RDA. The table on the inside back cover shows the U.S. RDA that are used on labels that make nutritional claims.

U.S. RDA—inside back cover.

For more about reading food labels, see Chapter 11.

Other recommendations. Different nations and international groups have published different sets of standards similar to the RDA. The Canadian equivalent to the RDA is the Dietary Standard for Canada, a table of Recommended Daily Nutrient Intakes (shown in Appendix I). The Canadian recommendations differ from the RDA in some respects, partly because of differences in interpretation of the data they were derived from and partly because conditions in Canada differ somewhat from those in the United States. The differences between the two sets of recommendations will be explained as the nutrients are discussed in the coming chapters.

Among the most widely used sets of recommendations are those of two international groups: the Food and Agriculture Organization (FAO) and the World Health Organization (WHO). The FAO/WHO recommendations are "considered sufficient for the maintenance of health in nearly all people."[4] They are generally lower than the RDA, not because the RDA are too high or the others too low but because different committees have applied slightly different judgment factors. FAO/WHO, for example, assumed a protein quality lower than that commonly available in the United States and so recommended a higher intake. The United States sets its calcium recommendation higher to keep it in balance with the higher phosphorus and protein intakes of its people. Nevertheless, the figures they arrived at all fall within the same range.

Evaluation of Nutritional Status

The RDA and other such standards for daily intakes of nutrients are based on determination of people's needs—and people's needs are discovered by seeing what happens when they don't get enough of the nutrients: They get sick, one way or another, and they exhibit the symptoms of nutritional deficiencies. A nutrient already used as an example in the last chapter is iron; iron can be used again here to illustrate the stages in development of an overt nutritional deficiency.

The overt, or outside, symptoms of an iron deficiency are pallor, weakness, tiredness, apathy, and headaches. These overt symptoms are the outward manifestations of an internal state of the blood—anemia—in which there is too little of the iron-containing protein hemoglobin to carry oxygen to the cells and enable them to get their energy.

In reality, however, the appearance of overt iron deficiency is the last of a long sequence of events, as shown in Figure 4. First, there is a deficiency of iron getting into the body—either because there is not enough iron in the person's food (a **primary deficiency**) or because the person's body cannot absorb enough of the iron taken in (a **secondary deficiency**). The body then begins to use up its own stores of iron, so there is a period of declining stores. At this point, a deficiency might be said to exist already, but there are no outward signs of it yet: The person hasn't started to feel bad. Finally, the stores are used up, and insufficient hemoglobin is available to fill the new red blood cells being made. At this point, the number of red blood cells declines, the cells shrink and their color fades, and every part of the body feels the effects of an oxygen lack. Weakness, fatigue, pallor, and headaches ensue.

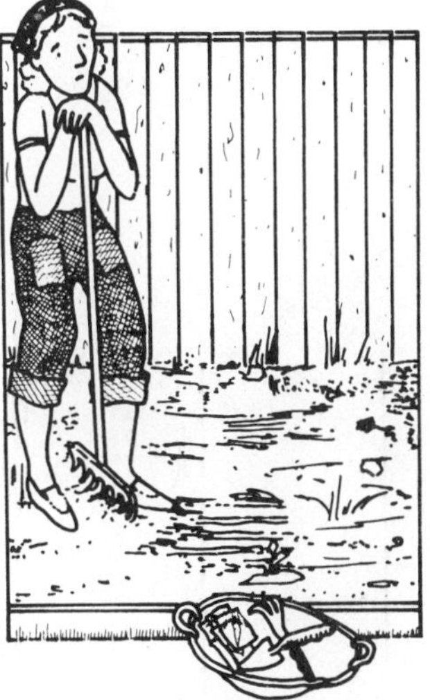

When the person feels bad, the iron deficiency has become obvious.

As Figure 4 shows, there are ways to get at the problem of deficiencies before the end stage is reached. One way that a deficient diet can be discovered is by means of a diet history. First a careful recording is made of all the foods a person eats over a period of time (say, three days or a week), with special attention to serving sizes. The foods are looked up in a table of food composition like Appendix H in this book. Then the calculated nutrient intakes are compared with recommended intakes like the RDA. This kind of study is recommended for you, the reader. The only cautions you have to exercise are to be aware that the

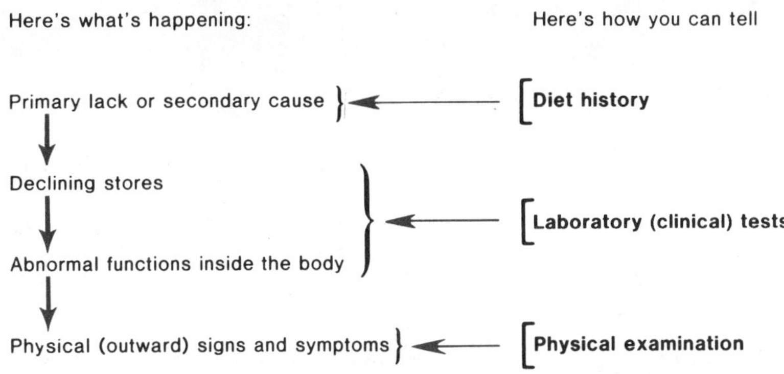

Figure 4. Stages in the development of a nutritional deficiency.

Adapted from H. H. Sandstead and W. N. Pearson, Clinical evaluation of nutrition status, in Modern Nutrition in Health and Disease, *ed. R. S. Goodhart and M. E. Shils, 5th ed. (Philadelphia: Lea and Febiger, 1973), p. 585.*

Appendix H values are not absolute (different oranges vary in their vitamin C contents), and that the values presented assume reasonable care was taken in the preparation of foods (for example, they weren't so seriously overcooked that vitamins were lost). You are also assumed to be healthy and to absorb and use the nutrients normally.

Another way to detect a developing deficiency is to take samples of body tissues (like blood or urine) and study them for the effects of a nutrient lack. If body changes are already occurring but are not yet obvious, such laboratory tests may reveal them. In the case of iron, for example, there are many tests to detect declining stores. A blood sample that shows a high level of the iron-carrier protein transferrin is an early indicator of a developing iron deficiency, because one of the body's first responses to such a deficiency is to increase its output of this protein in the effort to pick up more iron from the intestinal tract. A less sensitive but much more widely used test of iron status is the red blood cell count, which detects frank iron-deficiency anemia.

Another measure that may reveal nutritional deficiencies is the taking of height, weight, and other numerical determinations of body size. These **anthropometric measures** alert the clinician to such serious problems as growth failure in children and wasting or swelling of body tissue in adults, which may reflect severe nutrient or calorie deficiencies or imbalances.

In reading further, you may want to keep this example of nutritional assessment in mind. It illustrates several nutrition principles. For one thing, inside-the-body changes precede the outward signs of deficiencies. As a corollary, we do not have to wait for the signs of sickness to appear before doing something about it. There are tests that can be used to show deficiencies in the early stages or to confirm that nutrient stores are adequate. These principles underlie several later chapters about the vitamins and minerals. But the point of giving this example here was to lay the groundwork for answering another question: How well do we (the people of the United States and others like us, in Canada) actually meet our nutrient needs?

How Well Do We Eat?

The United States first became nutrition-conscious in the 1930s, when President Roosevelt expressed his concern that as many as a third of the nation's people might be poorly fed. A 1936 food-consumption survey confirmed his suspicions and led to national corrective programs. Significant among these were:

The Enrichment Act, which ensured that those who consumed refined bread and grain products would still obtain sufficient iron, thiamin, riboflavin, and niacin.

The National School Lunch Program, which guaranteed for every child in the public schools a lunch that would supply at least one-third RDA for all of the nutrients.

In the succeeding three decades, many surveys of the U.S. population were conducted. In general, the nutrition picture seemed to improve until 1955, when a broad survey yielded the finding that 60 percent of the households surveyed had good diets and only 15 percent had poor diets. Ten years later, in the broadest survey yet undertaken, the USDA collected data on food consumption of 15,000 households across the country and concluded that we had slipped. Only 50 percent of the households surveyed had good diets, and 21 percent had poor diets. As expected, people with limited incomes had the poorest diets, but even those with ample incomes often missed out on nutrients they needed. The nutrients most often lacking were calcium and iron, in all age groups; thiamin, in girls and women; riboflavin, in women and elderly men; vitamin A, in teenage girls and elderly men and women; and occasionally even vitamin C, in elderly men.

In 1969, public awareness of the nutritional status of U.S. citizens reached a new high. The White House Conference on Food, Nutrition and Health convened. The Senate's Poverty Subcommittee and the Select Committee on Nutrition and Human Needs held hearings that were widely broadcast on national television. They projected a picture of the poor family whose resources were inadequate to feed itself and its children. Hunger and malnutrition in the United States became a controversy and a political issue, disclaimed by some who said the findings were exaggerated, singled out by others who considered it a scandal and a national disgrace.

The Ten State (National Nutrition) Survey. In the period 1968 to 1970, the federal government authorized the National Nutrition Survey to determine the true extent of malnutrition in the United States. Dr. Arnold E. Shaefer, who had conducted many such surveys in other countries, was selected to head the project. Ten states (California, Kentucky, Louisiana, Massachusetts, Michigan, South Carolina, Texas, Washington, New York, and West Virginia) and New York City were chosen to represent geographic, ethnic, economic, and other features of the whole United States. In all, over 60,000 people were surveyed. While the findings from such a survey might be slightly different today, the kinds of information collected would be the same. Enough detail is given here to show how such a survey is conducted.

In the Ten State Survey, not only food intake but also other indicators of nutritional status were used:

Clinical tests. Blood and urine levels of many nutrients were determined and compared with standards deemed normal for the population.

Physical examination. The tissues of the skin, eyes, hair, teeth, tongue, and mouth were checked for the classical signs of nutrient deficiency, recognizable by the trained investigator. The examination also included anthropometric measures, in which body measurements such as height, weight, fatfold thickness, and x-ray measurements of bones were taken and compared with standards (such as the height-weight tables) deemed normal for the population.

Medical history. Interviews gave insight into conditions likely to precipitate nutritional deficiencies or to have been caused by them, such as the presence of intestinal parasites.

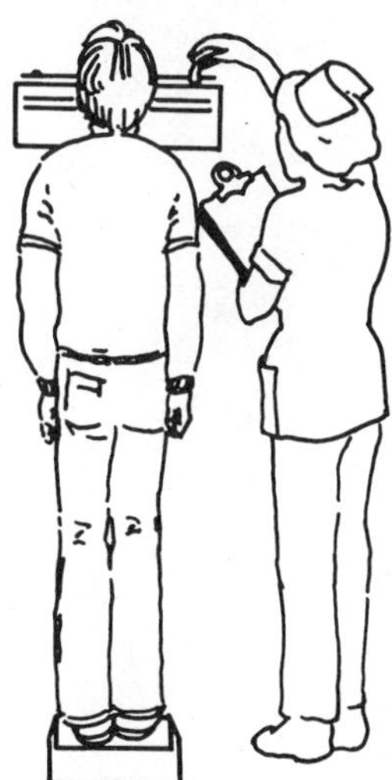

Findings from a physical examination can also reveal evidence of nutritional problems.

The subjects' educational and financial status was also determined, and information about food sources available to them was collected.[5] The results were reported in relation to age, sex, ethnic background, and location (whether the person resided in a low-income or high-income state).

The following is a brief summary of the Ten State Survey's findings:

Physical. Few severe deficiencies were identified by the physical examinations. This does not imply that there were no deficiencies present but, rather, that they were not prolonged or severe enough for the outward signs to have appeared.

Anthropometric measurements. People with higher income had greater height, weight, fatness, and skeletal weight; larger head circumference; earlier skeletal maturation; and earlier tooth eruption. Blacks were taller than whites and were more advanced in skeletal and dental development. Obesity was more prominent in adult women, especially in black women.

Persistence of childhood trends. One of the most significant findings was that the trends seen among the children persisted into adulthood, underscoring the effect of early poverty on later development.

Dental health. Among the children, Spanish and Mexican Americans were most in need of dental care. Among adults, Spanish Americans, Mexican Americans, and blacks had the greatest needs. There was a relationship between the intake of sugar and dental decay among adolescents and between low income and dental decay in all groups.

Hemoglobin and related measurements. Generally, higher dietary iron intakes correlated with higher hemoglobin levels, showing that food intakes do make a difference to this indicator of iron nutrition. Black populations, particularly, showed a prevalence of low hemoglobin in all income groups.

Protein. Deficient values for protein were not as widespread as for some of the other nutrients; the highest incidence was found among blacks and Spanish Americans. Protein deficiency correlated with low income level. Pregnant and lactating women exhibited more dietary deficiency and lower blood levels, but protein intake seemed to be generally adequate for most groups.

Vitamin A. The data show that vitamin A nutritional status was a major public health concern, particularly among adolescents and Spanish Americans, including Mexican Americans in the Southwest.

Vitamin C. There seemed to be no cause for concern regarding vitamin C intakes among the groups studied. There was a greater incidence of low values for blacks in the low-income states and generally a greater incidence among males than among females.

Riboflavin and thiamin. The B vitamin riboflavin appeared to be a potential problem among young persons of all ethnic groups and particularly among blacks and Spanish Americans in the low-income states. However, the B vitamin thiamin appeared to be no cause for concern in the populations studied.

Iodine. There did not seem to be a public health problem in regard to iodine. Iodized salt remains an important public health measure.

Multiple low biochemical values. Generally, blacks and Spanish Americans had a higher prevalence of multiple deficiencies. There was also a higher prevalence in the low-income states. One significant finding was that the fewer the years of school completed by the homemaker, the greater the prevalence of multiple low values in the family (see Figure 5).

Dietary intake. In all states, intakes of nutrients were generally lower for blacks than for whites and Spanish Americans, except that the latter had the lowest intakes of vitamin A. Foods rich in vitamin A were consumed on a daily basis by only 15 percent of all households, and 20 percent reported that they never or only rarely used them. Spanish Americans were the highest in their use of cereals and grains for calories; they received a substantially lower percentage of their calories from dairy products than did other groups. Over two-thirds of all the households used fresh milk as a beverage daily; over 80 percent of all households reported never using dry skim milk as a beverage. Evidently more education is needed in the use of economical dry skim milk.

In summary, then, target groups in need of help regarding their nutrition were obese people in all groups, blacks, Spanish and Mexican Americans, adolescents, and low-income families. The nutrients of greatest concern were iron, vitamin A, and riboflavin, with protein being a problem for pregnant and lactating women.

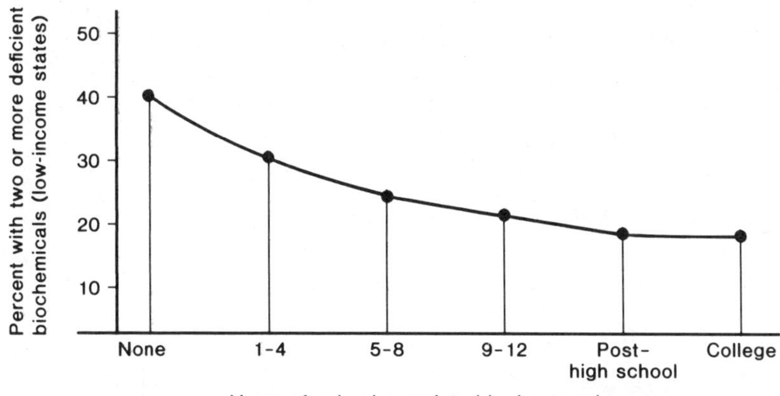

Figure 5. ***The figure shows that if the homemaker had less education, her family was more likely to have multiple deficiencies. Only data from the low-income states were used for this figure.—Ten State Survey (1968-1970)***

The Ten State Survey provided a disturbing answer to the question "How well do U.S. citizens eat?" Clearly, not as well as might be expected in the most prosperous nation in the world. But the resulting public awareness of the importance and imperfection of our nutrition led, in the 1970s, to many more questions. Which government programs should now receive top priority? Which groups of people should first receive nutritional assistance? In what form should assistance be offered: as nutrition education? as food supplementation programs? as direct financial contributions to increase the buying power of the poor? as feeding programs? The debate is likely to continue well into the 1980s and beyond. Meanwhile, priorities have been discussed and established and are being acted on. The identification of vulnerable groups has prompted the establishment of programs of many kinds intended to decrease the risk and incidence of nutritional deficiencies.

One of the greatest needs brought to light by the Ten State Survey is the need for better guidelines for all of us to follow in selecting foods. After all, nutritious foods are available and affordable, even to the poorest U.S. citizens. The RDA have been in existence since 1943, yet despite widespread familiarity with them and their use on labels they do not ensure the nutritional adequacy of our diets. The Four Food Group Plan and others like it have helped guide intelligent food selection by consumers but have sometimes had the unfortunate side effect of promoting overnutrition.

Another need is the need for better surveys. The Ten State Survey, for all the valuable data it reported, did not provide an accurate picture of the nutritional status of the people as a whole, partly because it was composed of an unbalanced sample containing a disproportionate number of low-income people. There is a need for continued surveillance, using improved techniques as they become available.

A model for action has been provided by our neighbor Canada, which conducted a massive survey during the early 1970s and kept it remarkably free from political debate.[6] Over 19,000 people of all ages and all economic levels had medical, dental, and anthropometric examinations and a dietary interview; most also provided blood and urine samples for analysis. Among the findings were:

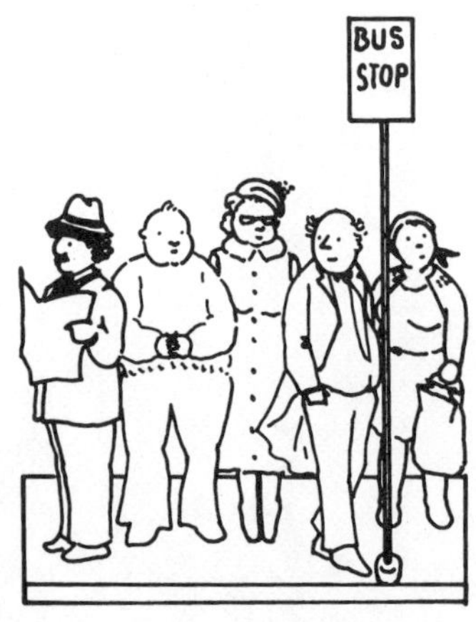

Obesity was found to be a problem among Canadians.

> The highest incidence of problems with nutritional status was found in lower-income middle-aged women and older men.
>
> A negative effect of low economic status on blood levels of certain nutrients, especially vitamin C and folacin, was seen.
>
> Evidence of iron-deficiency anemia in young and middle-aged women and elderly men was discovered.
>
> Evidence of low thiamin levels in adolescents and middle-aged adults was found.
>
> Considerable obesity was seen, especially in middle-aged adults.

The full report to the Canadian government appeared in thirteen volumes during 1974, and it led to the establishment of priorities for government action to improve the nutritional status of Canadians. These included improved food-supply monitoring, development of more complete nutritional standards for foods, consumer education programs, nutrition education for professionals, and continued surveillance of the nutritional health of the Canadian people.[7] The Canadian effort was praised by a critic who saw it as a model of "how to do a nutrition survey."[8]

At about the same time (1971-1974), the U.S. National Center for Health Statistics conducted a study of over 20,000 people, aged one to seventy-four, at sixty-five sampling sites in the United States. This study, known as the HANES (Health and Nutrition Examination Survey), avoided the bias of the Ten State Survey by adjusting for the effects of oversampling among vulnerable groups. Careful efforts were also made to evaluate protein and calorie intakes in relation to height, sex, and age on an individual basis.[9]

The HANES (Health and Nutrition Examination Survey). The investigators studied intakes of the same seven nutrients as had been used in 1965—protein, calcium, iron, vitamin A, thiamin, riboflavin, and vitamin C—as well as niacin and calories. Nutrient deficiencies were found only for protein, calcium, vitamin A, and iron. As expected, these were more extensive among people below the poverty line than among those above and generally more extensive in blacks than in whites. In particular:

> Protein intakes were low for low-income adolescents, women, and older men and for middle- and upper-income black women, older black men, and older white women.
>
> Calcium intakes were low for adult black women of all income groups.
>
> Vitamin A intakes were low for low-income white adolescents and young adult women and for adolescent black women of all income groups.
>
> Iron intakes were low for all women and for infant boys regardless of income.[10]

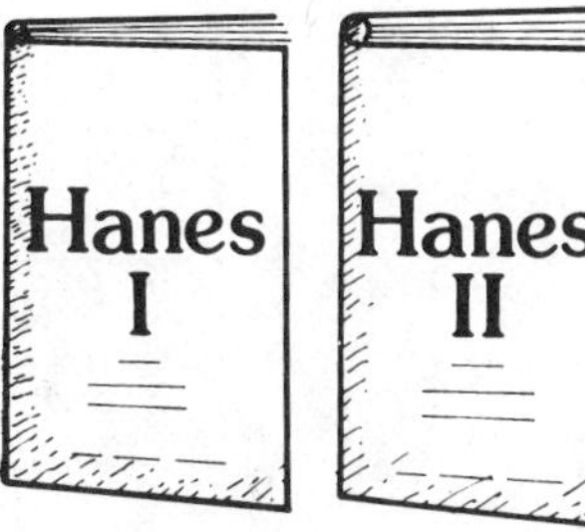

The HANES Surveys.

HANES II, undertaken in 1977 as a followup to HANES, was designed to collect biochemical and other data, with an emphasis on determining whether the low iron intakes so extensively found were reflected by a poor clinical picture.

Caution has to be exercised in interpreting the HANES survey. As the researchers themselves pointed out, "High mean intakes can mask the fact that a substantial proportion of individuals within a group may have usual nutrient intakes far below the recommended dietary allowances."[11] On the other hand, the extent of undernutrition in a single-day intake study can be overestimated. D. M. Hegsted notes: "All of us eat less than our usual intake half of the time. If we had an ideal survey of an ideal population . . . [it] would still show 50 percent below standard over any relatively short period of time."[12] These two limitations of the HANES tend to balance each other out. The survey's principal usefulness is in identifying the population subgroups most at risk of deficiency and the nutrients most in need of attention.

Further study is needed. In particular, according to Hegsted, the choice of indicator nutrients should be reexamined: "There is reason to believe that inadequate intakes of vitamin B_6, zinc, magnesium and folic acid [folacin] . . . may be more prevalent in our population than many of the nutrients usually covered in surveys."[13]

Considerable savings in the cost of surveys could be achieved if the number of indicators could be reduced without loss of valuable information. A retrospective analysis of the Ten State Survey data shows that this could be done and that folacin should be included among those included in any survey.[14] Folacin deficiency is probably the most common vitamin deficiency of all.[15]

Following HANES I, a Nationwide Food Consumption Survey was conducted in 1977-1978 to see how much and what kind of food people were eating at home and outside the home. A finding resulting from this survey confirmed suspicions that had existed from some time before: People are not eating large quantities of food calories. Although they are fat and getting fatter, their food consumption appears to be at a very low level. This must mean that they are extraordinarily inactive. The average woman consuming the foods typically available to her cannot obtain the RDA for several nutrients within the calorie allowance she obtains.[16]

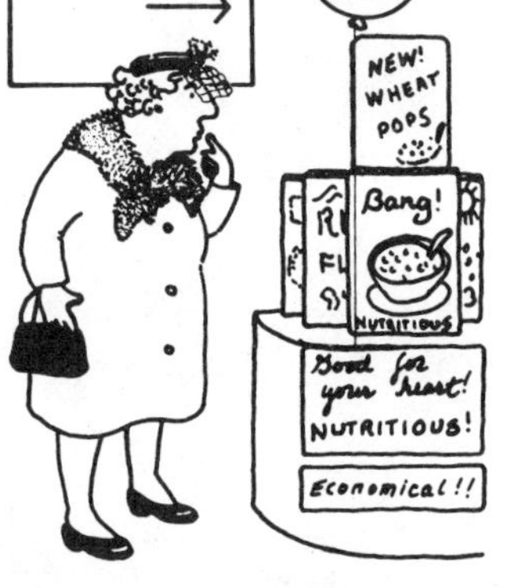

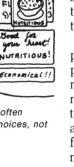

Poor nutrition today often reflects poor food choices, not poverty.

Only the major surveys have been discussed here. Many others have been conducted. It has been suggested that, wherever U.S. nutrition now is found to be poor, it is due to the greater variety of foods available, which has resulted in a "greater opportunity to make selection errors." A "short supply of nutrients in our society stems from inability to *pay* or to *choose* and, for most, it is *choose*."[17] This brings us back to the important subject of personal choices, which were the subject of Chapter 1 and which will be discussed again in the chapters to come after the individual nutrients are introduced and their importance is shown.

While surveys have revealed nutrient deficiencies in the diets of people in the United States and other developed countries, another problem has come to light that is equally serious: overconsumption of nutrients. Since the mid-1960s, there has been increasing concern that nutrition may be contributing to the illnesses our people suffer from today: heart disease, cancer, diabetes, liver disease, and others. These are not diseases of deprivation but may arise in part from excesses in fat, salt, sugar, even protein intake. Government authorities are now as much concerned to protect our people from consuming too much of these substances as they once were about our consuming too few nutrients. In the last decade, the governments of several of the developed countries have published recommendations that their people reduce their intakes of fat, salt, and sugar and turn back toward the more whole-food-based diets of their predecessors.

Among the new sets of recommendations have been the *Dietary Recommendations for Canadians* (1976), the *Dietary Goals for the United States* (1977), and the *Dietary Guidelines for Americans* (1980). These sets of guidelines differ somewhat from each other, but they generally suggest that people in the developed countries today are eating more fat, sugar, and salt than they need, and in some cases enough to harm their health. The controversies surrounding the guidelines are the subject of Controversy 3.[1]

[1]*Chapter Notes can be found at the end of the Appendixes.*

For Further Information

Recommended references on all nutrition topics are listed in Appendix J. This chapter's notes and the Controversy references also include readings that we highly recommend. The following provide further perspective.

The most recent RDA book is referred to in Appendix J.

To see how people are different from one another and how difficult this makes the task of setting standards like the RDA, turn to:

- Williams, R. J. Nutritional individuality. *Human Nature,* June 1978, pp. 46-53.

The RDA are for healthy people only. For people with disease conditions, much higher intakes of nutrients may be recommended, and the therapeutic diets necessitated by disease may not meet nutrient needs without careful planning. The topic of nutrition in disease is not covered in this book, but many excellent references are available. Among the best are:

- Williams, S. R. *Nutrition and Diet Therapy,* 3d ed. (St. Louis: Mosby, 1977)
- Mitchell, H. S., et al. *Nutrition in Health and Disease,* 16th ed. (Philadelphia: Lippincott, 1976).

For further reading on surveys of the nutritional status of people in the United States, we recommend:

- American Medical Association, Malnutrition and hunger in the United States and Iron deficiency in the United States. These reprints can be ordered from the American Medical Association (address in Appendix J).

The film *Hunger in America,* which attracted widespread publicity when broadcast on the nation's television screens in the late 1960s, can be ordered from AV Center, Indiana University, Bloomington IN, 47401. This is a humanistic documentary filmed entirely within the United States, and many viewers will find it an eye-opener with respect to the poverty it reveals. (The information given on food assistance programs is outdated, however.)

Controversy 3

Dietary Guidelines

Whose guidelines—if any —should we follow?

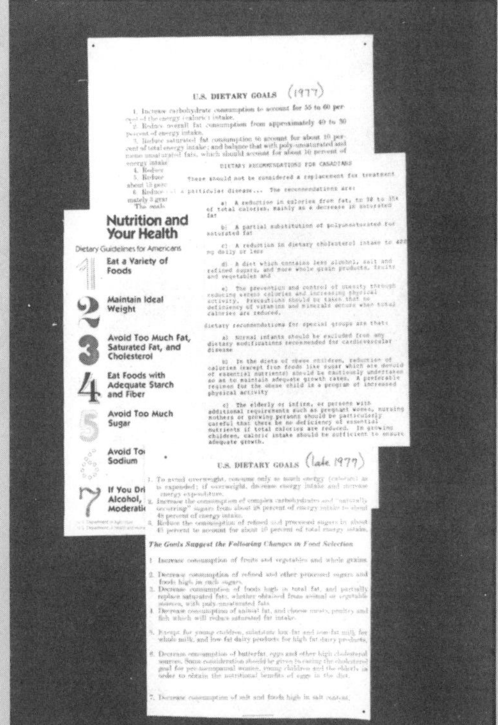

U.S. DIETARY GOALS (1977)

1. Increase carbohydrate consumption to account for 55 to 60 percent of the energy (caloric) intake.
2. Reduce overall fat consumption from approximately 40 to 30 percent of energy intake.
3. Reduce saturated fat consumption to account for about 10 percent of total energy intake; and balance that with poly-unsaturated and mono-unsaturated fats, which should account for about 10 percent of energy intake [illegible]
4. Reduce [illegible]
5. Reduce [illegible] about 15 perc[illegible]
6. Reduce [illegible] mately 3 gra[illegible]

The goals [illegible]

DIETARY RECOMMENDATIONS FOR CANADIANS

These should not be considered a replacement for treatment [illegible] a particular disease... The recommendations are:

a) A reduction in calories from fat, to 30 to 35% of total calories, mainly as a decrease in saturated fat

b) A partial substitution of polyunsaturated for saturated fat

c) A reduction in dietary cholesterol intake to 400 mg daily or less

d) A diet which contains less alcohol, salt and refined sugars, and more whole grain products, fruits and vegetables and

e) The prevention and control of obesity through reducing excess calories and increasing physical activity. Precautions should be taken that no deficiency of vitamins and minerals occurs when total calories are reduced.

Dietary recommendations for special groups are that:

a) Normal infants should be excluded from any dietary modifications recommended for cardiovascular disease

b) In the diets of obese children, reduction of calories (except from foods like sugar which are devoid of essential nutrients) should be cautiously undertaken so as to maintain adequate growth rates. A preferable regimen for the obese child is a program of increased physical activity

c) The elderly or infirm, or persons with additional requirements such as pregnant women, nursing mothers or growing persons should be particularly careful that there be no deficiency of essential nutrients if total calories are reduced. In growing children, caloric intake should be sufficient to ensure adequate growth.

Nutrition and Your Health

Dietary Guidelines for Americans

1 Eat a Variety of Foods

2 Maintain Ideal Weight

3 Avoid Too Much Fat, Saturated Fat, and Cholesterol

4 Eat Foods with Adequate Starch and Fiber

5 Avoid Too Much Sugar

6 Avoid To[illegible] Sodium

7 If You Dri[illegible] Alcohol, [illegible] Moderati[illegible]

U.S. DIETARY GOALS (late 1977)

1. To avoid overweight, consume only as much energy (calories) as is expended; if overweight, decrease energy intake and increase energy expenditure.
2. Increase the consumption of complex carbohydrates and "naturally occurring" sugars from about 28 percent of energy intake to about 48 percent of energy intake.
3. Reduce the consumption of refined and processed sugars by about 45 percent to account for about 10 percent of total energy intake.

The Goals Suggest the Following Changes in Food Selection

1. Increase consumption of fruits and vegetables and whole grains.
2. Decrease consumption of refined and other processed sugars and foods high in such sugars.
3. Decrease consumption of foods high in total fat, and partially replace saturated fats, whether obtained from animal or vegetable sources, with poly-unsaturated fats.
4. Decrease consumption of animal fat, and choose meats, poultry and fish which will reduce saturated fat intake.
5. Except for young children, substitute low-fat and non-fat milk for whole milk, and low-fat dairy products for high fat dairy products.
6. Decrease consumption of butterfat, eggs and other high cholesterol sources. Some consideration should be given to easing the cholesterol goal for pre-menopausal women, young children and the elderly in order to obtain the nutritional benefits of eggs in the diet.
7. Decrease consumption of salt and foods high in salt content.

The Canadian recommendations are taken from Report of the Committee on Diet and Cardiovascular Disease, *Health and Welfare Canada, 1976, pp. 81-82; the figure showing nutrition-sensitive and nutrition-resistant diseases is adapted from R. E. Olsen, Are professionals jumping the gun in the fight against chronic disease?* Journal of the American Dietetic Association *74 (1979): 543-550, Figure 2.*

The late 1970s and the early 1980s have seen more debate over health issues than ever before. Among the debaters are many nutrition authorities whose opinions and advice are cited often throughout this book. This Controversy is offered as a brief introduction to the principal debaters and to the issues they are struggling with.

The succession of goals and guidelines. In the 1960s, a select committee of the Senate —the Select Committee on Nutrition and Human Needs— was formed to study the nutritional status of the nation's people. For about ten years it held hearings on malnutrition and hunger in the United States and brought the people's nutritional problems to the nation's attention. Many national programs addressed to solving those problems resulted from the committee's efforts and from the publicity attending them, including feeding programs for preschoolers, school children, low-income pregnant women, and older adults. (Some details of these programs are presented later, in Part III.)

Then in the 1970s the committee's emphasis changed from a primary concern with undernutrition to a focus on overnutrition. Hearings were held on obesity, nutrition, and heart disease, the impact of dietary sugar on health, and the like. Seeing many connections between overnutrition and the diseases that disable and kill older people, the committee concluded that it would be desirable to issue some dietary guidelines to the nation's people. In February 1977, it published its *Dietary Goals for the United States*,[1] which emphasized sugar, fat, cholesterol, and salt as items to avoid.

In the next three years, there followed a flurry of activity. Critics reacted violently against the *Dietary Goals*, and the committee published a revised edition within the year that suggested weight reduction if necessary and the avoidance of alcohol overuse. Then the committee was disbanded. The Department of Health and Human Services (formerly Health, Education, and Welfare—DHEW) assumed the task of providing dietary advice to the people; the Department of Agriculture got into the act; and the two departments ended up sharing the job with occasional misunderstandings between them. In February 1980, they jointly issued a document entitled *Dietary Guidelines for Americans*, somewhat different from the *Goals* but still emphasizing the original four items as well as reduction of alcohol consumption and weight if necessary and the consumption of a variety of foods.

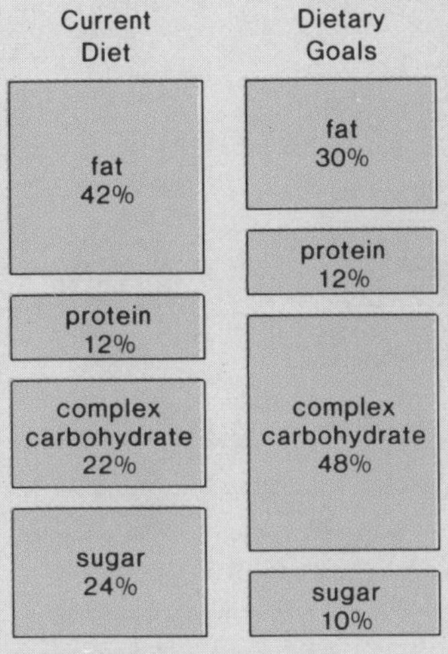

The American Diet

The current U.S. diet and the recommended diet, according to the Dietary Goals.

There were many differences of opinion among authorities in reaction to the *Goals* and *Guidelines*, and some were major ones; but there were also a few areas of agreement. Most seemed to think it was desirable to cut down on fat and cholesterol consumption.

Then the National Academy of Sciences' National Research Council (NAS/NRC) upstaged the others and wiped out this area of agreement. The NAS/NRC Food and Nutrition Board (the same agency that sets the RDA) published its statement in a document called *Toward Healthful Diets* that said almost nothing about fat and cholesterol. What it did say seemed to contradict most of the guidelines that had gone before. The popular magazine *Nutrition Today* compared the ensuing upset to the volcanic eruptions of Mount St. Helens that were occurring around the same time.

Still, there remained a last stronghold: weight control. Everyone agrees that we should achieve and maintain a weight on the slim side of average—right? Wrong: Actually this dogma too is being debated as statistics on the lifespans of Americans reveal a slight advantage (except for those with high blood pressure) to being a little *over*weight (see Controversy 8).

If the authorities can't agree, how can consumers decide whom to believe? The chapters and Controversies that follow will help you to make judgments on each of the issues the experts have been arguing about: carbohydrate and sugar, fats and cholesterol, salt, ideal weight. This Controversy sets the stage and presents the problems inherent in offering dietary advice to the public at all.

Risks of offering dietary advice. The dilemma of those who try to advise the public is revealed in the reactions of the many people who have responded to the various

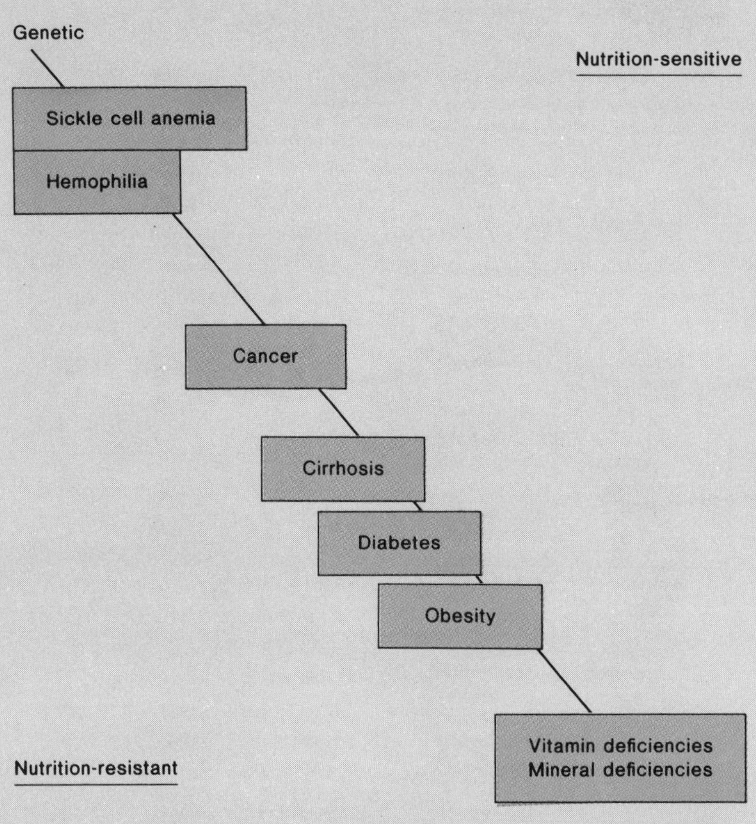

Not all diseases are equally influenced by diet. Some are purely hereditary, like sickle cell anemia. Some may be inherited (or the tendency to them may be inherited) but may be influenced by diet, like some forms of diabetes. Some are purely dietary, like the vitamin- and mineral-deficiency diseases.

Some authorities are concerned that the offering of dietary advice to the public may seem to exaggerate the power of nutrition in preventing disease. Nutrition alone is certainly not enough to prevent many diseases.

Adapted from R. E. Olsen, Are professionals jumping the gun in the fight against chronic disease? Journal of the American Dietetic Association *74 (1979): 543-550, Figure 2.*

documents mentioned above. Here are some of the problems.

(1) Do we know enough? The editor of *Nutrition Today*, C. F. Enloe, Jr., took a position against the *Goals*, arguing that to state such concrete guidelines before all the evidence was in was to overemphasize the power of nutrition, pretending to know more than we do. He believed that it was inappropriate for "politicians" to decide on nutritional issues and stated further that neither the risks nor the costs had been properly assessed. One of the risks, he said, was that public confidence in science might be undermined; another, that research funds might be cut if the public believed scientists already knew enough to make such concrete statements. Many other authorities agreed with Enloe, finding the *Goals* inexcusably premature: To adopt them would be to risk damaging public confidence, reducing support for research, and causing actual harm to health, as well as disrupting the food industry and disturbing the nation's economy.[2]

(2) Should they be so broad? There is some concern that recommendations made for the general public, while beneficial to most people, may harm some subgroups. For example the advice to cut down on fat may be suitable for most middle-aged adults but overlooks the young infant who could be harmed by such a measure.

Another concern is that the recommendations may benefit only a minority and may not be suitable for most. For example, reducing salt intake is generally agreed on as an important preventive measure for people whose family histories suggest they may inherit high blood pressure, but it may be unnecessary for other people. To suggest that everyone adopt this measure burdens those to whom it doesn't apply with unnecessary restrictions on their diets. Similarly, reducing fat or sugar intake may be advisable for people who are sensitive to these substances or already sick with heart disease but not for "normal" people.

(3) Are they farsighted enough? Those who offer dietary

advice to the public have their hearts in the right place; they are trying to do good, not harm. But they run the risk of overlooking important side effects. For example, the original *Dietary Goals* recommended cutting down on foods high in saturated fat and cholesterol, and this is taken to mean meat, milk, and eggs by most of the public. But it happens that meat is a major source of dietary iron, and one of the nation's most serious public health problems is iron-deficiency anemia. Cutting down on meat might make this problem worse, especially for vulnerable groups like children, women of childbearing age, and older people. Similarly, milk is an extremely nutritious food, and its calcium is needed by adults as well as by children. And eggs are one of the most economical, high-quality protein sources, especially valuable for low-income groups. Thus again, measures that might help some people would hurt others.

Years ago, in the 1940s, when the first study of diet and heart-artery disease in men was concluded, it was revealed that a high saturated-fat intake correlated with a high blood cholesterol level—and high blood cholesterol is a prominent risk factor for atherosclerosis. It was also clear that a high P:S ratio (ratio of polyunsaturated to saturated fat) appeared to protect against atherosclerosis. At that time, there were a few who suggested that a means of protecting oneself from risk would be to increase one's intake of polyunsaturated fat. But since then, population studies have shown high intakes of *any* kind of fat—and perhaps especially polyunsaturated fat—to be associated with certain kinds of cancers.[3] This is a striking example of prematurely offered dietary advice. The advice should have been to cut down on total fat first and only then—if at all—to alter the P:S ratio.

(4) What will it do to the food industry? Most vocal in opposition to the original *Goals* were the food people most likely to be hurt by them. In January 1978, the *New York Times* quoted the Salt Institute as saying it was "inappropriate" to reduce salt intake, the International Sugar Research Foundation as saying it was "unfortunate and ill-advised" to urge people to use less sugar, and the National Canners Association as taking exception to the select committee's stress on eating fresh fruits and vegetables—even while they were beginning to consider reducing the salt in their products.[4] These reactions are perhaps the least believable of the lot because they arise from a concern for corporate profits, not for the progress of science; but they reflect a real concern.

Benefits. Those who favor offering dietary advice to the public are more inclined to emphasize the positive. Among their views are the following.

(1) It can't hurt. D. M. Hegsted (professor of nutrition, Harvard School of Public Health, and a member of the select committee) introduced the *Goals* to the public and took a strong stand in their favor to the effect that they did not entail significant risks:

This diet which affluent people generally consume is everywhere associated with a similar disease pattern—high rates of heart disease, certain forms of cancer, diabetes, and obesity. These are the major causes of death and disability in the United States. . . . It is not correct, strictly speaking, to say that they are caused by malnutrition but rather that an inappropriate diet contributes to their causation. . . . Not all people are equally susceptible. Yet those who are genetically susceptible, most of us, are those who would profit most from an appropriate diet. . . . The diet we eat today was not planned or developed for any particular purpose. It is a happenstance related to our affluence, the productivity of our farmers and the activities of our food industry. The risks associated with eating this diet are demonstrably large. The question to be asked, therefore, is not why should we change our diet but why not? What are the risks . . . ? There are none that can be identified and important benefits can be expected.[5]

E. L. Wynder (president of the American Health Foundation) substantially agreed, saying, "The high-fat, high-cholesterol diet of most people in the Western world today is biologically and metabolically incompatible with man's sedentary way of life." Like Hegsted, Wynder admitted that more research would be necessary to pinpoint the exact relationships between diet and disease but said that in the meantime "it behooves us to act prudently. . . . In the words of Kant, 'It is often necessary to make a decision on the basis of knowledge sufficient for action but insufficient to satisfy the intellect.'"[6]

(2) It'll be good for the earth. As it happens (and perhaps this is no coincidence), most of the goals and guidelines offered to date have had a point in common: They tend to favor a return toward a more whole-food, plant-based diet. The Worldwatch Institute (a private organization) has taken the position that the only known risk of such a trend would be to the food industry, whereas important benefits to the economy would counterbalance this effect. An increase in the consumption of fruits, vegetables, and whole grains and a decrease in the consumption of empty-calorie fats, oils, and sugar would increase the nutrient density of our diet, thereby reducing both overnutrition and malnutrition. The shift from animal towards plant foods would also reduce the amount of land needed to produce food and so help solve the world's food shortage.[7]

Some have taken this idea a step further, urging that the effects on the earth should be a major factor affecting the choice of dietary advice offered to the public:

Raise chickens instead of beef and grass feed livestock. . . . Only one-half the energy required to produce beef protein is required to produce broiler protein. . . . Grass feeding of livestock . . . could save 135 million tons of grain per year (ten times as much grain as the U.S. human population consumes) and save up to 60 percent of the energy used. . . . The grain, valued at $20 billion, would be available for export.[8]

(3) It gets attention. Whatever ultimate good the offering of dietary advice may provide, calling attention to nutrition issues seems to be one guaranteed outcome, and there may be real benefits from this alone. As M. Winick (head of Columbia University's Institute of Human Nutrition) put it, the debaters have done "an incredibly good job of bringing awareness of nutrition as a major health problem to the people."[9]

Personal strategy: Informed tentativeness. While the folks in D.C. argue with those in Maryland who disagree with those in Illinois who criticize those in California (and so on through all the other states and Canada), what is the public to do—if anything—about their diets? They can't suspend eating until all of the answers are in. They'll be making choices three times a day or so, whether they want to or not.

Some disillusioned dieters are tempted to give up in disgust and ignore all dietary advice, figuring that the stress of worrying about it all may be worse than the risks of eating the wrong foods. Others are excruciatingly careful to avoid all suspect foods and substances, and they plan their whole lives around this objective. Still others switch from one strategy to another depending on their mood of the moment.

It is unwise to ignore the current dietary advice altogether—unless, perhaps, your family background suggests that you will live to be ninety no matter what you do. Where there has been so much ado, there is doubtless a reality: that nutrition does affect health, longevity, and the quality of life. The debaters aren't arguing this point. What concerns them is how strongly to put their advice—and to whom.

It makes sense, in fact, to follow the guidelines offered by these advisers and to follow most closely those that most probably apply to you. One that applies to all of us without exception is that we need to eat a balanced and varied diet. The human body hasn't been invented yet that can stay healthy without its needed nutrients. Beyond this basic advice, there are special factors. If some of your relatives have high blood pressure, for example, watch your salt intake. If they have early heart and artery disease, control your fat intake—until further notice. If you tend towards diabetes, avoid sugar. And so on. (The details of how to do these things are presented in the chapters to come.)

Meanwhile, keep your eyes and ears open—and also your mind. As new information becomes available, you may want to modify your food choices accordingly.

It is frustrating to have no hard-and-fast rules to follow, but the educated and mature person realizes that to ask for answers carved in stone is to ask too much, especially in science, including nutrition science. Scientific progress is not a series of revelations of new truths but a set of successive approximations of a picture of reality that fits the observed facts. As Editor Enloe puts it, "In science one has to be as ready to unlearn as to learn."[10] This doesn't make the scientist inferior to the dogmatist who has all the answers; it makes her or him superior, in the sense of being close enough to the borders of the unknown to be humble.

While it is frustrating to await solid statements on diet, it is equally difficult to perform the task of the scientist vis-a-vis the public: "to report accurately on scientific progress without at the same time fostering ideas that will later prove unsound." There is even an American Tentative Society whose goal is to try to do this.[11] This book takes the tentative line, and encourages you to do the same. It may not be comfortable, but it is challenging and growthful to await the latest nutrition news with a willingness to modify your views in its light.

The Controversy Notes and For Further Information follow the Appendixes.

PART TWO

THE NUTRIENTS

Chapters 4, 5, and 6 present the energy (calorie-containing) nutrients, show how the body handles them, and describe the foods that contain them.

Chapter 7 shows how energy is processed in the body, and Chapter 8 relates energy balance to the problems of overweight, obesity, and underweight.

Chapters 9 and 10 introduce and describe the noncalorie nutrients —vitamins, minerals, and water—and the foods in which they are found.

CHAPTER 4

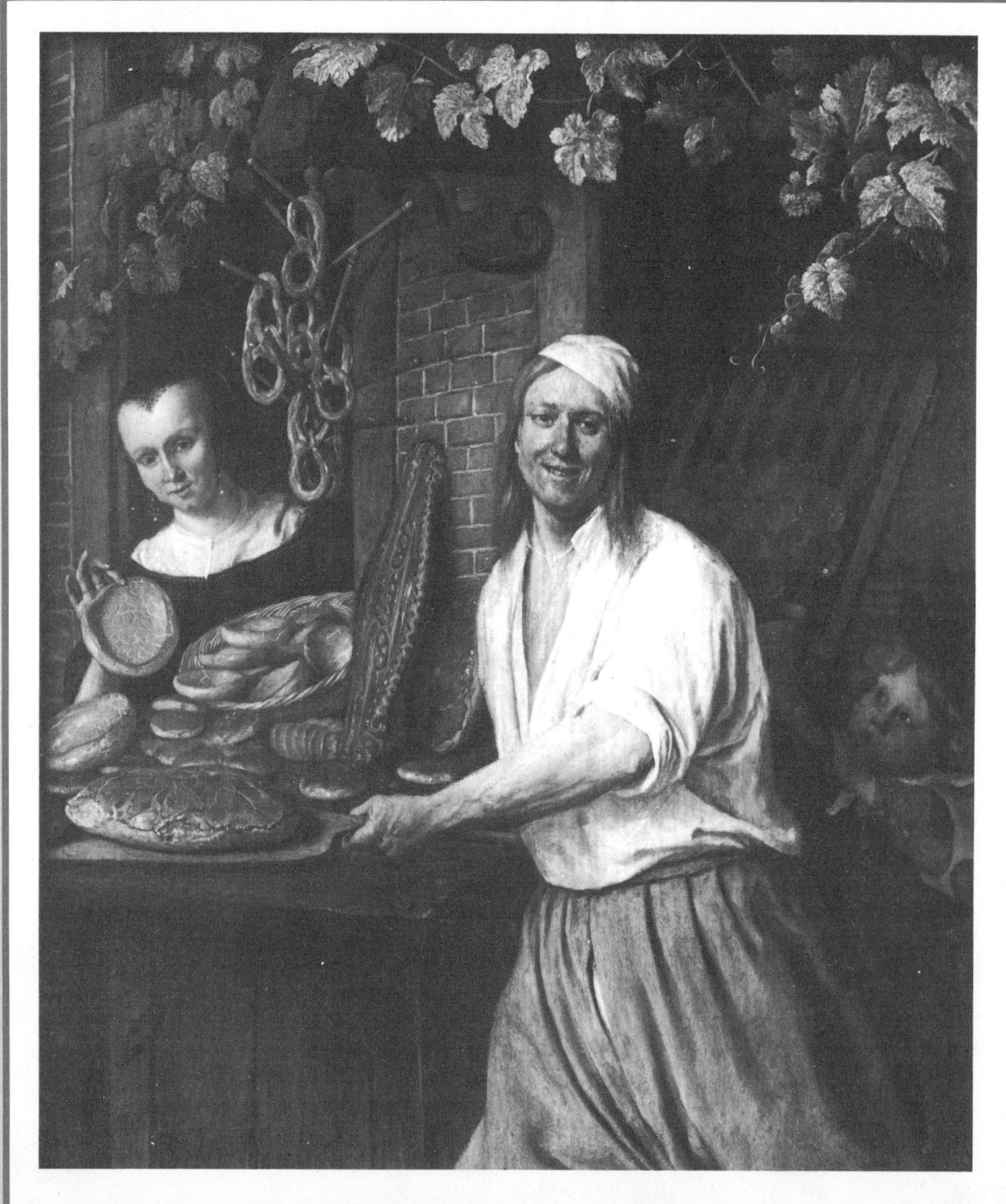

The Carbohydrates: Sugar, Starch, and Fiber

Carbohydrate has for years been wronged in the press. Its reputation as a fattening ingredient of foods doubtless comes from the fact that many foods high in carbohydrate are eaten with fat, such as butter on potatoes or bread. Carbohydrate, fat, and protein all supply calories. People who need to lose weight must avoid high-calorie foods, but they are ill advised to try to avoid all carbohydrate.

This chapter invites you to learn to distinguish between certain carbohydrates—such as starch and fiber—that are put to good use in the body and others—such as concentrated sugars—whose value is questioned.

***Carbohydrates*:**
Sugars.
Starch.
Fiber.

The Body's Need for Carbohydrate

Carbohydrate is the ideal dietary source of fuel for most body functions. There are only three alternative energy sources in the diet—protein, fat, and alcohol. Protein is expensive and, when used to make fuel for the body, provides no advantage over carbohydrate. Fat is less costly but can't be used efficiently by the brain and central nervous

Opposite: Baker Oostwaard *by Jan Steen. Used with the permission of the Rijksmuseum, Amsterdam.*

system. Alcohol has the same disadvantage, to say nothing of its well-known undesirable side effects. Thus, of all the possible alternatives, carbohydrate is the preferred calorie source.

Carbohydrate has always been a major fuel source for plant-eating animals, and it is believed that food starch has until recently been the main food source of human energy.[1] In fact, it seems that there had to be starchy plants before mammals and humans could even come into being.

Eons ago, the first green plants spread slowly over the earth and supported the gradual evolution of ponderous creatures like the dinosaurs of a hundred million years ago. While they were awake in the heat of the midday sun, these great beasts constantly ate masses of leaves and stems; but the plants contained no concentrated carbohydrate. The dinosaurs couldn't eat enough of them to store enough energy to keep their bodies moving or even warm during the cold nights. Their metabolic rate was slow, and their temperature changed with that of the air around them. Their brains were small and suffered from the lack of an energy supply when the temperature fell. In the face of cold, they helplessly went to sleep.

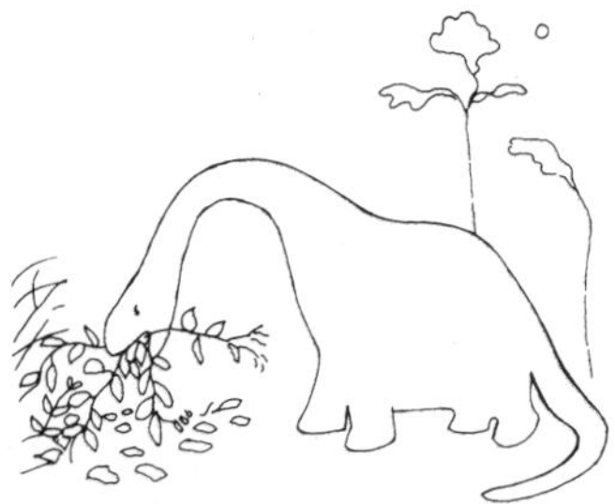

Dinosaurs had to eat masses of leaves and stems to obtain enough carbohydrate.

Then came the flowering plants. The earlier plants had reproduced by means of spores carried by the wind, but the flowering plants grew fruits containing sugars and seeds containing starch and oils. Thus they packaged each of their offspring with a case on the outside and enough energy food inside to sustain it until it could make a foothold in the earth. This advantage enabled the seed-bearing plants to replace the earlier plants as the earth's main form of vegetation.

The seeds and fruits of the flowering plants contained enough concentrated energy food to support animals whose expenditures of energy were greater than those of the dinosaurs. As the ages passed, the mammals evolved. These animals made significant advances in their use of plant carbohydrate. They developed the ability to store it and to use it between meals to keep their bodies warm and their blood sugar levels constant. A mammal doesn't need to eat constantly in order to think. A human being's large brain, supplied with constant warmth and fuel, doesn't have to turn off in winter or at night. Guaranteed of energy even between meals, the brain can occupy itself with matters other than the gathering of food. Thus, the ultimate evolution of human beings and the explosion of their civilization and technology are partly a result of these developments.

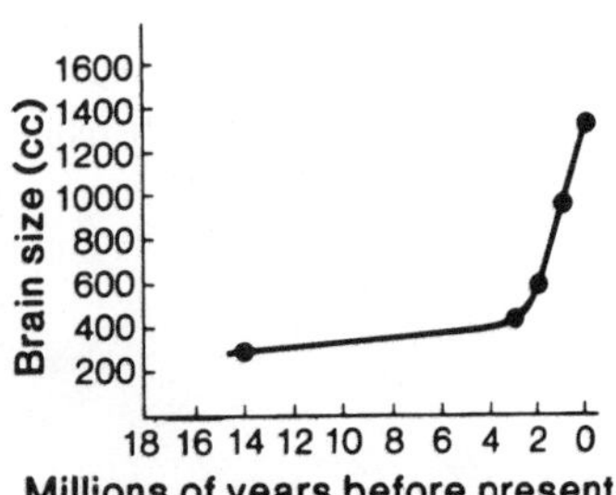

The graph shows that human brain size "suddenly" increased during evolution. The increase coincided with the development of flowering plants.

Adapted from D. Pilbeam, The Ascent of Man *(New York: Macmillan, 1972), as adapted by E. O. Wilson,* Sociobiology: The New Synthesis *(Cambridge, Mass.: Belknap Press, Harvard University Press, 1975), p. 548, with the permission of both publishers.*

The human brain still depends exclusively on carbohydrate for its energy whenever that fuel is available. And because the mind resides in the brain, to some extent your attitude toward life, the world, and other people is affected by the brain's blood glucose supply.

There are still other reasons why carbohydrate is thought to be our most valuable energy nutrient. A select committee of the U.S. Senate reviewed evidence and concluded that diets high in complex carbohydrates may reduce the risk of heart disease. Its report advocates high-starch diets, even for people with high blood fat. The report includes the observation that a young man's weight-reducing diet can include as many as twelve slices of bread in a day and still allow him to lose more than a pound a week;[2] it also recommends that we increase our consumption of potatoes. Even diabetics, who used to be thought unable to handle carbohydrates, are being exhorted to eat "liberal amounts of starch."[3]

The special energy needs of the endurance athlete, who uses both fat and carbohydrate during an endurance event, are described in Controversy 7.

The Senate committee's recommendations have generated much disagreement. Some people say the committee was guilty of jumping to conclusions. Its reasoning was: "We evolved using complex carbohydrate; therefore our bodies are not adapted to use sugar, and it may be damaging to our health." The reasoning seems sound and may very well point in the direction of good health, but it is only logic—logic without proof. To be acceptable as truth, the assumptions on which this logic is based must be subjected to experiments designed to test them objectively and thoroughly.

Many such experiments are reviewed in the committee's report, and they make interesting reading. The question of whether complex carbohydrate is "good" for you and simple carbohydrate is "bad" is also examined in depth in Controversies 4A and 4B, where other experiments are presented. As a general rule, however, you should be warned that logic, no matter how persuasive, can be used to mislead the unwary consumer. For example, it might be argued that you need energy, that sugar provides energy, and that therefore you need sugar. There are two true facts in this reasoning; and they have been used to sell cola beverages and candy bars, as any watcher of television is aware. However, the truths are bent to sell a product, the complete story is not told, and the conclusion is not based on evidence. Watch out for logic without proof.

In assessing the validity of statements about nutrition (or any other field), it also helps to know who the speaker is and what qualifies the speaker as an authority on the subject. Among the things to examine are the person's training, experience, credentials, and reputation. Some of the Controversies make rather heavy reading, because each authority is identified by a long list of titles and credentials. But when such information is supplied, even though it slows you down, you get an opportunity to weigh the statements being made.

Another question to ask is "What does the speaker stand to gain from having me believe the statement?" If the speaker has a direct financial interest—is, in fact, selling something—the statement may be suspect.

The title "Doctor" should—but doesn't always—identify a reliable authority.

If you have been exposed to as much anticarbohydrate propaganda as most people have been, these statements may be startling. Yet much evidence supports them. They are presented here not as absolute truths but as signs to alert you to think seriously about your own diet: You may want to make space in it for more carbohydrate-containing foods.

The Senate committee made two recommendations about carbohydrate, and the *Dietary Guidelines for Americans* include the same suggestions:

Eat foods with adequate starch and fiber.

Avoid too much sugar.

The Dietary Guidelines *are shown in full at the start of Controversy 3.*

The Canadian government has made similar recommendations to its people, as have the governments of several other countries. At this point, it becomes important to understand what starch and sugar are, and how the body handles them.

Actually, there are three categories of carbohydrates that we should think of separately: the complex carbohydrates, which include starch and fiber; the naturally occurring sugars like those in fruits; and the concentrated sugars like honey and the sugar in the sugar bowl. All of these carbohydrates have characteristics in common, but they are of different merit nutritionally. The sugar we are told to avoid is the concentrated kind, not the natural sugars in fruits and other plant foods.

Complex carbohydrates:
Starch.
Fiber.
Simple carbohydrates (sugars):
Naturally occurring sugars.
Concentrated sugars.

All of the carbohydrates are made partly or completely of the natural sugar glucose, and all but cellulose (fiber) can quickly be converted to glucose in the body, as the following section shows.

A Closer Look at Carbohydrate

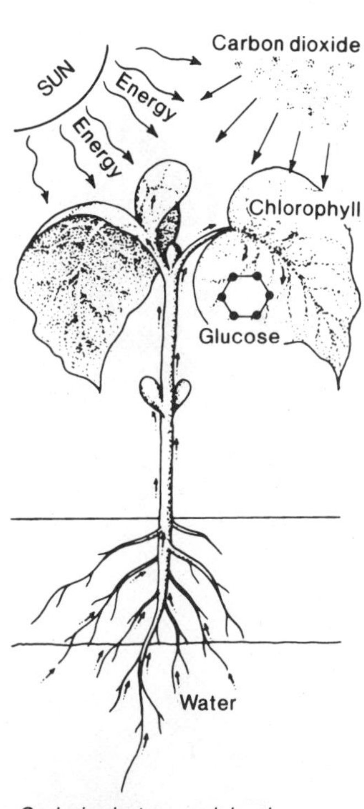

Carbohydrate—mainly glucose—is made by photosynthesis. The sun's energy becomes part of the glucose molecule—its calories.

When the sun beats down on the green leaf of an apple tree, the energy of its rays, with the help of **chlorophyll**, causes the carbon dioxide that the leaf takes from the air and the water that the roots bring up from the soil to combine into the simple sugar called **glucose**. This exceedingly complex reaction, **photosynthesis**, has never been reproduced in a laboratory. It has been analyzed, and scientists know in minutest detail most of the steps in the total chemical reaction, yet it has never been done from scratch; it requires the help of a green plant.

Some of the energy that the sun gives to the reaction is used to make it happen, and some is lost as heat, but some—and this is the part that is important to our survival—is trapped in the bonds that hold the atoms in the special configuration that is glucose. The energy so caught and held will remain there until some agent (perhaps an enzyme) breaks the bond, freeing the energy.

The glucose made in the leaf is sent throughout the entire apple tree to provide the energy for the work of its cells in the trunk, roots, and fruit. For example, in the roots, far from the energy-giving rays of the sun, each cell takes some of the glucose, breaks it down to carbon dioxide and water, and uses the energy thus released to fuel its own growth and water-gathering activities.

Some of the glucose units are linked together to form **cellulose** fibers, which make the supporting structures of the trunk, leaves, fruit, and roots of the tree. The bonds that hold these glucose units together can only be broken by certain enzymes. Ruminants, such as cattle, have bacteria in their stomachs that can synthesize the enzymes to break these special bonds, so ruminants can live on the energy from cellulose. Humans and some other animals can't synthesize the necessary enzymes and therefore can obtain no energy from the cellulose in plant foods. (But when we eat beef, we receive indirectly some of the sun's energy that was originally stored in the cellulose of the cattle's fodder.)

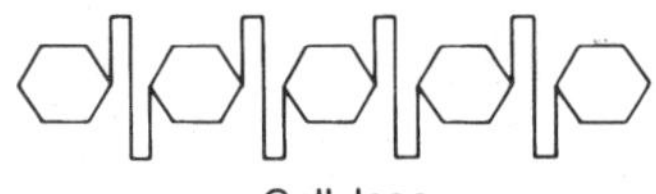
Cellulose

Glucose units are linked by bonds to form cellulose. We can't make the enzymes to break these bonds, so cellulose provides no energy for us.

Cellulose is a valuable part of the human diet, even though it provides no energy. It forms an indigestible bulk against which the muscles of the intestines can exercise and so retain their healthy tone. Cellulose is the **fiber** so highly praised in cereal advertisements today and the "roughage" of a generation ago.

roughage (RUFF-idge)

Some of the arguments for returning to a high-fiber diet are based on experiments that show that fiber does have certain beneficial effects. For example, it relieves constipation in some instances. However, other arguments, like the following, are based on logic without proof: (1) Certain African tribes eat a high-fiber diet, and they do not have diverticulosis; (2) people in Western countries eat much less fiber, and they do have diverticulosis; (3) therefore, we should eat more fiber. The first two statements are true and consistent with the fiber theory, but they don't prove it. Such evidence is sometimes called "correlational": A occurs with B, and this suggests but does not prove that A causes B.

Partial truths can be used to mislead a consumer into foolish actions. It takes practice to become alerted to them. In reading Controversy 4B you may want to try your skill at criticizing the evidence for and against the theory that we need more fiber in our diets.

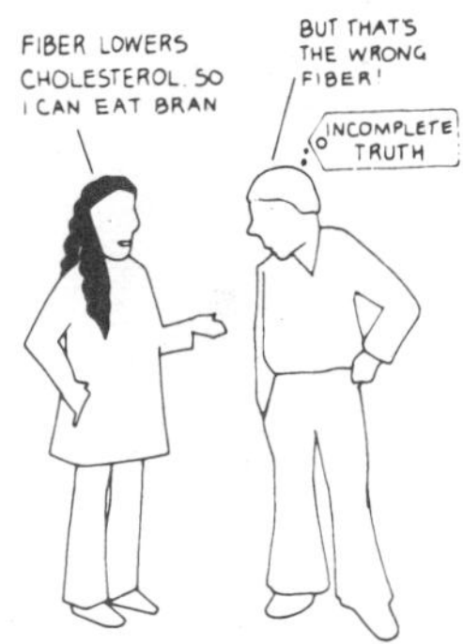
FIBER LOWERS CHOLESTEROL, SO I CAN EAT BRAN
BUT THAT'S THE WRONG FIBER!
INCOMPLETE TRUTH

The idea that all fibers lower blood cholesterol is an oversimplification.

As a plant matures, it provides not only for its own energy needs but also for food for the next generation. For example, after a potato plant reaches its full growth and has many leaves manufacturing glucose, it begins to store surplus energy for the growth of potatoes next season. It can't store the glucose itself, because glucose is soluble in water and would be washed away by the winter rains. Instead, it must form an insoluble substance, without a large outlay of energy, that will stay with the seed and nourish it until it puts out shoots with leaves to catch the sun's rays. This storage form of glucose is **starch**, packaged in the potato together with the seeds (eyes).

Starch, like cellulose, is made up of many (up to 1000) glucose units bonded together. Unlike cellulose, however, starch can be used by humans for energy; we can make the enzymes necessary to break the bonds in starch. Within the plant, starch molecules are found inside cells encased in cellulose (indigestible, insoluble) walls. Thus we must usually cook starchy foods to make them digestible. The cooking ruptures the cell walls and allows the starch to escape. While being cooked, the starch becomes soluble and can then be easily digested.

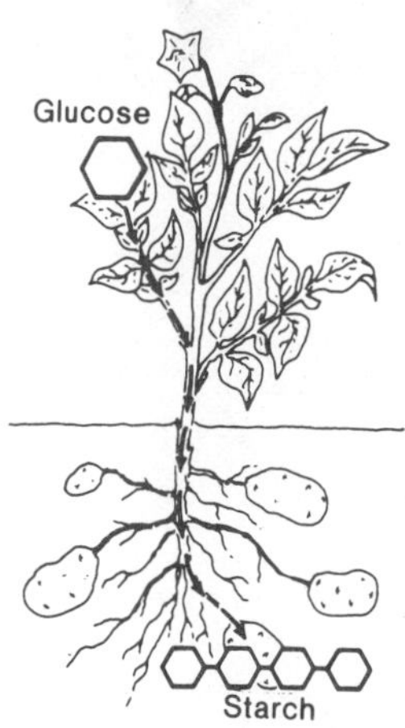

Glucose units link to each other to form starch. We can make the enzymes to break these bonds, so starch can provide energy for us.

The atoms of glucose can be rearranged by the plant to form another sugar, **fructose**, which is sweet to the taste. Fructose, as the name implies, is found mostly in fruits, berries, and honey. These two sugars, glucose and fructose, are the most common simple sugars in

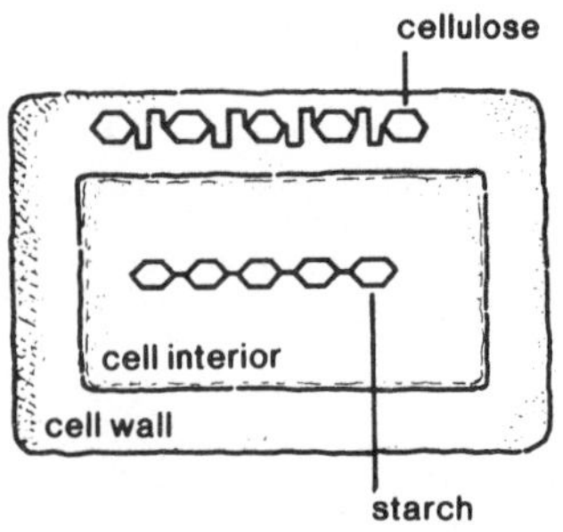

A plant cell. Plant foods provide glucose in both forms—as the indigestible fiber, cellulose, and as starch. Cooking them breaks open the cells and frees the starch.

nature. Another, **galactose**, has the same numbers and kinds of atoms, but they are arranged a little differently. Galactose does not occur free in nature; it is always bonded to something else. These three sugars are **monosaccharides**—single sugars that stand alone.

The monosaccharide fructose is now on sale in purified, crystalline form, billed as a "natural" sugar that—unlike the nasty unnatural sugar sucrose—won't cause ugly weight gain. The reader of Controversy 1 will easily recognize the fallacy in this sales pitch: What's natural about *any* purified, concentrated sugar? And the calories in fructose are used in exactly the same way as those in sucrose—to give you energy or to make you fat.

When glucose and fructose are bonded together, they form a **disaccharide**. This is the product most people think of when they use the term *sugar*. Ordinary white granulated table sugar is **sucrose**, a disaccharide whose sweet taste comes from the fructose in its structure. Its principal food sources are sugar cane and sugar beets.

Some people believe that honey is better than white sugar, because it's natural. As a matter of fact, chemically they are almost indistinguishable.

Table 1. Honey versus Sugar

	Protein (g)	Calcium (mg)	Iron (mg)	Vitamin A (IU)	Thiamin (mg)	Riboflavin (mg)	Niacin (mg)	Vitamin C (mg)
Sugar (1 tbsp)	0	0	tr	0	0	0	0	0
Honey (1 tbsp)	tr	1	0.1	0	tr	0.01	0.1	tr
1 tbsp honey's contribution to daily need of adult man	<1/100	<1/100	1/100	0	<1/100	<1/100	<1/100	<1/100

At first glance, honey looks more nutritious than sugar but when compared to a person's nutrient needs, neither contributes anything to speak of. Calculations are from Appendix H, Items 541 and 550, and the U.S. RDA.

Honey contains two monosaccharides, glucose and fructose, in approximately equal amounts. Sugar (sucrose) contains the same monosaccharides combined into the disaccharide sucrose. In the body, after digestion, sugar and honey are identical. Spoon for spoon, however, sugar contains fewer calories than honey, because the crystals of sugar take up more space.

Some people believe that fruit may be bad for you because it too contains the monosaccharides glucose and fructose. However, fruit differs in important ways from both table sugar and honey. Its sugars are diluted in large volumes of water, packaged in fiber, and mixed with many vitamins and minerals needed by the body.

From these two examples, you may see that the really significant difference between sugar sources is not between "natural" and "purified" sugar but between concentrated sweets and the dilute, naturally occurring sugars that sweeten nutritious foods.

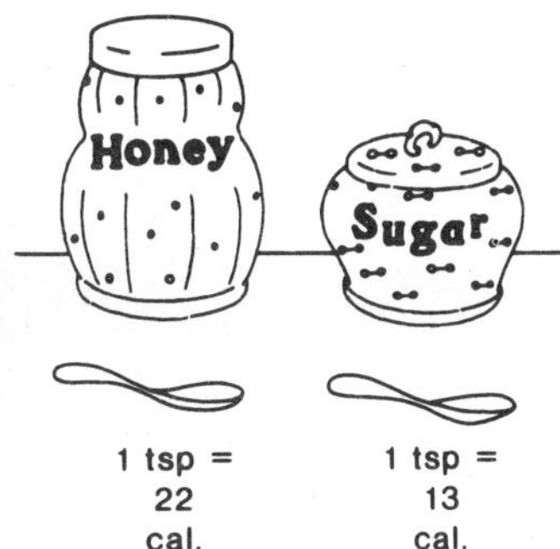

Honey and sucrose contain the same monosaccharides but in sucrose they are linked together.

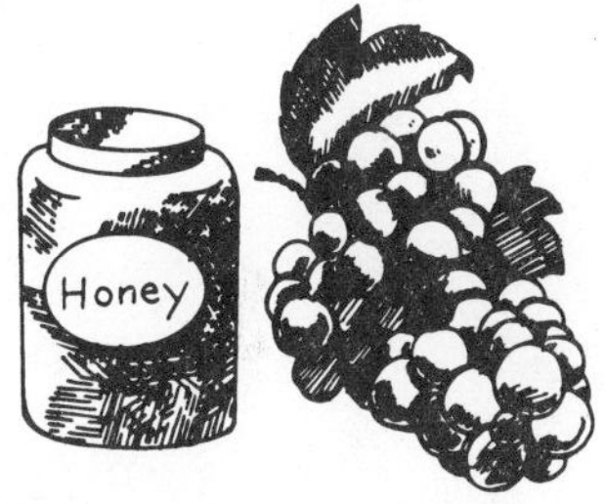

As compared to honey, fruit is truly nutritious.

Another disaccharide is **maltose**, which is found in the germinating seed. Maltose is a combination of two glucose units. Finally, there is the milk sugar, **lactose**, a disaccharide made in the mammary glands of mammals from a galactose unit and a glucose unit.

Some children become unable to digest lactose at about four years of age and so experience nausea and discomfort after drinking milk. This condition, known as lactose intolerance, is widespread, affecting about 80 percent of the world's population—including most Africans, Greeks, and Orientals. Because milk is an almost indispensable source of calcium for growing children, a milk substitute must be found in these instances. Sometimes yogurt or cheese make acceptable substitutes, because they contain no lactose; the bacteria use up the carbohydrate as they make these products.

Sometimes intolerance to milk is due not to lactose intolerance but to an allergic reaction to the protein in the milk. Children and adults with this problem often are intolerant to cheese and yogurt as well and have to find nondairy calcium sources such as greens and legumes to compensate.

The disaccharides, as well as the monosaccharides of which they are composed, are known as simple carbohydrates or simple **sugars** by nutritionists. This is because there is at most only one bond in each that must be broken by the digestive enzymes before the bloodstream can absorb them. In contrast, the **polysaccharides**, starch and cellulose, are complex carbohydrates.

In summary: If we include in our diet a variety of plant life, we will receive the monosaccharides glucose and fructose, the disaccharides sucrose and maltose, and the polysaccharides starch and cellulose. If we include the animal product milk, we will also receive the disaccharide lactose (see Table 2).

Table 2. The Carbohydrates

Complex carbohydrates (polysaccharides):

Starch
Glycogen
Cellulose

Simple carbohydrates, or sugars (monosaccharides and disaccharides):

Glucose Fructose Galactose[a]	Monosaccharides	
Sucrose Maltose Lactose	Disaccharides	**Glucose + fructose = sucrose.** **Glucose + glucose = maltose.** **Glucose + galactose = lactose.**

[a] Galactose is found only in lactose; it doesn't occur free in nature.

The Body's Use of Carbohydrate

This section refers to many body organs. If you want to review them, turn to Appendix A.

Just as glucose is the original unit from which the wide variety of carbohydrate foods are made, so also is glucose the basic carbohydrate unit that each cell of the body uses. Cells don't require fruits, vegetables, and cereals; they require glucose and other nutrients. The task of the various body systems, then, is to disassemble the disaccharides and polysaccharides to monosaccharides, to absorb these into the blood, to convert to glucose those that are not already in the form of glucose, and to transport the glucose to the cells. The process is diagramed in Figure 1. The cells may then use this glucose in any of several ways, as the following sections show.

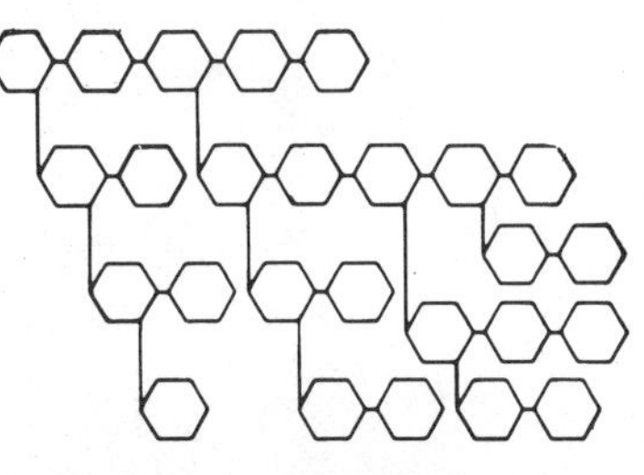

Glycogen is a branched chain of glucose units. Our enzymes can break these bonds (note the many "end" glucose units).

Storing glucose as glycogen. If the blood delivers more glucose than the cells need, the liver and muscles take up a certain amount of the surplus and build the polysaccharide **glycogen**. This carbohydrate is wondrously designed for its task. Instead of having long straight or branched chains like starch, which are slowly digested, it is highly branched, so that hundreds of ends extend beyond its central core. On the tip of each chain is a glucose whose attachment to the next glucose is easily accessible to the glycogen-splitting enzymes. When quick energy (glucose) is needed by the cells, a hormone (epinephrine, or what used to be called adrenaline), floods the bloodstream. The liver's responding enzymes can attack literally thousands of ends simultaneously, releasing a flood of glucose into the blood for use by all the other body cells. This response is part of the body's defense mechanism in time of danger.

For more about hormones, see Appendix A.

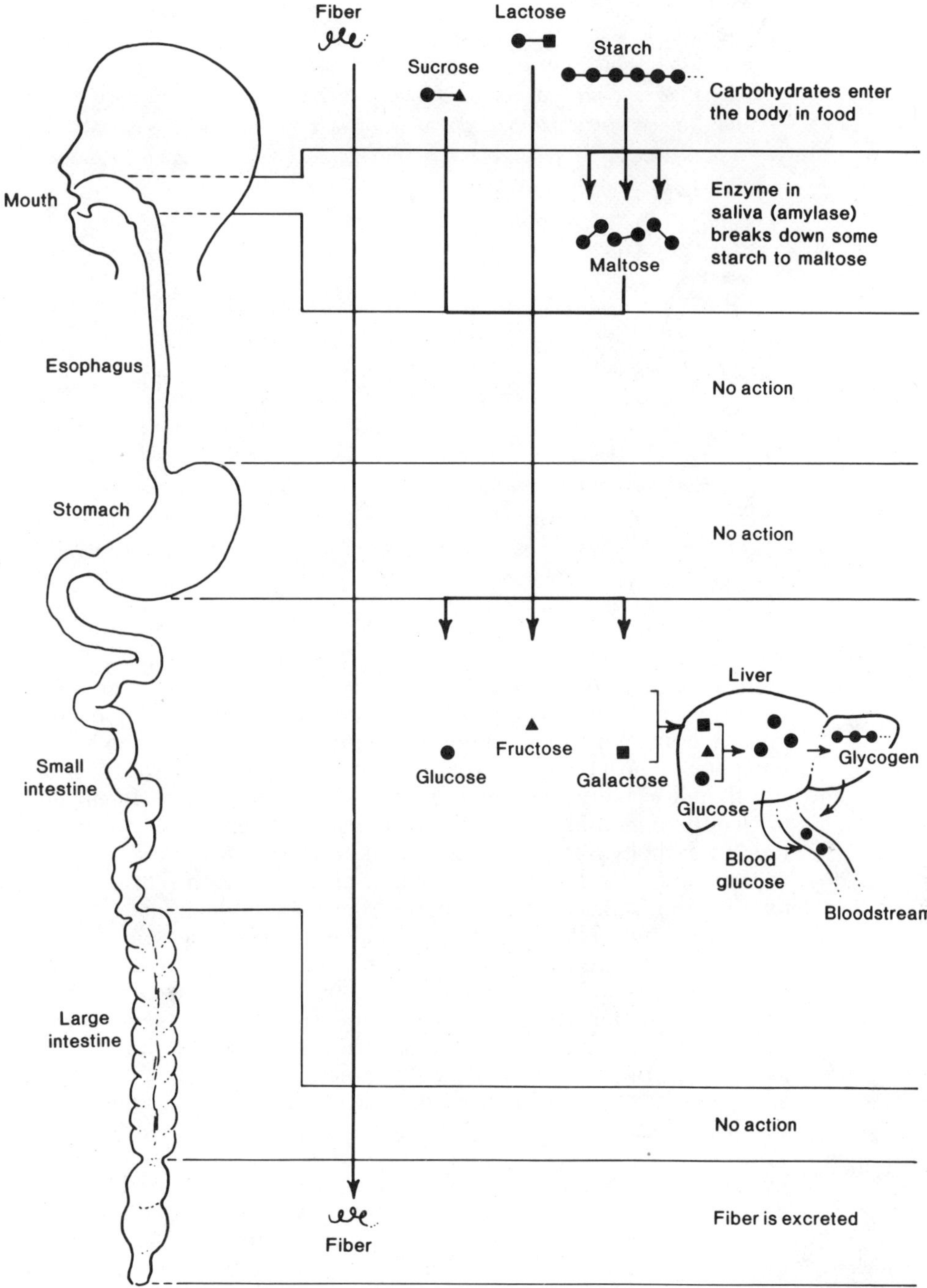

Figure 1. Digestion of carbohydrate. *Enzymes (amylase and the disaccharidases maltase, sucrase, and lactase) break down disaccharides to monosaccharides. These are absorbed and travel to the liver, where most are converted by enzymes to glucose. Glucose is then stored as glycogen or freed as blood glucose. (For further details, see Appendix A.)*

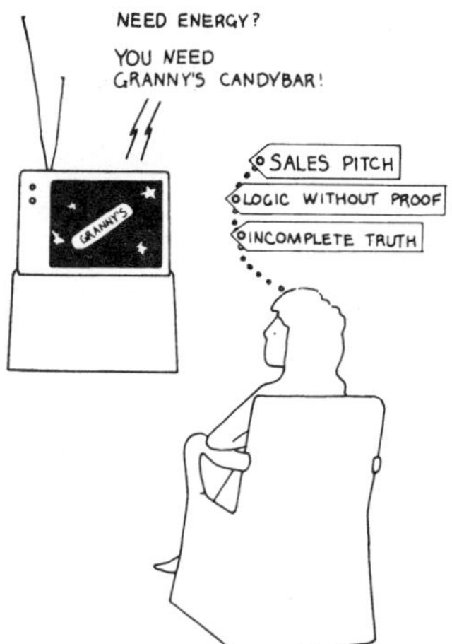
NEED ENERGY?
YOU NEED GRANNY'S CANDYBAR!
SALES PITCH
LOGIC WITHOUT PROOF
INCOMPLETE TRUTH

The implication that any kind of carbohydrate is a good energy food is often used to sell candy.

The advantage to the cave-dweller of having an internal source of quick energy is obvious. Life was fraught with physical peril; a cave-dweller who had had to stop and eat before running from the man-eating tiger might well not have survived to produce our ancestors. The quick-energy response in a stress situation works to our advantage today as well. It accounts for the energy you suddenly have to clean up your living room when you learn that a special person is coming to visit. To meet such emergencies, we are well advised to eat and store carbohydrate every four to six hours when we are awake.

You might rightly ask, "What kind of carbohydrate?" Knowing only that energy is needed, you might conclude that the best source of quick energy is a simple sugar food, such as a candy bar or a sugary beverage. These do supply sugar and energy quickly, but as you will see, they are not the best choices. Advertisements of quick-energy foods use a logic based on partial truth. Mindful of the facts presented so far, you might ask, "What does the speaker stand to gain from having me believe this statement?" The answer is obvious: The speaker is making a sales pitch and stands to gain whatever money you choose to spend on the product.

Splitting glucose for energy. When a cell splits glucose for energy, it performs an unbelievably intricate and sophisticated sequence of maneuvers that are of great interest to the chemist—and of no interest whatever to most people who eat bread and potatoes. There is only one fact that everybody needs to understand about the process. It may help to give the punchline before telling the story: There is no good substitute for carbohydrate. There is a point at which glucose is forever lost in the body, and this may be a matter of life or death. The following details are given only for the purpose of making this point clear.

Inside the cell, glucose breaks in half, releasing some energy. These halves have two pathways open to them. They can be put back together to make glucose, or they can be further broken apart into smaller fragments. If they are broken into smaller fragments, they can never again be used to form glucose. They can yield still more energy, and in the process break down completely to carbon dioxide and water; or they can be hitched together into units of body fat.

This body fat cannot later regenerate glucose to feed the brain. This is one reason why fasting can be dangerous and why low-carbohydrate diets are also dangerous. When there is a severe carbohydrate deficit, the body has two problems. Having no glucose, it has to turn to protein to make some, thus diverting protein from vitally important functions of its own. Protein's importance to the body is so great that glucose should be kept available precisely to prevent this use of protein for energy. This is called the **protein-sparing action** of glucose. For another thing, without sufficient carbohydrate the body can't use its fat in the normal way, even for the functions fat should be able to perform easily. The reason is that glucose (actually, a breakdown product of glucose) is needed to combine with the fat fragments so that they can be used for energy. So the body has to go into **ketosis** (using fat without the help of glucose), a condition in which unusual products of fat breakdown (**ketones**) accumulate in the blood. Ketosis during pregnancy can cause brain damage and irreversible mental retardation in the infant, but even in adults it is a condition to avoid.

More about the hazards of fasting and low-carbohydrate diets —Chapter 7.

The amount of carbohydrate needed to ensure complete sparing of body protein and avoidance of ketosis is around 100 grams a day in an average-size person; this has to be digestible carbohydrate, and considerably more than this minimum is recommended.[4]

Maintaining the blood glucose level. The maintenance of a normal blood glucose level depends on two types of safeguards. When the level gets too low, it can be replenished by drawing on liver glycogen stores. When it gets too high, it can be corrected by siphoning off the excess into liver and muscle glycogen.

The correction of a too-low level has already been mentioned: The hormone epinephrine is involved in bringing about the release of glucose from the liver glycogen. Other hormones also act in this manner, including some that promote the conversion of protein units into glucose, so that the body is well protected against a complete glucose deficit. However, there are limits. The liver can store only half a day's worth of glycogen; then the available supply is exhausted. As for protein, there is none that can be spared without cost. When body protein is used, it has to be taken from muscle, organ, or blood proteins—obviously a measure to avoid if possible. As for fat, you have already seen that it can't regenerate glucose.

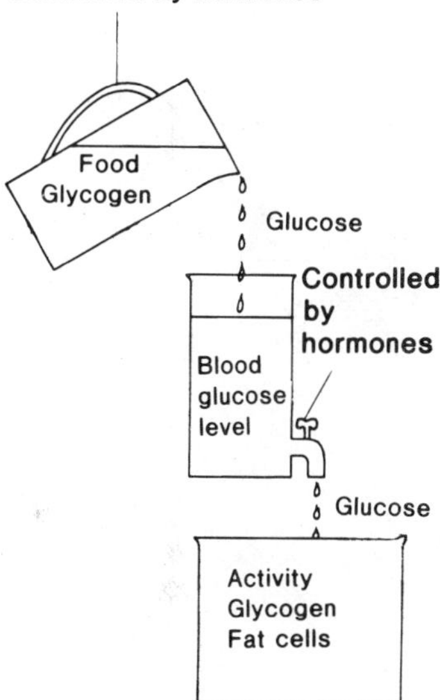

The close regulation of the blood glucose level shows how important a constant supply of glucose is to the body.

Obviously, when blood glucose falls, it has to be replaced sooner or later—a meal or a snack must be eaten. The question of what to eat becomes of greater interest than you might expect. You might think that the obvious solution is to eat a source of "quick energy," such as a candy bar or a cola beverage. Surprisingly, a more intelligent choice is to eat a complex carbohydrate food, such as crackers or bread. Even more suitable is a cracker with cheese (complex carbohydrate with some protein and fat). The reason for this has to do with the body's way of protecting itself against too *high* a blood glucose level.

When the blood glucose level rises, the body adjusts by storing the excess. The first organ to detect the excess glucose is the pancreas, which releases the hormone **insulin** in response. Many of the body's cells respond to insulin by taking up glucose from the blood. The liver stores glucose as glycogen, which can be returned to the blood when needed. The muscles store it as glycogen for their own use. The fat cells convert glucose to fat. Thus the blood glucose level is quickly brought back down to normal as the body stores the excess.

If you eat a meal or snack that is unusually high in carbohydrate, and especially if it consists mostly of concentrated sugar, your blood glucose concentration may rise too high, so that the pancreas overreacts, secreting too much insulin and driving too much glucose out of the blood into the cells. Then, unless glucose continues to pour in, the blood glucose level may fall too low or too fast. Some people then experience the symptoms of **hypoglycemia** described in the digression that follows. If you are such a person, you will benefit by learning that complex carbohydrate foods such as crackers or bread, which deliver less glucose over a longer period of time, elicit less of an insulin response and so help to avoid this rebound situation. A cracker with cheese is a better choice still: The fat slows down the digestion of the carbohydrate and the protein elicits the secretion of a hormone that opposes insulin, thus modulating its action. The protein can also provide some amino acids, from which additional glucose can be made when needed.

Suppose the blood glucose falls, the glycogen reserves are exhausted, and you choose *not* to eat. Gradually, your body will adjust to this situation by shifting into ketosis, breaking down its muscle protein to feed glucose to the brain and its body fat to fuel the other body cells. But before you have adjusted, there may be times when your blood glucose level falls rapidly or below normal, and you will experience symptoms of glucose deprivation to the brain: anxiety, hunger, and dizziness. Your muscles will become weak, shaky, and trembling, and your heart will race in an attempt to speed more fuel to your brain. These, the symptoms of **reactive hypoglycemia**, signify that you have let your system get out of balance. Reactive hypoglycemia occurs in about two to three out of every ten young women, more often in obese ones, less often in older people (over forty-five),[5] and is no great cause for concern. All of us experience low blood glucose levels at times; and if the symptoms are severe, it is easy to learn to eat promptly and properly. At such times, our best move is to obey the prompting and to eat a balanced meal or snack rather than a source of concentrated sugar.

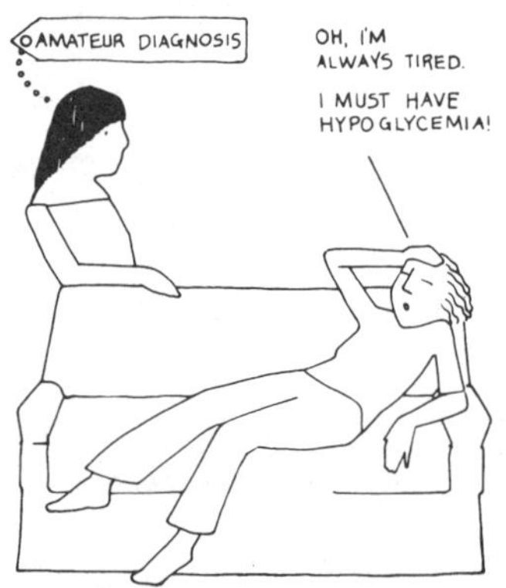

It's easy to think you have hypoglycemia but you may have something else.

There is another type of hypoglycemia, however—**spontaneous hypoglycemia**—which requires treatment. True spontaneous hypoglycemia is an extremely rare disease condition in which the pancreas habitually oversecretes insulin. As a result, the person's blood glucose is constantly too low. Such a person must eat high-protein foods frequently and exclude simple carbohydrates altogether. Few people are truly hypoglycemic in this sense.

The symptoms described above can be caused by a number of conditions other than hypoglycemia, such as oxygen deprivation to the brain. In fact, the effect of eating concentrated sweets sometimes is to attract large volumes of fluid from the bloodstream into the digestive tract, lowering the blood volume and so causing reduced blood flow to the brain. The same symptoms may also be psychologically caused, by an anxiety state. Nonmedical people, including nutritionists, who are not trained in the diagnosis of different conditions that present similar symptoms, are extremely unwise if they try to diagnose themselves. However, it will certainly do no harm to avoid the obvious unbalanced states caused by snacking on concentrated sweets and to choose balanced meals instead.

Converting glucose to fat. After (1) the glycogen stores are full and (2) the cells' immediate energy needs are met, the body takes (3) a third path for using carbohydrate. Say you have eaten. You are only sitting and watching a ball game on television. But you are eating pretzels and drinking beer. If your digestive tract is still delivering glucose to the liver, the liver will break the extra glucose into small fragments and put them together into the more permanent energy-storage compound—fat. The fat is then released, carried to the fatty tissues of the body, and deposited there. Unlike the liver cells, which can only store about half a day's worth of glycogen, the fat cells can store unlimited quantities of fat. Moral: You'd better play the game if you are going to eat the food.

The story of carbohydrate turns out to be a cycle. Carbon dioxide, water, and energy are combined in plants to form glucose; the glucose may be stored in the polysaccharide starch. Then, in the body, the starch becomes glucose again, and this may be stored as the body's polysaccharide, glycogen. Ultimately, the glucose delivers the sun's energy to fuel the body's activities and the waste products, carbon dioxide and water, are excreted to be used again by a plant.

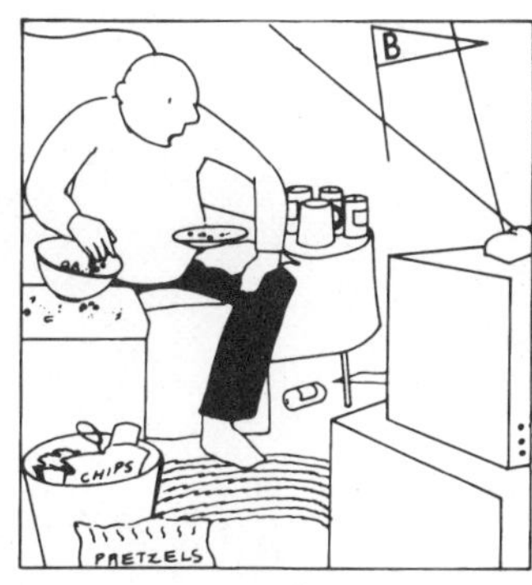

You'd better play the game if you are going to eat the food.

The diabetic and carbohydrate. Knowing how the blood glucose level is maintained, you can appreciate the problem of the person with **diabetes** whose insulin response is slow or ineffective. (Most adult diabetics fall into this non-insulin-dependent category.[6]) If the blood glucose level rises too high (**hyperglycemia**), it stays too high for an abnormally long time. The kidneys may respond by allowing some glucose to spill over into the urine. Hence the myth that the diabetic cannot handle carbohydrate. The diabetic must be exceptionally careful to eat balanced meals—providing a constant, steady, moderate flow of glucose to the bloodstream so that the pancreas will not be overwhelmed—and to avoid concentrated sugar altogether. But recent research indicates that diabetics actually do best on a diet that is high in complex carbohydrate foods—as high as that recommended for a normal, healthy person. The starch and protein in these foods help to regulate the blood glucose level as already described, while the fiber helps stimulate the prompt production of insulin in response to food.[7]

Both diabetes and hypoglycemia can be diagnosed by means of a glucose tolerance test, in which the pancreas is challenged to handle a large amount of glucose. After fasting overnight, the subject is fed a sudden large dose of pure simple carbohydrate (a glucose load), usually as a sweet drink. Four or six hours later, the hypoglycemic person is found to have an abnormally low blood glucose level, whereas the diabetic still has hyperglycemia.

There has been some serious discussion to the effect that fructose may be a desirable sugar substitute for use by diabetics, because it is sweeter (so they might use less), and because it doesn't raise the blood glucose level or require such an insulin response as glucose does.[8] However, early hopes that this might be true have been somewhat dampened. Fructose is not that much sweeter than sucrose (see Table 3); further, most of it becomes glucose after it enters the body, requiring insulin to be used. Anyway—perhaps most importantly—most non-insulin-dependent diabetics need to control their calorie intake and don't need the empty calories of fructose.[9]

Table 3. Relative Sweetness of Selected Sweeteners[a]

Sweetening Agent	Approximate Sweetness Relative to Sucrose
Sugars:	
Sucrose	1.0
Glucose	0.7
Fructose	1.2
Lactose	0.3
Maltose	0.4
Sugar alcohols:	
Xylitol	1.0
Mannitol	0.7
Sorbitol	0.5
Maltitol	0.7

[a] Adapted from D. B. Drucker, Sweetening agents in food, drinks and medicine: Cariogenic potential and adverse effects, *Journal of Human Nutrition* 33 (1979): 114–124. The authors point out that the sweetness of these agents depends on the foods they are used in. Others, too, have found this to be true. Fructose, in particular, is not found to be as sweet in baked goods (basic) as sucrose, although it is sweeter in lemonade (acid): S. L. Hardy, C. P. Brennand, and B. W. Wyse, Fructose: Comparison with sucrose as sweetener in four products, *Journal of the American Dietetic Association* 74 (1979): 41–46.

Food Sources of Carbohydrate

Glucose is vital to the functioning of every cell of the body, especially the cells of the nervous system; and the body is equipped with exquisitely designed systems to acquire, transport, and conserve it. Protein, in time of need, can provide glucose, but the body normally depends mostly on starch and sweet foods for this valuable commodity—that is, it depends on plants.

We eat all parts of plants—stems, leaves, roots, tubers, fruits, blossoms, and seeds—one part from one plant, a different part from another. Stems and leaves provide mostly cellulose, from which we cannot extract the glucose, and so they are energy poor (low in calories). Higher sugar concentrations are present in fruits and berries, and higher starch concentrations are found in roots, tubers, and seeds.

Throughout the world, seeds play the most important role in the human diet; within them are not only starch for energy but also the vitamins and minerals the new plant will need until it can put down its roots and spread its leaves to the sun. Peas and beans (legumes) may come to mind as seeds you enjoy eating; but worldwide it is cereal grains, such as wheat, rice, oats, millet, barley, and corn—the seeds of grasses—that supply over 50 percent of human energy.[10] The Modified Four Food Group Plan recommends that you have four servings of these grains (bread and cereal products) a day and two of legumes.

Humans have lived with the same complex carbohydrate plants for thousands of years. In fact, no important new plants of any kind (except tomatoes and coffee) have been domesticated in the last 2000 years. Thai farmers were cultivating rice 12,000 years ago; North American natives ate beans and squash at least 9000 years ago; wheat and barley were under cultivation 7000 years before the Christian era began. In contrast, the purification of simple carbohydrate into table sugar is a process only 100 years old. We have had no time to adapt to it.

Every culture has a favorite traditional food source of starch. Those who live in areas of the world where the monsoon seasons bring drenching rains eat rice almost exclusively and obtain up to 70 percent of their calories from it. Latin Americans depend on corn as their staple, whereas in Western Europe and North America, wheat is the predominant cereal. These grains are often ground into flours used to make bread, pudding, or porridge.

Some parts of the world depend on roots and tubers rather than grains as a staple food source of starch. White potatoes, sweet potatoes, and yams are the major plant foods in such countries as Ghana and Nigeria; cassava, in parts of Latin America and Africa. Elsewhere it is not starch but sugar that supplies more calories than any other food. This sugar may come from the fleshy stem of the sugar cane, from the root of the sugar beet, or from such fruits as the banana. The diagram in the margin shows the percentage of calories provided for human needs by various foods around the world.

Much world misery is caused by loyalty to one carbohydrate source. The Irish suffered a protein deficit during the potato famine because they would not eat meat without potatoes. Starving children won't accept an unfamiliar cereal. The elderly in our country may abandon all sources of variety by sticking resolutely to one staple, such as rolled oats.

As the wealth of a people increases, more of their available plant food is fed to animals, and a larger proportion of the people's calories comes from livestock. In North America, the world's wealthiest continent, 31 percent of the people's daily food energy comes from animal flesh and animal products — meat, milk, eggs, and fish.[11] Elsewhere, these products supply only 12 percent of people's food energy, and in Asia they represent less than 5 percent of the calories in the diet. The figure in the margin shows the changes that take place with increasing national wealth.

In the United States, there has been a shift away from complex carbohydrate foods since 1900. Today's diet derives 42 percent of its calories from fat, 12 percent from protein, and the remaining 46 percent

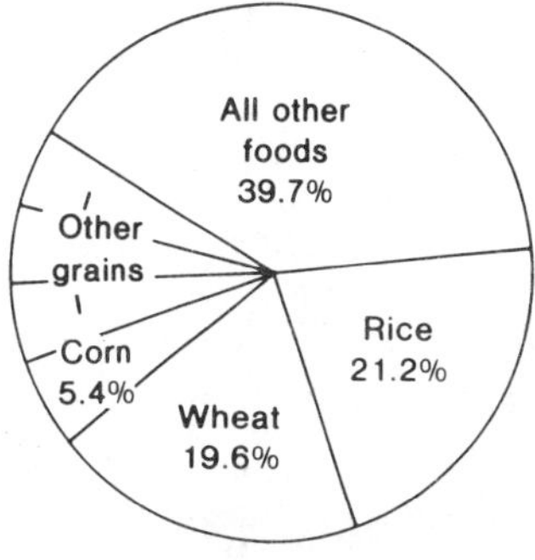

Grains provide more than half of the world's food energy.

Adapted from L. R. Brown and G. W. Finsterbusch, Man and His Environment: Food *(New York: Harper & Row, 1972), p. 32, and used with the permission of the authors and publisher.*

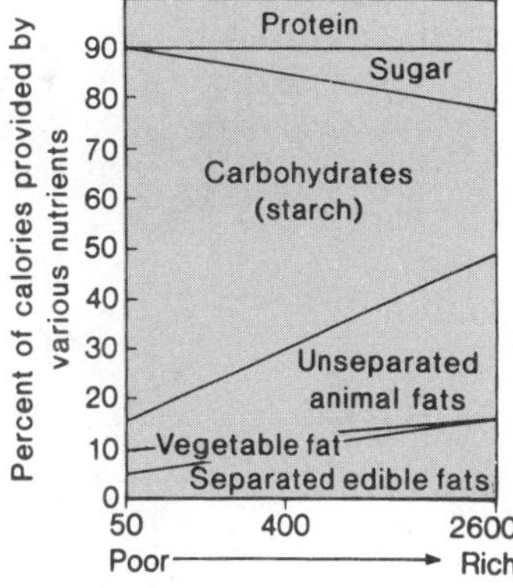

As a nation grows richer, its people derive more of their energy from sugar and meat, less from starch.

Adapted from D. F. Hollingsworth, Translating nutrition into diet, Food Technology *31 (February 1977): 38-41. Based on material in J. Prissé, F. Sizaret, and P. Francois,* FAO Newsletter *7 (1969): 1. Used with permission of the author and publisher.*

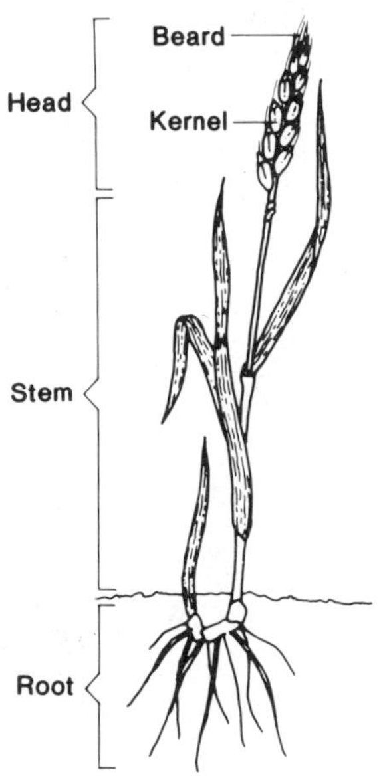

A wheat plant.

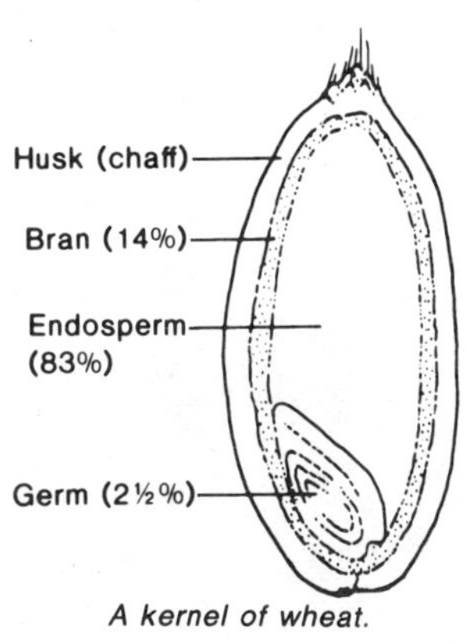

A kernel of wheat.

from carbohydrate—22 percent from complex carbohydrate and 24 percent from sugar.[12] It has been recommended that we shift our pattern to double our consumption of complex carbohydrate and cut our sugar intake in half. (Controversy 3, Figure 2, shows how the proportions would change.) To do this, we need to become aware of the foods available to us that contribute carbohydrate to our diet.

The staple complex carbohydrate food in the United States and Canada is bread made from wheat. As the main contributor of carbohydrate to the diet, it deserves some special attention. If it assumes a place of greater prominence, it will become imperative to make sure that it contributes the nutrients we need.

Food Feature: Refined, Enriched, and Whole-Grain Bread

Consumers often want to know what kind of bread is the most nutritious and what are the meanings of words—refined, enriched, and whole grain—associated with the wheat flour that makes up the bread.

Wheat, a grass-type plant, is the staple cereal of most of the world and covers more of the earth's surface than any other crop. (Other cereals are rice, oats, corn, barley, and rye.) The part of the wheat plant that is made into flour and then into bread and other baked goods is the kernel. About fifty kernels cluster in the head of the plant, on top of the stem, where they stick tightly until fully ripe. These kernels are first separated from the stem and then further broken apart by the milling process.

The wheat kernel (**whole grain**) has three main parts: the germ, the bran, and the endosperm. The germ is the part that reproduces when planted, and so it contains concentrated food to support the new life. It is especially rich in vitamin E and the B vitamins niacin and thiamin. The bran, a protective coating around the kernel similar to the shell of a nut, is also rich in nutrients. In addition, the bran is a source of valuable fiber. The endosperm is the soft inside portion of the kernel containing starch and proteins (including gluten, which is used for making white flour). The husk, commonly called chaff, is unusable for most purposes.

Most discussion about bread among people concerned with good nutrition has to do with the loss of nutrients from the wheat kernel during the milling process. In earlier times, people milled the kernel by grinding it between two stones to expose the endosperm and then blowing or sifting out the inedible chaff. Much of the bran and germ were included in the final product. As improvements were made in the machinery for milling, a whiter, smoother-textured flour resulted, and it became more desirable than the crunchy, dark brown, "old-fashioned" flour. But where whole-wheat flour uses the entire wheat kernel, white flour uses only the endosperm. During the further processing of **refined**, white flour for the market, additional nutrients are lost. The bran layers and other parts of the kernel that remain after white flour is milled are used as livestock and poultry feed. Actually, these parts of the grain contain more protein, minerals, and vitamins than the endosperm does.

As white flour became more popular for making breads, bread eaters suffered a tragic loss of needed nutrients. A survey that took place in the United States in 1936 revealed that many people were suffering from the loss of the nutrients iron, thiamin, riboflavin, and niacin, which they had formerly received from unrefined bread. The Enrichment Act of 1942 required that these lost nutrients be returned to flour. Thus, in **enriched** bread, iron and the vitamins thiamin and niacin are restored to the levels found in whole wheat; riboflavin is added to a level higher than that in whole grain. This doesn't make a single slice of bread "rich" in these nutrients, but people who eat several or many slices of bread a day obtain significantly more of them than they would from plain, refined white bread.

To a great extent, the enrichment of white flour eliminated the deficiency problems that had been observed in people who depended on bread for most of their calories but who were unwilling to use the whole-grain product. Today, you can almost take it for granted that all bread, grains like rice, wheat products like macaroni and spaghetti, and cereals like farina have been enriched. The law requires that all grain products that cross state lines must be enriched. A look at the food composition tables in Appendix H shows to what levels whole-grain bread, unenriched white bread, and enriched white bread contain the four nutrients mentioned above.

But the food composition tables don't tell the whole story. When the grain is refined, many nutrients not listed in the tables are also lost. As more and more foods other than bread are refined and processed, other nutrients may begin to be lost from our diet. Evidence is piling up that our fiber needs are increasing as fiber is lost from many refined foods, not just from bread and cereal. Recently, many new cases of diabetes have been appearing, caused not by failure of insulin responsiveness but by deficiency of chromium. Some have attributed these cases to our increased use of processed foods. Therefore, although the enrichment of wheat and other cereal products restores four of the lost nutrients, there is increasing evidence that we should return to the use of the whole grain in order to restore trace minerals

Table 4. Nutrient Levels of One-Pound Loaves of Bread

Item Number	Type of Bread	Iron (mg)	Thiamin (mg)	Riboflavin (mg)	Niacin (mg)
368	Whole wheat	13.6	1.36	0.45	12.7
346	Italian, unenriched	3.2	0.41	0.41	3.6
345	Italian, enriched	10.0	1.32	1.32	11.8

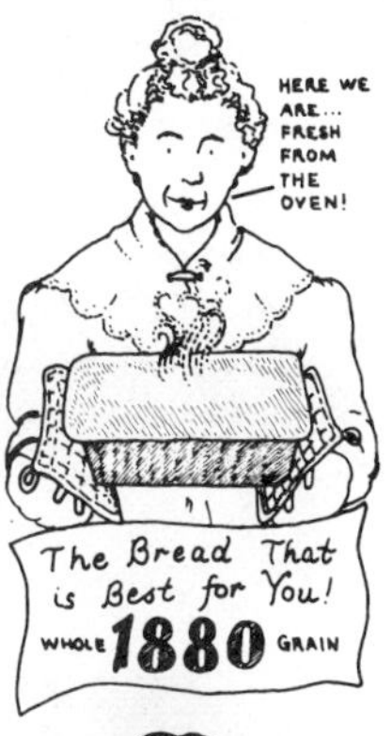
HERE WE ARE... FRESH FROM THE OVEN!
The Bread That is Best for You!
WHOLE 1880 GRAIN

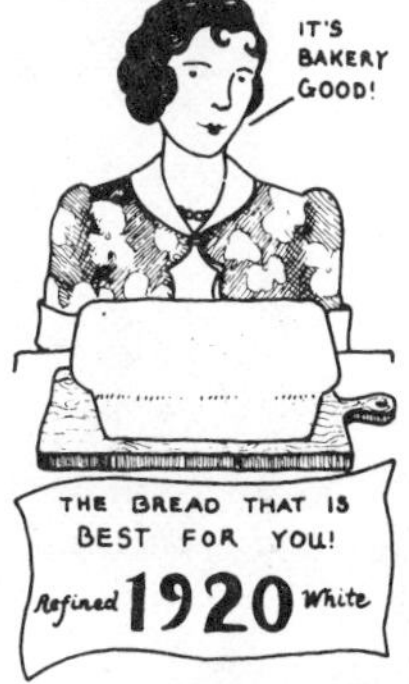
IT'S BAKERY GOOD!
THE BREAD THAT IS BEST FOR YOU!
Refined 1920 White

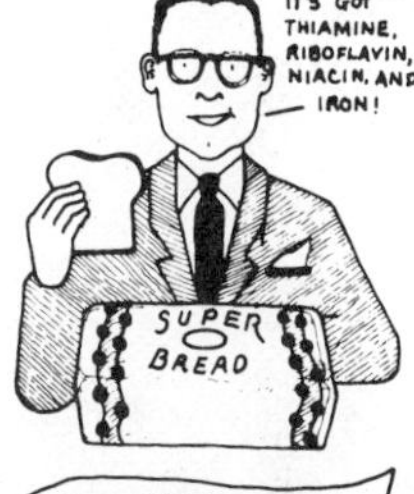
IT'S GOT THIAMINE, RIBOFLAVIN, NIACIN, AND IRON!
SUPER BREAD
THE BREAD THAT IS BEST FOR YOU!!
Enriched 1950 White

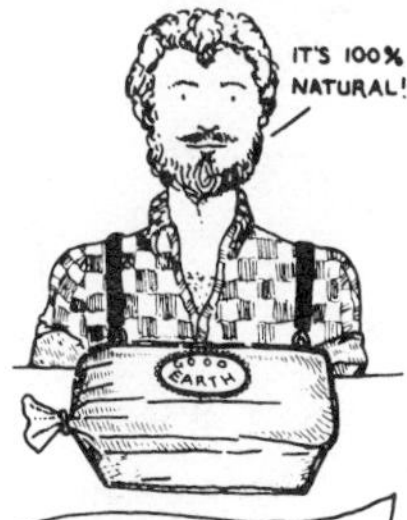
IT'S 100% NATURAL!
GOOD EARTH
The bread that is best for you!!
TEN 1980 GRAIN

A hundred years later, we've realized that whole-grain bread is best.

and fiber to our diet. *Nutrition and the MD* reports: "Whole grain items are preferred over enriched products because they contain more magnesium, zinc, folate, and vitamin B_6 than enriched bread and cereals."[13]

Carbohydrate in the Food Groups

The food-grouping system that pays special attention to the carbohydrate amounts in foods is the exchange system. (It groups foods according to their carbohydrate, fat, protein, and calorie contents.) Almost every carbohydrate-containing food in common use has a place in one of four of its groups: the milk, vegetable, fruit, or bread and starchy vegetable group. (Foods in the meat and fat groups contain no carbohydrate.) If you want to take seriously the advice to increase complex carbohydrate and to reduce concentrated sugar intake, it will help to review Figure 1 in Chapter 2 and to remember the following facts.

More about the exchange system—Chapter 2 and Appendix L.

Milk group. A cup of skim milk or the equivalent is a generous contributor of carbohydrate, donating 12 grams as the milk sugar lactose. It also contributes protein (a point in its favor) and no fat (another point). Like milk in these respects are the other members of its group:

1 cup buttermilk.

1 cup yogurt (plain).

⅓ cup powdered, nonfat dry milk (before adding liquid).

½ cup canned evaporated milk (before adding liquid).

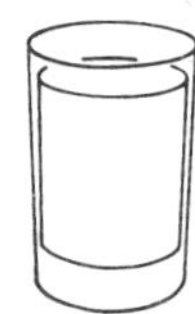

12 g carbohydrate.

Cream and butter, although dairy products, are *not* members of the milk group, because they contain little or no carbohydrate and insignificant amounts of the other nutrients important in milk. They are found on the fat list instead.

Vegetable group. A half-cup serving of green beans contains 5 grams of carbohydrate as a mixture of starch and sugars. Any other vegetable serving that fits this description is called a vegetable exchange. The vegetable exchanges include tomatoes, greens, okra, onions, beets, carrots, and others. Each of these foods also contributes a little protein and no fat.

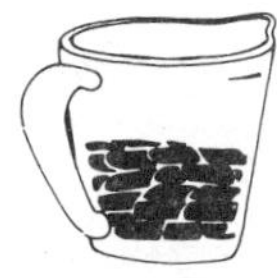

5 g carbohydrate.

Some vegetables are so low in carbohydrate and calories that dieters call them "free foods." Among these are lettuce, parsley, and radishes.

Fruit group. A half cup of orange juice contains 10 grams of carbohydrate, mostly as simple sugars including the fruit sugar, fructose. Fruits vary greatly in their water content and therefore in the concentrations of sugar they contain. Serving sizes of different fruits can be adjusted so that each contains 10 grams of carbohydrate. With this adjustment, a dieter can "exchange" any fruit for any other without altering the amount of carbohydrate in the diet. Among the fruit exchanges are ⅓ cup pineapple juice, ½ cup applesauce, and half of a small banana. The fruits contain insignificant amounts of fat and protein.

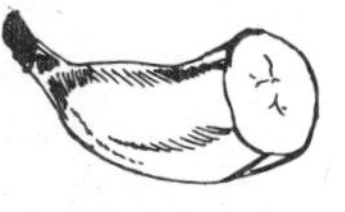

10 g carbohydrate.

Bread and starchy vegetable group. A slice of white bread contains 15 grams of carbohydrate as starch. Equivalent foods are other breads, potatoes, rice, pasta, corn, lima beans, and many other foods that are predominantly complex carbohydrate. It is very useful in diet planning to be aware that starchy vegetables such as corn are actually more bread-like than vegetable-like in this respect. Diet planners who enjoy using these foods are happy to learn that the new view encourages their generous inclusion in the diet. If calories are a problem, cut out fat, not complex carbohydrate foods.

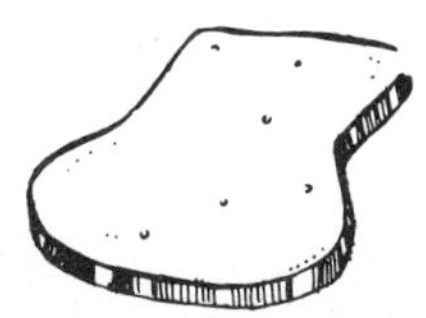

15 g carbohydrate.

Sugar. The carbohydrate item that the exchange groups do *not* include is concentrated sugar (not surprisingly, since the exchange system was originally designed for use by diabetics). But to get a complete picture of the places carbohydrate can come from, it is necessary to consider these items:

1 teaspoon brown sugar.	1 teaspoon jam.
1 teaspoon molasses.	1 teaspoon jelly.
1 teaspoon corn syrup.	1 teaspoon candy.
1 teaspoon honey.	1 teaspoon maple syrup.

Each of these teaspoons is equivalent in sugar content to a teaspoon of pure white sugar. (We repeated the "1 teaspoon" with each item to emphasize that each of them is like *pure* white sugar, in spite of many people's belief that they are different or "better.")

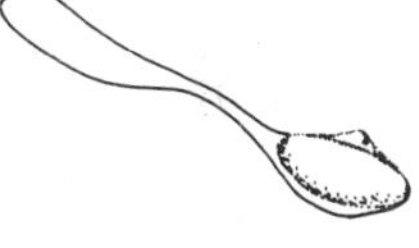

5 g carbohydrate.

For a person who uses catsup liberally, it may help to remember that a tablespoon of it contains a teaspoon of sugar. And for the soft-drink user, a 12-ounce can of a cola beverage contains about 9 teaspoons of sugar.

Sugar contents of common foods are shown in Appendix F.

This chapter began with the statement that carbohydrate is the ideal fuel for most body functions. Authorities recommend that we consume a diet high in carbohydrate, especially from grains and tubers. The sample diet shown above fits this recommendation, because most of the foods—the ten bread items—have to be selected from the bread and starchy vegetable list, which includes all the cereal grains and such tubers as potatoes, sweet potatoes, and yams.

Many a reader will likely be surprised at the idea that the "ideal" diet includes so much starch. But newer understanding of people's nutrient needs has brought the once-maligned nutrient starch to new favor. Carbohydrates will appear again in later chapters. Meanwhile, the next chapter will show you that the fats, too, are being reassessed in light of new health findings.[1]

For Further Information

Recommended references on all nutrition topics are listed in Appendix J. This chapter's notes and the Controversy references also include readings that we highly recommend.

On the question of hypoglycemia—who actually experiences it, at what blood glucose level, and with what symptoms—a researcher in

[1] *Chapter Notes can be found at the end of the Appendixes.*

the area has published a monograph that the advanced student might find interesting:

- Danowski, T. S. The hypoglycemia syndromes. Pittsburgh, Pa. (15234): Harper Printing Service, 1978.

Controversy 4A

Sugar

Is sugar "bad" for you?

This controversy first presents logical arguments that sound good but that may not be true. You are advised to withhold judgment until the evidence is presented.

Logic: Six arguments against sugar. Sugar stands accused of several crimes and indiscretions. The arguments against it are summed up briefly in the following list:

(1) If you eat a lot of sugar, you will have to eat a lot less of something else that would have contained essential nutrients. Therefore, sugar causes malnutrition by displacing nutrients in the diet.

(2) If you eat a lot of sugar *without* eating less of something else, you will get too many calories. Used this way, sugar causes obesity.

(3) Sugar taken in excess of the body's glycogen-storage capacity will be converted to fat and so can cause high levels of fat in the blood (hyperlipidemia). This is a known risk factor for heart and blood-vessel disease (atherosclerosis).

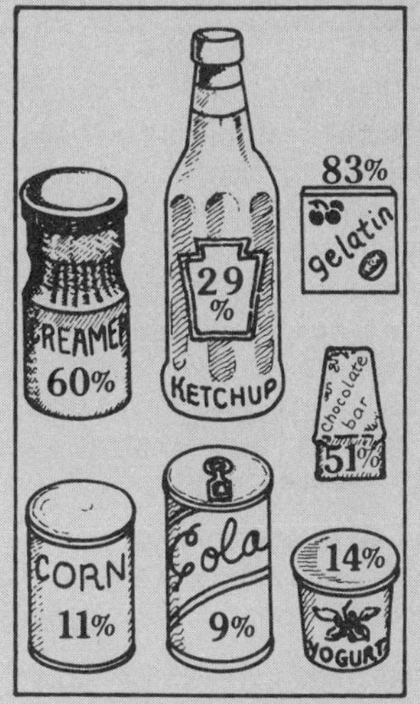

Here's the amount of sugar in some common products.

Adapted from Too much sugar,* Consumer Reports, *March 1978, pp. 137, 139.

(4) Concentrated sugar is new in the human diet. The human species evolved without it and does not need it. It isn't a nutrient, it's an additive. As such, it is not natural, and anything not natural is dangerous.

(5) If you dump a lot of sugar into your bloodstream, your pancreas will overstrain itself trying to produce insulin to handle the load and will wear out. Thus excessive sugar consumption leads to diabetes.

(6) Sugar also causes tooth decay.

So go the arguments of those who claim we should eliminate sugar from our diets.

Evidence. (1) Does sugar displace nutrients in the diet? Purified, refined white sugar—sucrose—is a fifty-fifty mixture of glucose and fructose. In the body it becomes equivalent to pure glucose. As such, it differs in no way from the glucose that comes from starch; but (as we have seen) it is absorbed more rapidly because its units can be

Comparison of the Nutrients in Potatoes and Sugar

Nutrient	From 400 Calories Potatoes	From 400 Calories Sugar
Protein	12 g	0
Complex carbohydrate	84 g	0
Calcium	36 mg	0
Vitamin C	80 mg	0

digested simultaneously rather than sequentially like those of starch. Sugar contains no other nutrients—protein, vitamins, or minerals—and so can be termed an empty-calorie food. If 400 calories of sucrose are eaten in place of 400 calories of starch-containing food like potatoes, the nutrients and fiber of the potatoes are lost. It is theoretically possible, however, with very judicious food selection, to obtain all the needed nutrients within a calorie allowance of about 1500 calories. If a teenage boy needs as many as 4000 calories to get all the energy he needs and eats some very nutritious foods, perhaps even the "empty calories" of cola beverages are acceptable. (Many teenage *girls* eat only 1200 calories or even less, however, so they can't afford any but the most nutrient-dense foods.)

(2) Does sugar cause obesity? Excess calories from any energy nutrient, even protein, are stored in body fat. Evidence from population studies shows that in many countries obesity rises as sugar consumption increases. But sugar cannot be singled out as the sole cause. Where sugar intake increases, usually fat and total calorie intake also rise.[2] Simultaneously, physical activity decreases. Obesity also occurs where sugar intake is low, and in one society it appears that fat people eat less sugar than thin people.[3]

The consensus of opinion, as summed up by one nutritionist, is that it "appears virtually impossible to separate the effects of sugar ingestion from the effects of increased calories and associated obesity."[4]

(3) Does sugar cause atherosclerosis? (More about atherosclerosis and its causes appears in Controversy 5A.) The same population studies that show increased obesity with high sugar intakes also show

Miniglossary

Terms that mean "sugar" on labels include the following.[1] In terms of nutritional value, these are all very much the same.

brown sugar: Sugar crystals contained in molasses syrup with natural flavor and color, 91 to 96 percent pure sucrose. (Some refiners add syrup to refined white sugar to make brown sugar.)

corn sweeteners: A term that refers to corn syrup and sugars derived from corn.

corn syrup: A syrup produced by the action of enzymes on cornstarch. High-fructose corn syrup may contain as little as 42 percent or as much as 90 percent fructose; dextrose makes up the balance.

dextrose: The technical name for glucose.

honey: Invert sugar formed by an enzyme from nectar gathered by bees. Composition and flavor vary, but honey usually contains fructose, glucose, maltose, and sucrose.

invert sugar: A mixture of glucose and fructose formed by the splitting of sucrose in a chemical process. Sold only in liquid form, sweeter than sucrose, invert sugar is used as an additive to help preserve food freshness and prevent shrinkage.

levulose: The technical name for fructose.

natural sweeteners: A term that refers to any of the sugars listed here.

raw sugar: The residue of evaporated sugar cane juice, tan or brown in color. Raw sugar can only be sold in the U.S. if the impurities (dirt, insect fragments, and the like) have been removed.

sorbitol, mannitol, maltitol, xylitol: Sugar alcohols, that can be derived from fruits or produced from dextrose.

sucrose: Table sugar or powdered (confectioner's) sugar, 99.9 percent pure.

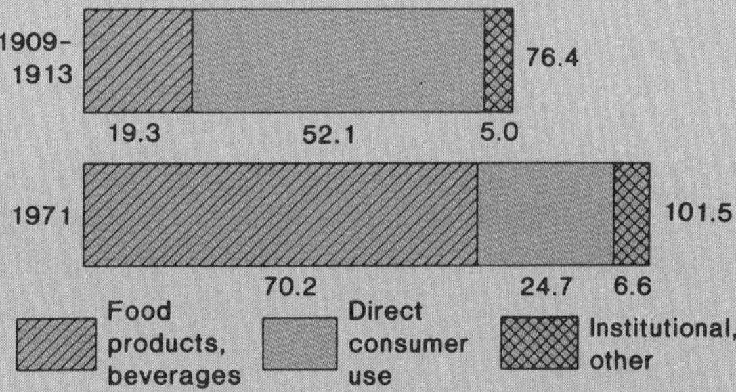

Use of refined sugar (pounds per person). The graph shows the rise in sugar consumption since 1909-1913 and the large contribution made to that rise by already-added sugar.

From L. Page and B. Friend, Level of use of sugars in the United States, in Sugars in Nutrition, *ed. H. L. Sipple and K. W. McNutt (New York: Academic Press, 1974).*

increased blood fat levels and deaths from heart disease. It is found, however, that the closest correlation is between obesity and atherosclerosis, not between sugar intake and atherosclerosis. Animal experiments implicating sugar in heart and artery disease have used diets so high in sugar that they are "unphysiological." No one has yet shown that moderate amounts of sugar (10 to 20 percent of total calories) affect the disease process. "The inevitable conclusion on the basis of evidence to date is that sucrose in the amounts usually consumed has no discrete, untoward effects upon hyperlipidemia, atherosclerosis and coronary heart disease."[5] *To date* means, of course, that it still is possible that experiments will show such effects.

(4) Is sugar not essential in the human diet? The same nutritionist who finds no correlation between dietary sucrose or carbohydrate and the development of atherosclerosis agrees that sugar is new in the human environment and that we are not adapted to cope with it biologically.[6] Dr. J. Mayer, whose newspaper column can be considered a reliable reference, says, "While we require dietary carbohydrates, the body has absolutely no need for sugar as such."[7] Apparently we did evolve without it, as the beginning of Chapter 4 showed. "The sugar derived from cane and beets is a comparatively new substance in our diets."[8] In the United States, sugar consumption had reached seventy-six pounds per person per year by 1913 and over a hundred pounds per person per

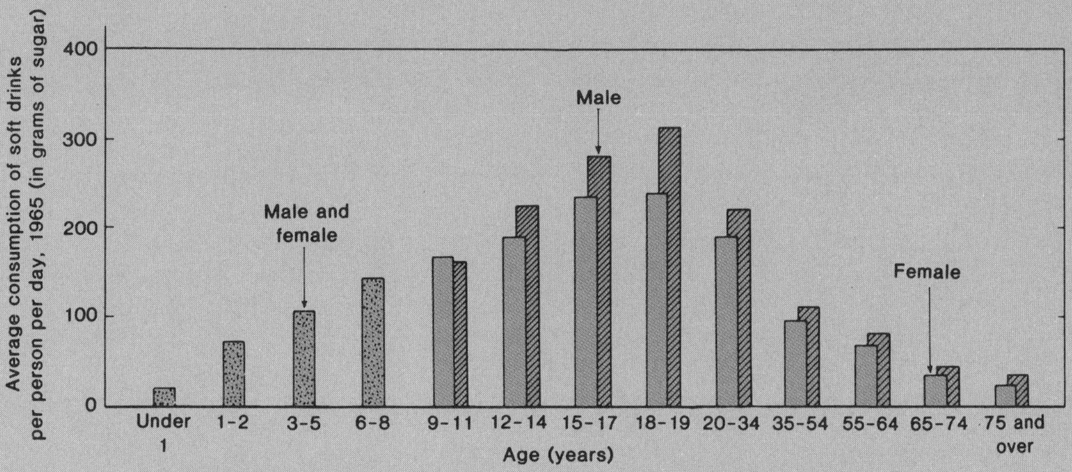

Teenagers consume large quantities of sugar in cola beverages. One pound is 454 grams, and some of these bars reach almost 400 grams a day.

From L. Page and B. Friend, Level of use of sugars in the United States, in Sugars in Nutrition, *ed. H. L. Sipple and K. W. McNutt (New York: Academic Press, 1974).*

year in the 1970s. It has been estimated that over a third of the calories in our diet now come from sugars and visible fats,[9] and sugar is the leading ingredient added to foods today.[10] Our consumption of it is not entirely voluntary; of the hundred-plus pounds that we eat in a year, seventy-some pounds come already added to foods during processing.[11]

Carbohydrate has an important role to play in sparing protein. If the only carbohydrate available or acceptable is sugar, then it may perform a much-needed function. For example, children with advanced kidney disease often lack appetite, and concerned nutritionists are eager to see that they receive as much protein as they can tolerate. One way to ensure that the protein is not wasted by being used for energy is to feed popsicles and hard candy to these children as a delectable carbohydrate source.[12] Although sugar is not an essential nutrient, it is certainly not a poison, as some hysterical headline-makers have made it out to be. (The question of whether sugar has adverse effects on those special children who are diagnosed as hyperactive is the subject of Controversy 13.)

(5) Does sugar cause diabetes? Here, the evidence is conflicting and interesting. First of all, it should be pointed out that diabetes is not one, but several disorders (see Chapter 4). The predominant type, and the one being discussed here, is non-insulin-dependent diabetes, which may develop only in people who have the genetic tendency for it. (Another type of diabetes is insulin-dependent, and is less common. Still another type, caused by chromium deficiency, is described in Chapter 10.) Being careful to make this distinction, we can ask whether those who are prone to the major type of diabetes should eliminate sugar from their diets.

In vast areas of the world, as the diet has changed in the direction of increased sugar consumption, a profound increase—by as much as tenfold—in the incidence of diabetes has occurred. This is true for the Japanese, Israelis, Africans, Native Americans, Eskimos, Polynesians, and Micronesians. Yet in other populations, no relation has been found between sugar intake and diabetes. Wherever starch (or is it the fiber or the chromium that goes with it?) is a major part of the diet, diabetes is rare, and "high rates of diabetes have not been reported in any society where obesity is rare."[13] (Sometimes one wishes that the science of population studies had never been invented.)

When we turn to animal experiments, we also find conflicting evidence. The idea that large amounts of glucose "overstrain" the pancreas appears overly simple in light of the fact that mixed meals stimulate much greater insulin production than sugar alone.[14] Diabetes can be induced in experimental animals by feeding them diets high in fat, protein, *or* sugar and can be reduced by lowering total food intake. From these facts, it is tempting to conclude that excess energy intake—obesity—causes diabetes; however, diets very high in sugar can cause the disease even if the animals do not become obese.[15] One extensive and well-designed study on rats clearly implicated sugar as the cause of diabetes. In this study, one set of animals was fed a starch-based diet, the other a similar, but sugar-based diet. Those fed starch did not develop symptoms; those fed sugar did.[16] The fairest conclusion that can be drawn is that obesity is a major factor but that sugar has not been proven innocent as a special factor in the causation of diabetes.

One of the earliest symptoms of diabetes is excessive hunger. In the most common form of diabetes (the adult-onset, or non-insulin-dependent, type), the person typically next becomes obese, and finally the diabetes appears. Thus sugar may contribute, not to diabetes, but to the obesity that brings the disease into the open. Obesity then aggravates the situation by causing resistance to insulin.[17] In fact, in this type of diabetic there may be too much, rather than too little, insulin, but the tissues fail to respond to it.[18] Both weight control and avoidance of sugar are therefore recommended for the potential and overt diabetic.[19]

(6) Does sugar cause cavities? Cavities (or dental caries) are a serious public

health problem, afflicting nearly everyone in the country, half of them by the time they are two years old. One of the most successful measures taken to reduce the incidence of dental decay is fluoridation of community water (see Controversy 10B). But sugar may have something to do with cavities, too.

Cavities are actually caused by the acid byproduct of bacterial growth in the mouth. Bacteria thrive on food particles, especially if they contain carbohydrate,[20] and so it is logical to implicate sugar as the cause of cavities. However, any carbohydrate, including starch, can support bacterial growth.[21] Equally important is the length of time the food stays in the mouth, and this depends on whether you brush your teeth and how sticky the food is. Milk or water drunk with a meal will help wash the carbohydrate off the teeth.[22] In this matter, as in the others, sugar may not be the extreme villain that some have made it out to be. One large (979 children) and well-controlled two-year study showed that presweetened cereals eaten for breakfast did not increase cavities, probably because they were eaten at mealtimes and with milk.[23] Mechanically disturbing bacteria by flossing every twenty-four hours may effectively prevent formation of cavities, regardless of carbohydrate content of the diet. And some people may *never* get cavities because they have inherited resistance to them. Still, if sugar is guilty of any of the six accusations listed at the start, it is guilty of contributing to tooth decay.[24]

Dietary Guidelines for Americans

THE USDA/USDHHS Guidelines offer the following pointers for those who wish to avoid excessive sugars:

- **Use less of all sugars, including white sugar, brown sugar, raw sugar, honey and syrups.**
- **Eat less of foods containing these sugars, such as candy, soft drinks, ice cream, cakes, cookies.**
- **Select fresh fruits or fruits canned without sugar or in light syrup rather than heavy syrup.**
- **Read food labels for clues on sugar content—if the names sucrose, glucose, maltose, dextrose, lactose, fructose, or syrups appear first, then there is a large amount of sugar.**
- **Remember, how frequently you eat sugar is as important as, and perhaps more important than, how much sugar you eat.**

Personal strategy. Should we eliminate sugar from our diets? Moderation in its use is probably the course to adopt. Totally eliminating sugar seems unnecessary, even if it were possible. But those who consume large amounts of sugar should reduce their intake, and potential diabetics should probably avoid it altogether.

Should we switch to saccharin in place of sugar? The question whether saccharin use incurs any risks is still open (see Controversy 11B); but if it does, those risks have to be weighed against the risks of consuming the sugar you would otherwise use. An interesting calculation was presented by B. L. Cohen in *Science*: Assuming (1) that saccharin users consume less sugar than they would otherwise, and (2) that consuming less sugar entails consuming fewer calories, and (3) that leanness promotes longer life, Cohen figures that the risk from using saccharin is far less than that from consuming sugar would be.[25] All three of these assumptions may be false, however,[26] so it is more prudent to reduce sugar intake without substituting saccharin.

Recommendations on ways to reduce sugar consumption flood the scientific journals. Recipes for sugarless confections have been published in the *Journal of the American Dietetic Association*.[27] Sweet beverage and dessert substitutes are suggested in the *Journal of Nutrition Education*:

Try water, mineral water or club soda with or without a slice of fresh lime or lemon. With a little persistence, unsweetened tea, hot or cold, with a twist of lemon, tastes fine. The same is true of coffee—except maybe a stick of cinnamon might be preferred to the lemon slice! . . . Enjoy fresh fruit in season. Try canned fruits packed in their own juice. . . . Try apple slices (unpeeled) with fresh grapefruit sections tipped with a sprinkling of nuts. . . .[28]

The *Journal of School Health* suggests that the snack foods available in vending machines be changed to more nutritious, less sugary snacks.[29] The preference for sugary foods is to some extent conditioned. It can be altered with enough motivation.

Others make similar recommendations. Films are available to teach children more nutritious snacking habits.[30] An American Friends Service Committee publication points out that alternatives to desserts might be "cheese and whole grain crackers and yogurt" and that snacks for children need not be sugar-water drinks. Instead, they can have "fruits, raw vegetables, popcorn, unsalted nuts, home made fruit juice popsicles and other wholesome foods."[31]

Many recommend substituting raw or brown sugar or honey for white sugar, because they contain some minerals essential for human health. They contain chromium, for example, although the amount is miniscule. It would be absurd to rely on any kind of sugar for its nutrient contributions, because one would have to eat so much to obtain significant amounts. (There is only one significant exception: Blackstrap molasses contains over 3 milligrams of iron per tablespoon and so, if used frequently, can make a major contribution of this important and, for women, hard-to-get nutrient. It's not as sweet as the other sweeteners, however, and so doesn't satisfy the "sweet tooth" of people who like sugar.) Rather than go to the extreme of eating large quantities of any sweetener, it makes sense to ensure that the diet is otherwise adequate and then use sugar for its taste appeal in whatever form one prefers. You might then choose honey, correctly, not for its nutrient contributions but for its sweetness. Perhaps the most important thing to remember about sugar in any of its forms (brown sugar, white sugar, honey, and all the other forms listed at the start) is that it is an empty-calorie food. Its "emptiness" can be tolerated as long as the diet is otherwise adequate, balanced, and nutritious; but it does dilute the nutrients in the diet. It reduces nutrient density. As for its calories, they can be tolerated as long as the total energy budget is balanced. Potential diabetics, however, should probably avoid sugar (and honey) altogether.

The Controversy Notes and For Further Information follow the Appendixes.

Controversy 4B

Fiber

Does fiber deficiency cause intestinal diseases?

Many of the arguments in favor of increasing our fiber intakes are logical. However, what is logical does not always stand up to testing. Only the most discerning person can see the flaws in arguments like some of those that follow. You are advised to read the logical arguments with an open and skeptical attitude and pay close attention to the evidence that follows.

Logic. If you don't eat enough fiber, enthusiasts say, the contents of the intestine will move sluggishly and create local regions of high pressure. Blood trying to force its way through blood vessels in the intestinal walls of these regions will encounter this pressure, and the result will be varicose veins. In the rectum, these are known as hemorrhoids.

If you don't eat enough fiber, the theory is that your intestinal muscles will become weak from lack of stimulation. This weakness, especially in the colon where the fecal matter is solid, will make portions of the colon wall balloon out (diverticulosis) which will lead to irritation or infection (diverticulitis) and possibly a rupture. About one in every six people in Western countries develops diverticulosis in middle or later life.[3]

Fiber also holds some water, yielding a soft stool. Because of this, the fiber people reason that if you don't eat enough fiber, the colon contents may become dry and hard, and this together with their sluggish

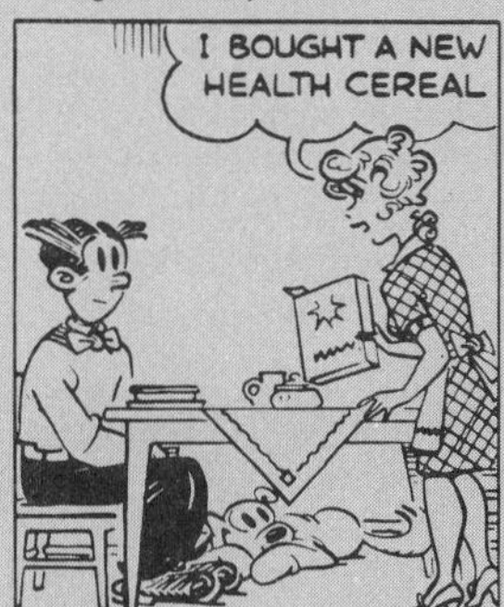
I BOUGHT A NEW HEALTH CEREAL

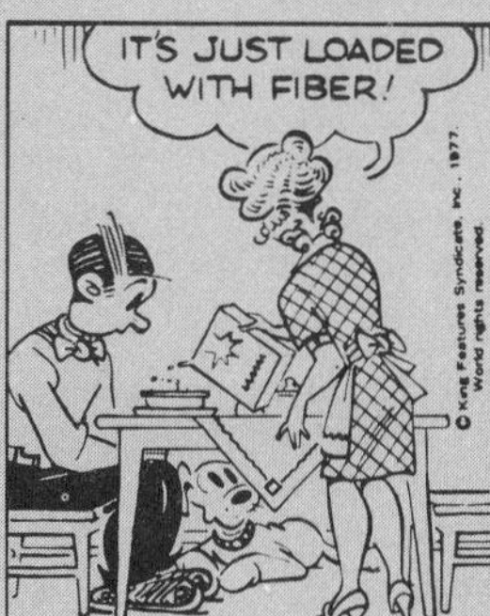
IT'S JUST LOADED WITH FIBER!

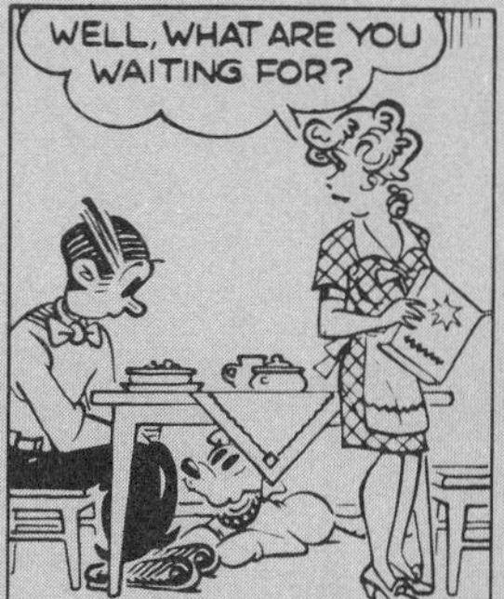
WELL, WHAT ARE YOU WAITING FOR?

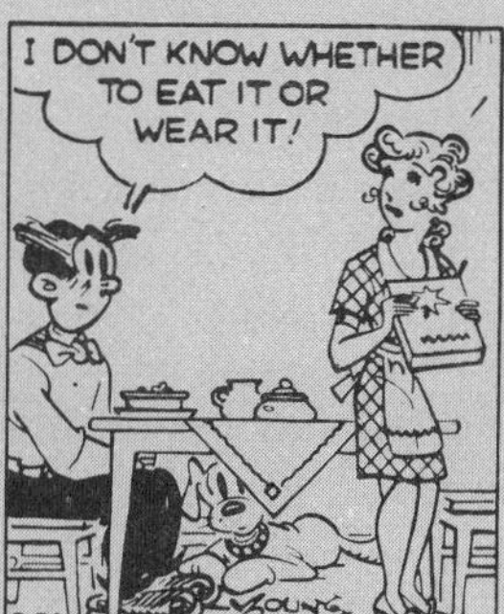
I DON'T KNOW WHETHER TO EAT IT OR WEAR IT!

passage and the weakness of the intestinal muscles will cause a long transit time and constipation. If there are cancer-causing agents present, the colon will be exposed to these agents for longer than necessary, thus increasing the likelihood of colon cancer, the second-ranked killer among cancers in the United States.[4]

If you choose to believe this logic, then, you had better eat plenty of fiber to avoid getting hemorrhoids, diverticulosis, constipation, and cancer of the colon. Other intestinal disorders (appendicitis, gall bladder disease, deep-vein thrombosis, and hiatal hernia) have also been linked by logic to a lack of fiber in the diet.[5] (What fiber might have to do with cardiovascular disease is presented in Controversy 5A).

Evidence. The proponents of these hypotheses advance several kinds of evidence to support their claims. Much of the most persuasive evidence comes from studies of populations. Wherever a country's wealth has increased, the "modern diseases" have been seen to emerge in the same order: first, appendicitis; then hemorrhoids and varicose veins; then colon cancer, diverticulosis, and hiatal hernia.[6] This is the same order in which these diseases are likely to appear in one person's lifetime, implying that they are related to the time of exposure to some factor, such as lack of fiber in the diet.

Opponents of the fiber theory point out, however, that

Miniglossary

Terms relating to fiber:

bran: The fiber of wheat, notable for its effectiveness against constipation and also notable for *not* being effective in lowering blood cholesterol. Its principal constituent is cellulose.

cellulose: The indigestible polysaccharide composed of glucose (see Chapter 4); it is the principal constituent of bran (the fiber of wheat) and is also found in fruits and vegetables.

crude fiber: The indigestible material found in food when it is subjected to a laboratory procedure; more technically, "the residue of plant food left after extraction by dilute acid followed by dilute alkali." Sometimes abbreviated CF.

dietary fiber: The indigestible material actually remaining when food passes through the intestinal tract; more technically, "the residue of plant food resistant to hydrolysis 'splitting' by human 'digestive' enzymes."[1] Sometimes abbreviated DF.

fiber: The indigestible part of plant food, including pectin, cellulose, hemicelluloses, mucilages, and lignin.[2] See also crude fiber, dietary fiber.

hemicellulose: A carbohydrate fiber that occurs in the same foods as cellulose.

lignin: A noncarbohydrate fiber that occurs in grains, especially wheat and rye, cabbage and other vegetables, apples and strawberries and other fruits, and nuts.

pectin: The fiber of apple, citrus fruits, and other fruits, notable for its effectiveness in lowering blood cholesterol.

residue: A term not used here, residue is sometimes confused with fiber but actually refers to whatever material still remains solid when the intestinal contents reach the colon. Milk, for example, contains no fiber, but its curds form a residue in the intestines.

Terms relating to intestinal diseases:

appendicitis: Inflammation and/or infection of the appendix, a sac protruding from the large intestine.

constipation: Hardness and dryness of bowel movements, associated with discomfort in passing them.

deep-vein thrombosis (throm-BOH-sis): Clot formation inside an interior vein in a body organ.

diverticulitis (dye-ver-tic-you-LYE-tiss): Inflammation or infection of diverticular pockets in the intestine; a disease condition which can lead to rupture.

diverticulosis (dye-ver-tic-you-LOCE-iss): Outpocketings of weakened areas of the intestinal wall; can lead to diverticulitis.

hemorrhoids (HEM-or-oids): Varicose veins in the rectum, sometimes caused by the pressure resulting from constipation.

hiatal hernia (hye-AY-tal): An outpocketing at the top of the stomach at the point of entry of the esophagus. Such a hernia can slide up and down through the diaphragm (see Figure 3 in Appendix A), becoming irritated, and can be most uncomfortable when the stomach is full and when a person is lying down so that the stomach contents put pressure on it.

spastic colon: A condition in which the colon is irritable and tends to tighten, causing constipation. Stimulation by fiber makes this kind of constipation worse, not better.

varicose veins (VAIR-ih-kose): Veins that have become hard and knotted because of high pressure in them.

the lack of fiber itself may not be responsible for these phenomena. As fiber disappears from the diet, such nutrients as fat, sugar, and protein increase and it may be these nutrients that account for the increased disease incidence.[7] Colon cancer, especially, correlates far better with high intakes of dietary fat and animal protein than with low intakes of fiber.[8] Another possibility is that the increasing incidence of the diseases may be caused by lack of such trace elements as chromium and zinc, which disappear with fiber when cereal is refined.[9] But the fiber-theory proponents score a logical point when they retort that these are colon diseases and that fiber is the only food constituent that reaches the colon.[10]

Not all the evidence from population studies supports the fiber theory. Constipated people do not have more colon cancer than nonconstipated people.[11] In northern India, where the diet is high in fiber, colon cancer is more common than in southern India, where fiber is almost completely lacking in the diet.[12] Opponents of the fiber theory also point out that appendicitis has decreased in the United States by 40 percent in the past twenty years,[13] whereas fiber intakes have simultaneously decreased.

Controlled experiments yield specific findings that help to clarify the confusion somewhat. Hospital tests show that high-fiber foods do help to relieve constipation, and older people who use high-fiber foods have less need for laxatives.[14] Fiber absorbs water and so softens the stools (1 gram of fiber increases stool weight by 15 grams of water.[15]) The extent to which fiber affects intestinal transit time is unsettled; it may be that some fibers (like pectin) slow it down while others speed it up[16] or it may be that it shortens transit time in people with constipation and lengthens it in people with diarrhea.[17] The consensus among gastroenterologists (digestive tract specialists) at a 1977 conference was that "significant amounts of high-fiber foods *may* protect the colon from diverticulosis and cancer."[18]

The evidence just described comes from experiments using fiber from different foods. Not all fibers are the same. In the future it will help greatly to clarify the role of fiber if experimenters distinguish among the many different fibers found in foods. For example, bran (wheat fiber) holds five times its weight in water, whereas carrot fiber holds twenty to thirty times its weight.[19] Experiments with bran show that it does not have the same effect as many other fibers; unfortunately, this is the product most often bought by consumers jumping prematurely onto the fiber bandwagon. The distinction between bran and the other fibers becomes especially important when the effect on blood lipids is considered, because bran is notable for *not* lowering blood cholesterol.[20]

To unmuddy the waters surrounding the term *fiber*, it is also important to be aware that the fiber in the gut is not the same as the fiber found in foods when they are analyzed in the laboratory. When you look up the fiber content of a food in a table (for example, in Appendix C), you are told its crude fiber content, but the fiber that works in your intestine is dietary fiber.[21]

Personal strategy. Tentativeness is obviously the attitude to adopt toward the fiber hypothesis at present, as all the authorities seem to agree. But while awaiting more evidence, what course of action would be prudent? One author recommends increasing crude fiber in the diet to 12 grams a day, which would effectively increase total dietary fiber to 20 to 36 grams a day.[22] Some books have recommended as much as 28 grams crude fiber, on the basis that the African populations noted for their freedom from colonic disease average 25 grams a day.[23] Diets in the United States presently provide an average of about 4 grams a day, as compared with 6 grams back in 1900.[24] The digestive tract specialists already mentioned recommend 5 to 6 grams a day.[25] Burkitt offers a simple guideline: "Dietary intake is sufficient," he says, "if the feces are soft and they float; more fiber is needed if the stools are hard and sink."[26]

Before jumping to any conclusions, an important question to ask is: What are the risks? A proponent of dietary fiber says, "There is nothing to lose. . . . It is easier to increase the size of stools passed than to build larger hospitals."[27] An opponent argues that fibrous foods are unappealing: "A constant awareness of bowel activity is hardly conducive to a serene state of mind. Fiber may stir the gut but is unlikely to stir the imagination!"[28]

In a more serious vein, several studies suggest that large amounts of fiber may have ill effects. It can aggravate, rather than alleviate, constipation due to spastic colon.[29] It can also produce a deficiency of trace elements.[30] In one study, in which eight subjects consumed 16 grams of fiber a day for three weeks, they excreted significantly higher amounts of sodium, potassium, and magnesium than did control subjects.[31]

High-fiber foods may also be high in phytic acid, a substance that can combine with important minerals like zinc and carry them out of the body with the stools. There are upper limits beyond which the consumption of these foods would not be prudent.[32] It has also come to light that some fibers, notably pectin and hemicellulose, may be digested by colon bacteria, yielding glucose, from which the human body can then actually derive calories after all.[33] The dieter who relies on high-fiber foods to be low in calories would be disappointed to learn this, but the amount of energy anyone derives this way is probably very small.[34]

We might also consider some further proposed benefits of fiber. One theory holds that bacteria flourishing in the colon produce waste products that may cause cancer and that high-fiber diets might change the colon bacterial population in a favorable direction. But an experiment designed to test this hypothesis showed no effect of fiber on colon bacteria.[35] Fiber may also reduce the toxicity of certain substances in the colon,[36] but experimental evidence shows that this effect is not uniform.[37]

It seems that the indiscriminate use of fiber, especially in purified form (bran) added to recipes would be ill advised. On the other hand, there is no apparent risk in shifting toward the use of more *foods* high in natural fiber, such as whole-grain breads and cereals and fresh fruits and vegetables (see Appendix C). You might also want to know that foods high in fiber are not necessarily coarse in texture. The Japanese foods miso (bean paste) and tofu (bean curd) are smooth and soft but very high in fiber.[38] Adopting a dietary pattern similar to that of our farm ancestors would bring us in line with the current recommendations like the *Dietary Guidelines* and, while increasing our consumption of fiber and complex carbohydrate, would also decrease our sugar and fat intake, a move heartily endorsed by most authorities.

The Controversy Notes and For Further Information follow the Appendixes.

CHAPTER 5

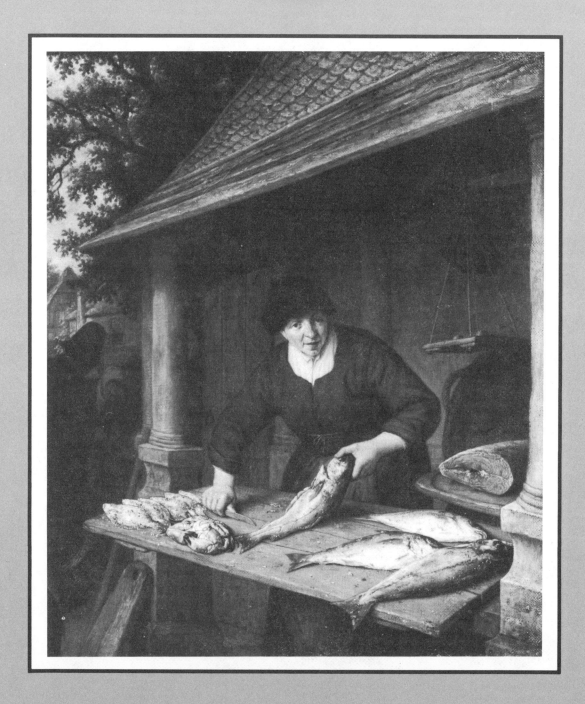

The Lipids: Fats and Oils

"Your triglycerides are up," reports the doctor. "Take off that ugly fat," shouts the ad for a diet pill. "Blood lipid profile—$85," states your bill from the medical laboratory. "My doctor says my cholesterol level is high," says your friend when refusing an egg. "Use lecithin to lower your blood cholesterol," recommends an ad in a health food store window. Triglycerides—fat—blood lipid profile—cholesterol—lecithin. It is reasonable for you to ask the meaning of these words that are so casually tossed about.

You know more than you think you do about the lipids, more commonly called the fats or **fats** and **oils**. You know that butter, coffee cream, and salad oil are fats; that a ham is covered with fat that you usually choose to cut away because of the calories; that the odors of fat identify the meat that is cooking (recall the odor in the house when bacon is frying); and that you have layers of fat under your skin, perhaps more than you would like to have. In addition, you may already have a smattering of food science information—say, that egg yolks contain cholesterol or that the marbling of expensive steaks is really fat, which carries many extra calories. However, you may be confused by much of the terminology used in discussing diet changes that might improve the health of your arteries. Let's look at some of these terms.

Oil: Fat in liquid form.

Opposite: A detail from The Fish Seller *by Adrian van Ostade. Used with the permission of the Rijksmuseum, Amsterdam.*

Terminology

Lipid is the general term for fats. It includes naturally occurring substances that generally cannot be dissolved in water but can be dissolved in solvents like fingernail polish remover (acetone) or paint thinner (turpentine). Most of the time, when we refer to fat—whether it is the fat in the middle-age spread or on our toast or trimmed off our steaks—we would more correctly speak of lipid. About 95 percent of the lipids in food and in our bodies are **triglycerides**. Other members of the lipid family are the **phospholipids** (of which lecithin is one) and the **sterols** (cholesterol is the best known of these). "Blood lipid profile" refers to the results of a test conducted by a medical laboratory, which reveals the amounts of various lipids—especially triglycerides and cholesterol—found in your blood. The results of this study can help a doctor assess your risk of heart and artery disease.

Lipids:
Triglycerides.
Phospholipids.
Sterols.

Fat in food includes visible fats and oils, such as butter, margarine, safflower oil, and the fat you trim from a steak. It also refers to some you can't see, such as the fat that "marbles" a steak or that is hidden in foods like nuts, cheese, pastries, avocados, and processed foods.

Because triglycerides are the chief form of fat found in foods, the following four sections are mostly devoted to them. A brief section at the end of the chapter presents a few details about lecithin and cholesterol. Cholesterol, which is at the heart of a major dispute over cardiovascular disease, is discussed in Controversy 5A at the end of this chapter, and the relation of fat to cancer is described in Controversy 5B.

Usefulness of Fats

You have heard and read so much about the bad effects of too much fat and about the increase in the amount of fat in the typical diet that you may decide that fat is bad for you. It may come as a surprise that these lipids are valuable. More than valuable, they are absolutely necessary, and some must be present in the diet for you to maintain good health.

Triglycerides are the body's storage form for food energy eaten in excess of need. This was described in Chapter 1 as being a valuable evolutionary mechanism for people who must live a feast-or-famine existence. It enables them to remain alive during the famine period. In addition, it is an asset in time of illness and high fever. Suppose two infants, one thin and the other fat, contracted a disease such as typhoid fever. The high fever would create a need for more calories. Nausea and discomfort would make it difficult for these babies to consume enough food to deliver those calories. Both infants then would have to draw on their more permanent storehouse of calories—their fat stores. Naturally, the fat baby would have a longer-lasting energy supply to draw on while battling the disease. The longer survival under such circumstances of fat babies in earlier times may account for the common belief persisting today that a fat baby is a healthy baby. (But in today's world, where most childhood diseases have been controlled, this belief is not valid.)

Fat is a concentrated energy food, in contrast to carbohydrate, and valuable in many situations for this reason. A gram of fat or oil from the diet delivers over twice as many calories as a gram of carbohydrate. A hunter or hiker needs to consume a larger number of calories to travel long distances or to survive in very cold climates. It is difficult in such a situation to carry enough carbohydrate food to provide these calories; but the same number of calories can be carried in the form of fat in a smaller and lighter package. On the other hand, high-fat foods may deliver many unneeded calories to the person who is not expending much energy in physical work.

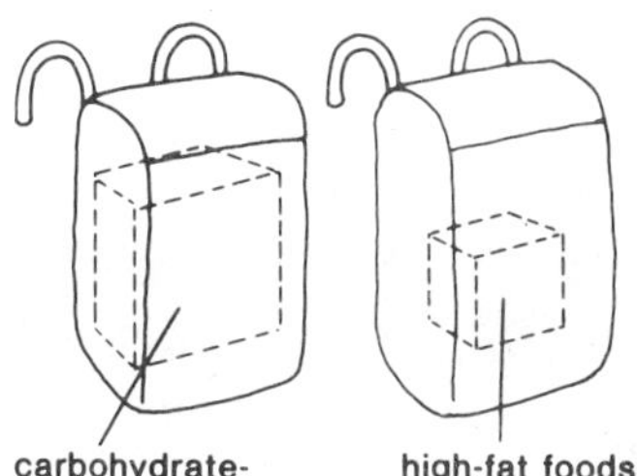

Both lunches contain the same number of calories.

1 g carbohydrate = 4 calories
1 g fat = 9 calories
1 g protein = 4 calories
1 g alcohol = 7 calories

Fat surrounds and pads all the vital organs, protecting them from blows and from temperature variations. This padding enables you to ride a horse or a motorcycle for many hours with no more serious damage than sore muscles.

Fat is important for another reason. Some essential nutrients are soluble in fat and therefore are found mainly in foods that contain fat. These nutrients are linoleic acid (an essential fatty acid) and the fat-soluble vitamins—A, D, E, and K. Fat also carries many compounds that give foods their aroma and flavor. This accounts for the delicious smell associated with foods that are being fried, such as bacon or french fries. When a person has lost the desire to eat, foods flavored with some fat, such as margarine, may awaken the appetite.

Fat is an important component of the membranes surrounding the cells of your body. Many of the household chemicals that we keep out of the reach of small children do their deadly work on the fat in cell membranes. Kerosene, gasoline, and paint thinners are a few of the substances that dissolve fat. When a child swallows these, the fat in the membranes is dissolved, destroying the cells lining the mouth, esophagus, and stomach. Another illustration of fat's presence in the membranes of cells is the effect some substances have on the skin of the hands. A harsh soap, such as a mechanic might use, has an excess of alkali. This combines chemically with the fat of the skin cells, forming soap which washes away. The loss of fat leaves the hands dry and cracked. Oily salves must then be put on the hands in an effort to return the lost fat.

To sum up, lipids not only provide energy reserves but also play many other roles. They protect the body from outside forces, are constituents of all cells, help maintain body temperature, add flavor to foods, and carry the fat-soluble nutrients.

A Chemist's View of Triglycerides

The bulk of the fats in our diet come from animal flesh or animal products. Animal fat, in turn, may have come from the carbohydrates in plants, as you learned in the last chapter, or from protein, which will be discussed later. You may recall the fragments into which glucose is broken on its way to becoming energy. When this energy is to be stored as fat, these fragments are linked together into chains known as **fatty acids**. Fatty acids are packaged in threes with glycerol to make triglycerides, the material of fat.

Fatty acids may differ from one another in two ways: in chain length and in degree of saturation. Chain length has an effect on their solubility in water; the shorter chains are more soluble. Saturation, a term that you hear very often, refers to the chemical structure—specifically, the number of hydrogens the fatty acid chain is holding. If every available bond from the carbons is holding a hydrogen, we say the chain is a **saturated fatty acid**—filled to capacity with hydrogen.

Sometimes, especially in the fatty acids in plants, there is a place in the chain where hydrogens are missing. This is a **point of unsaturation**, and such a chain is an **unsaturated fatty acid**. (An example is **oleic acid**.) If there are two or more points of unsaturation, then we say it is a **polyunsaturated fatty acid**. (You sometimes see polyunsaturated fatty acids abbreviated on food labels as PUFA.) Most polyunsaturated fatty acids are made in plants, where they help form the protective coating of leaves and the skin of seeds.

The human body can synthesize all the fatty acids it needs from carbohydrate, fat, or protein, except one—**linoleic acid**. Linoleic acid cannot be made from the breakdown of other substances and so must be provided in the diet. It is, therefore, considered an **essential fatty acid**. Linoleic is a polyunsaturated fatty acid, widely distributed in plant oils, and is readily stored in the adult body. Infants are especially in need of linoleic acid, and it is no coincidence that human breast milk has a much higher percentage of it than cow's milk.

Points of unsaturation are like weak spots in that they are vulnerable to the attack of oxygen. This is why polyunsaturated oils, such as safflower oil, should be refrigerated and not stored for long periods. The unsaturated points easily undergo chemical change, and when they do, the oil becomes rancid.

There are two ways of handling this spoilage problem. One is to change the oil chemically (**hydrogenation**), but this causes it to lose its polyunsaturated character and the health benefits that go with it. A second alternative is to add a chemical that will compete for the oxygen and thus protect the oil. Such an additive is called an **antioxidant**. Examples are the well-known BHA and BHT seen on bread labels and the natural antioxidants vitamin C (ascorbic acid) and vitamin E. A third alternative is to keep the product refrigerated. Cold temperatures retard chemical action.

When fats are hydrogenated, they form some trans-fatty acids, implicated in cancer causation; see Controversy 5B. And for more about additives, turn to Chapter 11.

One interesting result of the presence of unsaturated fatty acids in a fat is that they affect the temperature at which the fat melts. The more unsaturated a fat, the more liquid it is at room temperature. In contrast, the more saturated a fat (the more hydrogens it has), the firmer it is. Thus, of three fats—lard, chicken fat, and safflower oil— lard is the most saturated and the hardest (it comes from pork); chicken fat is less saturated and somewhat soft (chicken is recommended over pork in a heart patient's diet); and safflower oil, which is the most unsaturated, is an oil at room temperature (and the only one of the three that comes from a plant). If your doctor tells you to use polyunsaturated fats, you can judge by the hardness of the fat which ones to choose.

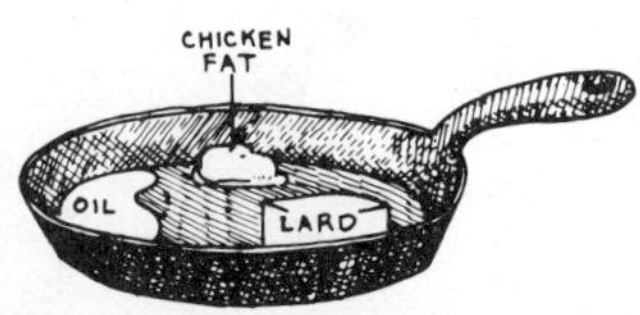

The most polyunsaturated fat is the softest.

Generally speaking, vegetable and fish oils are rich in polyunsaturates, whereas the harder fats—animal fats—are more saturated. But beware. Not all vegetable oils are polyunsaturated. If you are looking for a substitute for cream, you may choose a nondairy creamer. But many nondairy creamers substitute coconut oil for butterfat (cream). Coconut oil is actually more saturated than cream and therefore is no better for you. Palm oil, also used frequently in food processing, is also highly saturated. Another exception to the rule is olive oil, widely used in salad dressings and in the cooking of Greek and Italian foods. The predominant fatty acid in olive oil is a *mono*-unsaturated fatty acid, oleic acid. Thus olive oil can claim to be unsaturated, but not to be polyunsaturated.

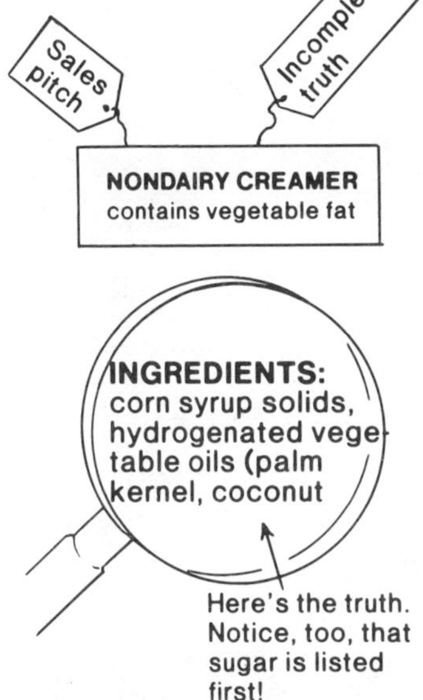
Sales pitch
Incomplete truth
NONDAIRY CREAMER
contains vegetable fat
INGREDIENTS:
corn syrup solids,
hydrogenated vege-
table oils (palm
kernel, coconut
Here's the truth.
Notice, too, that
sugar is listed
first!

People sometimes think nondairy creamers are better for them, because they contain no animal fat. But the fat is saturated, and sugar is the major ingredient.

When food producers want to use a polyunsaturated oil such as corn oil to make a spreadable margarine, they use the hydrogenation process. Hydrogen is forced into the oil, some of the unsaturated fatty acids accept the hydrogen, and the oil becomes harder. The spreadable margarine that results is more saturated then the original oil. If you, the consumer, were looking for polyunsaturated oils to include in your diet, these hydrogenated oils would not meet your need. This does not imply that they are "bad" for you. It depends on what you want. Were you trying to buy polyunsaturated fat because your doctor ordered you to? Or were you looking for something you could spread on toast? The hydrogenated oils are easy to handle, store well, have a high smoking temperature, and are a perfectly suitable product for some purposes. But they are more saturated. Margarines that list liquid oil as the first ingredient are usually the most polyunsaturated.

There are very few free fatty acids found in the body or in foods. Usually, the fatty acids have been incorporated into large, more complex compounds such as triglycerides. Most of the time when you speak of fat—"I am fat" or "That meat is fat"—you are speaking of triglycerides. The name almost explains itself: Three fatty acids (*tri*) are attached to a molecule of **glycerol**.

Any combination of fatty acids can be incorporated into a triglyceride—long-chain or short-chain, saturated or polyunsaturated. Each type of animal (including humans) has its own characteristic kinds of triglycerides, but animals raised for food can be fed certain diets in order to give them softer or harder fat, whichever is demanded by the consumer.

The Body's Use of Triglycerides

When you partake of carbohydrate or protein, some of it can be made into fat in the body, as you have already seen. The carbohydrate is first digested to monosaccharides, mostly glucose. Some is stored as glycogen, and the remainder is broken down to fragments. Some of these fragments are used for energy; some are joined together to make fatty acids. The fatty acids are attached to glycerol to make triglycerides. Finally, these are transported to the fat depots—muscles, mammary glands, the insulating fat layer under the skin, and others.

When you partake of animal flesh (meat, fish, poultry) or animal products (milk, cheese, eggs), you are eating animal protein and fat. Of the fat, 95 percent is triglyceride that has been made this way from carbohydrate. This fat can end up being used the same way as body fat, but first it has to be digested, absorbed, and transported to its cell destinations.

Separation. When we eat fat-containing foods, one of the first steps in digestion is a physical separation of the fat from the other nutrients. Some of this is done by subtraction. That is, as carbohydrate and protein digestion begins, the fat is left behind and merges into large globules, as oil does on street puddles. When the acid of the stomach touches the complex food, the fat is separated even more and clumps together in larger drops that float to the top of the contents of the stomach. Fat is the last of the foodstuffs to leave the stomach and enter the small intestine. Some enzyme activity on fats takes place in the stomach, but not much. The digestive system seems to give first preference to carbohydrate and protein—because they alone can supply significant amounts of glucose—and to hold back the concentrated energy food in the stomach until the other nutrients are out of the way. When fat finally gets to the small intestine, we want to give it our undivided attention, the system seems to say, underscoring nature's conservation of valuable calories.

Whatever the reason, it is true that the fat stays behind in the stomach and that muscular action is slowed. This accounts for the fact that fat in the diet lends a longer-lasting feeling of satisfaction and fullness—**satiety**—than the other energy nutrients.

Before emulsification:

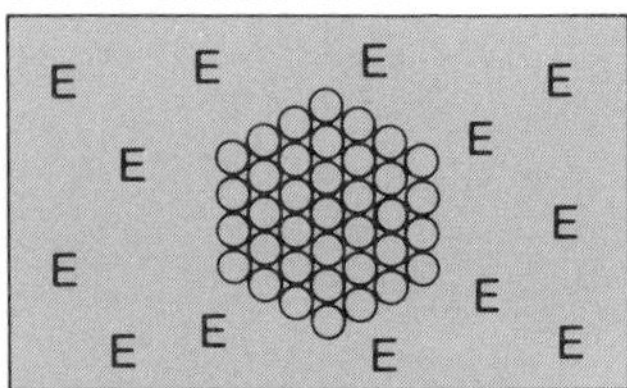

Fat-splitting enzymes can only reach the fat molecules on the outside of the fat globule.

After emulsification:

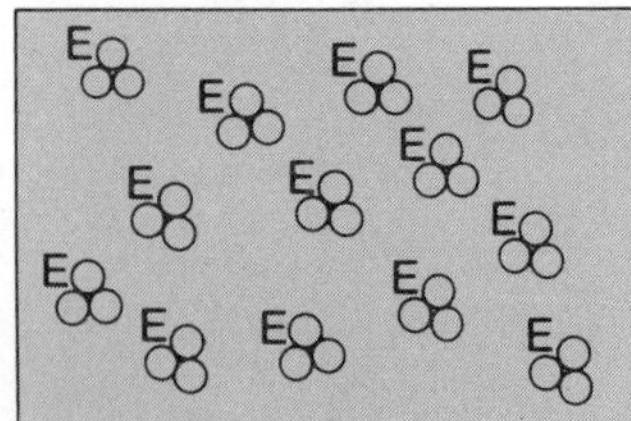

Fat-splitting enzymes can make physical contact with fat molecules.

Emulsification. When the fat finally reaches the small intestine, **bile** salts are squirted into the mixture to break up the fat globules. Bile contains no enzymes but is an **emulsifier**—that is, a compound that can separate the fat globules into smaller and smaller droplets. This enables the enzymes that are going to attack the bonds to get next to them. Emulsification resembles the method you use to remove a grease spot from your clothes. You pour detergent onto the grease spot and rub it between your hands to get the detergent in close contact with every part of the grease; the detergent molecules then return to the water solution, drawing grease along with them. In the upper intestine, the bile salts act as the detergent, and the muscles of the digestive tract do the agitating.

Digestion and absorption. Once the fat has been emulsified, the enzymes can chemically attack the bonds that hold the triglycerides together. The enzymes are made in the pancreas and flow into the intestine through the pancreatic duct when the message is received that fat is present. Strangely, these enzymes sometimes free the two fatty acids on the ends and allow the middle fatty acid to remain attached, forming a **monoglyceride**.

At this point, most of the triglycerides that entered the body in food have been digested to their components—fatty acids, glycerol, and monoglycerides. They are moved continuously through the small intestine and must be absorbed into the bloodstream if they are to be of any use to the body's cells. If not absorbed, they will continue on their way and be excreted. But one difficulty must be overcome before the fat can be absorbed. Fats are insoluble in water, and both lymph and blood are watery. The way this problem is solved is the subject of much current research. As of this date, the following seems to be the most widely accepted theory.[1]

The shortest free fatty acids pass by simple diffusion through the membranes of the cells that reside in the tips of the villi. Because these short-chain fatty acids are somewhat water soluble, they can, without any further processing, leave the cells on the other side and enter the capillaries inside the villi. From these capillaries the short-chain fatty acids are transported through collecting veins to the capillaries of the liver. There they are removed and remade into whatever substances the body needs.

The glycerol follows the same path as the short-chain fatty acids, because it too is water soluble.

The longer-chain fatty acids are also absorbed through the cell membranes at the tips of the villi, but there they are reconnected with glycerol or with monoglycerides. This forms *new* triglycerides. But triglycerides are insoluble in water and must be specially packaged for transport before they can leave the cells (see Figure 1).

Formation of lipoproteins and transport to liver. Triglycerides are insoluble in water, but both of the body's transport systems—lymph and blood—are filled with water. Clearly, if the triglycerides were dumped "as is" into the bloodstream, they would clump together to form globs of fat that would clog the arteries. You are familiar with this effect if you have ever carelessly dumped greasy foods down the kitchen sink; the drain becomes clogged and the grease has to be removed at great expense to you. The body is "smarter" with triglycerides than you may be with your kitchen grease. Pure, unadulterated grease never travels through the body's arteries, although they sometimes clog for other reasons.

A cell of the intestinal wall allows a cluster of triglycerides and other lipids to form, then wraps the cluster with a protein coat to form a **chylomicron**, one of the five types of **lipoprotein**. The sketch in the margin shows that the fatty acids position themselves as far away from the water as they can get; then a small skin of protein forms around the fat globule. In this ingenious configuration, the water-soluble protein skin protects the fat and carries it through the lymph until it reaches a connecting duct through which it can enter the blood.

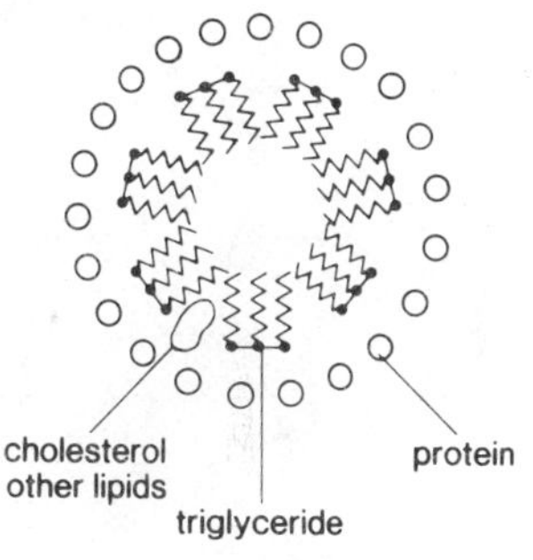

A chylomicron—lipids surrounded by a protein coat—is made in the intestinal wall cells.

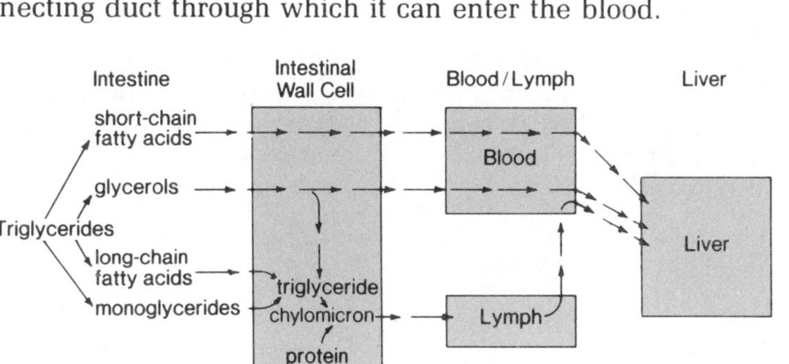

Figure 1. *Path of lipids from intestine to liver.*

The special function of the chylomicrons is to carry the fat you have eaten to the liver, where it will be dismantled and reassembled into other fats. The presence of these chylomicron particles in the bloodstream following a meal containing fat gives the blood a milky appearance. This cloudy look remains until the liver cells have selected and disposed of most of the fat within the particle.

This description of the intestine's processing of fat has omitted the few other dietary fats, like phospholipids and cholesterol, that may have entered the body in food. These are absorbed similarly and are also packaged in chylomicrons. After transport, they too end up in the liver.

Transport within the body. Within the body, fats always travel from place to place wrapped in protein coats—that is, as lipoproteins. Lipoproteins are very much in the news these days. In fact, the doctor who measures your blood lipid profile is interested not only in the types of fat in your blood (triglycerides and cholesterol) but also in the types of protein coats in which they are wrapped.

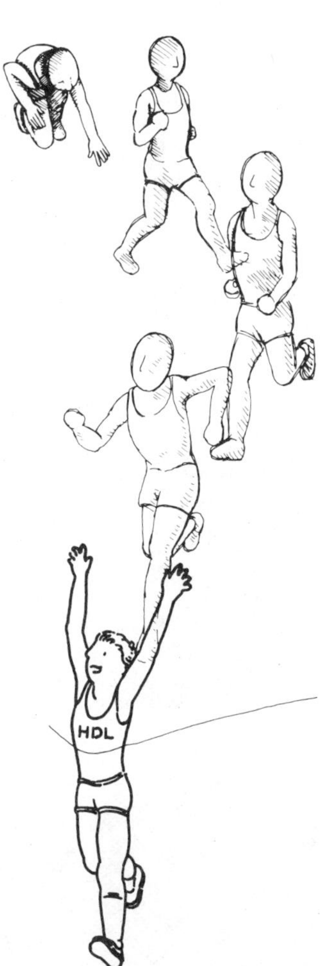

Endurance athletes have higher HDL levels than other people.

One distinction among types of lipoproteins is of great interest because it has implications for the health of the heart and blood vessels; that is the distinction between low-density lipoproteins (**LDL**) and high-density lipoproteins (**HDL**). Raised LDL concentrations in the blood are a sign of high heart-attack risk. Raised HDL concentrations are associated with a low risk.[2]

Actually, there are, at last count, five types of lipoproteins circulating in the blood:

Chylomicrons—made by the intestines for transport of just-eaten fat to the liver and other organs. These carry mostly triglycerides.

VLDL (very-low-density lipoproteins)—made by both intestine and liver for transport of fats around the body. These, too, carry mostly triglycerides.

IDL (intermediate-density lipoproteins)—an intermediate class not recognized by all researchers, formed as cells remove fat from VLDL.[3]

LDL (low-density lipoproteins)—made by the liver. These carry cholesterol (much of it synthesized in the liver) to the body's cells.

HDL (high-density lipoproteins)—small particles of uncertain origin, perhaps what's left after fat is removed from the other lipoproteins. These particles are believed to pick up and carry unused cholesterol *back* from the body tissues to the liver for dismantling and disposal.

Research presently is directed toward asking whether the HDLs are truly protective, and if so, how we can raise them. One way seems to be by increasing our physical activity.

Storage of fat. Any cell can take triglycerides out of a lipoprotein and use them for energy or store them. Most cells can store only a limited amount, but the fat cells can store a virtually infinite amount of triglycerides. In an adult, the number of fat cells seems to be fixed, but their size can expand indefinitely. The more triglycerides they store, the larger they grow, until a very obese person's fat cells may be a hundred times as large as a thin person's.

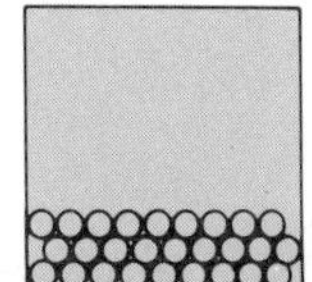
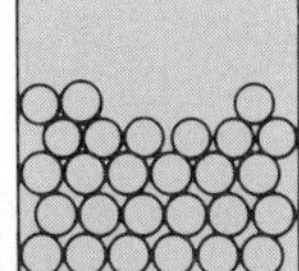

Fat cells enlarge.

Use of fat for energy. When the body uses this stored fat for energy, it breaks it down the same way as already described in the last chapter. The fatty acids are cleaved from the glycerol backbone, and then each is chopped into fragments. To be completely broken down, each fragment has to be combined with a fragment made from glucose. In other words, carbohydrate is necessary for the complete metabolism of fat. Without carbohydrate, ketosis will occur, characterized by the appearance of incomplete fat-breakdown products in the blood (ketones). Because it is so important for dieters to understand this, the whole sequence of events is described in greater detail in Chapter 7.

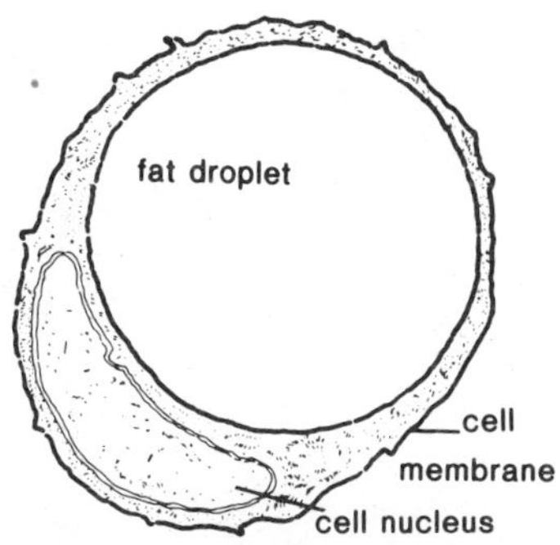

Within the fat cell, lipid is stored in a globule. This globule can enlarge indefinitely and the fat cell membrane will grow to accommodate its swollen contents.

Lecithin and Cholesterol

Lecithin and other phospholipids play key roles in the structure of cell membranes. Because of the way they are constructed, they have both water-loving and fat-loving characteristics, which enable them to help fats into and out of the watery insides of cells. Magical properties are sometimes attributed to lecithin, and people are admonished to supplement their diets with it. But lecithin is widespread in food and is also made by the body in abundant quantities. It is not an essential nutrient.[4]

One of the claims made for lecithin is that it helps to lower the cholesterol in the body. Factors that actually lower blood cholesterol are described in Controversy 5A, and lecithin is not significant among them. If it has any effect, it is probably due to the fact that it has polyunsaturated fatty acids as part of its structure; any other polyunsaturated fat would work equally well.

Another claim made for lecithin is that it helps improve people's memory. If only this were true, we could all benefit by eating lecithin; but it seems to be true, if at all, only for people with a specific kind of memory disorder. Even there, high doses are needed, suggesting that the effect is like that of a drug, not a nutrient. Lecithin probably works by contributing choline, which has been found to help in several neurological disorders. But memory weakness is not a sign of "lecithin deficiency."[5]

More about choline—Chapter 9.

As for **cholesterol**, it is an important compound. It has many functions in the body. It is a part of the bile acids, which are necessary in the digestion of fats. It is a forerunner of the sex hormones. It is an important lipid in the structure of brain and nerve cells. In fact, cholesterol is a part of every cell. Like lecithin, cholesterol can be made by the body or can be obtained in the food we eat. But while it is widespread in the body and necessary to its function, it also is the major part of the plaques that narrow the arteries in the killer disease atherosclerosis.

Cholesterol's reputation as a harmful compound is addressed further in Controversy 5A, but the main points of that discussion should be stated here, too. Cholesterol in *foods* does not appear to be the villain some have made it out to be. It is cholesterol in the *blood*—

especially in the LDLs—that forecasts heart and artery disease. And this blood cholesterol is made not from food cholesterol but from triglycerides—that is, plain old fat, and saturated fat in particular. People who need to try to lower their blood cholesterol levels by means of diet can take three precautions, of which the first is by far the most important:

Reduce total fat intake.

This strategy is called "increasing the P:S ratio." For fats with high P:S ratios, see Appendix D.

Increase the proportion of polyunsaturated fat relative to saturated fat—the **polyunsaturated:saturated fat ratio (P:S ratio)**.

Reduce cholesterol intake.

Some say all adults should take these measures; others say only those specially identified as "at risk" for heart disease should take them. The question remains open, but it seems likely that most people need not make efforts to reduce their intakes of food cholesterol very stringently. Eggs, shellfish, and other cholesterol-containing foods are extremely nutritious and have little or no blood-cholesterol-raising effect. Cholesterol is unlike salt and sugar in this respect: you can't omit it from the diet without omitting nutritious foods.

Fat in the Diet

At the turn of the century in this country, people were eating about 125 grams each of fat per day, according to a survey of the period 1909-1913. By 1972, they were eating 159 grams each, but by 1975, they were eating less: 147 grams a day.[6]

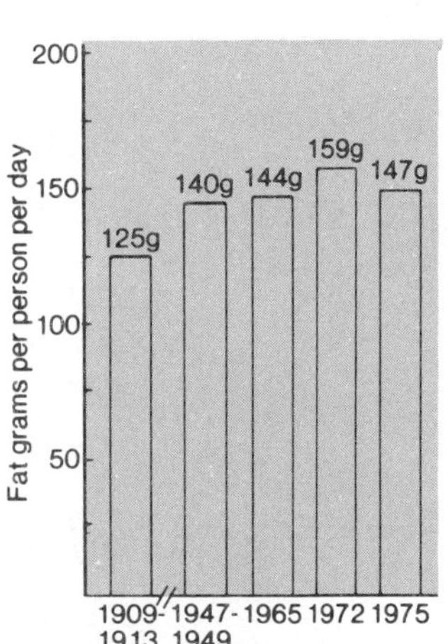

Recently, people have been eating less fat.

This recent downturn in the consumption of total fat has been greeted with joy by nutritionists. They would like to believe that it has come about as a result of an intensive campaign to show the public the relationship between dietary fat and the development of cardiovascular disease. Another benefit is that a lowered fat consumption may mean a reduced risk of certain kinds of cancer, for fat has been implicated in the causation of this disease as well (see Controversy 5B). In the meantime, there is still much concern over the fact that today's fat consumption is one-sixth higher than it was in the 1913 survey and that, until recently, heart and blood vessel diseases and cancers have also been increasing.

Food disappearance studies and diet surveys have both produced the same finding: People in the United States probably do eat about 40 to 50 percent of their calories as fat—more than perhaps they should. Those who wish to adopt the measures just suggested need to know where the fats are found in foods.

Three food groups—fats and oils; meat, poultry, and fish; and dairy products—account for about nine-tenths of the fat in the U.S. diet. However, there has been a shift from animal fats to fats of vegetable origin. The rising consumption of vegetable fats and oils has come about because of three factors: their increased use by fast-food chains serving fried foods like french fries and chicken, a shift away from the use of lard, and a shift from butter to margarine.[7]

A look at the food groups used in the exchange system will show exactly where fats are found in our diets. Two groups always contain fat—the fats and the meats—and two sometimes contain fat—the milks and the breads.

The fats. One fat exchange is considered to have 5 grams of fat, donating 45 calories and negligible protein and carbohydrate. Examples are:

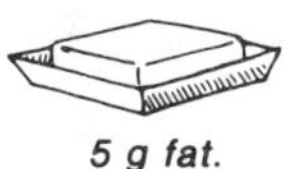

5 g fat.

1 teaspoon of butter or margarine.

1/8 of an avocado.

5 small olives.

2 large whole pecans.

1 tablespoon of french dressing.

2 tablespoons of sour cream.

1 tablespoon of heavy cream.

1 strip of bacon.

Many are surprised to find bacon listed with the fat group. They expect to find bacon fat included but think of crisp bacon as meat. It is classified as a fat, however, because its protein content is negligible, even if it is fried crisp and the melted fat is drained away.

The meats. The meat exchanges probably conceal most of the fat that people unwittingly consume. Many laypersons, when choosing a serving of meat, don't realize that they are electing to eat a large amount of fat. To help people "see" the fat in meats, the exchange system divides the meats into three categories according to their fat content. Table 1 shows the protein and fat content of the three categories of meat.

Users of the exchange system must be aware that a meat exchange is 1 ounce of meat. This is a very small amount of meat and is not a serving size. A small fast-food hamburger, for example, weighs about 3 ounces (three exchanges), and 4 ounces of meat is thought of as a normal serving size for meal planning. Of course, your judgment of what is normal differs from other people's, and you might have to weigh your meat to discover the size of your servings.

1 oz = 28.4 g.
1 oz meat = 28.4 g meat (but only 7 g protein).

Among the lean meats are:

Leaner cuts of beef, such as tenderloin, chuck steak, or roast.

Table 1. Protein and Fat Content of Meat Exchanges

Exchange	Size	Protein (g)	Fat (g)	Energy (cal)
Lean meat	1 oz	7	3	55
Medium-fat meat	1 oz	7	5½	80
High-fat meat	1 oz	7	8	100

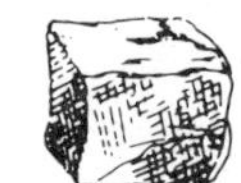
1 oz lean meat = 3 g fat.

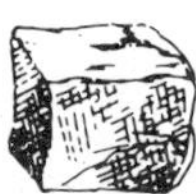
1 oz medium-fat meat = 5½ g fat.

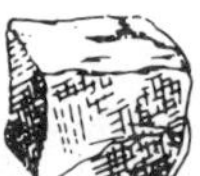
1 oz high-fat meat = 8 g fat. The complete meat exchange lists are in Appendix L.

Chicken or turkey without skin.

Leg of lamb.

Fresh or frozen fish.

Dry cottage cheese.

In the medium-fat group are:

Canned corn beef.

Commercially ground round steak.

Boston butt (pork).

Liver.

Heart.

Kidney.

Egg.

Creamed cottage cheese.

The high-fat group includes:

Commercially ground hamburger.

Club or rib steak.

Breast of lamb, duck, or goose.

Cold cuts.

Hot dogs.

Cheddar cheese.

People think of meat as protein food, but calculation of its nutrient content shows a surprising fact. A quarter-pound hamburger contains 28 grams of protein and 23 grams of fat. Because protein offers 4 calories per gram and fat offers 9, the hamburger provides 112 calories from protein and a whopping 207 calories from fat! The total is over 300 calories. From this, you might predict that overeaters of meat would tend to be overweight. (In fact, obesity probably is an occupational hazard of butchers.) This is because so much of the energy in a meat eater's diet is hidden from view—unrecognized.

Other foods. Meat and fat are not the only contributors of fat to the diet. Some milk exchanges also contain fat. The exchange system defines the basic milk exchange as 1 cup of skim milk, which contains no fat. A glass of whole milk, then, contains the protein and carbohydrate of skim milk but, in addition, contains 10 grams of fat. (A glass of low-fat milk is halfway between whole and skim, with 5 grams of fat.) The exchange system thus encourages people to view whole milk as milk with added fat. The small volume of added fat more than doubles the calories in the milk.

Not all dairy products are found on the milk list in the exchange system. Today's consumer is well advised to distinguish between the calcium- and protein-contributing dairy products, like milk and cheese, and those containing mostly fat. The "fat" dairy products are cream, whipped cream, sour cream, cream cheese, and butter. These are grouped with the fats.

Bread exchanges also sometimes contain fat. Notable are biscuits, corn bread, french-fried potatoes, potato chips, snack and party crackers, pancakes, and waffles. People are often surprised to learn of the high fat content of these snack items.

A useful feature of the exchange system is that it separates the polyunsaturated fat items from the saturated fat items. Of course, which of these you eat makes no difference in the total calories coming from fat, but it may make a difference in the unseen condition of your arteries.

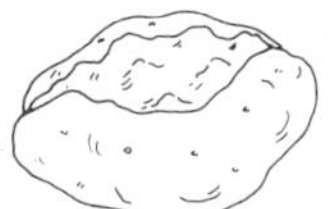

Plain potato 100 cal

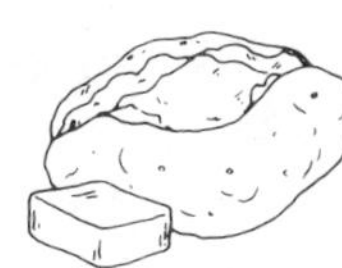

Potato with 1 tbsp butter and 1 tbsp sour cream 260 cal

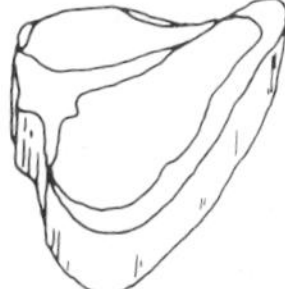

Pork chop with ½ inch fat 260 cal

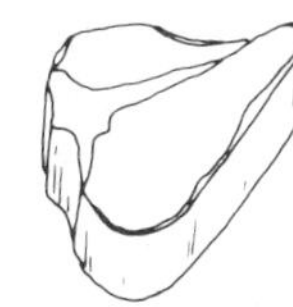

Pork chop with fat trimmed off 130 cal

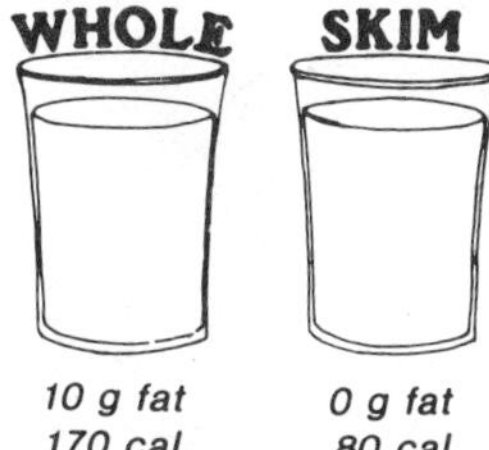

10 g fat 170 cal

0 g fat 80 cal

It's the fat in foods that makes the calories add up.

Food Feature: Cutting Fat While Dining Out

There is ample evidence that people in the developed countries are consuming a high-fat diet. Strong indications are accumulating in the reliable literature that this high-fat diet is causing an increase in some of the modern diseases. But perhaps you are not convinced that the diet you and your friends eat is actually high enough in fat for you to be concerned about, say, developing atherosclerosis. If you are not convinced, you certainly won't make the recommended changes.

To help you discover for yourself what foods deliver the fat, let's analyze a menu considered typical in the United States: a steakhouse dinner. Travelers report that this same meal is available to tourists in any large city of the world. The menu:

An 8-ounce rib steak.

A large baked potato served with butter and sour cream.

A mixed green salad with french dressing.

Hot rolls with butter.

Coffee with cream and sugar.

Table 2 shows the menu as exchanges. Your first observation of this analysis is probably surprise at the number of calories in this one meal. Habitually eating over 1600 calories at one meal would lead to obesity in a person who was not engaged in very hard physical labor. Your next observation more than likely is that most of the calories come from fat—1100 out of 1600, or over 67 percent. Observe, too, that virtually all the fat calories come from the beef and dairy products and thus are saturated fats. A calculation like this shows how it is that 42 percent of the calories in the U.S. diet come from fat. When you drive past steakhouses around dinnertime each night and notice the packed parking lots and long waiting lines, remember that all those people are probably eating meals in which over 60 percent of the calories come from fat, saturated fat at that. Of course, the

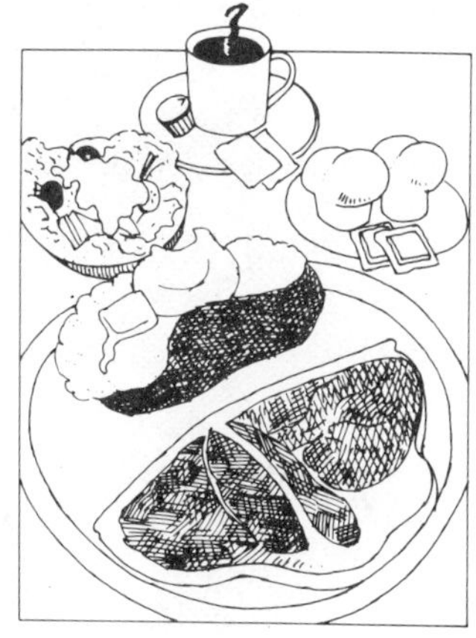

Before

Table 2. Fat Content of a Typical Steakhouse Meal

Food	Serving Size	Exchanges	Fat (g)	Fat Energy (cal)	Total Energy (cal)
Rib steak	8 oz	8 high-fat meat	64	576	800
Baked potato	1 large	2 bread	0	0	140
Butter	1 tbsp	3 fat	15	135	135
Sour cream	2 tbsp	1 fat	5	45	45
Mixed green salad	1 cup	Free	0	0	0
French dressing	3 tbsp	3 fat	15	135	135
Dinner roll	2	2 bread and 2 fat	10	90	230
Butter	2 tsp	2 fat	10	90	90
Coffee	2 cups	Free	0	0	0
Cream, light	2 tbsp	1 fat	5	45	45
Sugar	2 tsp		0	0	40
Total			124	1116	1660

Most of the total calories (67 percent) come from fat. Most of the fat calories (more than 90 percent) come from saturated fats.

meal analyzed here is a typical evening meal, and so it is probably common to include extra meat. On the other hand, it might also be the meal at which a person could, instead, include vegetables.

Let's now apply some recent dietary recommendations to this meal. We are choosing the *Dietary Goals* because, of their seven recommended changes in diet, five have to do directly or indirectly with decreasing fat or with shifting from saturated fat to polyunsaturated fat.[8] (The other two concern consumption of salt and sugar.) The USDA *Guidelines* are similar in spirit but not as specific (see Table 3).

(**1**) Increase consumption of fruits and vegetables and whole grains. In this meal there are two vegetable items (the potato and salad), no fruit, and two dinner rolls. If the vegetables were increased, the meat could easily be decreased, because this is already a large meal. We could add a yellow and a green vegetable—squash and green beans—and then cut the size of the serving of meat so that there would not be too much food. The dinner rolls could be changed to sliced whole-wheat bread. Fruit could be added at another meal or eaten for an evening snack.

(**2**) Decrease consumption of animal fat and choose meats, poultry, and fish that reduce the intake of saturated fats. The meat selection could be changed to poultry or fish, both of which contain a greater percentage of polyunsaturated fats than beef. However, if this person is especially fond of beef, another alternative might be to choose a

Table 3.

The USDA/USDHHS *Guidelines* offer the following pointers for those who wish to avoid too much fat, saturated fat, and cholesterol:

- Chose low-fat protein sources such as lean meats, fish, poultry, dry peas, and beans.
- Use eggs and organ meats in moderation.
- Limit intake of fats on and in foods.
- Trim fats from meats.
- Broil, bake, or boil—don't fry.
- Read food labels for fat contents.

low-fat cut of beef. Eating 4 ounces of round roast beef ground to order and broiled would decrease the meat calories from 800 to 220, quite a saving.

(**3**) Decrease consumption of foods high in total fat and partially replace saturated fats, whether obtained from animal or vegetable sources, with polyunsaturated fats. The items high in fat are steak, butter, sour cream, french dressing, and the cream in the coffee. All but the dressing are saturated fats. The high-fat steak has already been changed to a lean meat and reduced in amount; margarine high in polyunsaturated fats can be substituted for the sour cream and the butter; the amount of margarine and dressing can be lowered; the coffee can be drunk black. A person who could not give up coffee lightener might drastically cut some other saturated fat instead.

(**4**) Except for young children, substitute low-fat and nonfat milk for whole milk and low-fat dairy products for high-fat dairy products. (Had milk been part of the meal, this would have been an obvious change to make.)

(**5**) Decrease consumption of butterfat, eggs, and other high-cholesterol foods. Cholesterol is synthesized in the body from the fragments derived from any energy nutrient—carbohydrate, fat, protein, or alcohol. Saturated fatty acids are good sources of these fragments. Thus the changes that have been made to lower the amount of saturated fat have probably reduced the cholesterol level in the blood. Margarine has been substituted for butter, and it is assumed that this margarine will be made from 100 percent corn oil or some other polyunsaturated vegetable oil that does not contain cholesterol.

The alternative menu:

A 4-ounce serving of ground round steak, broiled.

A large baked potato served with margarine.

Squash.

Green beans.

Mixed green salad with french dressing.

Whole-wheat bread with margarine.

Black coffee.

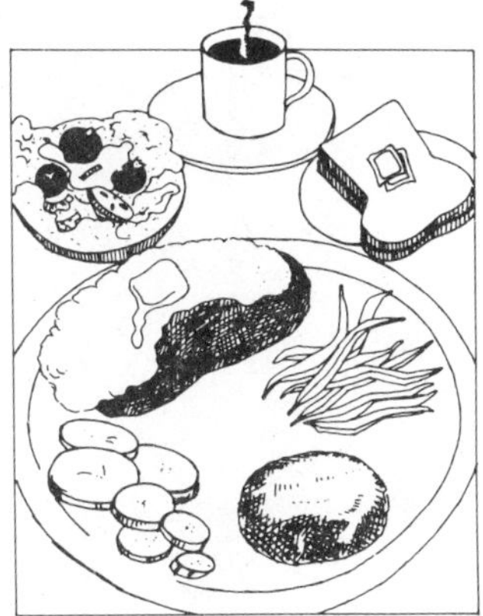

After

The new menu has about 800 fewer calories from fat. Of these, about 30 percent are from beef, as compared with almost 100 percent in the original menu. The total calories have dropped from over 1650 to under 800—a drop of about 900. The second menu is much bulkier (providing more fiber) and should be equally satisfying.

You will observe that the fat calories in this altered menu are still above the recommended 30 percent of total calories. With a full day's meals,

Table 4. Fat Content of Altered Menu

Food	Serving Size	Exchanges	Fat (g)	Fat Energy (cal)	Total Energy (cal)
Ground round steak	4 oz	4 lean meat	12	108	220
Potato	1 large	2 bread	0	0	140
Margarine	1 tsp	1 fat	5	45[a]	45
Squash, summer	½ cup	1 vegetable	0	0	25
Green beans	½ cup	1 vegetable	0	0	25
Mixed green salad	1 cup	Free	0	0	0
French dressing	2 tbsp	2 fat	10	90[a]	90
Whole-wheat bread	2 slices	2 bread	0	0	140
Margarine	2 tsp	2 fat	10	90[a]	90
Coffee, black	2 cups	Free	0	0	0
Total			37	333	775

42 percent of total calories from fat; 30 percent of fat calories from saturated fats.

[a]Polyunsaturated fat. To analyze the ratio of polyunsaturated to saturated fat, see this chapter's self-study.

which might include cereal at breakfast and a salad for lunch, dilution may bring the calories from fat under the desired 30 percent.

In summary, lipids—the fats and oils—serve as a major energy reserve and also provide nourishment and structural support for many tissues. All but five percent of them are triglycerides, compounds of glycerol with three fatty acids attached. The fat may be saturated, in which case the triglycerides contain saturated fatty acids, or may be mono-unsaturated or polyunsaturated, in which case the triglycerides contain unsaturated or polyunsaturated fatty acids. The other five percent of food fats come as phospholipids, which include lecithin, and sterols, of which cholesterol is the best known.[1]

For Further Information

For practical guidelines on diet, useful in helping to control fat intake, we especially recommend this paperback:

[1]*Chapter Notes can be found at the end of the Appendixes.*

- Mayer, J. *Fats, Diet & Your Heart.* Norwood, N.J.: Newspaperbooks, 1976.

The American Heart Association also puts out a multitude of useful and informative materials on both prevention and treatment of heart and artery disease. Check your phone book for the local office or write to the National Center, 7320 Greenville Avenue, Dallas, TX 75231.

Controversy 5A

Atherosclerosis

What causes it, and can we prevent it?

More than half of the people who die in the United States each year die of heart and blood vessel disease.[1] The underlying condition that contributes to most of these deaths is atherosclerosis, which is so widespread it has been called an epidemic.[2] What are its causes? How can it be prevented? Can it be reversed?

Atherosclerosis is the most common type of hardening of the arteries. It is a "soft" hardening in which mounds of lipid material, mixed with smooth muscle cells and calcium, accumulate in the inner artery walls.[3] These mounds, called plaques, grow larger and larger. Eventually, they may completely stop the flow of blood; or they may cause turbulence in the blood flow at that point, setting in motion the formation of a blood clot. The clot then may shut off the flow of blood. If this happens in an artery that supplies blood to a part of the heart muscle (a coronary artery), that part of the heart muscle will die and be replaced by scar tissue. If it happens in an artery in the brain, that part of the brain will die.

Sudden death also becomes more likely. A growing clot (thrombus) may break loose, becoming a traveling clot—and of course such a clot is most likely to catch and lodge in an artery that has been narrowed by atherosclerotic plaques. In a coronary artery, this causes sudden death of part of the heart muscle—a "coronary" or "heart attack." In a cerebral artery, it kills a part of the brain—"cerebral thrombosis" or "stroke."

Atherosclerosis begins early. Fatty streaks have been observed in the aortas of infants less than a year old, and plaques are well developed in most individuals by the time they are thirty. No one is free of the condition.[4] The question is not whether you have it but how far advanced it is and what you can do to retard or reverse it.

Risk factor studies. A host of factors has been linked to atherosclerosis. A smoker has a statistically greater chance of developing CVD (cardiovascular disease) and dying of a heart attack or stroke than does a nonsmoker, and smoking has therefore been labeled a "risk factor" for CVD. Other factors associated with greater risk are gender (being male), heredity (including diabetes), high blood pressure, lack of exercise, obesity, stress, high blood cholesterol and triglyceride concentrations, and some thirty others less thoroughly investigated.

The risk factors are powerful predictors of heart disease. If you have none of

Table 1. Your Risk for Heart Disease

H E A R T

Everyone plays the game of health whether he wants to or not. What is your score? Add up the numbers in each category that most nearly describe you.

Heredity	**1** No known history of heart disease	**2** One relative with heart disease over 60 years	**3** Two relatives with heart disease over 60 years	**4** One relative with heart disease under 60 years	**6** Two relatives with heart disease under 60 years
Exercise	**1** Intensive exercise, work, and recreation	**2** Moderate exercise, work and recreation	**3** Sedentary work & intensive recreational exercise	**5** Sedentary work & moderate recreational exercise	**6** Sedentary work & light recreational exercise
Age	**1** 10-20	**2** 21-30	**3** 31-40	**4** 41-50	**6** 51-65
Lbs.	**0** More than 5 lbs below standard weight	**1** ±5 lbs standard weight	**2** 6-20 lbs overweight	**4** 21-35 lbs overweight	**6** 36-50 lbs overweight
Tobacco	**0** Nonuser	**1** Cigar or pipe	**2** 10 cigarettes or fewer per day	**4** 20 cigarettes or more per day	**6** 30 cigarettes or more per day
Habits of eating fat	**1** 0% No animal or solid fats	**2** 10% Very little animal or solid fats	**3** 20% Little animal or solid fats	**4** 30% Much animal or solid fats	**5** 40% Very much animal or solid fats

Your risk of heart attack:

4-9 Very remote	16-20 Average	26-30 Dangerous
10-15 Below average	21-25 Moderate	31-35 Urgent danger—reduce score!

Other conditions—such as stress, high blood pressure, and increased blood cholesterol—detract from heart health and should be evaluated by your physician.

Courtesy of Loma Linda University

them, the statistical likelihood of your developing CVD may be only one in a hundred. If you have three, the chance may rise to over one in twenty. Table 1 shows one way of calculating your risk score.

Three factors have emerged as the major predictors of risk:

- Smoking.
- High serum cholesterol.
- High blood pressure.

From statistics pooled from many studies on these risk factors, the American Heart Association has published a Coronary Risk Handbook, a small portion of which is shown in Table 2. Evidently, the chances of having a healthy heart and arteries are greatest if you don't smoke and your serum cholesterol and blood pressure are low.

Millions of dollars and decades of effort by hundreds of researchers have yielded many positive findings from risk factor research. Still, the ultimate causes of CVD are unknown. The kind of problem that repeatedly hinders research is illustrated by the story of an investigation conducted in Britain.

The researchers, who wanted to relate physical activity to heart attack risk, chose to study bus drivers and bus conductors. They did find, as

Table 2. Risk of Developing CVD within Six Years for a Forty-Five-Year-Old Man. (This table from the Coronary Risk Handbook, shows the effect of the three major risk factors alone and in combination.)

	Smoker	Cholesterol (mg/100 ml[a])	Risk (per 100)
No	185	105	1.5
No	185	195	4.4
No	335	195	16.7
Yes	335	195	23.9

[a] Milligrams of cholesterol per 100 ml of blood.

[b] The first of the two numbers recorded (for example, 105/70). The silver column that rises on a blood-pressure instrument is a column of mercury; the height to which it is pushed is marked off in millimeters.

U. S. Senate, Select Committee on Nutrition and Human Needs, Diet Related to Killer Diseases II: Part 1. Cardiovascular Disease (Hearings) *(Washington, D.C.: Government Printing Office, 1977).*

expected, that the more active people—the conductors—suffered fewer heart attacks than did the sedentary ones—the drivers. They might have been tempted to conclude that they had found the relationship they were looking for: "Less activity leads to more heart attacks." But they looked further and found that the drivers were also fatter than the conductors. Perhaps the relationship was: "Less activity leads to more obesity leads to more heart attacks." They checked further still, however, and found that the drivers had already been fatter than the conductors when they had started work years before. The conclusion had to be rephrased: "Fatter people choose less active work." But what, then, caused the heart disease? Conceivably, these people might have already been headed for CVD as children, even before they became obese. What comes first? Inactivity? No, obesity (in this study). What comes before obesity?[5]

The problem illustrated by this study is one that plagues the researcher who is trying to untangle a chain of events and find its beginning. You can see that conclusions drawn from research like this are always somewhat shaky. They can always be criticized on the basis that they are "retrospective" (looking back), so that the researcher cannot tell whether the people who developed the condition might have been self-selected—might have gotten onto the track headed toward heart disease long before the differences (in occupation, for example) were observed. To be free of this criticism, such a study should be "prospective": A matched group of people should be selected for study and then followed through time to see what differences develop. Understanding this sampling problem in research will help you evaluate the results of other studies like this one.

Another complicating factor has already been mentioned in connection with the sugar-and-diabetes relationship discussed in Controversy 4: the problem of interpretation of population studies. It can be demonstrated that in many countries where the diets are low in fat the incidence of heart and artery disease is much lower than it is here. But to attribute the difference in disease rates to the differing diets would be naive. Many other factors that are also present in developed countries may play a role: urban life, lack of exercise; indeed, lifestyles that differ in many, many respects.

It can be argued that the risk factors all reflect an underlying prior condition. Psychologists point to personality type, and especially the way the person responds to stress, as a potent predictor of risk.[6] People of the personality type called "Type A" are notorious for

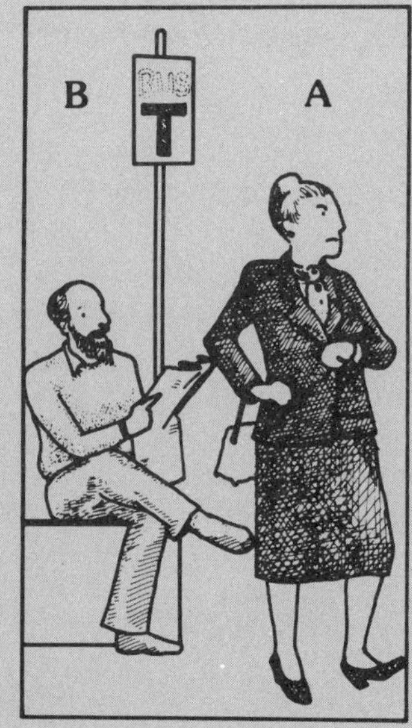

Miniglossary

Not all of the terms shown here are used in the text, but people often want to know what they mean.

aneurysm (AN-yoo-rism): The ballooning out of an artery wall where the wall is weakened by deterioration and the pressure is high (ana means "throughout"; *eurus* means "wide").

angina (an-JYE-nuh; some people say ANN-juh-nuh): Pain in the heart region caused by lack of oxygen.

atherosclerosis (ATH-er-oh-scler-OH-sis): The most common kind of hardening of the arteries, characterized by plaque formation in their inner walls (*athero* means "porridge"; *scleros* means "deterioration"). (The general term for hardening is **arteriosclerosis** (ar-TEER-ee-oh-scler-OH-sis.)

CAD (coronary artery disease): Another term for CHD.

CHD (coronary heart disease): Atherosclerosis in the arteries feeding the heart muscle.

CVA (cerebrovascular accident): A stroke or aneurysm in the brain.

CVD (cardiovascular disease): A general term for all diseases of the heart and blood vessels. Atherosclerosis is the main form of CVD.

embolus (EM-boh-lus): A clot (thrombus) that has broken loose from one location and traveled until it has lodged in a small artery cutting off the blood flow. Once the embolus has lodged (embolism) it has the same effect as a thrombosis.

hypertension : High blood pressure (*hyper* means "too much"; *tension* means "pressure").

ischemia (iss-SHE-me-uh): The deterioration and death of tissue (for example, of heart muscle), often caused by atherosclerosis. Ischemic heart disease (IHD) is another term for atherosclerosis and its relatives.

myocardial infarct (MI) (my-oh-CARD-ee-ul in-FARKT): The sudden shutting off of the blood flow to the heart muscle by a thrombus or embolism; the same as a heart attack (*myo* means "muscle"; *cardium* means "heart"; *infarct* means "blocking off").

occlusion (ock-CLOO-zhun): Shutting off the blood flow in an artery.

plaque (PLACK): A mound of lipid material, smooth muscle cells, and calcium that accumulates in the inner artery wall, causing atherosclerosis.

plasma (PLAZ-muh): Unclotted blood with only the cells removed. The terms *blood*, *plasma*, and *serum* mean about the same thing when referring to concentrations of substances in the blood like glucose or cholesterol, but they refer to different laboratory procedures used to measure those concentrations.

serum (SEER-um): The watery portion of the blood that remains after the cells and clot-forming material have been removed. See *plasma*.

thrombosis (throm-BOH-sis): The closing off of an artery by a growing clot. A cerebral thrombosis is such an event in the brain—a stroke (*cerebrum* means "brain"). A coronary thrombosis is such an event in the arteries that feed the heart muscle—a heart attack (*coronary* means "crowning" the heart).

thrombus (THROM-bus): A clot that forms in an artery. See also *embolus*.

A note on normal blood values: People sometimes ask about "high cholesterol." How high is too high? Blood cholesterol levels considered normal in the United States range from 140 to 260 mg per 100 ml plasma, with younger people having lower values—but while these values are "normal," they may not be desirable; the whole U.S. population may have abnormally high blood cholesterol levels compared with those of healthier peoples. Triglycerides range from 10 to 200 mg per 100 ml, depending on the individual and on the time that has elapsed since he or she last ate a fat-containing meal.[9]

being heart-attack prone. A Type A person is competitive, strives for achievement, has a sense of time urgency, is inclined to be hostile, suppresses the feeling of fatigue—in short, is uptight, as compared with the more easygoing Type B person. It has been demonstrated that people can be scored A or B first and then followed up and that the Type A's will have more than twice the rate of heart disease as the B's.[8] This is prospective research, and the A-versus-B difference shows up even when the three major risk factors already mentioned are taken into account.

Type A people's heart disease seems to arise in the classic way: by blockage of the arteries. The way they react physically to stress may account for the damage. The stress hormones affect blood pressure and blood lipid levels, so they may put the strain on the arteries that leads to atherosclerosis. The key to prevention may lie in study of the hormones or of the stress response.

Intervention studies. But while research goes on, people want to know what to do *now* to prevent this devastating disease that kills one out of every two people. To find out what to do, researchers design intervention studies. An intervention study involves tinkering with a cluster of factors (like the obesity—inactivity—smoking—high blood pressure—cholesterol cluster), altering the items one by one, and seeing if any of these interventions leads to reduction in deaths from CVD. A successful intervention study is a major step forward in research; it helps to demonstrate that a risk factor not only accompanies but causes a disease.

Some massive intervention studies are under way as of the early 1980s, but few findings have been released. So far the results seeking causes of CVD are frustratingly inconclusive, but it looks as if at least some people can reduce their risk of CVD by:

- Quitting smoking.
- Reducing their serum cholesterol.
- Reducing their blood pressure.

But much more research will need to be done before all the gaps and loopholes in the evidence are closed up.

The decline in heart disease. Meanwhile, a spontaneous change in the U.S. population has been observed. There was an impressive downturn in the rate of deaths from CVD between the late 1960s and the late 1970s. Something seemed to have happened in that ten-year period that saved 200,000 lives.[10] At a major conference held in 1979, the experts who had been following the lifestyle changes and trends among Americans reported that as a people:

(1) We are smoking less.[11]

(2) We are controlling our blood pressure better.[12]

(3) Our serum cholesterol levels have fallen slightly.[13]

(4) We are exercising more.[14]

In analysing all the data, Dr. J. Stamler reported that:

This, of course, does not prove that the recent changes in risk factor status of the population have led to— caused—the decline in mortality rates. But the data do fit. They certainly are consistent with—and lend support to—the hypothesis that the reduced mortality rateş are a result of the changes in risk factor status of the population.[15]

He also emphasized that the reduction of risk factors seems advisable for all members of the population, not just for the most heart-attack prone. If you divide the population into five groups from the lowest to the highest risk, more than half of the preventable heart disease deaths appear to be in the *middle* three groups.

Which of the risk factors is most important? According to Dr. Stamler, the balance sheet may look like this:

- A fourth of the reduced risk comes from a moderate reduction in serum cholesterol.
- A fourth comes from better control of high blood pressure.
- Half comes from a decrease in the prevalence of cigarette smoking.[16]

Personal strategy. The answers are not all in, but we have to make daily choices anyway. What shall we do?

The smoking question is not strictly nutritional, but the answer is quite obvious: Stop. As for high blood pressure, there are two means of reducing it: by drugs or by diet (weight reduction if necessary and reduction of salt intake). Drugs used to reduce blood pressure have been shown to be life-saving; the biggest problem with their use seems to be to persuade people who need them to keep on taking them. The matter of dietary control of blood pressure is examined in Chapter 10. It will be wise, too, to exercise more and to learn to handle stress.

This leaves the question of serum cholesterol. Should efforts be made to lower it? Can it be lowered by diet? This in itself is a controversial question, and a short discussion may be helpful. Before getting into it, let us clarify one point: which cholesterol we are talking about. The public has been very much confused by a failure to distinguish between *dietary* cholesterol and *serum* cholesterol. We are talking about *serum* cholesterol.

Two kinds of fat in foods are emphasized when people talk about CVD:

- Dietary fat (triglycerides, and these can be saturated or polyunsaturated).
- Dietary cholesterol.

Similarly, two kinds of lipid in the blood (serum) are traditionally talked about in connection with CVD:

- Serum triglycerides.
- Serum cholesterol.

(There are also phospholipids, but these don't often receive much attention.) We might call the first pair "the fat on the plate" and the second, "the fat in the blood." The question to ask, then, is "What fat on the plate contributes most to the fat in the blood?" And the answer is not dietary cholesterol (that in eggs, shellfish, liver, and the like). The important relationship is: Saturated fat (on the plate) raises cholesterol (in the blood). People often fail to understand this point and the question arises again and again: "Should we eat cholesterol?" When told, "It doesn't matter much," the questionner often jumps to the wrong conclusion: "Cholesterol doesn't matter." It does matter: High *serum* cholesterol is an indicator of risk for CVD, and the main food factor associated with it is a high saturated *fat intake*.

Figure 1 shows how a plaque is formed and the role blood cholesterol is thought to play in the process. As you can see, many factors are involved in plaque formation other than the cholesterol passing by in the arteries. In spite of the strength of the association between high serum cholesterol and CVD, it may turn out in the end that the blood condition does not cause the disease but rather that both are caused by some third factor (stress?).

Still, let's assume that we want to lower blood cholesterol. Remember, there are two

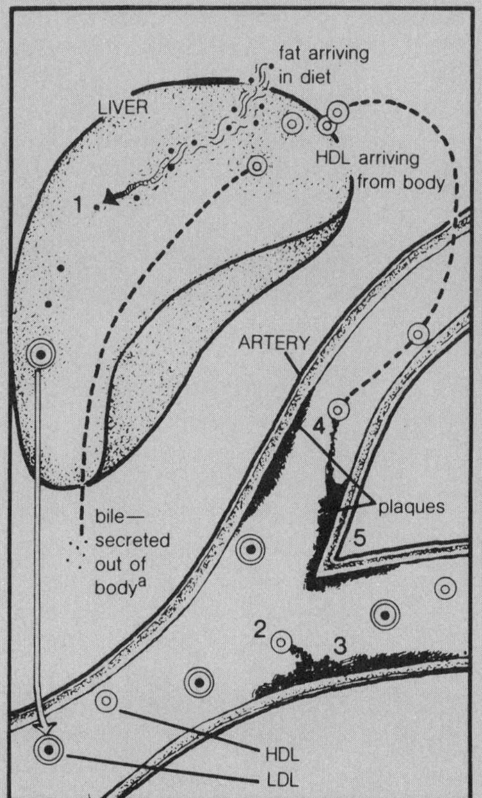

Figure 1. Factors influencing plaque formation. ***These are a few of the more important factors thought to contribute to atherosclerosis.***

(1) The liver makes cholesterol from saturated fat. The higher the saturated fat intake, the more cholesterol it makes.

(2) LDLs carry cholesterol to the plaques.The higher the LDLs, the greater the likelihood of plaque formation.

(3) Smooth muscle cells from the middle wall of the artery invade the inner wall and help form plaques. This process may be started by mutation in a smooth muscle cell (caused by some factor from cigarette smoke carried in the blood? or by a virus carried in the cells' genes and made to emerge by some stress like high blood pressure or cigarette-smoke derivatives?).

(4) HDLs carry cholesterol away from plaques. The higher the HDLS, the lower the likelihood of plaque formation.

(5) Plaques usually form at branch points where mechanical stresses on the artery are greatest: The higher the blood pressure, the greater the stress. Lack of oxygen and failure to repair injuries at branch points may also play a role.

[a] Goes to gall bladder, to be squirted into intestine.

vehicles in the blood that carry this substance, the low-density lipoproteins (LDL) and the high-density ones (HDL). It is the low-density ones that we want to lower. As it turns out, in general, the changes in diet that reduce serum cholesterol concentrations do so by reducing LDL, not HDL.[17]

How to lower serum cholesterol (LDL). Practically every dietary factor that has been studied—carbohydrate, fat, protein, vitamins, minerals, and fiber—has an effect on serum cholesterol, but by far the most influential would appear to be:

- Saturated fat—which raises it.

Next comes:

- Polyunsaturated fat—which lowers it.

And then comes:

- Cholesterol itself—which raises it slightly, depending on the amount already being eaten and on the body's ability to compensate by making less.

Much farther down the list come other items:

- Deficiency of vitamin C—which raises it.
- Fluoride or chromium deficiency—which raises it.
- Copper or iron or sodium excess—which raises it.
- A high-animal-protein, low-vegetable-protein intake—which raises it.
- Fiber, especially the fiber of legumes and apples (pectin), but not bran, the fiber of wheat—which lowers it.
- A high sugar intake in people with a certain inherited abnormal blood lipid pattern—which may raise it.[18]

For years, the American Heart Association has been publishing guidelines focussing on the top three factors:

- Lower your **S**aturated fat intake.
- Partially compensate by raising your **P**olyunsaturated fat intake.
- (These two measures will increase your **P:S** ratio.)
- Reduce your cholesterol intake.

Most recently, however, the Food and Nutrition Board has reviewed the research and concluded that the evidence is not convincing enough to warrant recommending that the general public undertake these measures. It recommends only that healthy people adjust their total fat intakes to a level appropriate for their calorie intakes and never mind the P:S ratio or the cholesterol.[19] The Canadian Health Protection Branch had already made a similar statement to the Canadian people.[20] One of the arguments against the measures is that to adopt them involves the loss of benefits, a problem that makes them different from the recommendation to reduce sugar intake discussed earlier. To cut down on fat intake means to reduce our meat consumption, and meat is a food that contributes many valuable nutrients to the diet: high-quality protein, B vitamins, iron, and other minerals. To reduce cholesterol intake people might choose to limit their consumption of eggs and liver, two of the most high-nutrient-density foods available. (Eggs don't seem to affect cholesterol anyway, if eaten as whole eggs rather than as purified cholesterol, so they have been exempted from the recommendations by some nutritionists for several years.)

The board singled out people at high risk, however, and gave special advice to them: "Persons with a positive family history of heart disease and other risk factors, such as obesity, hypertension, and diabetes" should be screened to determine their blood lipid and lipoprotein profiles. If these are abnormal, they should be given dietary advice in the attempt to normalize them.[21]

There are about five or six classes of lipid disorders (depending who's doing the diagnosing); they are given roman numerals (Type I, Type II, and so on) and called the hyperlipidemias or lipid transport disorders. Each involves a characteristic alteration in the normal pattern of lipoprotein forms and concentrations. For each, there is a corresponding dietary treatment which is often successful all by itself in restoring the normal pattern. The treatments have features in common; several involve controlling weight and fat intake, and four require that dietary cholesterol be restricted. "Diet is the cornerstone of therapy for each of the primary lipid transport disorders," reads an authoritative textbook in diet therapy.[22]

There has been a to-do over the difference of opinion between the Food and Nutrition Board, quoted here, and other authorities, like the American Heart Association and the Senate's *Dietary Goals*, which have given highly specific advice to the whole population regarding fat and cholesterol intakes. The board only recommends these dietary measures to people at high risk. But if you stop and think that half of the persons who die every year die of heart disease, that at least a third of adults are obese, and that high blood cholesterol itself is one of the risk factors, it seems as if what the board has said is in essence similar to what has been said before: A large number of adults would be prudent to curtail their fat intakes. And no one is forbidden to do so.

How to raise HDL. While most of the blood cholesterol is carried in the LDL and correlates *directly* with CVD risk, some is carried in the HDL and correlates *inversely* with risk. In fact, for men over fifty, the most potent single predictor of heart-attack risk may be the HDL level—the higher, the better.[23] While we must exercise the same caution here as formerly (since we don't know for sure if it will have any beneficial effect), we can examine the question how to raise HDL levels.

One way (although you can't do much about this) is to be female: Women have higher HDLs than men. Another, interestingly, seems to be to stop smoking. Smokers have uniformly lower HDLs than nonsmokers. Still another is to be in the process of losing weight.

If there are dietary factors of any significance, one may be the use of fish rather than meat;[24] another may be the use of certain fibers (which lower LDL selectively and leave HDL unchanged).[25] A few reports have appeared in which the consumption of moderate amounts of alcohol appeared to raise HDL; however, it is becoming apparent that there is more than one kind of HDL,[26] and that the kind of HDL affected by alcohol may not be the "good" kind. But by far the most powerful influence on HDL levels is not a nutritional factor at all, but exercise—prolonged, intense, and frequent.

The discovery that exercise raises HDL has given great impetus to the physical fitness movement of the 1970s and 1980s, and especially to the popularity of running as a national pastime. The earliest reports were of raised HDL in long-distance runners.[27] At first it was thought that only long-distance, endurance-type running had any significant effect, but subsequent reports have suggested that even moderate exercise may both lower LDL[28] and raise HDL[29] if consistently pursued. Evidently, then, it is beneficial even for very sedentary people to become only moderately active.[30]

It seems that the factors affecting health are all tangled together. The exact relationships among them all have not yet been worked out; but although we don't know which causes what, all evidence points in the same general direction. For good health and to avoid CVD, stop smoking; reduce blood pressure and weight if necessary; eat a balanced, adequate, and varied diet; reduce fat intake, especially saturated fat; increase activity; and—now that you have it all under control—enjoy life.

Although diet and nutrition are the focus of attention in the discussions to follow, it seems important to take a broad view of the problem of CVD. Nutrition is obviously not the only factor involved. People die of heart attacks and strokes for many reasons: urbanized living, breakup of the family, alienation, air pollution, and many others. And CVD deaths are falling while others are on the rise: deaths from accidents, homicides, suicides, lung cancer, liver disease. The lifestyle of the whole society is implicated in these deaths—it is an urbanized, competitive, industrial society with built-in stresses that have major impact on health. While we continue focussing on this book's central concern, nutrition, we must acknowledge that society itself may need to change in fundamental ways to arrive at ultimate solutions to some of these problems.

The Controversy Notes and For Further Information follow the Appendixes.

Controversy 5B

Nutrition and Cancer

What's the connection?

You probably know someone who has cancer, or who has recovered from it, or who has died of it. It is our second most prevalent disease (after heart disease) and can be expected, in one form or another, to affect one out of every four persons living today. If there is a connection between nutrition and cancer, we are well advised to learn what it is, because unlike so many factors in our environment, the food we choose to eat is a factor we can to a great extent control. Is there a connection? If so, what is it?

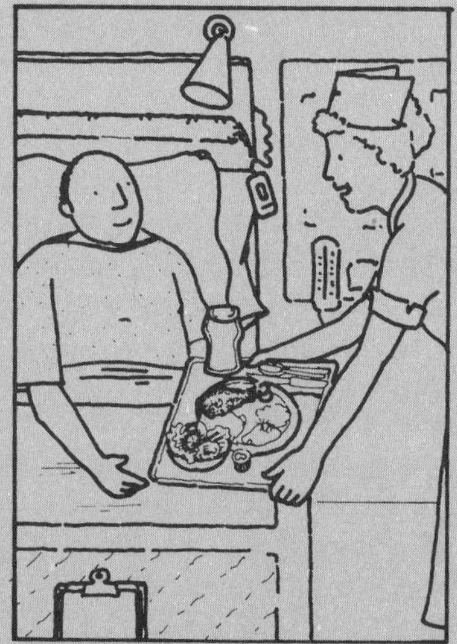

How cancer starts. Any cell in the body can become a cancer cell. One thing (but not the only thing) that has to happen is that the cell has to be exposed to a carcinogen, such as the tars in cigarette smoke or the UV rays of the sun. Not surprisingly, there is a connection between the areas most exposed to a carcinogen and the cancers that develop. Smoking affects the lungs; sunbathing, the skin.

The largest area of the body that is exposed to the environment is the GI (gastrointestinal) tract. The skin has a surface area of about 1½ meters (if you stretched it out flat like a bear rug you'd see); but the GI tract, because of all its folds and velvety, hairlike projections, has an enormous area of about ¼ acre. Moreover, the skin and lungs are exposed to gases, in which the molecules are far apart, whereas the GI tract is fed concentrated liquid solutions several times a day. It is natural to suspect that carcinogens in food would affect the GI tract, causing stomach or colon cancer or the like. The GI tract is also an absorbing surface, one that lets things into the body, so that carcinogens in food can reach other internal organs, perhaps causing breast cancer, liver cancer, cancer of the pancreas, and others.

The public has understood these concepts, and it also has a greater horror of the disease cancer than of any other common disease of today. The thought that there might be cancer-causing agents in food frightens and angers people who want themselves and their loved ones to be protected from this threat. If they think that food companies might knowingly allow cancer-causing substances to be added to foods or that a regulatory agency such as the FDA might overlook such additions, they are outraged. Controversies have raged over the additives that have been suspected of causing cancer, and the names of banned additives are familiar to everyone: red dye no. 2, cyclamate, DES, and, more recently, saccharin and nitrites.

The arguments over these additives and the laws relating to them are the subjects of Controversy 11A (FDA) and 11B (Saccharin and Nitrites). This Controversy is devoted to a factor that looms far larger in the causation of cancer than any additive: food itself.

An expert in population studies has estimated that as many as half of all cancers in humans are related to food factors.[1] For example, there is an extraordinarily close correlation between populations' total fat consumption and the incidence of certain kinds of cancers, especially those of the colon, the breast, the uterus, the ovaries, and the prostate gland.[2] The *Journal of the American Medical Association* states that 100,000 new cases of cancer of the colon and rectum are diagnosed each year in the U.S. alone, and that no risk factors have been linked to these cancers other than age (the patients are mostly over forty) and a high-fat diet.[3] (In contrast, not one case of human cancer of any kind has ever been traced to an additive.) Furthermore, animal experiments have shown that, while fat doesn't initiate cancers, and therefore doesn't qualify as a carcinogen, it does enhance them somehow. Animals fed a high-fat diet after exposure to a carcinogen develop more cancers than animals fed a low-fat diet.[4] Just plain overeating, in fact, makes animals much more susceptible to cancer than they are otherwise.[5]

Miniglossary

carcinogen (car-SIN-oh-jen): A cancer-causing substance (*carcin* means "cancer"; *gen* means "gives rise to").

cocarcinogen: A carcinogen helper; see *promoter*.

promoter: A substance that does not initiate cancer but that favors its development once the initiating event has taken place.

prostate gland: A gland associated with the male reproductive organs.

***trans*-fatty acid**: An unsaturated fatty acid that has assumed an unusual shape, often as a result of heat processing (*trans* means "opposite sides" and refers to the arrangement of the parts of the molecule around one of the double bonds.) The natural form is *cis* ("same sides").

The onset of cancer is a multistep process, and knowing what the steps are can help you understand how different factors may affect the process. This understanding, in turn, may help you work out preventive strategies. The steps seem to include:

(1) Exposure to a carcinogen.
(2) Entry of the carcinogen into the cell.
(3) Initiation, probably by the carcinogen's altering the cellular DNA somehow.
(4) Tumor formation (probably several more steps before the cell begins to multiply out of control).

You can imagine a "stop" before each of these steps. Not being exposed (stopping Step 1) is the only one most people think of. But being exposed is not enough to cause a cancer. The cell may still resist entry of the carcinogen, stopping Step 2. Or the carcinogen may get in but be prevented from reaching or altering the DNA, stopping Step 3. Or the initiating event may occur, but the cell may repair itself and correct the change in the DNA, stopping Step 4. Even after a tumor has begun to form, the body's defenses may detect it as unwanted foreign tissue and wall it off or attack it, rendering it harmless. One of the characteristics of people who *don't* get cancer may be healthy defenses, including cell membranes that don't let carcinogens in, intracellular machinery that destroys them if they do get in, efficient repair systems that detect and fix alterations in the cellular DNA before they can affect the cell's behavior, and a fully functioning immune system that destroys baby tumors before they get established.

Fat and cancer. Dietary fat might have something to do with these processes in several ways. For one thing, diets high in fat change people's hormone levels so that their cells behave differently. The higher incidence of breast cancers in women who eat diets high in fat may be related to a difference in the hormones in these women that promote breast development. (Women who have breastfed their babies or who start menstruating at late ages or who stay thin also have fewer breast cancers.) Body hormone levels affected by fat may also make a difference in women's cancers of the uterus and in men's cancers of the prostate gland.

Fat may affect cancer incidence in another way, too. Fats are a major part of cell membranes, and some of the fats you eat are used unchanged as building blocks for the membranes in cells all over your body. The next chapter will show that this is not as true of protein. The body dismantles and remakes proteins to its own very precise specifications; it uses ready-made pieces from the proteins you eat only when they fit those specifications exactly. But with fats, the body may not be so discriminating. As Chapter 5 explained, it takes triglycerides in, removes some or all of their fatty acids from the glycerol backbone they are attached to, and absorbs the parts separately. But it may then end up using some of the fatty acids without further alteration. Cell membranes made of the usual fatty acids may exclude carcinogens easily, but cell membranes made of unusual fatty acids may discriminate less successfully. Unusual fatty acids (called *trans*-fatty acids) are formed when fat is processed (hydrogenated), so processed fat, in particular, may be to blame for carcinogens getting into cells.[6]

Curiously, another connection of fat with cancer has to do with the HDLs, already familiar to many as the "good" lipoproteins that are associated with low rates of heart and artery disease. It may be that there is some connection between having a *high* HDL level early in life and getting cancer later. But the study that revealed this connection involved only a very small sample (284 men) as such studies go and can't be taken too seriously unless its findings are confirmed by other investigators with other, larger populations.[7]

A food factor that contains fat and that has been accused of contributing to cancer causation is beef. It has been said that "no example exists of a population that has a high beef consumption and a low rate of bowel cancer."[8] But it takes considerably more than a statement like this to prove a causal connection. The idea that beef is guilty has been pretty well shot down,[9] although the charcoal-broiling or long-time cooking of beef may cause substances to form that are carcinogenic.[10]

Whatever it is doing, whether altering hormone levels, altering cell membranes, or affecting some other body system, fat is clearly not carcinogenic: Its role is not to initiate cancer but to favor its initiation or enhance its growth once it has gotten started. Fat has therefore been called a cocarcinogen, or cancer promoter, to distinguish it from the compounds known as carcinogens.[11] Also, whatever it may have to do with cancer, it is clear that saturated fat is not so especially noteworthy for its ill effects as it is with artery disease. In fact, polyunsaturated fat—or *processed* polyunsaturated fat (because of the *trans*-fatty acids in it)—may be the principal offender.[12]

Other nutrients and cancer. Of all the components in foods, fat is the main one, but not the only one, connected with cancer. Animal protein is also implicated,[13] and some investigators believe there is evidence showing a protective effect of fiber against colon cancer. For example, bile—secreted in response to fat—might be carcinogenic, and fiber, by binding bile acids and carrying them out of the body with the feces, might counteract the carcinogenic effect. Or fiber might speed up the transit time of all materials through the colon, thus reducing the period of exposure of the colon walls to cancer-causing substances. Another possibility is that the kind of fat and fiber in the diet influence the kind of bacteria present in the lower colon—and the bacteria in turn influence the colon chemistry leading to more, or less, carcinogenesis. Colon bacteria do act on the fecal matter, producing substances that may be carcinogenic or that may be (according to some indications) anticarcinogenic. Obviously, it's a complicated business, and one in which continuing research will be important.

All three energy nutrients, then—carbohydrate (including fiber), fat, and protein—may play a role. What about the vitamins and minerals? A reviewer finds that "deficiencies of protein, iron, vitamin A, riboflavin and vitamin C have been incriminated in cancers in various sites in the body."[14]

Of particular interest, because much is now known about it, is the role of vitamin A. Long known to be involved in maintaining the health of the skin, the vitamin is now known to protect against skin cancer. It is not the familiar form, retinol, that provides this protection, but another form, retinoic acid—and retinoic acid is normally produced in the body from retinol with the help of zinc and other nutrients. (Chapters 9 and 10 explain these relationships in more detail.) In any case, it is now clear that a vitamin A deficiency can increase the likelihood of your getting skin cancer, and that an adequate vitamin A intake can reduce that chance. Not only the skin but other body tissues may be similarly protected, notably the bladder, the lungs, and the breasts. Experiments are in progress to see if synthetic forms of vitamin A (which are less toxic than the natural form) can protect against these cancers.[15]

These findings constitute another of the many reasons why people who cherish their health must take care of themselves nutritionally. But they don't suggest what to do in the event that cancer strikes. Once you have skin cancer, for example vitamin A won't cure it, no matter how high a dose you take; it will only poison you if you overdose. Does nutrition help at all in therapy for any kind of cancer?

Nutrition and cancer therapy. If a cancer is caught early enough it may be eradicated by prompt treatment: radiation, chemotherapy, or surgery. But if it spreads, untreated, its effect on the body is dramatic. It speeds up the metabolism so that energy needs are greatly increased. It disturbs many metabolic processes so that nutrients can't be used in the normal way, and it devours the body's tissues so rapidly that the changes can be seen from one day to the next—especially if nutritional support is not provided. It is estimated that a third of all terminal cancer patients die not of cancer but of malnutrition caused by the cancer.[16] Because cancer is so widespread in our society, it is important for people to know that aggressive nutritional support is an indispensable ally to physicians in the battle against cancer. No diet and no nutrient can, by itself, cure cancer; but frequent, nourishing meals can maintain a patient's strength and resistance during the treatments necessary to defeat the cancer. Doctors who are engaged in the battle against cancer are emphatic in urging families and hospital staff not to allow cancer patients to become malnourished, because it is much harder to bring them back from a debilitated state than to prevent their becoming debilitated in the first place.[17] Cancer often destroys the appetite and causes changes in taste sensations so that foods are less appetizing; thus, the patients must be helped to understand why it is urgent to try to eat in spite of an aversion to food. For the reader who wants to pursue this subject further, some of the selected references at the end of this Controversy provide helpful information.

Personal strategy. Many of the relationships between nutrition and cancer have not been described here, but some concepts have emerged that point to actions we can take to promote our health and resistance to cancer. We can *not* help being exposed to carcinogens: the sun, the natural radiation in the environment, particles in the air, naturally occurring compounds in the foods we eat, and even possibly (very rarely) an occasional food additive (as Controversy 11B explains). But exposure to a carcinogen is only the first of a sequence of events that can lead to cancer. We can stop the sequence at any later step along the way.

Eating a low-fat diet is probably the smartest of

preventive measures relating to nutrition. While the heart people say it is prudent to derive fewer than 30 percent of our calories from fat, some of the cancer people have suggested that it may be wise to go even lower: 20 percent or less. This means avoiding fats and oils of all kinds as well as fat-rich meats and products like cream, gravies, sauces, and the like. Among fats, if there are any to be especially avoided, they might be the ones containing *trans*-fatty acids. In Canada, these are taken into account in the way fats are listed on labels;[18] in the United States you have to watch for the words *hydrogenated*, *partially hydrogenated*, and *processed* fat.

The earnest reader who follows these suggestions is not guaranteed that they will really be helpful. They are a sort of insurance, an "in case" measure undertaken while research continues to probe the relationships between fat and cancer. As of 1980, the Food and Nutrition Board was still advising the public that "no direct cause-effect relationship has been observed for nutrition and cancer in humans" and was advising against anyone's being alarmed or changing their food habits drastically.[19] Still, in view of the fact that fat is implicated in cardiovascular disease as well, and is the richest of all nutrients in calories which most people don't need, it seems we really would be wise to learn to eat more of the more nutrient-dense, lower-calorie foods in the low-fat food groups: vegetables, fruits, and whole grains.

If a low-fat diet is protective at all, it is at Step 2 of the sequence outlined earlier. It may help cells keep initiators out, and it may support the hormonal environment most likely to defend against cancer. You can also strengthen your defenses at Step 3 by making sure that your cells possess all the ingredients to keep them functioning normally—that is, by eating an adequate diet. And at Step 4, you can strengthen your immune system the same way. The immune system is very sensitive to malnutrition and is severely weakened by nutrient deficiencies. But interestingly, it is also weakened by overdoses such as those of vitamin C or E that people take in the hope of protecting themselves from various hazards. All things in moderation, then, and nothing in excess, would seem to be the watchwords in the nutritional vigil against cancer as well as in many other aspects of lifestyle.

The Controversy Notes and For Further Information follow the Appendixes.

CHAPTER 6

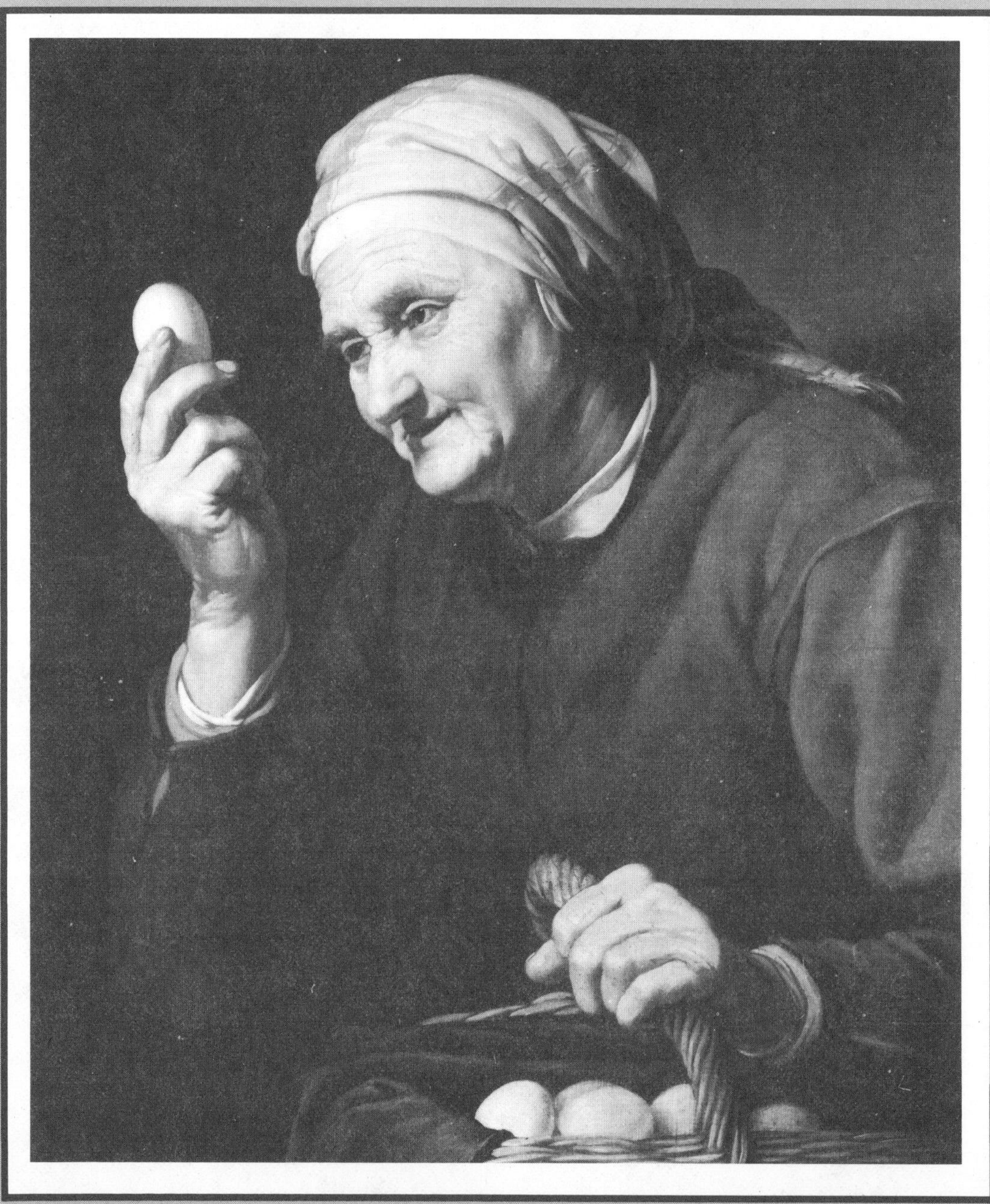

The Proteins: Amino Acids

For nearly 140 years, protein has been recognized as a nitrogen-containing substance necessary to the life of all cells and tissues of the body. It was named after the Greek word *proteios* meaning "of prime importance." We now know that protein is built of amino acids. Whether in a mouse or an elephant, a weed or a stalk of wheat, a flowering plant, a giant sequoia, or the ultimate in creation—a human being—life is possible only because there is protein to provide the necessary amino acids.

The prime importance of the amino acids is reflected by their uses in the body. They are required to make body tissues for new growth and replacement of worn-out cells; to build such body proteins as hemoglobin, enzymes, hormones, and antibodies; to form proteins for the transport of fats and other nutrients; to construct proteins that maintain the proper amount of fluid in the blood and tissues and serve as buffers against changes in the composition and acidity of tissue fluids; and to provide energy if there is a shortage of the other energy nutrients.

Only within the last several decades have new laboratory techniques unlocked the mystery of the specific design of protein. They have revealed how the body can recognize a particular protein, how the cells can repeat the building of that protein to exact specifications, and how alteration of the design can have disastrous effects on health.

Opposite: The Egg Seller *by H. Bloemaert. Used with the permission of the Rijksmuseum, Amsterdam.*

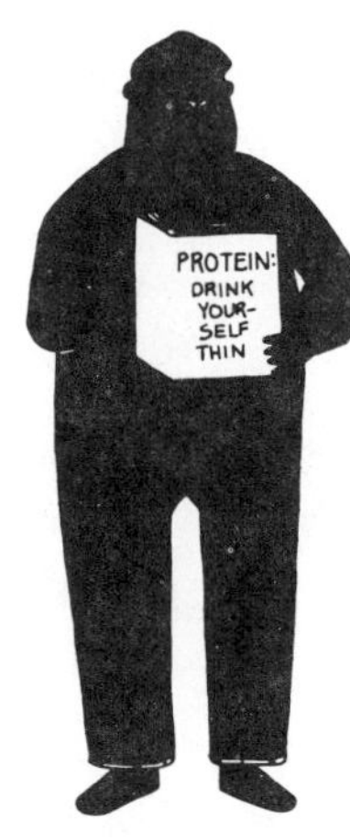

This new knowledge of protein has developed at such a fast pace that textbooks in the science-related fields have had difficulty remaining up to date. Meanwhile, the consumer, through constant exposure to the news media, has become familiar with scientific vocabulary without at the same time gaining an understanding of the exact meaning of the terms. For example, the popular press discusses the "protein-sparing fast" for treatment of intractable obesity, using terms like "predigested protein," "hydrolyzed amino acids," and "liquid protein."

These phrases are also used in advertisements for weight-reducing regimens based on amino acid mixtures. The scientific ring of the ads gives the average person a false sense of security in the use of the products. Only a person knowledgeable in nutrition understands that liquid protein products are not a food and that anyone using one of these regimens for losing weight is in reality fasting. Fasting is a method of reducing that requires close medical supervision in a hospital.

For more on liquid protein, see Controversy 6. Fasting, particularly the protein-sparing fast, is discussed in Chapter 7.

Another example of the use of protein terminology in the press is found in discussions of world food policies. Because it is general knowledge that the lack of protein in the diet is the basic cause of death during a famine, we may assume that providing protein-rich foods to starving people is the solution to the problem. As a matter of fact, the nutritional problems of a starving population are much too complex for such a simple solution as, for example, distributing dried milk or promoting the eating of meat. Some of the reasons for this will be clear after the body's handling of protein is discussed in this chapter.

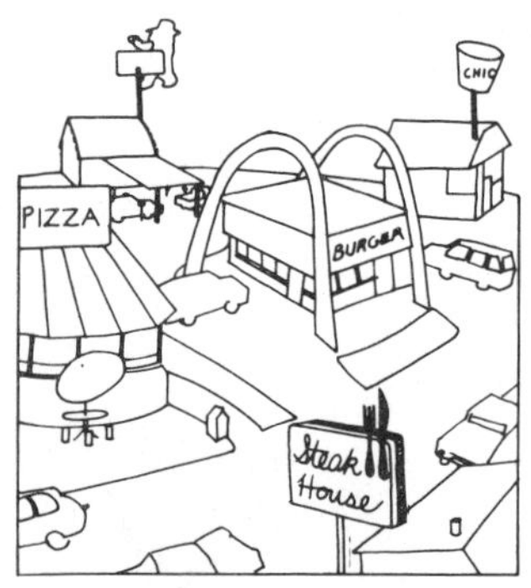

In developed countries like the United States, animal foods provide a substantial portion of the calories.

In the United States, the knowledge that protein is of prime importance has probably contributed to an increase in the consumption of meat and meat products. It has been estimated that about 31 percent of the total calories in our diet now come from livestock, as contrasted with 12 percent worldwide.[1] The increase in consumption of animal protein, as well as of animal fat, may be a factor in the development of the diseases of modern humans.

This is an exciting era in which to study protein. Such a study can help consumers to judge fad reducing diets and to buy the needed protein without spending money unnecessarily or endangering their own good health.

Structure of Protein

To appreciate the many vital functions of protein, we must understand its structure. A key difference from carbohydrate and fat, which contain only carbon, hydrogen, and oxygen atoms, is that protein contains nitrogen atoms. These nitrogens are found in the **amine groups** that give the name *amino* to the amino acids.

Amino acids and their side chains. A **protein** is a chain of units called **amino acids**. You will recall that carbohydrates are chains of glucose units and that the fatty acids are chains of fragments from glucose or fat. In contrast to the carbohydrates and fatty acids, however, in which the repeating units—glucose or fragments—are identical, the amino acids in a strand of protein are different from one another.

All amino acids have a simple backbone similar to the fragments derived from glucose or fat—but with an amine group at one end. At the other end is an acid group. Attached to the backbone of each amino acid is a distinctive structure, the side chain. It is the nature of the side chain that gives identity to each amino acid. Twenty amino acids with different side chains make up the proteins of all living tissue. (Two other rare amino acids appear in a few proteins.)

The side chains vary in complexity from a single hydrogen atom (like that on glycine) to a complex ring structure (like that on tryptophan). In addition to differing in composition, size, and shape, these structures differ in electrical charge. Some are negative, some are positive, and some have no charge. These side chains determine many of the characteristics of protein.

Essential and nonessential amino acids. The body can make most of the amino acids for itself, given the needed parts: nitrogen in the form of an amine group and fragments derived from carbohydrate or fat. But there are eight amino acids that the adult body can't make. These are the **essential amino acids**

The amino acids are often listed on food labels. Their names are:

glycine
alanine
*valine**
*leucine**
*isoleucine**
serine
*threonine**
aspartic acid
glutamic acid
*lysine**
arginine
cystine
cysteine
*methionine**
tyrosine
*phenylalanine**
*tryptophan**
proline
histidine
glutamine
asparagine

**Those marked with an asterisk are the essential amino acids.*

Amino acid strands of protein. In a protein, each amino acid is hooked to the next. The bond is formed between the amino group of one and the acid group of the next. In bonding to each other, amino acids release hydrogen and oxygen, which form water. As the chain lengthens, say to four amino acids, there develops a strand like this:

Three free molecules of water are released, and the side chains stand out from the backbone of the structure, retaining their identity.

A strand of protein is not a straight chain, however, as this description seems to imply. Proteins are made of many amino acid units, perhaps as many as 300, and these may be in several strands. The amino acids are attracted or repelled by the charges they carry, so the strands tangle into intricate shapes. Amino acids of adjoining strands interact, forming bonds of various strengths that hold the strands together. The charged amino acids are attracted to water, and in the body fluids, they orient themselves on the outside of the structure. The neutral amino acids are repelled by water and attracted to one another; these tuck themselves into the center, away from the body fluid. All these interactions among the amino acids and the surrounding fluid result in a protein whose architecture is entirely unique.

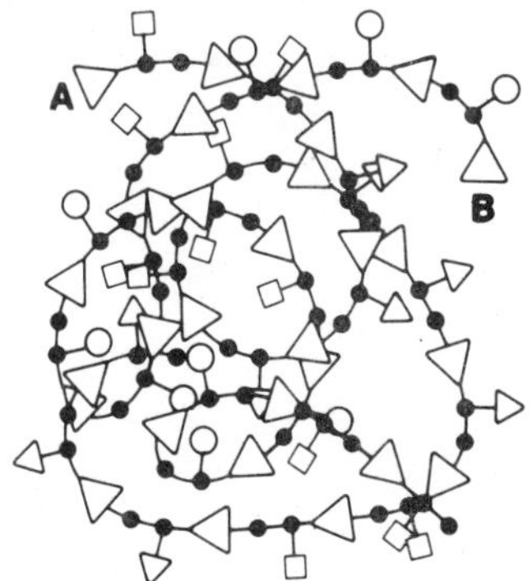

Fanciful drawing of a protein.

Proteins have dramatically different shapes, which enable them to perform different tasks in the body. Some are more than ten times as long as they are wide, forming stiff, rodlike structures that are somewhat insoluble in water and very strong. These proteins provide support to tissues. Examples are the collagen in connective tissues like

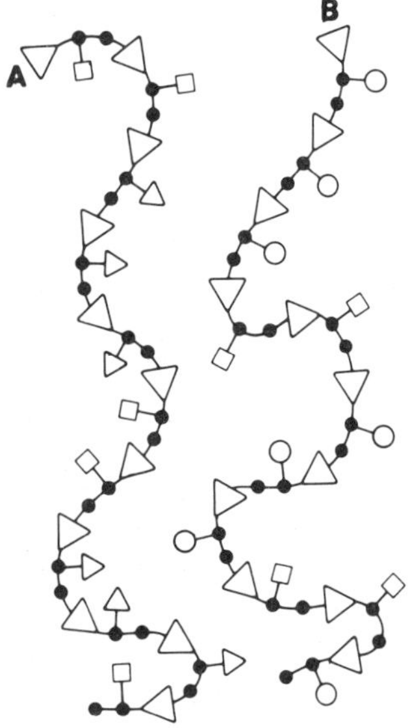

Protein strands A and B have uncoiled and come apart.

The first eight amino acids in one of the chains of human hemoglobin:

Normal	*Sickle-Cell Disease*	
valine	*1*	*valine*
histidine	*2*	*histidine*
leucine	*3*	*leucine*
threonine	*4*	*threonine*
proline	*5*	*proline*
glutamine	*6*	*valine*
glutamine	*7*	*glutamine*
lysine	*8*	*lysine*

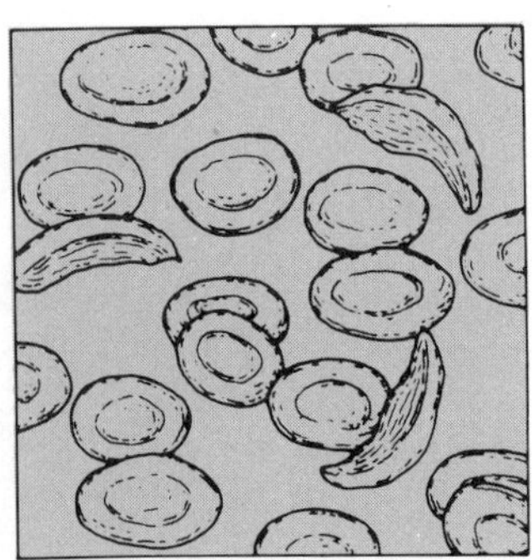

Normal cells and sickle cells.

bones, tendons, and ligaments, the fibrin of blood clots, and the keratin in hair. Other proteins are almost perfectly spherical and are more soluble and easily deformed. These are more often present in fluid tissues. Examples are the hemoglobin in red blood cells, the albumins and globulins in blood fluid, the casein in milk, and the enzymes within cells.

Denaturation of proteins. Proteins can undergo **denaturation** (that is, alteration) by heat, alcohol, acids, or the salts of heavy metals. Many everyday reactions are useful or harmful because of their effects on protein. For example, cooking an egg denatures the proteins of the egg and makes them more appetizing and digestible. Alcohol is an effective agent for sterilizing the skin in preparation for a medical procedure; the alcohol penetrates the proteins of the bacteria, alters their structure, and thus destroys them. The principal protein in cow's milk, casein, is altered by the hydrochloric acid of the stomach so that it becomes accessible to digestive enzymes. Many of the well-known poisons are salts of heavy metals like mercury and silver; these alter the structure of protein wherever they touch it. The common first-aid remedy for swallowing a heavy-metal poison is to drink milk. The poison then acts on the protein of the milk rather than on the protein tissues of the mouth, esophagus, and stomach. (Then vomiting is induced to expel the poison.)

Specificity of protein structure. The great variety of proteins in the world is due to the infinite number of sequences of amino acids that is possible. If you consider the size of the dictionary, in which every word is constructed from just twenty-six letters, you can visualize the variety of proteins that are designed from twenty or so amino acids. Unlike the letters in a word, which must alternate between consonant and vowel sounds, the amino acids in a protein need follow no such rules. Also, there is no restriction on the length of the chain of amino acids. Thus, there are many more possible proteins than possible English words.

The sequences of amino acids that make up a protein molecule are specified with exquisite order and precision. For each protein there is only one proper sequence. If the wrong amino acid is inserted or if one is out of place, the result may be disastrous.

Sickle-cell disease—in which hemoglobin, the oxygen-carrier protein of the red blood cells, is abnormal—is an example of a mistake in the amino acid sequence. Normal hemoglobin contains two kinds of chains. One of the chains in sickle-cell hemoglobin is an exact copy of that in normal hemoglobin. But in the other chain, the sixth amino acid, which should be glutamine, is replaced by valine. The altered protein is unable to carry and release oxygen. If too many of these abnormal hemoglobins appear in the blood, the result is illness and death. One of the methods of detecting the disease is to observe the altered shape of the red blood cells. Normal red cells are flat and disk-shaped, but those containing the abnormal hemoglobin are shaped like a crescent or sickle.

Each species of animal (including humans) has proteins particularly designed for it. There may be great similarities; for example, the sequence of amino acids in insulin is nearly identical in most animals.

But there are also some differences that make each insulin most suitable for the animal it belongs to. When an animal eats protein, the digestive and absorptive systems break it down and deliver the separated amino acids to the body cells. The cells then put them together in the order necessary to produce the particular proteins the animal needs.

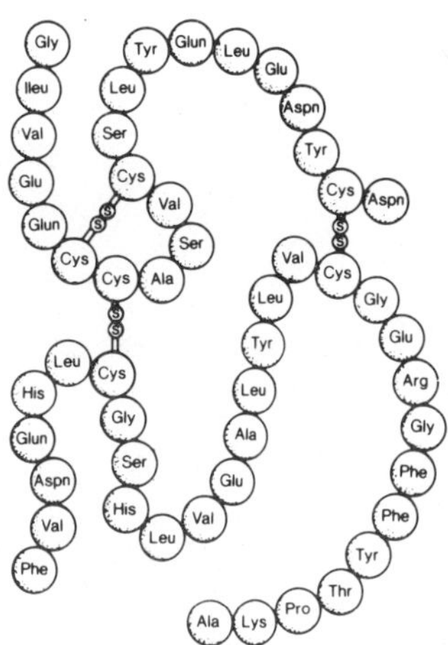

The hormone insulin is a protein composed of these 51 amino acids in this sequence.

The Roles of Protein

Only a few of the many roles of protein will be described here, to give an appreciation of its versatility and importance.

Growth and maintenance. One function of protein in the diet is to ensure that amino acids are available to build the proteins of new tissue. The new tissue may be in an embryo; in a growing child; in the blood that replaces that lost in burns, hemorrhage, or surgery; in the scar tissue that heals wounds; or in new hair and nails. Not so obvious is the protein that helps replace worn-out cells. The red cells of the blood are useful for about a month and then must be replaced by new cells that have been manufactured in the bone marrow. The cells that line the intestinal tract live less than a week and are constantly being shed and excreted. You may have observed that the cells of your skin die and rub off and are replaced from underneath. Nearly all cells are constantly being replaced, and for this new growth, amino acids must be supplied constantly from food.

Enzymes and hormones. Enzymes are among the most important of the proteins formed in living cells. Enzymes are protein catalysts—they help reactions take place. There may be as many as 1000 enzymes inside a single cell, each one enabling two substances to come together to form a new substance or making it possible for a substance to break apart.

One of the mysteries that has been partially explained in recent years is how an enzyme can be specific for a particular reaction. The surface of the enzyme is contoured so that the enzyme can recognize the structures it works on and no others. The surface provides a site where two substances may become attached, first to the enzyme itself, then to each other. The new substance is then expelled by the enzyme into the fluid of the cell. The margin diagram shows compounds A and B parking for a moment on the enzyme, then leaving it as the new compound AB. It could be that A and B, because they were both swimming around in the cell fluid, would have eventually discovered each other and combined without help. However, the enzyme attracted them and made them snap into the exact position for bonding. In this way, the enzyme speeded up the reaction time. A single enzyme can facilitate several hundred such reactions in a second.

Similar to the enzymes—small molecules with profound effects—are the **hormones**. However, these differ from the enzymes in that not all of them are made of protein and in that they don't catalyze specific reactions. They regulate overall body conditions, such as the blood glucose level (insulin) and the metabolic rate (thyroxin).

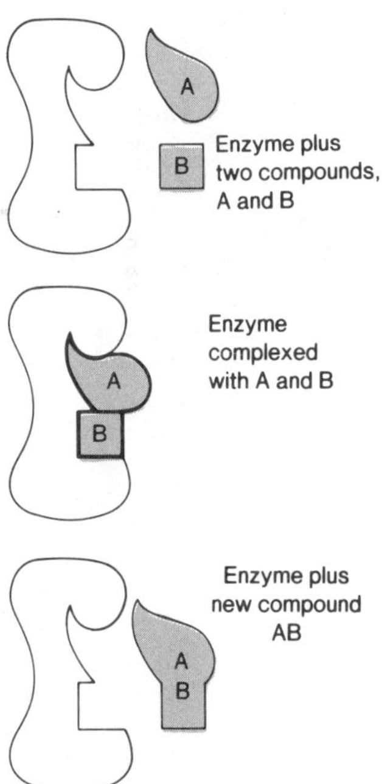

Enzymes are proteins. Each enzyme facilitates a specific chemical reaction.

Development of immunity.

(1) Body is challenged with foreign invaders.

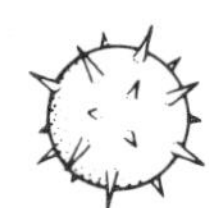

(2) Body makes "machine" for manufacturing antibody:

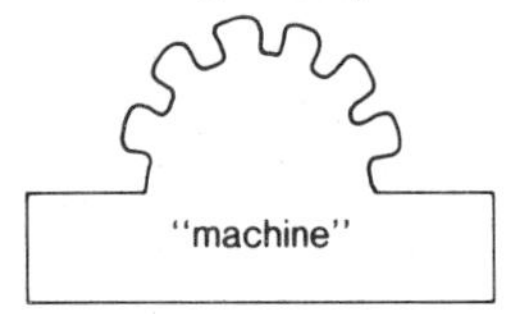

(3) "Machine" makes antibody.

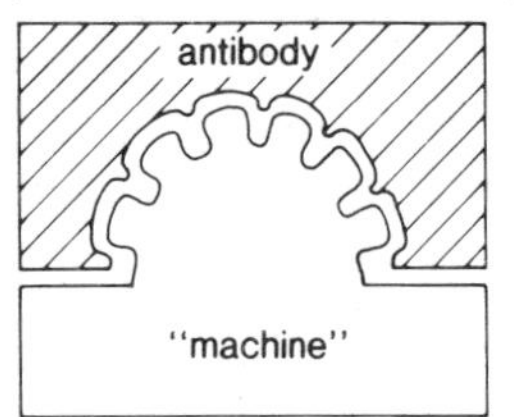

(4) Antibody inactivates foreign invader.

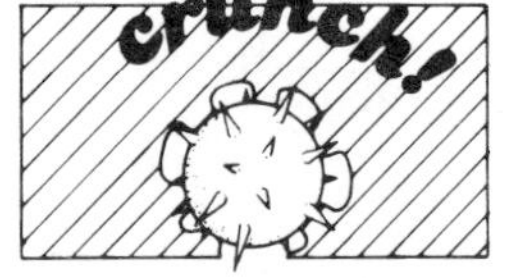

(5) "Machine" remains to make antibodies faster the next time a foreign invader attacks.

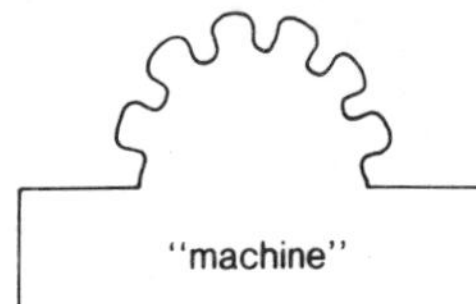

Antibodies. Of all the great variety of proteins in living organisms, the **antibodies** best demonstrate that proteins are specific for one organism. Antibodies are formed in response to the presence of foreign particles (usually proteins) that invade the body. The foreign protein may be part of a bacterium, a virus, a toxin or may even be present in food that causes allergy. The body, after recognizing that it has been invaded, manufactures antibodies, and they inactivate the foreign protein.

One of the most fascinating aspects of this response is that each antibody is designed specifically to destroy one invader. An antibody that has been manufactured to combat one strain of influenza would be of no help in protecting a person against another strain. Once the body has learned to make a particular antibody, it never forgets; and the next time it encounters that same invader, it will be equipped to destroy it even more rapidly. In other words, it develops an **immunity**. This is the principle underlying the vaccinations and antitoxins that have almost eradicated childhood diseases in the Western world.

In some cases, the immune response can cause harm. If a transfusion should accidentally deliver the wrong blood type, the body would make antibodies to inactivate the foreign blood proteins. The first time this happened, the body might be able to tolerate or get rid of the gradual accumulation of inactivated foreign blood cells. But with a second transfusion of the wrong type, the body would be overwhelmed by an immediate, massive immune response, and death would result.

Fluid balance. Proteins help regulate the quantity of fluids in the compartments of the body to maintain the **fluid balance**. To remain alive, a cell must contain a constant amount of fluid. Too much might cause it to rupture, and too little would make it unable to function. Although water can diffuse freely in and out of the cell, proteins cannot—and proteins attract water. By maintaining a store of internal proteins, the cell retains the fluid it needs (it also uses minerals this way). Similarly, the cells secrete proteins (and minerals) into the spaces between them to keep the fluid volume constant in those spaces. The proteins secreted into the blood can't cross the vessel walls and thus maintain the blood volume in the same way.

Salt balance. Not only the quantity but also the composition of the body fluids is vital to life. Transport proteins in the membranes of all the cells respond sensitively to small changes in the circulating fluids and work to maintain equilibrium by pumping substances into and out of cells. Thus, for example, sodium is concentrated outside the cells, and potassium is concentrated inside—a condition that is critical to the functioning of nerve and muscle cells. A disturbance of the **salt balance** (the electrolyte balance) can impair the action of the indispensable heart, lungs, and brain, triggering a red-hot medical emergency.

Acid-base balance. Normal processes of the body continually produce acids and their opposite, bases, which must be carried by the blood to the organs of excretion. The blood must do this without allowing its own **acid-base balance** to be affected. This magical feat is another trick of the proteins in the blood, which act as **buffers**. They pick up hydrogens (acid) when there are too many and release them again when there are too few. The secret is that the negatively charged side chains of the amino acids can accommodate additional hydrogens (which are positively charged) when necessary.

The acid-base balance of the blood, called the **pH** by chemists, is kept between 7.35 and 7.45—one of the most rigidly controlled conditions in the body. If these limits are exceeded, the dangerous condition **acidosis** or the opposite basic condition, **alkalosis**, can cause coma or death. The hazard of these conditions is due to their effect on proteins. When the proteins' buffering capacity is exceeded—for example, when they have taken on board all the acid hydrogens they can accommodate—additional acid deranges their structure by pulling them out of shape; that is, it denatures them. Knowing how indispensable the structures of proteins are to their functions and how vital their functions are to life, you can imagine how many body processes would be halted by such a disturbance.

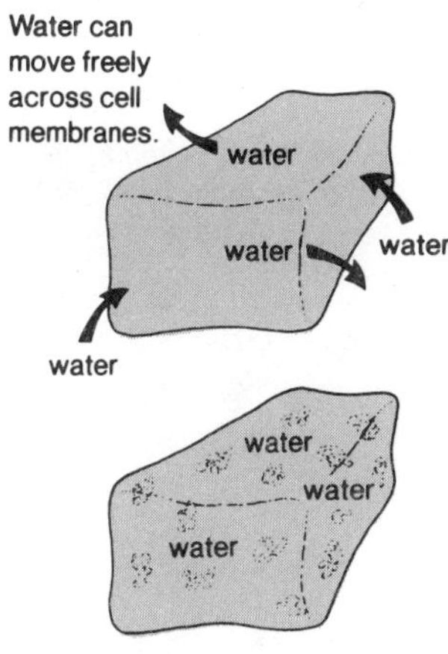

Proteins inside cells help keep the correct amount of water inside.

These are but a sampling of the major roles proteins play in the body but should serve to illustrate their versatility, uniqueness, and importance. No wonder they are said to be the primary material of life.

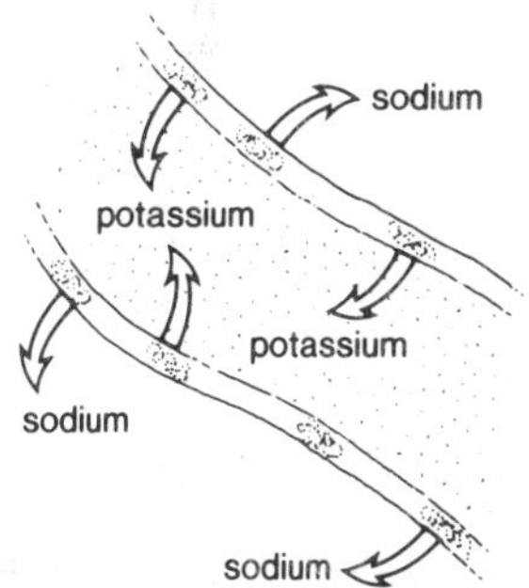

Proteins push potassium into and sodium out of nerve cell.

Energy. Only protein can perform all the functions described above, but it will be sacrificed to prove needed calories if insufficient fat and carbohydrate foods are eaten. The body's top priority need is the need for energy. All other needs have a lower priority.

When amino acids are degraded for energy, their amine groups are usually incorporated by the liver into **urea** and sent to the kidney for excretion. The fragments that remain are composed of carbon, hydrogen, and oxygen, as are carbohydrate and fat, and can be used to build those substances or be metabolized like them.

Not only can amino acids supply energy, but also half of them can supply that energy as glucose, as fat can never do. Thus, if need be, protein can help maintain a steady blood glucose level and so serve the brain.

A perspective on the three energy nutrients—their similarities and differences—now should be clear. Carbohydrate offers energy; fat offers concentrated energy; and protein, if needed, can offer energy plus nitrogen.

Only if the protein-sparing calories from carbohydrate and fat are sufficient to power the cells will the amino acids be used for their most important function—making proteins. Thus energy deficiency (starvation) is always accompanied by the symptoms of protein deficiency.

If amino acids are oversupplied, the body has no place to store them. It will remove and excrete their amine groups and then convert the residues to glucose and glycogen or to fat for storage. At this point, only their energy value can be retrieved. Amino acids are only stored in the sense that they are present in all the tissues. In case there is a great shortage of amino acids, tissues like the blood and skin have to be degraded so that their amino acids can be used to maintain the heart, brain, and lungs. The body's wisdom in its choice of priorities is reflected in the precise and orderly way it handles protein from the moment that protein enters it in food.[2]

The Body's Handling of Protein

If you want to review the body systems relevant to the study of the body's handling of protein, turn to Appendix A.

Each protein is designed for a special purpose in a particular tissue of a specific kind of animal or plant. When a person eats food proteins, whether from cereals, vegetables, beef, or cheese, the body must break them down into amino acids in order to rearrange them into its own unique sequences.

Cooking and chewing. Some proteins are folded in such a way that the digestive enzymes of the stomach can't get at the bonds to attack them. The protein-rich foods, especially the meats, thus require more tenderizing through cooking—which denatures their coils—and more thorough chewing—to mechanically separate them—than most other foods. One of early humankind's giant steps was acquiring control of fire, because this permitted the cooking of meats and thereby greatly expanded the choice of foods. No doubt, too, the difficulty of chewing raw meats made the arrival in adulthood of four grinding teeth a valuable evolutionary asset. The four so-called wisdom teeth bring mostly pain to modern humans, because they come into a mouth already crowded with teeth. However, our ancestors needed these extra grinders to replace lost molars and to enable them to continue obtaining good-quality protein.

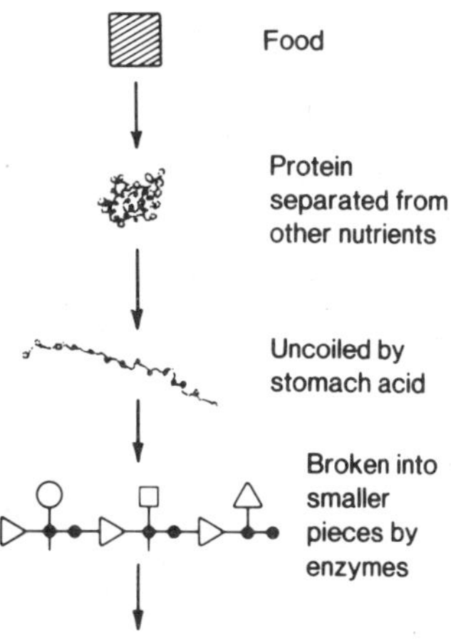

Protein digestion begins.

Digestion in the stomach. Other than being chewed and mixed with saliva, nothing happens to protein until it reaches the very strong acid of the stomach. There, the acid helps to uncoil (denature) the protein's tangled strands so that the stomach enzymes can attack the bonds. You might expect that the stomach enzymes themselves, being protein, would be attacked, but these are the only proteins in the body whose design protects them and allows them to become most active in strong acid. Their job is to break apart the food protein strands into smaller pieces. The stomach lining, which is also made partly of protein, is protected by a coat of mucus, secreted by its cells.

Another active participant in this reaction is water. When the bonds holding the amino acids together are originally put in place, a molecule of water is taken out. When the bonds are broken, water must be replaced so that the amino acids can separate.

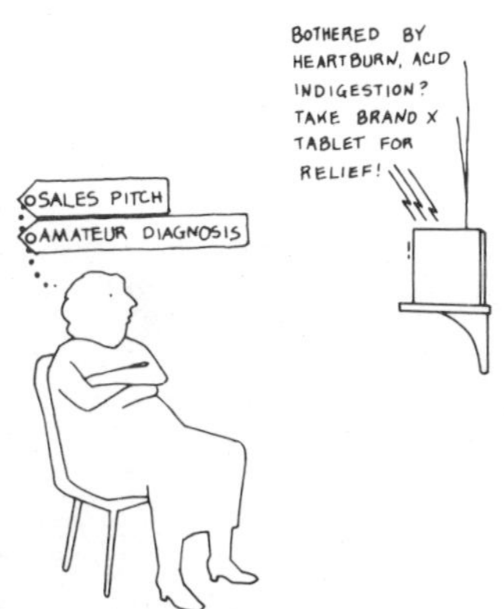
BOTHERED BY HEARTBURN, ACID INDIGESTION? TAKE BRAND X TABLET FOR RELIEF!
SALES PITCH
AMATEUR DIAGNOSIS

Knowing how the body works helps people see through false claims made for medicines.

The whole process of digestion is an ingenious solution to a complex problem. Proteins (enzymes), made active by acid, digest proteins (food) denatured by acid, and the mucous coating of the stomach wall protects *its* proteins from being affected by either acid or enzymes. The acid in the stomach is so strong (pH 2) that no food is acid enough to make it stronger. It is obvious from this that the stomach is supposed to be acid to do its job.

Taking antacids, promoted by TV commercials for relief of "acid indigestion," only puts the burden on the stomach to produce even more acid to restore its normal balance. Antacids have their uses but are not appropriate for use by normal, healthy people. A person who thinks he has an acid stomach is probably right and should be grateful.

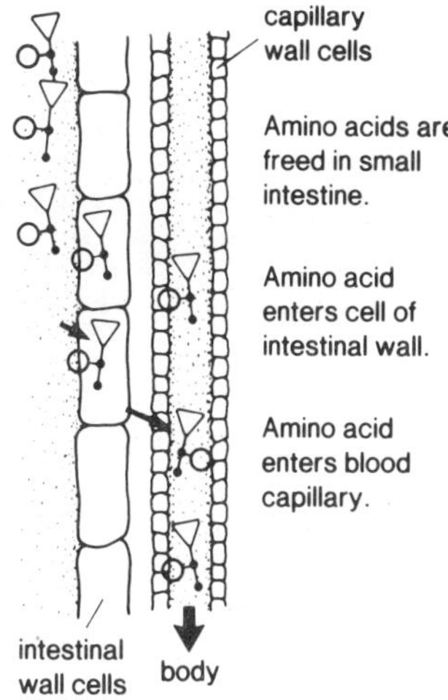

Protein digestion proceeds.

Digestion in the small intestine. By the time proteins slip into the small intestine, they are already broken into different-sized pieces. There will be some single amino acids, to be sure, but many will still be joined together in strands of two, three, or more amino acids (**dipeptides, tripeptides**, and larger peptides). In the small intestine, the acid delivered by the stomach is neutralized by alkaline juice from the pancreas. The raising of the pH (to about 7) enables the next enzyme team to accomplish the final breakdown of the strands. Digestion continues until almost all pieces of protein are broken into small fragments and more free amino acids.

Absorption across intestinal wall cells into blood. Absorption takes place all along the small intestine. Recent research shows that the cells lining the small intestine absorb dipeptides and tripeptides as well as amino acids and then separate them into amino acids to let them cross the capillary walls.[3] It is thought that some food allergies may be due to a reaction against particular dipeptides and tripeptides that slip across the barriers and enter the bloodstream whole.

There are specific sites along the small intestine for the absorption of amino acids. Different carriers help neutral, basic, and acid amino acids across the cell membranes. Within each class, amino acids compete for the carriers.

The presence of specific sites for the absorption of amino acids explains why nutritionists advise against supplementing the diet with specific amino acids, as is recommended by some food faddists. Nutritionists believe that, if one amino acid floods the absorptive carriers, another similar one will travel by the site without having a chance to be absorbed. Competition for transport will cause loss by excretion of that amino acid, even though it is present in the diet. The best guarantee of having a good balance of amino acids is to supply the dietary protein from foods.

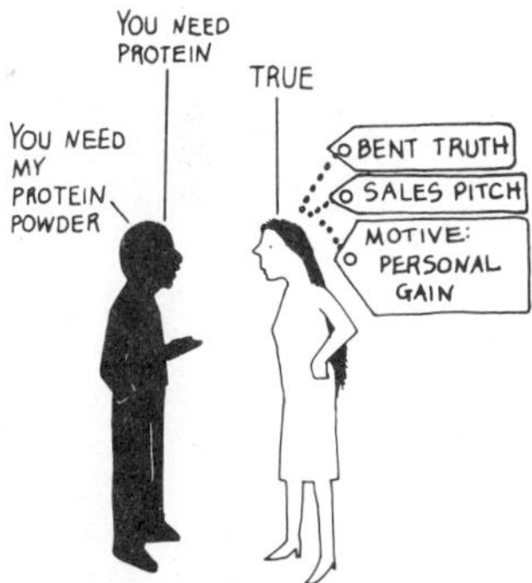
YOU NEED PROTEIN
TRUE
YOU NEED MY PROTEIN POWDER
BENT TRUTH
SALES PITCH
MOTIVE: PERSONAL GAIN
While protein is immensely important in nutrition, there is no need to take it in powder or liquid form.

Use of amino acids inside cells. Once they are circulating in the bloodstream, the amino acids are available to be taken up by any cell of the body. The cells can then use them to make proteins, either for their own use or for secretion into lymph or blood for other uses. The discovery of the way **protein synthesis** is accomplished inside a cell is one of the exciting new chapters in genetics and biochemistry. The details are very well known but beyond the scope of a basic nutrition

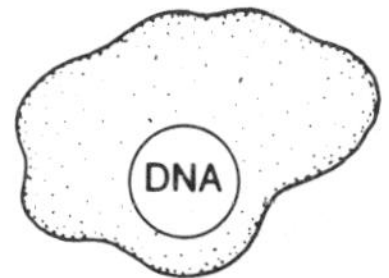

1. DNA is in the nucleus of each cell.

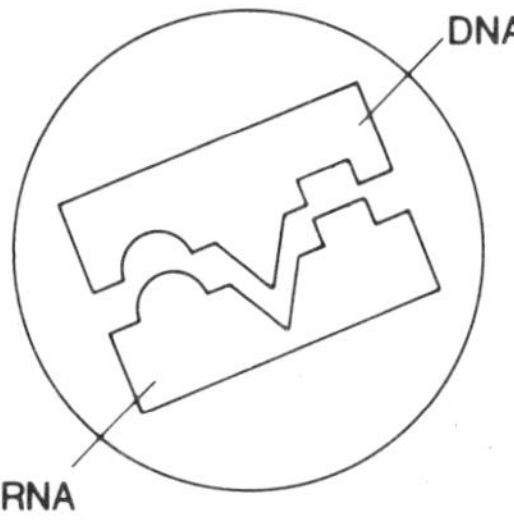

2. DNA makes a complementary copy of that portion of itself that has the instructions for the protein the cell needs.

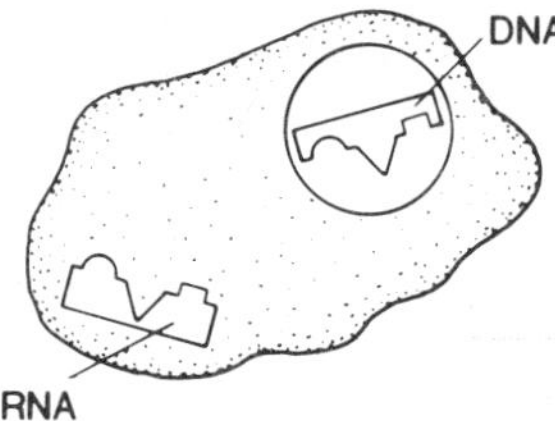

3. RNA leaves the nucleus.

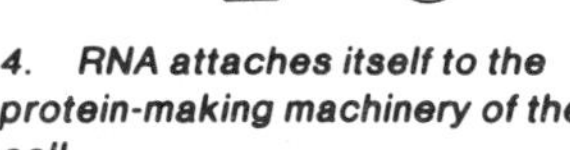

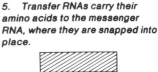

4. RNA attaches itself to the protein-making machinery of the cell.

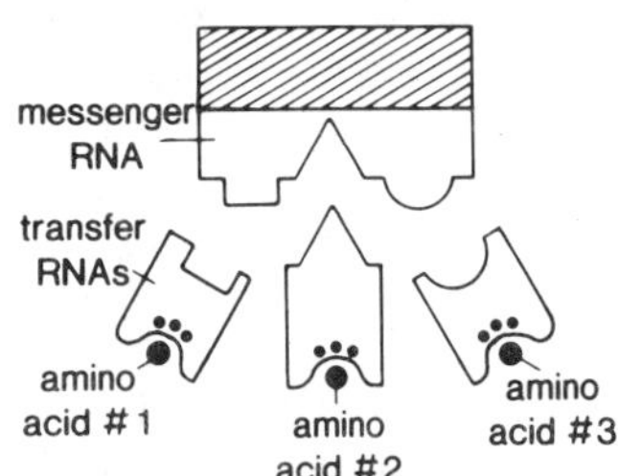

5. Transfer RNAs carry their amino acids to the messenger RNA, where they are snapped into place.

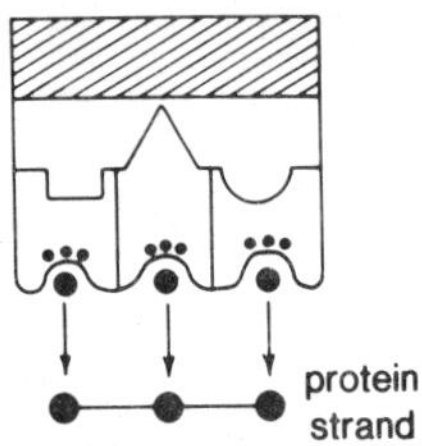

6. The completed protein strand is released, and the messenger RNA is degraded.

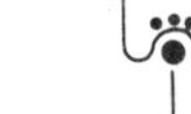

Figure 1. *Protein synthesis.*

The instructions for making every protein in a person's body are transmitted in the genetic information he or she receives at conception. This body of knowledge is filed away in a master file in the nucleus of every cell. The master file is the DNA (deoxyribonucleic acid), which never leaves the nucleus. The DNA is identical in every cell and is specific for each individual. Each specialized cell has access to the total inherited information but calls on only the instructions needed for its own functions.

In order to inform the cell of the proper sequence of amino acids for a needed protein, a "xerox copy" of the appropriate portion of DNA is made. This copy is messenger RNA (ribonucleic acid), which is able to escape through the nuclear membrane. In the cell fluid, it seeks out and attaches itself to one of the ribosomes (a protein-making machine, itself composed of RNA and protein). Thus situated, the messenger presents the specifications for the amino acids to be linked into a protein strand.

Meanwhile, another form of RNA, called transfer RNA, collects amino acids from the cell fluid and brings them to the messenger. For each amino acid there is a specific transfer RNA. Thousands of these transfer RNAs, with their loads of amino acids, cluster around the ribosomes, like vegetable-laden trucks around a farmer's market awaiting their turn to unload. When an amino acid is called for by the messenger, the transfer RNA carrying it snaps into position. Then the next and the next and the next loaded transfer RNAs move into place. Thus the amino acids are lined up in the right sequence. Then an enzyme bonds them together.

Finally, the completed protein strand is released, the messenger is degraded, and the transfer RNAs are freed to return for another load. It takes many words to describe these events, but in the cell, forty to a hundred amino acids can be added to a growing protein strand in only a second.

book. However, Figure 1 may aid in your understanding some of the dietary recommendations for protein.

If a *non*essential amino acid (that is, one the cell can make) is unavailable for a growing protein strand, the cell will synthesize it and continue attaching amino acids to the strand. If an essential amino acid (one the cell can't make) is missing, the building of the protein will be halted. Partially completed proteins are not held for later completion (for example, on the next day). Rather, the partial structures are dismantled, and the surplus amino acids are returned to circulation to be made available to other cells. If they are not soon inserted into protein, their amine groups will be removed and excreted, and the residues will be used for other purposes. Whatever the need that prompted calling for a particular protein, that need will not be met.

It follows that all the essential amino acids must be eaten within the same time period, probably about four hours.[4] This presents no problem to people who regularly eat **complete proteins**, such as those of meat, fish, poultry, cheese, eggs, or milk. The proteins of these foods contain ample amounts of all the amino acids essential for humans. An equally sound choice is to eat two protein foods, each of which supplies the amino acids missing in the other. This strategy is called **mutual supplementation,**[5] and the two protein foods chosen are **complementary proteins.** People who subsist on proteins from cereal or plant foods that do not supply the complete assortment of needed amino acids may suffer a serious deficiency of one or more of them.

Complete protein: protein containing all the essential amino acids.

Complementary protein combinations:
Peanut protein—wheat, oats, corn, rice, coconut.
Soy protein—corn, wheat, rye, sesame.
Legumes—cereals.
Leafy vegetables—cereals.

Traditional protein combinations:
Soybeans—rice (Indochina).
Peas—wheat (Fertile Crescent).
Beans—corn (Central and South America).

More about vegetarian diets in this chapter's Food Feature.

Figure 2. *Mutual supplementation. Each of these two proteins is of relatively low quality by itself, but the two are complementary. They lack different amino acids. Together, they provide a balanced assortment.*

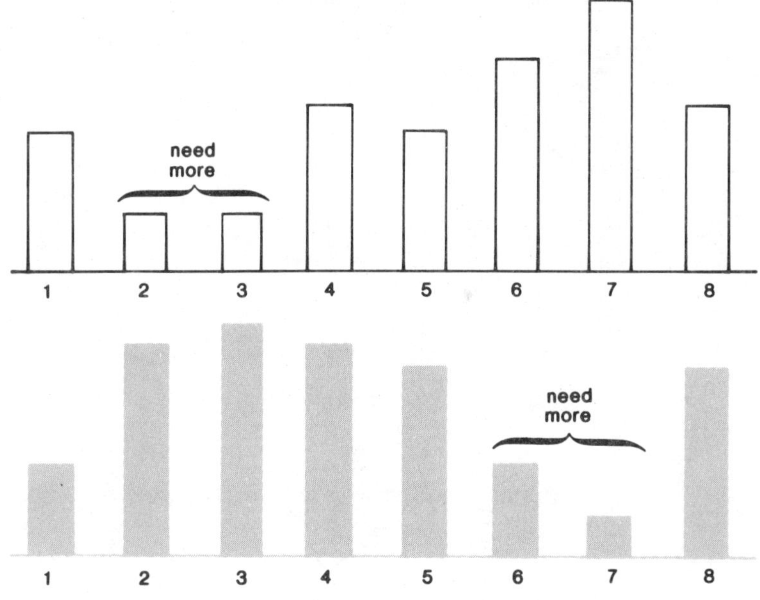
This protein lacks amino acids 2 and 3 but has plenty of 6 and 7.
need more
1 2 3 4 5 6 7 8
need more
1 2 3 4 5 6 7 8
This protein lacks amino acids 6 and 7 but has plenty of 2 and 3.

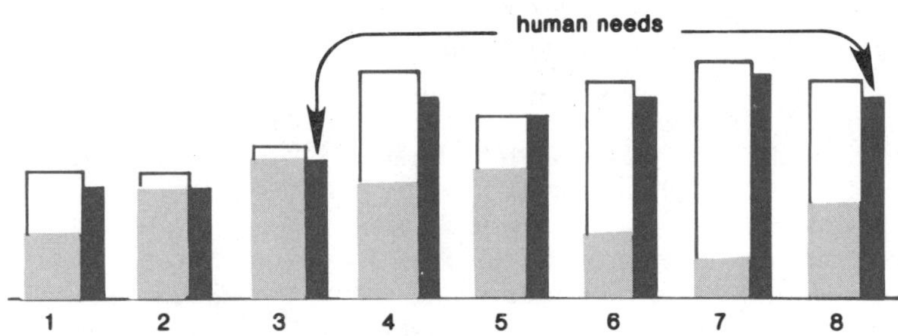

Put them together in a half-and-half mixture, and the balance of amino acids meets human needs quite well.

Repeat, with applications. The preceding description of the body's handling of amino acids provides a basis for wise selection and use of protein food for the diet. It will be helpful to put the story together here and show its relevance before turning to other topics. Let's follow the fate of an amino acid that was originally part of a protein-containing food. When it arrives in a cell, it may be used in several different ways, depending on the needs of the cell at the time.

The amino acid may be used as is and become part of a growing protein. But if the cell has need of a nonessential amino acid, the cell may take the newly arrived amino acid, dismantle it, and use its amine group to build the needed amino acid. The remainder of the amino acid may be used in building a new amino acid or may be used as if it were a carbohydrate or a fat. The carbohydrate or fat energy then will be used as fuel or, if not needed, stored as glycogen or fat.

Obviously the highest-quality proteins are animal proteins, because their essential amino acid composition most closely matches that of human protein. But the cell can use animal proteins as they are only if it has an abundance of all the other amino acids to go with them. Otherwise, it must destroy some of the essential amino acids to make the others. It follows that a good way to support the efficient use of high-quality animal protein is to eat plenty of plant protein along with it. Recent research has shown that expensive meat protein is far more efficiently used when ample bread, cereal, and vegetable protein accompanies it. An adult needs only 20 percent of total protein as essential amino acids.[6]

People engaged in solving the world food crisis are working to encourage cultures that depend on a single staple food to diversify their household crops. Education in this field is being directed at the women of the culture, who are usually the ones who tend the family garden; the men often garden for a cash crop. If a family that normally eats rice can be persuaded to add one of the legumes, it gains a much improved balance and use of the essential amino acids.

Nearly the same fate awaits the amino acid if it arrives at a cell that is screaming for fuel but has no glucose or fatty acids. Even though this amino acid may be needed to build a vital protein, the energy need will be given top priority. Without energy, the cell dies. Therefore, this valuable amino acid will be stripped of its amine group, and the remainder of its structure will be used for energy. The amine group will be excreted from the cell and, finally, from the body in the urine.

Another circumstance in which amino acids are used for energy is

The tendency to sacrifice amino acids for their energy in a crisis is why the protein-sparing action of carbohydrate and fat is so vital. It is pointless to eat expensive protein alone when energy needs are not being met. It is like using dollar bills as fuel for a fire when newspaper would do. At the beginning, this chapter mentioned the problem of the world's starving people and stated that this problem is too complex to be solved by distributing powdered milk or teaching the people to eat meat. One reason for this is now apparent. Only after energy needs are met can protein play its unique and vital roles.

A person deprived of food shows all the symptoms of protein deficiency. Not only food protein but also body tissues made of protein are broken down to meet the body's energy needs. But this kind of protein deficiency must be remedied by feeding adequate *calories*. The person needs energy, which usually can be supplied most inexpensively from carbohydrate. Possibly, given enough energy food, the person will be able to eat enough protein to meet the body's amino acid needs. Thus the protein-deficiency problems arising during food shortages can usually be solved least expensively by supplying more of the local carbohydrate food.

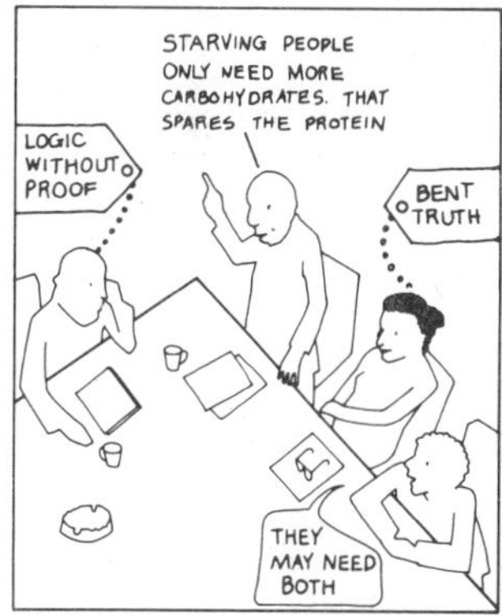
STARVING PEOPLE ONLY NEED MORE CARBOHYDRATES. THAT SPARES THE PROTEIN
LOGIC WITHOUT PROOF
BENT TRUTH
THEY MAY NEED BOTH

It takes advanced nutrition knowledge to make correct policy decisions.

Nutritionists have made a great effort to convey this fact to policy makers whose task is to solve their countries' malnutrition problems. Unfortunately, however, sometimes the message has been oversold. Promoting the use of expensive protein food is often a mistake, but policy makers can err in the other direction, too. It is not true that *all* malnutrition problems can be solved by "using more of the local carbohydrate food." The economists sometimes say, "Let them eat beans; we'll export the ground nuts," on the assumption that more beans (calories) will allow the protein in the beans to remedy the protein-deficiency problems, and the nation's economy will profit from the export of ground nuts (protein-rich food). But sometimes the local carbohydrate food is so poor in protein or contains protein of such poor quality that it will not support the growth of children or the health of pregnant women or working men. And sometimes the victims can be protected from the most devastating effects of malnutrition by eating a very small quantity of very high-quality protein. Tragic and avoidable errors arise when policy makers oversimplify the nutrition problems their countries face.[7]

when there is a surplus of amino acids and energy. In this case, the body does not waste this resource. It takes the amino acid apart, excretes the amine group in the urine, converts the rest to fat, then stores it in the fat cells. In this way, valuable, expensive, protein-rich foods can contribute to obesity.

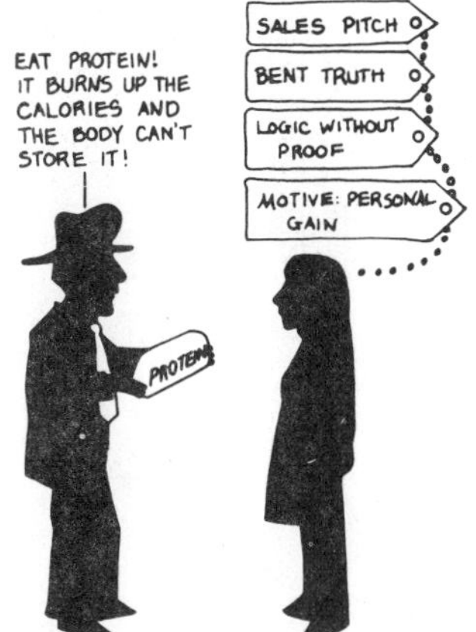
EAT PROTEIN! IT BURNS UP THE CALORIES AND THE BODY CAN'T STORE IT!
SALES PITCH
BENT TRUTH
LOGIC WITHOUT PROOF
MOTIVE: PERSONAL GAIN
PROTEIN

High-protein diets don't make you burn more calories.

Promotion of trying to lose weight by eating only protein is based on the idea that the body doesn't store protein. The truth is that the body doesn't store the amino acid as such, with its nitrogen, if there is a surplus. The body excretes the nitrogen. But it retains the remainder of the molecule. It converts it to fat, which is stored in the fat cells.

Another reason often heard for eating only protein in order to lose weight is that it takes more calories to digest protein than to digest the other energy nutrients. This is not true. In fact, it is truer to say that it is pointless to eat any protein at all on a diet of less than 900 calories a day, because only the energy value can be salvaged from such a ration.[8]

The rationale for supplying protein during a medically supervised fast for weight loss has a sound basis, and the procedure has met with some success in the hands of competent physicians. But it is hazardous when undertaken impulsively without supervision.

In summary, amino acids in the cell can be used to:

Synthesize protein.

Provide glucose (at least, half of them can).

Provide nitrogen in the form of amine groups to build nonessential amino acids.

Provide energy if there is a scarcity of energy nutrients.

Increase the stored energy in glycogen and fat.

Amino acids are wasted (not used to build protein) whenever there is:

Not enough energy from carbohydrate and fat.

An imbalance, with not enough essential amino acids (low-quality protein).

Too much protein so that not all is needed.

Factors that must be supplied in the diet for the body to be able to synthesize protein include:

All essential amino acids simultaneously and in the proper ratio (because they cannot be synthesized and the ratio influences their utilization).

An adequate total amount of protein (to supply amine groups to synthesize the nonessential amino acids).

Adequate carbohydrate and calories (to spare the protein and to supply energy for the synthetic reactions).

Food Proteins: Quality and Use

The body responds to different protein foods in different ways, depending on many factors: the body's own state of health, the food source of the protein, its digestibility, the other nutrients taken with it, and its amino acid assortment. To know whether, say, 30 grams of protein is enough to meet a person's daily needs, it is necessary to know how all these other factors affect the body's use of the protein.

Health or physiological state. A person in good health can be expected to use dietary protein efficiently. However, malnutrition or infection can seriously impair digestion (by reducing enzyme secretion), absorption (by causing degeneration of the absorptive surface of the small intestine or losses from diarrhea), and the cells' use of protein (by forcing amino acids to be used to meet other needs). Most statements on protein requirements for human beings come from research on the needs of healthy subjects. Malnutrition or infection may greatly increase the needs while making it harder to meet them.

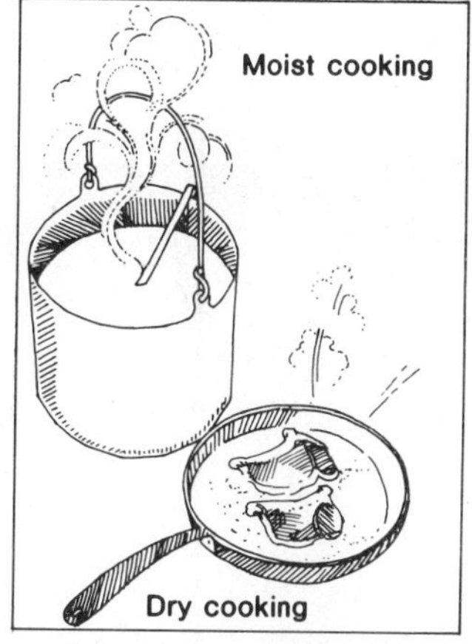

Cooking with moist heat improves protein digestibility.

Food source and digestibility. Amino acids from animal proteins are best absorbed (over 90 percent). Those from legumes follow (about 80 percent), and those from cereal and other plant foods vary (from 60 to 90 percent). Cooking with moist heat generally improves protein digestibility, whereas dry heating may impair it.

Other nutrients present. As already mentioned, protein will be used as such only if the protein-sparing calories supplied by carbohydrate are adequate to meet the energy need. Certain vitamins and minerals must also be present to ensure the absorption of protein.

Protein quality. All other conditions being equal, the prime consideration in evaluating protein quality is its essential amino acid composition. A protein that supplies all the amino acids needed by the body in exactly the right ratio will be more completely used for protein synthesis than one that supplies only a limited quantity of one or more essential amino acids. If an essential amino acid is not present in adequate quantity, it limits the utilization of all the other essential amino acids, so that they will have to be wasted. A protein that almost entirely lacks an essential amino acid can't be used for protein synthesis at all unless that amino acid is supplied from some other source.

When amino acids are wasted, their amine groups (which contain their nitrogen) can't be stored. Therefore, the efficiency of a protein can be assessed experimentally by measuring the amount of nitrogen retained by the body. This is the basis for determinations of the **biological value (BV)** of proteins by the Food and Agriculture Organization of the United Nations, which sets world standards. The higher the amount of nitrogen retained, the higher the quality of the protein.

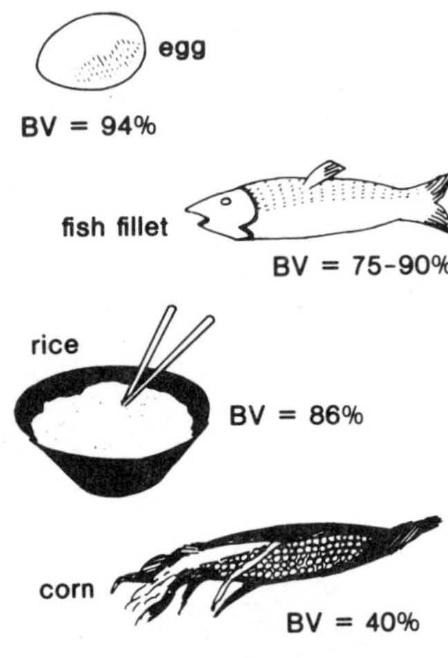

The biological values attached to proteins indicate their quality.

The most perfect protein by this standard is egg protein (biological value 94 percent on a scale of 100); this has been designated the **reference protein**, against which other proteins are measured as good sources of amino acids in human nutrition. Other animal proteins such as milk, meat, and fish compare favorably. Rice protein is well balanced, but other plant proteins are of poorer quality (down to about 40 percent). Generally, a biological value of 70 percent or above indicates acceptable quality.

Another measure of protein quality is based on the efficiency with which a protein supports growth. Testing the protein source involves seeing how many pounds a growing animal will gain on a fixed amount of dietary protein. This measure, the **protein efficiency ratio (PER)**, is the measure of quality that provides the basis for statements about our daily protein requirements and is the one used on food labels. As it happens, the number 70 is chosen to draw a line with respect to PER, too, although PER and BV are quite differently determined. You are assumed to eat protein with a PER of 70 or above; if the PER is lower, you need more protein. Thus the U.S. RDA for protein is 45 grams; but if the PER is less than 70, then the U.S. RDA is 65 grams (see inside back cover).

For those who choose not to tangle with the formulas for BV and PER, a convenient way to distinguish among proteins is to use the following guidelines:

Complete protein foods include all meat, fish, poultry, milk, milk products, and eggs.

Complementary protein foods are grains, nuts, legumes (beans/peas).

No significant protein is found in other vegetables or fruits.

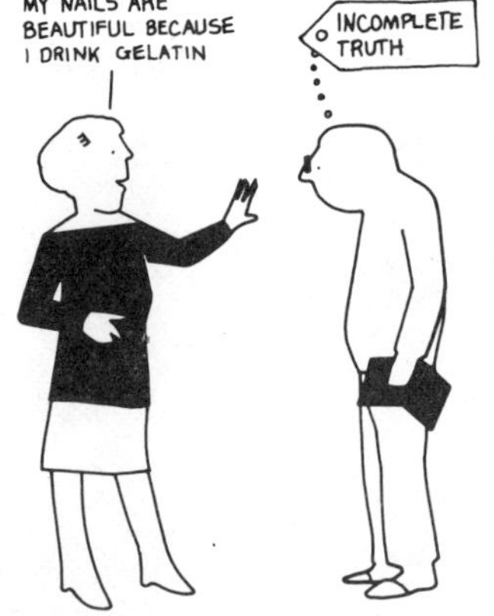

MY NAILS ARE BEAUTIFUL BECAUSE I DRINK GELATIN
INCOMPLETE TRUTH

It just happens that gelatin lacks the essential amino acid tryptophan.

As always, a little knowledge can be a dangerous thing. One animal protein that is not complete is gelatin (it lacks tryptophan, one of the essential amino acids). Ironically, this is the protein often recommended for correcting cracked nails and dull or brittle hair. The logic is that because these tissues are made of protein, a drink of protein will improve their texture. Even if this were the case, however—and a symptom is not a deficiency disease—gelatin supplements would help only if protein containing tryptophan had already been supplied—and if that protein were complete, the gelatin would not be needed!

The Protein RDA

Protein is the first nutrient we have discussed for which there is an RDA (Recommended Dietary Allowance). The amount of protein needed daily depends on the many factors already mentioned and also on the stage of growth and the amount of body tissue that needs constant repair or replacement (therefore it depends on the size of the person). There are continuous daily losses of body protein due to the constant processes of repair and maintenance.

Underlying the protein RDA are **nitrogen balance** studies. The basis of these studies is that nitrogen lost by excretion must be replaced by nitrogen taken in food; nitrogen-in must equal nitrogen-out. The laboratory scientist measures the body's daily nitrogen losses in urine, feces, and sweat under controlled conditions and can then estimate the amount of protein needed to replace these losses. As a rule of thumb, the weight of the nitrogen as determined in these lab studies can be multiplied by 6.25 (representing the average weight of an amino acid) to determine the amount of protein that contained the nitrogen.

Under normal circumstances, healthy adults are in nitrogen equilibrium, or zero balance—that is, they have at all times the same amount of total protein in their bodies. When nitrogen-in exceeds nitrogen-out, they are said to be in positive nitrogen balance; this means that somewhere in their bodies more proteins are being built than are being broken down and lost. When nitrogen-in is less than nitrogen-out, they are said to be in negative nitrogen balance.

Growing children add to their bodies new blood, bone, and muscle cells every day. These cells contain protein, so children must have in their bodies more protein (and therefore more nitrogen) at the end of each day than they had at the beginning. A growing child is therefore in positive nitrogen balance. Similarly, when a woman is pregnant she is, in essence, growing a new person; she too must be in positive nitrogen balance. When she is lactating, she may be in equilibrium again, but it is a sort of enhanced equilibrium. She is eating more protein than before to make her milk and is secreting it whenever the baby nurses.

Negative nitrogen balance occurs when muscle or other protein tissue is broken down and lost. Consider the situation when people have to rest in bed for a period of time. Their muscles degenerate and they suffer a net loss of protein. One of several problems faced by the nutritionists responsible for the welfare of astronauts was that of the negative nitrogen balance that occurred when they were lying down for days in the space capsule. Their muscles failed to receive enough exercise to maintain themselves.

It is commonly believed that athletes need more protein than others because their bodies contain more muscle tissue. But once they have conditioned their bodies and are maintaining a fixed amount of muscle tissue, they need no more protein to replace losses than does any other person.

For healthy adults, the RDA for protein has been set, at present, at 0.8 grams for each kilogram (or 2.2 pounds) of ideal body weight. Ideal weight, rather than actual weight, is used because the amino acids are needed by the lean body tissues, not by the fat cells. For children who are growing, the RDA is higher per unit of body weight; for infants it is highest of all.

In establishing the RDA for protein, the Committee on RDA took into consideration that the protein in a normal diet would be mixed—that is, a combination of animal and plant protein. An allowance was also made for the fact that not all proteins are used with 100 percent efficiency and that individuals vary in the efficiency with which they

RDA for Protein

Age (yr)	RDA (g/kg)
0 – ½	2.2
½ – 1	2.0
1 – 3	1.8
4 – 10	1.1
11 – 14	1.0
15 – 18	0.9
19 and up	0.8

The RDA increases by 30 g per day during pregnancy and by 20 g during lactation.

Protein RDA (adult) = 0.8 g/kg.

To figure your protein RDA,

1. *Look up your ideal weight on the inside back cover.*
2. *Convert pounds to kilograms (pounds ÷ 2.2 lb/kg = kilograms).*
3. *Multiply by 0.8 g/kg to get your RDA in grams per day.*

For example,

1. *Ideal weight = 110 lb.*
2. *110 lb ÷ 2.2 lb/kg = 50 kg.*
3. *50 kg × 0.8 g/kg = 40 g.*

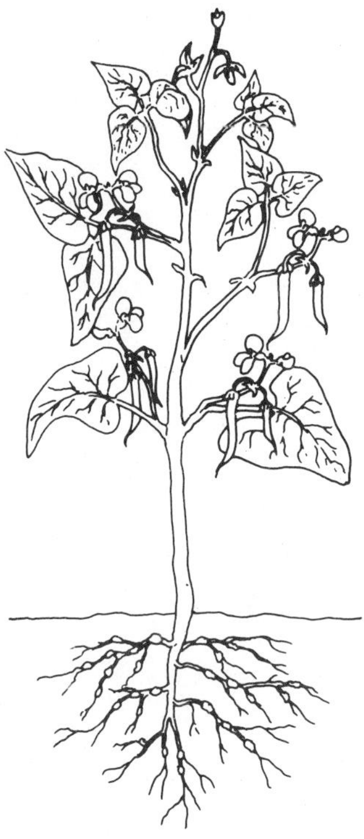

The pods of legumes contain seeds high in protein content. The roots can "fix" nitrogen, contributing to the soil more nitrogen than the plant takes out. For the uses of legumes in cooking, see Figure 1 in Chapter 2.

use protein. With these safeguards built into the recommendation, most individuals can consume two-thirds of the RDA for protein and be assured of meeting their bodies' needs. What this means in terms of food is presented in the Food Feature in this chapter.

The RDA must be interpreted with caution. For the present, perhaps the most important point to be made is that they are generous recommendations and that there is no need for the healthy person to exceed them. A look at food sources of protein will show that it is abundantly supplied in the foods normally consumed by people in the United States.

Food Sources of Protein

In the exchange system, two groups contribute an abundance of high-quality protein—the milk and meat groups. Two others—the vegetable and grain groups—contribute smaller amounts and lower-quality proteins.

An important class of foods included among the meat exchanges is the plant family known as the **legumes**, sometimes called the poor man's meat. If in the future, as some predictions have it, the world's developed countries shift to a more vegetarian economy and the use of animal food declines, the alternative sources of high-quality protein will become important. We will then become much more familiar with the legumes.

The legumes are the seeds of such plants as the kidney bean, soybean, garden pea, lentil, black-eyed pea, and lima bean. These plants have nodules on their roots containing bacteria that can "fix" nitrogen; that is, they can capture nitrogen from the air and soil and use it to make amino acids and protein. Farmers often grow legumes in rotation with other crops. They plow the roots under at the end of the season and restore nitrogen to the soil in a form that other plants can use.

Legumes are very rich in protein, and the protein is of quality almost comparable to that of meat. They are also good sources of many B vitamins and iron. Meat is presently the major contributor of these three nutrients in the Western diet; legumes not only offer these but are rich in natural fiber too. A cup of cooked legumes supplies 31 percent of the protein and 42 percent of the iron recommended daily for an adult male. Long scorned by middle-class people because of their supposedly fattening, high-carbohydrate content, legumes are coming into their own as an inexpensive, land-sparing, low-fat, nutritious source of good-quality protein.

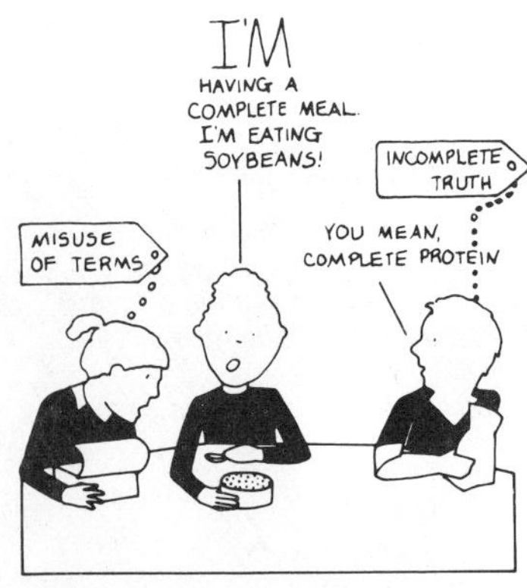
I'M HAVING A COMPLETE MEAL. I'M EATING SOYBEANS!
MISUSE OF TERMS
YOU MEAN, COMPLETE PROTEIN
INCOMPLETE TRUTH

Legumes are nutritious but they aren't that nutritious.

Not long ago, a speaker was heard to remark, at a public meeting on world hunger, "I've just read that soybeans make a complete meal." Having read the kind of high praise about legumes that has just been presented, she had reached an erroneous conclusion. Many people are choosing to include soybeans in their diets, and even to build their diets around them, and this choice probably benefits both the health and the pocketbook. However, the

Table 1. Protein Content of the Exchange Groups

Exchange	Serving Size	Protein (g)	Energy (*k*cal)
Skim milk	1 cup	8	80
Lean meat	1 oz (meat)	7	55
	½ cup (legumes)		
Vegetable	½ cup	2	25
Bread	1 slice	2	70

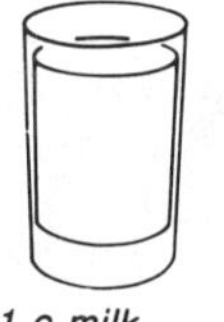
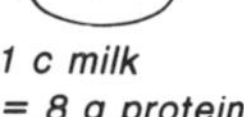
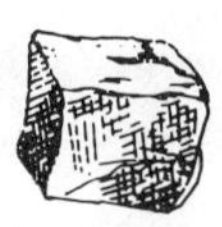

1 c milk = 8 g protein.

1 oz meat = 7 g protein.

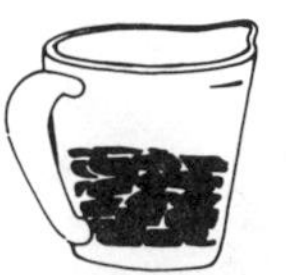
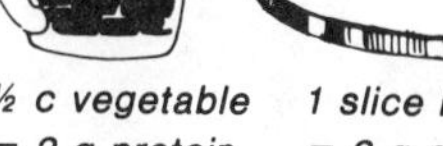

½ c vegetable = 2 g protein.

1 slice bread = 2 g protein.

trend could be taken too far. Soybeans contain good-quality protein, but they do not make a complete meal by themselves. They contain no vitamin A or vitamin C, and their balance of amino acids can be improved by using other vegetables with them. An adequate diet provides not only protein but also carbohydrate, fat, vitamins, minerals, and water.

The protein values assigned to each of the exchange groups permit us to estimate the protein content of some possible menus. For comparison purposes, remember that the U.S. RDA for protein is 45 grams (of high-quality protein) a day. The Food Feature in this chapter shows that this recommendation is extraordinarily easy to meet.

Food Feature: Meeting Daily Protein Needs

A breakfast of 1 ounce of cereal with ½ cup of milk would provide 6 grams of protein, 4 grams of it high-quality, complete protein. An alternative breakfast consisting of 2 eggs, a 3-ounce slice of ham, a glass of milk, and 2 slices of toast would contribute 47 grams of protein. This would be abundant protein for a 120-pound woman for an entire day.

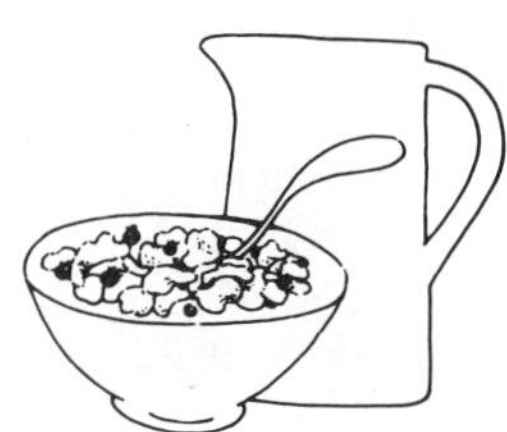

Breakfast: 6 g protein.

For lunch, a quarter-pound hamburger with a slice of cheese would contribute 40 grams of protein. This lunch alone would provide more than two-thirds of the RDA; it is unnecessarily high in protein. As an alternative, you could eat a chef's salad, which usually contains, in addition to a variety of salad greens, a hard-cooked egg and about 1 ounce each of cheese, turkey, and ham. These four meat exchanges total 28 grams of protein.

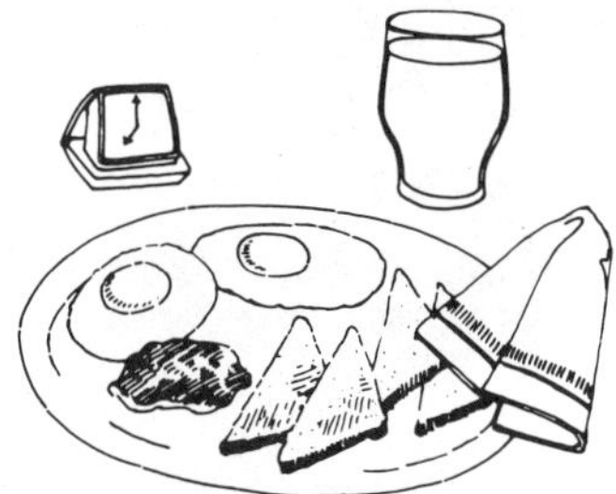

Breakfast: 47 g protein.

It seems that, after almost any kind of breakfast and lunch, it is hard not to exceed the protein allowance at dinnertime. The steak and potatoes meal described at the end of Chapter 5, for example, provided 56 grams of protein from the 8-ounce steak alone, to say nothing of the additional 8 grams or so (depending on size) from the potato and rolls. After revision in

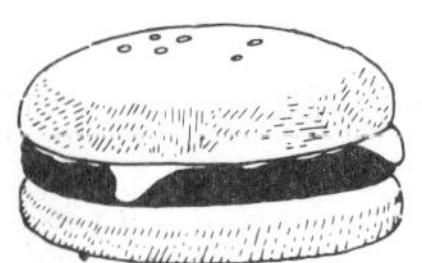

Lunch: 40 g protein.

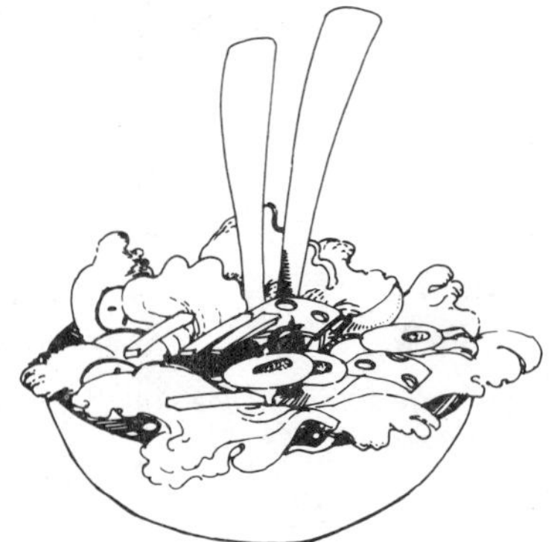

Dinner: 28 g protein.

accordance with the recommendations for balance, the dinner still provided 28 grams of protein from the 4 ounces of ground beef and more than 10 grams of protein from the potatoes, bread, and vegetables.

Obviously, with the great availability of animal foods and nutritious grains and vegetables, most of us have little trouble meeting or exceeding the protein RDA. Protein is of prime importance, but its importance may have been so overemphasized that the nutritional problems of meat eaters now more often reflect overnutrition than undernutrition.

For the vegetarian, the problem of meeting daily protein needs takes on another dimension. The lacto-ovo-vegetarian (who includes dairy products in the diet) can manage perfectly well by substituting two servings of legumes for the two servings of meat the Four Food Group Plan recommends, as shown on page 30. For the strict vegetarian, who uses only plant foods, legumes take on greater importance, but if these are appropriately complemented (for example, with grains eaten at the same time), they can provide a combination of amino acids equivalent to that of complete protein. Other products, newly available and very useful to the vegetarian, are meat analogs—fabricated foods made to resemble meat but using vegetable protein.

Complementary protein combinations for the vegetarian:
- *Peanut-butter sandwich (legume with grain).*
- *Macaroni and cheese (grain with milk).*
- *Black bean and rice soup (legume with grain).*

Curiously, the vegetarian has to eat more calories to meet protein needs than the meat eater does. A cup of cooked legumes provides only about half as much protein as a serving (3 ounces) of meat, so you have to eat 2 cups of legumes to equal the protein of a meat serving. If you choose nuts, you are choosing a food with as high a fat content as meat. Thus you have to eat 600 bulky calories of legumes or nuts to get the same amount of protein as from 300 to 400 calories of lean meat. This leaves you with fewer calories to spend on the other needed nutrients.

Paradoxically, however, vegetarians tend to consume fewer calories and to be thinner than meat eaters. This is because the bulk of the vegetarian protein food is so filling that the vegetarian cannot physically accommodate much more food and so is likely to eat fewer total calories than the meat eater.

Guidelines for the lacto-ovo-vegetarian:
- *Decrease empty calories.*
- *Replace meat with eggs, legumes, nuts, seeds, and meat analogs.*
- *Use lowfat or nonfat milk and milk products.*
- *Select grain products from whole-grain foods only.*
- *Include a variety of fruits and vegetables.*

The fact that more calories have to be spent on protein makes it necessary to adopt a guiding principle. You can't afford to waste calories, and so you are advised to stay away from empty-calorie foods. In fact, even the relative emptiness of enriched bread is not recommended. The calories invested in grains should go for whole grains, with all the nutrients they provide.

More about vitamins D and B_{12} in Chapter 9.

Following these guidelines, even the strict vegetarian can plan a diet that is adequate in calories, protein, and most other nutrients. The task is not finished, however, for there remain two vitamins that demand special attention: vitamin D and vitamin B_{12}. The plant-food sources of vitamin D are unreliable (depending on how long and under what conditions the plant has been in the sun), and there are no plants that contain vitamin B_{12}. For these reasons, nutritionists try hard to persuade young vegetarians to include milk and milk products in the diets of their children. The pure vegetarian diet is acceptable "for adults only."

Additional guidelines for the vegetarian will be presented in later chapters. So far, you can see that the educated vegetarian can plan a perfectly acceptable diet, as far as protein is concerned, around plant foods alone.

Protein Deficiency: Kwashiorkor

In most of the world, the poor have trouble obtaining protein-rich food. Even when there is an abundance of food to eat, it usually is a single plant food composed largely of carbohydrate and a low-quality protein. The poor, depending on this staple, develop a protein deficit.

The disease resulting from protein deficit has been given the name **kwashiorkor**, after the Ghanaian word for "the evil spirit that infects the first child when the second child is born." In countries where kwashiorkor is prevalent, there is a custom of giving the newly weaned child a thin gruel rather than the food eaten by the rest of the family. The child has been receiving breast milk from the mother containing high-quality protein designed beautifully to support the body's growth. Suddenly the child receives only a watery carbohydrate drink with scant protein of very low quality. Small wonder the just-weaned child sickens when the new baby arrives.

The child who has been banished meets this threat to life by engaging in as little activity as possible. Apathy is one of the earliest signs of protein deprivation; the body is collecting all its forces to meet the crisis and so cuts down on any expenditure of protein not needed for function of the heart, lungs, and brain. As the apathy increases, the child will finally not even cry for food. All growth ceases; the child will

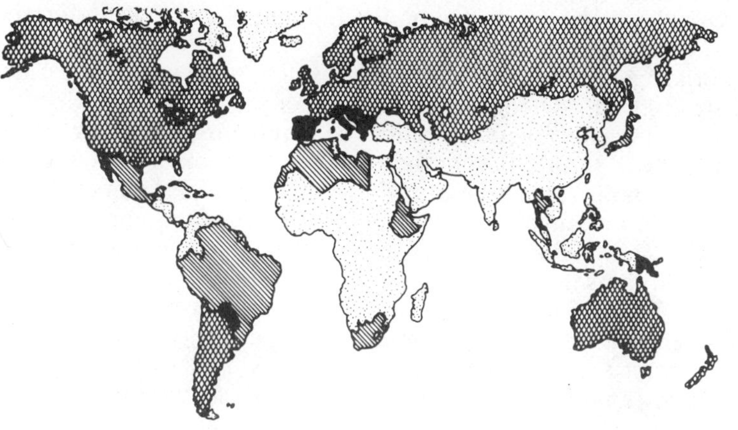

World protein-calorie malnutrition.

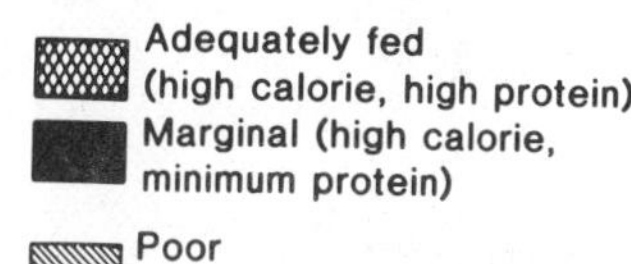

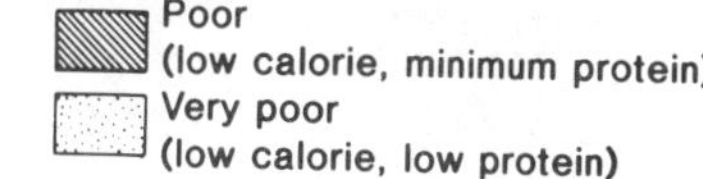

UN Food and Agriculture Organization, 1965.

be no larger at four than at two. New hair grows without the protein pigment that gave it its color. The skin also loses its color, and when sores open, they fail to heal. Enzymes for digesting foods are in short supply, the cells that line the intestinal wall to absorb nutrients are not renewed, and the carriers to transport nutrients out of the intestine into the blood are no longer made. This deterioration of the digestive system causes what food is eaten to be digested and absorbed poorly, worsening the condition. Proteins and hormones that previously kept the fluid in the compartments of the body now are diminished, so that fluid leaks out into the tissues (**edema**). The fluid usually accumulates in the belly and legs, because the weakened child is sitting down most of the time. Blood proteins, including hemoglobin, are not synthesized, so the child becomes anemic; this increases the weakness and apathy. The kwashiorkor victim often develops a fatty liver, caused by lack of the protein carriers that transport fat out of the liver. Antibodies to fight off invading bacteria are degraded to provide amino acids for other uses; the child becomes an easy target for any infection. Then dysentery, an infection of the digestive tract that causes diarrhea, further depletes the body of nutrients, especially minerals. Measles, which might make a healthy child sick for a week or two, kills the kwashiorkor child within two or three days.

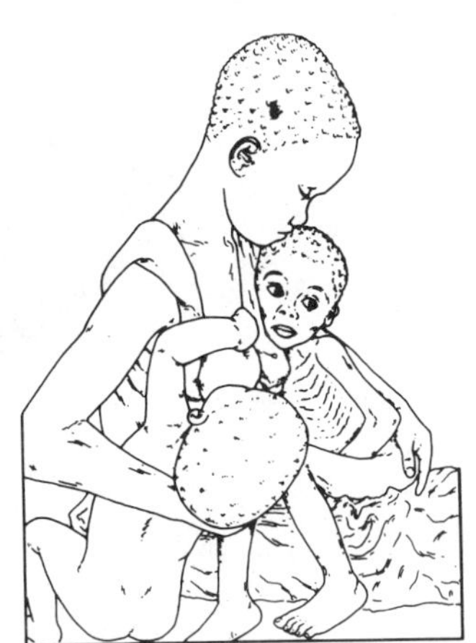

Kwashiorkor.

If the child is taken into the hospital, this starved condition may not be obvious. Water in the tissues may cause the body to look almost fat. Only when the fluid balance is restored will it be seen that the child is just a skeleton thinly covered with skin.

If caught in time, a kwashiorkor victim may be rehabilitated by careful nutritional management. The first consideration is to correct the fluid balances. Diarrhea will have depleted the body's potassium stores and upset other salt balances. Careful remediation of these critical balances will prevent sudden death from heart failure about half the time. Only later can skim milk, containing protein and carbohydrate, be safely given; then comes fat, when body protein is sufficient to provide carriers, and finally vitamins, when the tissues are ready to use them.

Kwashiorkor occurs not only in Ghana but in other African countries, in Central America, South America, the Near East, and the Far East. Cases have been reported on the Indian reservations and in the slums of the United States.

In practice, a deficiency of just one nutrient, such as protein, is not generally seen. More likely, a combination of protein and calorie malnutrition will occur. Overt starvation, or **marasmus**, has other symptoms of its own, in addition to those caused by protein deficiency: a lowered metabolic rate and reduced body temperature from the sheer energy deficit. Protein and calorie deficiency go hand in hand so often that public health officials have given a name to the whole spectrum of disease conditions that range between the two—"**protein-calorie malnutrition" (PCM)**. This is the world's most widespread malnutrition problem, killing millions of children every year.[9]

Nutritionists are concerned over a growing trend away from breastfeeding among the world's poor. Breast milk guarantees that the child will receive high-quality protein and the accompanying carbohydrates to protect it during the period of most rapid growth. If the insult of protein deficiency occurs during the time of cell division in the central nervous system, the number of brain cells will forever be limited. Brain cells increase in number up to the age of about fourteen months in humans, after which no new cells are formed. Protein deprivation during this critical period could therefore limit intelligence. Another argument for continuing breastfeeding until about one year of age is that breastfeeding suppresses the hormones that promote ovulation, thus acting as a natural contraceptive. Although not reliably effective (some women conceive a next baby while breastfeeding one), this effect helps to delay the conception of the next child until the mother has replenished her own body stores.[10]

More on breast versus bottle—Chapter 12 and Controversy 12.

Kwashiorkor is only one of several diseases associated with protein deficiency. Another that is closer to home for most of us is the nutritional liver disease associated with alcoholism. The alcoholic, like the kwashiorkor child, consumes abundant calories, but up to three-fourths of the calories come from alcohol, a nonprotein energy source. Among the symptoms of protein deficiency seen in the alcoholic are edema, which shows up in the abdomen and in the hands and feet, and fatty liver, resulting from the lack of protein for transporting fat to the fat cells. This eventually causes the death of liver cells that can't receive nourishment because they are clogged with fat. If the condition progresses, the result is hardening and death of the liver cells (cirrhosis), which is irreversible. Cirrhosis is now the sixth leading cause of death in the United States.

More about alcohol—Chapter 14.

Protein Excess

Many of the world's people struggle to obtain enough food and enough protein to keep themselves alive, but in the developed countries protein is so abundant that the opposite problems are seen. There are risks associated with the overconsumption of protein. Infants and children do not adjust well to diets containing large amounts of protein; their body composition is altered.[11] Animals fed high-protein diets experience a "protein overload effect," seen in the hypertrophy of their livers and kidneys. There are evidently no benefits to be gained by consuming a diet that derives more than 15 percent of its calories from protein, and there are possible risks.[12] The higher a person's intake of such protein-rich foods as meat and milk, the more likely it is that fruits, vegetables, and grains will be crowded out of the diet, making it inadequate in other nutrients. And diets high in protein necessitate higher intakes of calcium as well, because they increase the body's losses of calcium by way of excretion.

Overconsumption of protein can also cause dehydration, because water is needed to help excrete the wasted nitrogen—a problem the athlete should be warned about, because water balance is of such great importance to athletic performance (see Controversy 7). And animal protein may be one of the many dietary factors associated with a high risk of atherosclerosis (see Controversy 5A). In a world where protein deficiency is such a threat to so many, it is ironic that the people of developed countries should be overconsuming protein.[1]

[1]*Chapter Notes can be found at the end of the Appendixes.*

For Further Information

The recommended references listed in Appendix J contain abundant additional information on protein.

Controversy 6

Liquid Protein

Is predigested, powdered, or liquid protein "bad" for you?

Protein can be delivered to the body by foods as long chains of amino acids linked and tangled together. Or it can be digested in the laboratory to single amino acids and sold as pure-protein powders, pills, or liquid preparations for use as dietary supplements or food substitutes. (The merits of liquid meals like Metrecal or Sego are not being discussed here.) Which is better for the body? Some say the natural way: The body is best adapted to handle whole proteins. Others say that eating pre-separated amino acids spares the digestive system the work of having to digest protein, so that the body will not wear out so fast.

A nutrition principle. The theory that whole proteins are better was best expressed by W. H. Griffith, who said in 1965:

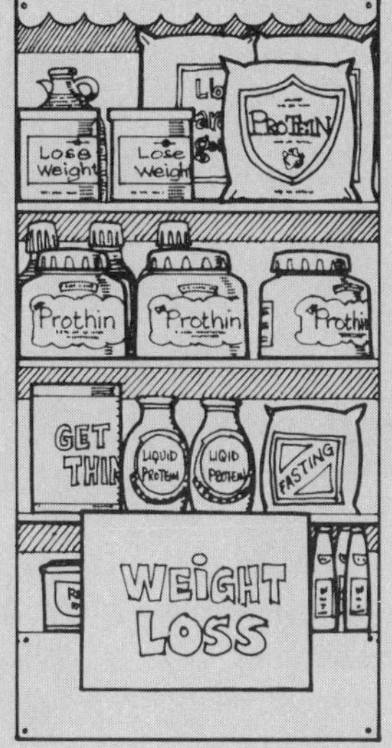

I have always chosen to believe that for the digestion of protein . . . the stages of digestion in the stomach and in the respective parts of the small intestine are considerably more significant than is ordinarily assumed. This special significance is believed to insure the orderly liberation of the twenty amino acids in accordance with their individual rates of absorption so that when the entire process is functioning normally the individual amino acids arrive at protein-building sites in tissues in the right amounts and proportions and at the right time. If this is true, then the administration of a mixture of amino acids, even if patterned after a specific protein, could never be used as efficiently as the intact protein subjected to normal digestion and absorption.[1]

This is a beautiful theory, but it must be subjected to the test of experimentation before it can be accepted. Does the body use whole proteins from foods more efficiently than amino acid mixtures?

After a whole protein is eaten, its amino acids remain in the intestine, mostly as dipeptides and tripeptides, for more than three hours. Only when these contact, and in many cases enter, the cells of the intestinal wall do they split into single amino acid units. This enables them to bypass the bottleneck of transport into the cells, where they would otherwise have to compete with one another for entry sites.[2] Research reports dating from 1968 show that amino acids are more efficiently absorbed when they are part of dipeptides or tripeptides than when they are free. In fact, one way to speed up intestinal absorption of amino acids is to add whole protein pieces to them.[3]

When hospital patients must have liquid feedings, they can be given whole protein, perhaps from milk, in the formula. If they can't digest whole protein, perhaps because they have a disease affecting the supply of digestive enzymes from the pancreas, the next-best choice is partially digested protein rather than individual amino acids.[4] If the pancreas can secrete digestive enzymes at all, it is stimulated to do so by whole proteins more effectively than by mixtures of single amino acids.[5]

These findings suggest that Griffith's belief is well founded. At least the digestive system seems better equipped to handle whole protein than amino acid mixtures. But what about after the amino acids get into the body? Surely, once they have entered the bloodstream, the body can't tell where they have come from. Amino acid units from predigested protein would be just as well used as those from whole protein, would they not?

Apparently not, although experimentation on this question has just begun. For example, one experiment showed that human subjects retained more nitrogen when fed diets of rice and wheat than they did when fed the same amino acids in crystalline form.[6] It seems the body can tell the difference after all, probably because the amino acids are liberated from the whole protein in an ordered time sequence that better matches the timing of protein synthesis in the cells.

Even if whole protein is better used, this does not necessarily mean that amino acid mixtures are bad for you. They apparently do have some disadvantages, however. Because amino acid mixtures are much more attractive to water than whole proteins, they draw fluid into the intestine, causing cramping and diarrhea. Absorbed simultaneously, they can't all be used, and some are wasted. Then, if they reach too-high levels in the blood, they can cause nausea and vomiting.[7] One writer has said that amino acid preparations are "expensive, unpalatable, irritating, impractical, and an inefficient source of available nitrogen."[8]

The available evidence, on the whole, thus strongly supports the view that the body is better adapted to handling protein from natural food, as Griffith believed. In this instance, logic has been borne out by experimentation. The findings to date illustrate a general principle that pervades nutrition science, and one that has been a theme of this book from the first chapter onwards: Our bodies are best equipped to deal with the foods they evolved with—plants, animal products, and animal flesh. The farther removed a food is from its natural state, the more it should be tested before being made available for human use. The events of the late 1970s relating to the protein-sparing fast provide a telling example of what can happen when this principle is ignored.

The principle ignored. A person who is starving loses not only body fat but also precious lean tissue made largely of protein (Chapter 7 explains why this happens). Physicians, concerned about the wasting of lean tissue in hospital patients who can't eat, have been working for a decade to learn how to prevent this wasting. One of the answers they have come up with is to feed protein-rich foods in order to "spare" body protein. Cautious experimentation based on this idea was beginning around 1973.[9] By 1977 several reports had been published and a promising application had been found. Not only could lean tissue be preserved during involuntary starvation but also during fasting undertaken for the purpose of losing weight.

Not surprisingly, a popular book came out that hailed this preliminary work as "a revolutionary new approach to weight loss." The paperback edition of *The Last Chance Diet* by Dr. Linn[10] soon became a best-seller, and thousands of people in the United States and Canada launched themselves on the "protein-sparing fast." But there was at least one crucial difference between Dr. Linn's diet and the previous efforts of the hospital physicians. The Last Chance Diet required that patients purchase and use only a predigested liquid protein product named Prolinn while they were fasting. By October of 1977 two deaths had been tentatively linked to the diet; one reportedly involved a woman about thirty-five years old who had used the diet to lose about fifty pounds. Shortly after her first meal of solid food, the woman's heart stopped beating.[11] Half a year later, several similar deaths had occurred in people using the protein-sparing fast, and most of them seemed to be due to degeneration of the heart muscle. The *Journal of the American Medical Association* reported, "To date, death has occurred only in individuals using protein in the liquid or powder form and not as lean meat or fish."[12] By October 1978, forty-six people had died after engaging in the fast, they had used a multitude of different liquid protein products that had proliferated in response to the popularity of the original one, Prolinn.[13] The Center for Disease Control and the Food and Drug Administration (FDA) were investigating and had found several factors in common among those who had died:

- They typically were consuming 300 to 600 calories a day, all of it from protein.
- The proteins were generally modified proteins or hydrolysates of collagen or gelatin.
- Eight of the deaths were known to have been caused by abnormal heart rhythms.
- Some patients had been under their doctors' supervision during the fast.[14]

Since 1977, the mechanism by which the liquid proteins and fasting cause death has been very much discussed, and a number of different elements have been suspected. Among the possibilities:

- That potassium deficiency causes the deaths.[15]
- That potassium deficiency does *not* cause the deaths.[16]
- That potassium deficiency causes the deaths but that it can't be corrected until a magnesium deficiency is first corrected[17] (this possibility is still being discussed in 1980.[18])
- That a deficiency of sulfur-containing amino acids is responsible.[19]
- That it's a copper deficiency.[20]
- That selenium might have something to do with it.[21]

By now the FDA has arrived at a ruling that "liquid protein" and other protein products promoted for use in weight reduction or as dietary supplements have to carry warning labels. Three types of warning are required, depending on how the product is promoted:

Food products deriving more than 50 percent of their calories from protein and promoted for weight reduction must carry the following label: "Warning: Very low calorie protein diets (below 800 Calories per day) may cause serious illness or death. DO NOT USE FOR WEIGHT REDUCTION WITHOUT MEDICAL SUPERVISION. Use with particular care if you are taking medication. Not for use by infants, children, or pregnant or nursing women."

Protein products promoted as part of a nutritionally balanced diet plan providing 800 Calories or more must declare: "Warning: Use only as directed in the diet plan described herewith. Do not use as the sole or primary source of calories for weight reduction."

Food products intended for dietary supplementation that derive more than 50 percent of their total caloric value from protein for purposes other than weight reduction must state on their labels: "Warning: Use this product as a food supplement only. Do not use for weight reduction."[22]

A hard lesson has been learned at great cost.

The moral. The protein-sparing fast, as promoted in *The Last Chance Diet*, looked good. A caution on the back cover read, "The diet and the products recommended in this book should be used only under medical supervision," and many patients did consult their doctors about it; but medical supervision was not enough to protect them. The bibliography of the book contained five pages of references to reliable authorities' works as published in reputable journals. The author, a physician, was a member of the American Medical Association. When you ask yourself "How can I tell when a product or a diet may be dangerous?" remember, it may be harder to tell than you think. But there were three clues here that might have helped. One was that the product and the diet had not been tested. No matter how good the logic on which an idea is based, the proof is in the actual application of the idea.

A second clue was that the book was a popular book written for the public, to make money. Book writers cannot be punished by law for publishing misinformation unless a court case shows that they have caused bodily harm. Seeing a statement in black and white on the pages of such a book is no guarantee that it is a fact. In fact, "because of the protection afforded by the First Amendment (Freedom of the Press), those who prey on the public do so not with products, but with books."[23]

A third clue was that the book was written by a physician. This may seem a strange criticism, but Controversy 14B: Doctors will show why physicians cannot be assumed to be reliable authorities on foods and diets.

Personal strategy. The story of the protein-sparing fast is the last in a long series of hoaxes perpetrated on the public by self-styled experts in nutrition who have something to gain by being believed. This particular diet has been exposed as a fraud and a hazard, and its popularity has been dying out. But this story has left unanswered the question of the person who is most likely to turn to this diet (or to the next one of its kind): the person who has tried everything else and despairs of losing weight except by drastic means.

A person who is motivated strongly enough to carry out such a plan would more profitably mount a massive attack on a weight problem on several fronts (see Chapter 8). Adopt a balanced, nutritious, low-calorie diet. Devote time and energy to intensive self-retraining, knowing that the first three weeks will be the hardest. Obtain family support. Join a reputable weight-loss group. Learn and use behavior modification techniques, possibly with the help of a specialist like a registered dietitian (R.D.). Start a regular exercise program. In short, mobilize all resources to maximize the chances of permanent success. The next two chapters provide an abundance of information that will be useful in such an effort.

The Controversy Notes and For Further Information follow the Appendixes.

CHAPTER 7

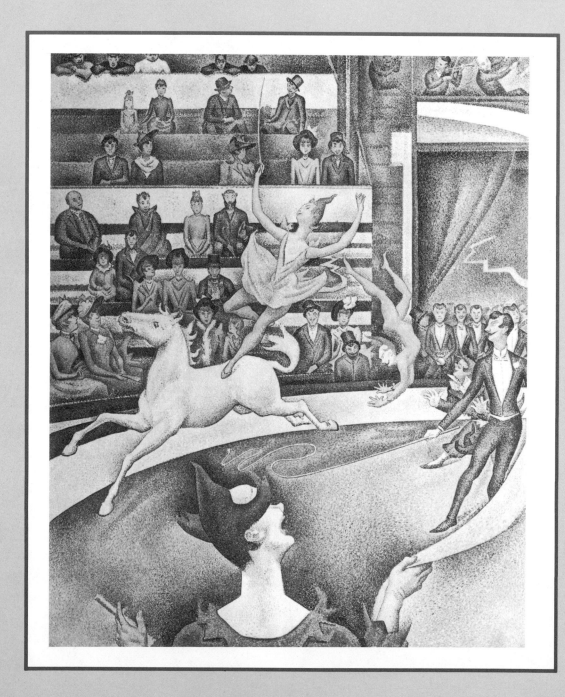

Energy Balance: Feasting, Fasting, Loafing, Exercise

When you eat too much you get fat; when you eat too little you get thin. When you exercise hard you gain muscle mass and may lose weight from fat deposits; when you loaf you may gain weight by increasing fat deposits even while you lose muscle mass. Everyone knows these simple facts, but nobody knows exactly how to account for them. The mission of this chapter is to shed some light on what we do know and to provide answers to some of the questions dieters and athletes often ask. What makes a person gain weight? Are carbohydrate-rich foods more fattening than other foods? What's the best way to lose weight: fasting? low-carbohydrate diets? The answers to these and many other questions lie in an understanding of **energy metabolism**—the processes by which the body stores or releases the energy from nutrients.

The last three chapters introduced and described the three kinds of nutrients the body uses for energy: carbohydrate, fat, and protein. These (and alcohol) are the only substances that give energy to the body. This chapter shows what the body does with these nutrients.

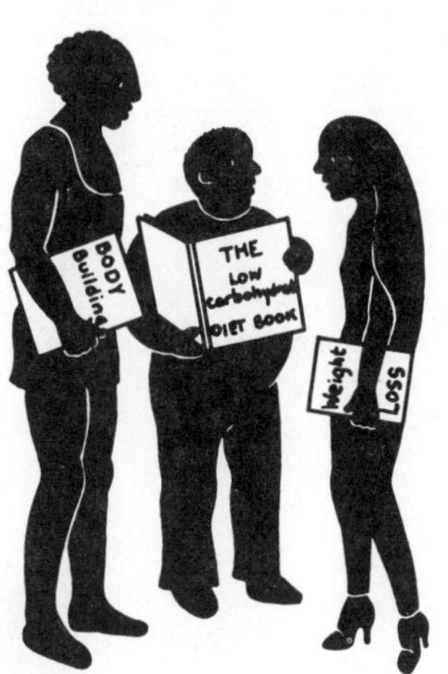

Diet rumors are everywhere.

Starting Points

A brief review of the facts already presented about the energy nutrients follows, to provide background.

Opposite: Le Cirque *by Georges Seurat, at the Musées Nationaux de Louvre, Paris. Used with permission.*

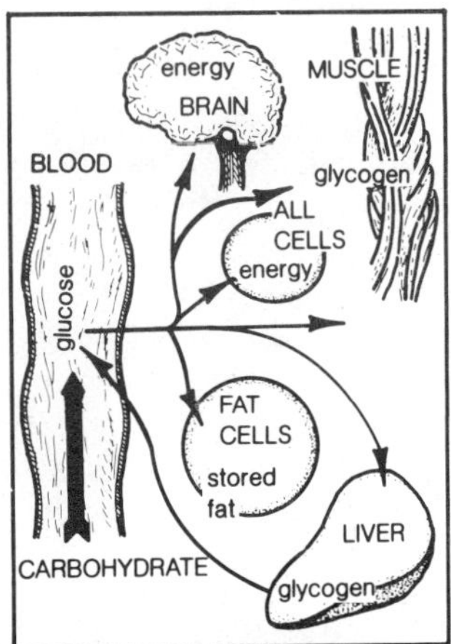

Main sources and uses of glucose under normal conditions. *Note that only two arrows point to glucose. All cells use glucose for energy; the brain is emphasized here because it tends to use only glucose. In these diagrams, the brain stands for all cells of the central nervous system.*

Carbohydrate. A carbohydrate is made of glucose or of monosaccharides that the body readily converts to glucose. Glucose is one of the two major fuels used by cells for energy (the other is fatty acids) and is the preferred, and usually the only, fuel for the cells of the brain and nervous system. In times of intensive exercise it becomes the preferred fuel of the muscles as well. Circulating at all times in the blood, and stored in the liver and muscles as glycogen, it is drawn upon continuously by the cells and oxidized within them.

The blood level of glucose is maintained by periodic eating of foods containing carbohydrate, by release of glucose from glycogen stored in the liver, and—if necessary—by conversion of amino acids from muscle and other tissue proteins. Excess glucose in the blood is drawn off and stored in liver and muscle cells as glycogen; if these stores become full, further excess is converted to fat and stored in fat cells.

Fat. Fats are mostly triglycerides: Each triglyceride is a trio of long fatty acids attached to a glycerol molecule. These enter the body and are stored by way of the complicated transport system described earlier (in Chapter 5), but this system does not concern us here. In the body, the fatty acids of triglycerides can be broken off at their attachment point to glycerol and then used as the cells' other major energy fuel. Fatty acids can be used for energy by all the body's cells except the brain, nerve, and red blood cells; and they are the preferred fuel for voluntary muscles, including the heart muscle, under conditions of low to moderate exercise. To maintain the fatty acid level in the blood, the fat cells can dismantle stored fat and release its fatty acids into the bloodstream.

The muscles' fuel during moderate activity is a mixture of glucose and fat, which requires oxygen to be burned. During intensive exercise, especially of long duration, the muscles shift to using only glucose from their stored glycogen, because oxygen isn't supplied fast enough to support fat oxidation.

MUSCLE FUEL:
Moderate exercise: glucose and fat.
Intensive exercise: glucose.

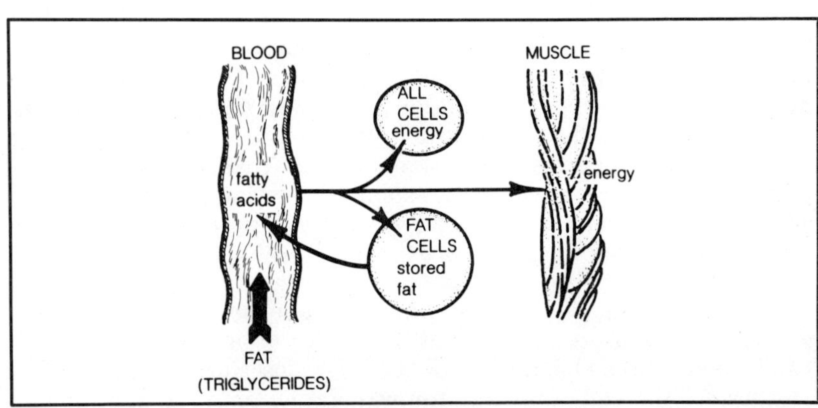

Fatty acid sources and uses. *All cells except brain, nerves, and red blood cells can use fatty acids for energy. Muscles are the principal users of this fuel. The fatty acid supply can be replenished by the diet or from fat stores (two arrows point to fatty acids).*

Protein. Protein is not normally used as fuel because it has important jobs to do, and no other nutrient can substitute for protein in doing those jobs. But energy is the body's top-priority need, and energy is needed in the form of both glucose and fatty acids. If the cells run out of glucose, body proteins will begin to break down, yielding amino acids which are stripped of their nitrogen-containing amine groups and used as fuel. About half of the amino acids can be converted to glucose and so can enter the brain and nerve cells and give up their energy to keep those cells going. The other half are converted to fragments like those from fatty acids, and these are used by the cells of the muscles and other tissues.

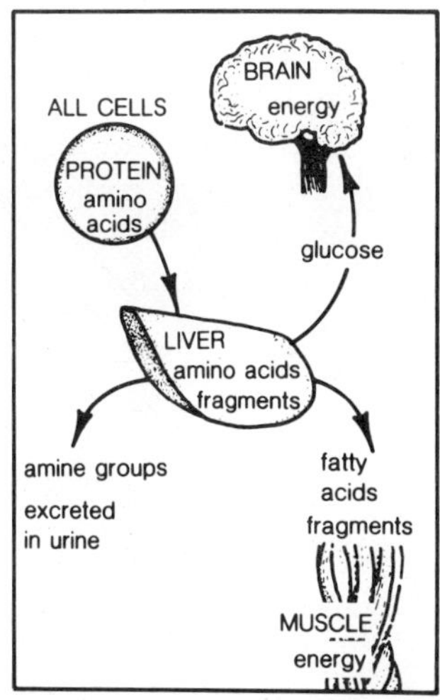

Fate of protein during energy deprivation. *Body protein breaks down, losing its nitrogen-containing amine groups, to provide energy for the body's cells. Fat fragments can also form ketones (see below).*

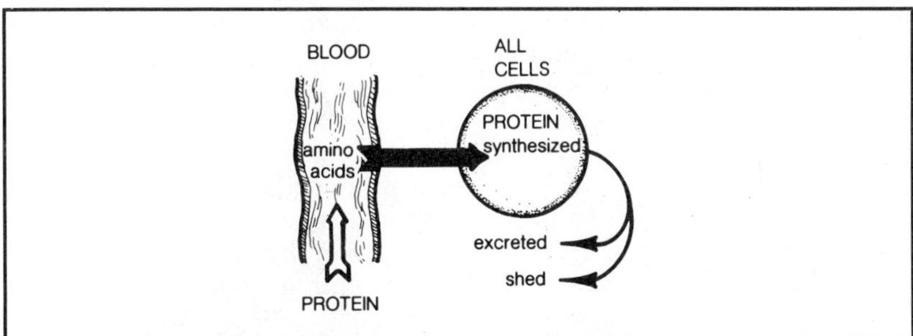

Principal use of protein: *To supply amino acids to build cell proteins. The arrows are shown going one way because cell proteins don't necessarily return amino acids to the blood. The reason you need to keep eating protein every day is because your body loses whole cells (for example, those that are shed from the GI tract lining and the skin) and because the cells secrete proteins that are lost from the body (such as hair, the proteins of sweat, and some of the enzymes from the digestive system). See Chapter 6 for more details.*

The body's balanced state. After a normal mixed meal, the body handles the nutrients in all of the ways just described. The carbohydrate yields glucose. Some is stored as glycogen, and some is taken into brain and nerve cells and oxidized for energy. Later, the glycogen is gradually released to keep the energy flow going. When it is used up, it is time to eat again.

At the same time, the fat consumed in the meal is partly stored as fat and partly broken down and used for energy. Several hours after the meal, fat is being returned from storage and used for energy. If you are achieving perfect energy balance, then by the time you eat again, you have used the same amount of fat you have taken in.

Meanwhile, if the protein amount in the meal was neither too much nor too little, the balance works out evenly for this nutrient, too. The protein yields amino acids, these enter cells to be incorporated into cell proteins, and the amounts made are sufficient to replace protein lost by way of shed cells (Chapter 6). Excess amino acids, beyond those needed for protein synthesis, lose their amine groups and are used as an energy source.

Of course this description of the balanced state is oversimplified. The glycogen you are drawing from stores may not be exactly the same glycogen that you just put away after the last meal (it could be yesterday's glycogen). And no one eats so perfectly on time that stores empty and fill to the same levels at every meal. But over many days' time such balances are achieved. The average person consumes more than a

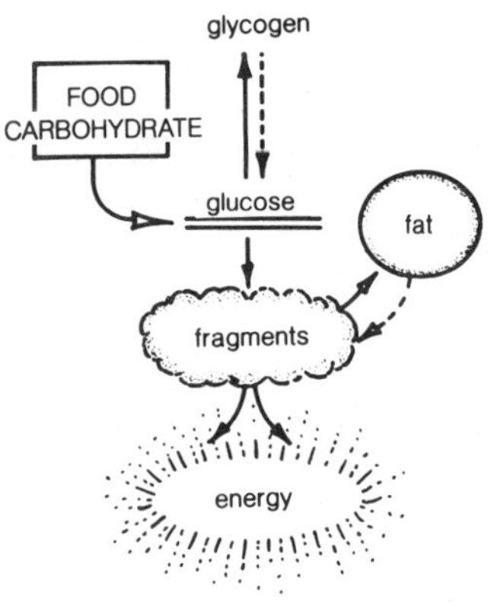

Feasting.

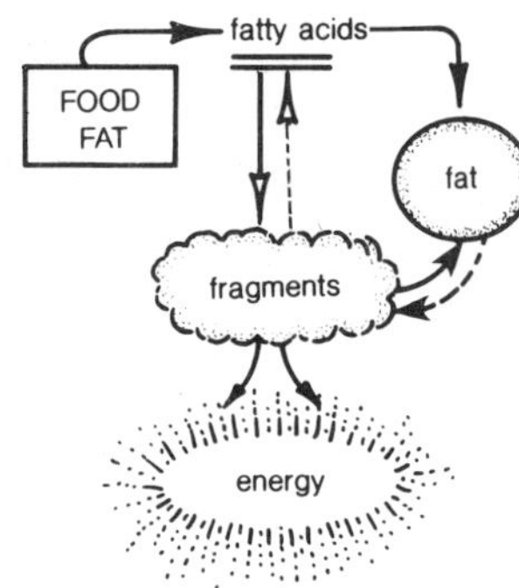

Feasting.

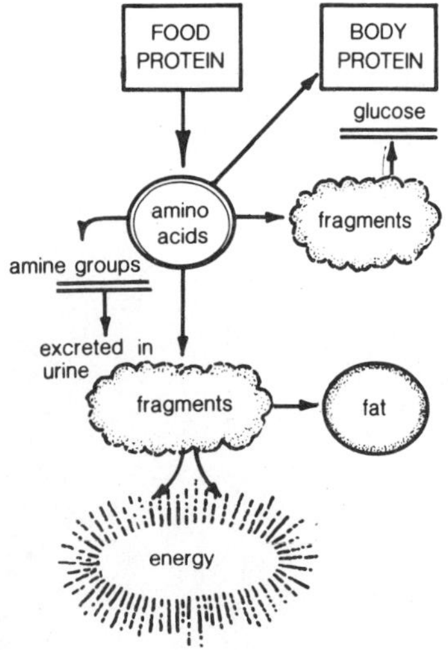

Feasting.

million calories a year and expends more than 99 percent of them, maintaining a stable weight for years on end.[1]

Still, some people get fat, others get too thin. The possible reasons *why* people may eat too much or too little are explored in the next chapter. What happens inside the body when they do is discussed here.

Feasting

The pathways of metabolism just described make it clear why consuming too much of any energy nutrient can make you fat. Surplus carbohydrate (glucose) can be stored as glycogen but there is a limit to the capacity of the glycogen-storing cells. Once glycogen stores are filled, the overflow is routed to fat. Fat cells expand as they fill; in a growing baby or child they multiply *and* expand. Thus excess carbohydrate, above and beyond the energy need, can contribute to obesity.

Of course, surplus fat in the diet can also contribute to the body's fat stores. It may break down to fragments on the way to oxidation for energy, but if energy flow is already rapid enough to meet the demand, these fragments will not enter the energy-yielding pathway. They will be diverted back again to the assembly of triglycerides and stored in the fat cells.

Surplus protein may encounter the same fate. If not needed to build body protein or to meet present energy needs, amino acids will lose their amine groups and become fragments indistinguishable from those used to build glucose and fat. These will fill the glycogen stores if needed, and the excess will be converted to triglycerides and stored in the fat cells, adding to the body's bulk and weight.

These facts have been repeated several times in different ways out of a mindfulness that information learned in the classroom often fails to transfer to life situations and that nutrition education in particular seldom operates at the dinner table. To help effect the transfer, it is necessary to think once more in terms of foods: Eating high-protein foods does not make you immune to gaining weight, nor does it force the body to build up more muscle mass. The most common error in the use of protein-rich foods in diets is to overlook their fat contents: Beef, ham, pork, and cheese are higher in fat than many people think they are. But there is another error people make—to think that lean meats and low-fat cheeses are not fattening. They are—if you eat enough of them or enough calories along with them.

High-protein, low-carbohydrate diets often advertise themselves as "eat-all-you-want" diets, as if protein calories didn't "count." Some people lose weight on these diets, but most regain the weight quickly. Those who do lose weight do so because they so soon find a constant diet of meat and fat unappealing that they wind up eating less food and so fewer calories. Those who don't lose weight don't lose it because they manage to keep on

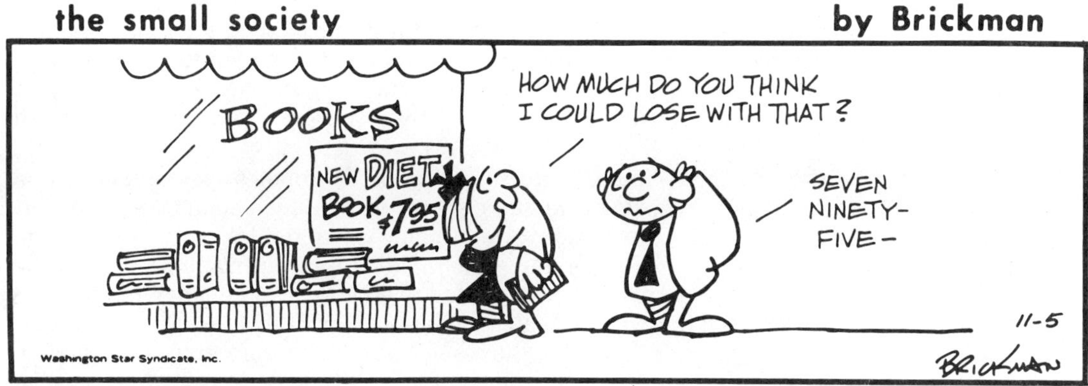
the small society
by Brickman
BOOKS
NEW DIET BOOK $7.95
HOW MUCH DO YOU THINK I COULD LOSE WITH THAT ?
SEVEN NINETY-FIVE -
11-5
Washington Star Syndicate, Inc.
BRICKMAN

eating the same number of calories as before, even without carbohydrate-containing foods.

The low-carbohydrate diet is based on many fallacies. This is one of them: that only carbohydrate calories "count." Others will be revealed in the pages that follow.

Fasting

Even when you are asleep and totally relaxed, the cells of many organs are hard at work spending energy. In fact, the work that you are aware of, that you do with your muscles during your waking hours, represents only about a third of the total energy you spend in a day. The rest is the metabolic work of the cells, for which they constantly require fuel.

Fuel must be delivered to every cell. After a meal, as a fast begins, both glucose and fatty acids are flowing into cells, breaking down, and delivering energy to power the cells' work. Several hours later, however, most of the glucose is used up, the available glycogen has been withdrawn from storage to replenish it, and this source in turn is being exhausted.

At this point, most of the cells are depending on fatty acids to continue providing their fuel. But the brain and nerve cells cannot; they still need glucose. (The problem is that the only nutrient that can get through their membranes is glucose. Once inside, this glucose breaks down and is processed the same way as in other cells.) Normally the brain and central nervous system consume about two-thirds of the total glucose used each day.

The brain's special requirement for glucose poses a problem for the fasting body. The body can use its stores of fat, which may be quite generous, to furnish most of its cells with energy, but for the brain it must supply energy in the form of glucose. This is why body protein tissues, such as liver and muscle cells, always break down to some

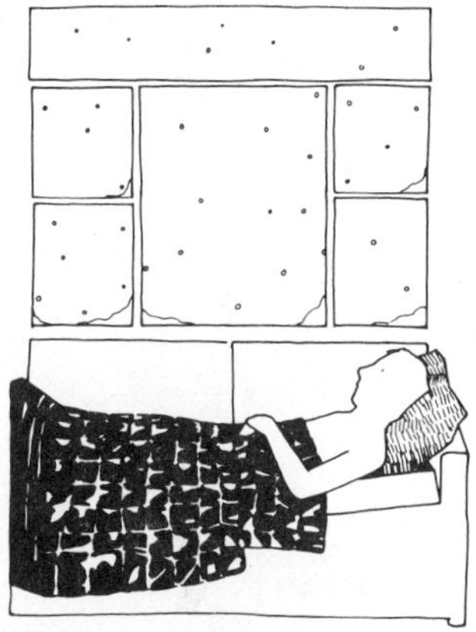

The body at rest spends many calories on metabolism.

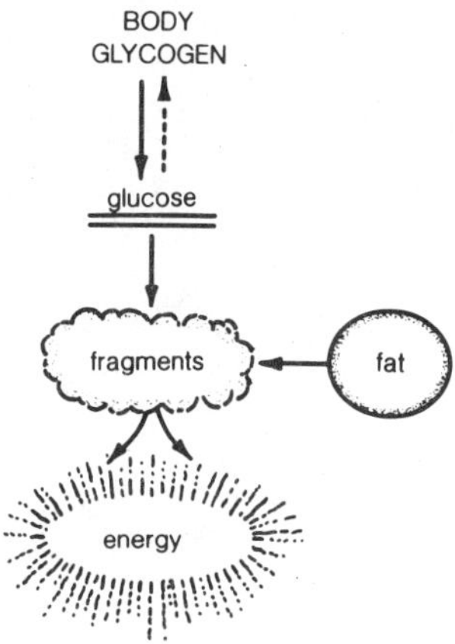

Fasting (early).

extent during fasting. Only half of the amino acids, after giving up their amine groups, yield skeletons that can be put together to make glucose; but to obtain them, whole proteins must be dismantled and the other half of the amino acids have to be disposed of. This is wasteful of protein.

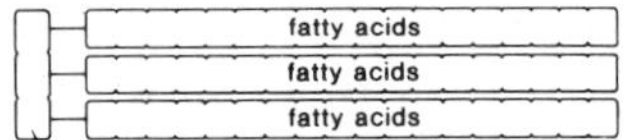

A triglyceride.

Only the tiny glycerol backbone in each giant triglyceride molecule can be converted to glucose, and it takes two glycerols to make a single glucose unit. This is why the fats are such an inefficient source of glucose. To get rid of the fatty acids released from the glycerol, the body has to make ketones.

To make matters worse, body fat is hopelessly inefficient as a glucose source: only the tiny glycerol backbone in each giant triglyceride molecule can be converted to glucose, and it takes two glycerols to make a single glucose unit. Fatty acids, representing 95 percent of the weight of fat, cannot be converted to glucose at all. Using the glycerols from fat in this way obligates the body to dispose of the large quantities of fatty acids released at the same time. Furthermore, in order for the energy from fatty acids to be released, carbohydrates (glucose) must be entering the energy cycle simultaneously. During fasting, after glycogen stores are exhausted, there is no available glucose in the body for this function. Therefore, the fatty acid fragments are converted into **ketone bodies**, eventually resulting in **ketosis**

In the first few days of a fast, body protein provides about 90 percent of the needed glucose, and glycerol about 10 percent. But if body protein loss were to continue at this rate, death would ensue within three weeks. Ketosis seems to be a state of adaptation to an undesirable situation (starvation), which serves as the better of two evils.

As the fast continues, then, the body adapts by condensing the fragments derived from fatty acids into ketones. Meanwhile, an adaptation takes place in the brain as well. Some of the nerve cells become able to use the ketones as fuel. Ketone production rises until, at the end of several weeks, it is meeting about half or more of the brain's energy needs. Still, many areas of the brain rely exclusively on glucose, and body protein continues to be sacrificed to produce it.[2] A hazard of ketosis is that ketones may be produced in greater quantities than can be used or excreted in the urine, so they accumulate in the blood. Because they are organic acids, their accumulation leads to acidosis, which can disturb many body functions.

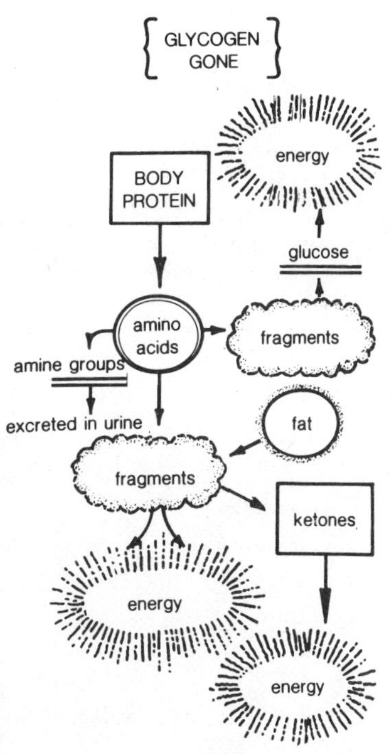

Fasting (ketosis).

Simultaneously, the body drastically reduces its energy output in order to conserve both its fat and lean tissue. As the lean (protein-containing) organ tissue shrinks in mass, it performs less metabolic work, reducing energy needs. As the muscles waste, they do less work, enhancing this effect. Because of the slowed metabolism, the loss of fat falls to a bare minimum—less, in fact, than the fat that would be lost on a low-calorie diet. Thus, although weight loss during fasting may be quite dramatic, fat loss may be less than when at least some food is supplied.

Marasmus. The adaptations just described also occur in the starving child and help to prolong its life. The severe malnutritional state resulting from starvation is termed *marasmus.* Together with protein deficiency, it is the most widespread malnutrition problem in the world. Children with marasmus suffer symptoms similar to those of children with the protein-deficiency disease *kwashiorkor*, since both cause loss of body protein tissue; differences are that kwashiorkor children retain some of their stores of body fat (because they are still consuming calories), accumulate fat in their livers (because they can't make protein to carry it away), and develop edema (from protein lack). Marasmus children experience ketosis to conserve body protein, while kwashiorkor children do not, because they are receiving some carbohydrate; so kwashiorkor is actually a less balanced state and a more fatal disease than marasmus for children at any given age.

A marasmic child looks like a wizened little old person—just skin and bones. The child is often sick, because its resistance to disease is low. All the muscles are wasted, including the heart muscle, and the heart is weak. Metabolism is so slow that body temperature is subnormal. There is little or no fat under the skin to insulate against cold. The experience of hospital workers with victims of this disease is that their primary need is to be wrapped up and kept warm. They also need love, because they have often been deprived of maternal attention as well as food.

Unlike the kwashiorkor child, who is fed milk until weaning, the marasmic child may have been neglected from early infancy. The disease occurs most commonly in children from six to eighteen months of age in all the overpopulated city slums of the world. Since the brain normally grows to almost its full adult size within the first two years of life, marasmus impairs brain development and so may have a permanent effect on learning ability.

Marasmus also occurs in adults in countries where calorie deficiency is prevalent and in recent years has also been seen to occur in many undernourished hospital patients. Adults also bring it on themselves when they fast or eat too little food for too long a time, whether to lose weight or for religious, philosophical, or political reasons.

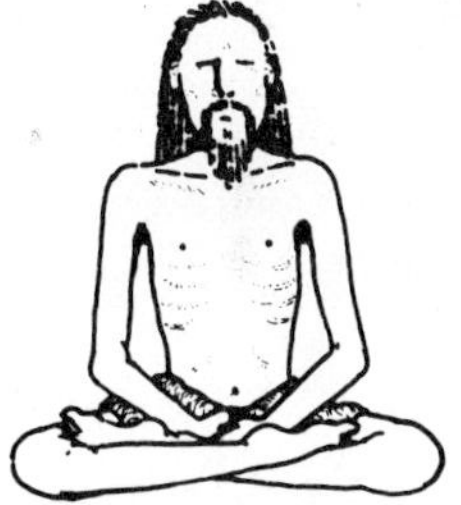

Marasmus = consuming your body's protein and fat.

The low-carbohydrate diet. A similar economy prevails if a low-carbohydrate diet is consumed. Advocates of the low-carbohydrate diet would have you believe that there is something magical about ketosis which promotes faster weight loss than a regular low-calorie diet. In fact, however, the low-carbohydrate diet presents the same problem as a fast. Once the body's available glycogen reserves are spent, the only appreciable source of energy-in-the-form-of-glucose is protein. The low-carbohydrate diet provides a little protein from food, but some protein must still be taken from body tissue to meet the demand for glucose. The onset of ketosis is the signal that this wasting process has begun.

Another problem with the low-carbohydrate diet is that it is necessarily a high-fat diet, too, because high-protein animal foods donate about half of their calories as fat. These fat calories, just like those from body fat, require glucose for their entrance into the energy cycle and so contribute to the ketone load. The advocates of the diet would have you believe that all this helps you lose weight because ketones excreted in urine carry calories with them out of the body, and it is true that ketones represent unused calories from body fat. However, the amount of energy lost in ketones seldom approaches even 100 calories a day and so could not promote weight loss at a rate faster than a pound every one or two months.

Low-carbohydrate diet = eating protein and fat.

In case you are wondering what "the" low-carbohydrate diet is, it should be explained here that *any* diet that has certain characteristics qualifies as a low-carbohydrate diet. The diet has masqueraded under many different names for fifty years or more, ever since weight loss became fashionable. One of its most often used aliases is the "Mayo" diet (which has nothing to do with the famous and highly respectable Mayo Clinic, but is said to have been invented by a man whose last name was Mayo and whose first name —on his birth certificate—was "Doctor"). Other names are the Air Force diet, the Drinking Man's diet, the "Calories Don't Count" diet, the grapefruit diet, the Atkins diet, the Ski Team diet, the Stillman diet, the Scarsdale diet —the list is endless. Under all of these guises, it can be recognized as a diet that restricts carbohydrates, either by requiring that carbohydrate grams be counted; by forbidding the use of breads, potatoes, pasta and other starchy foods; or by limiting the foods permitted to a list of meats, high-fat items, and alcoholic beverages consisting of hard liquor but not wine or sugar-containing mixers. By whatever name, the diet is to be avoided.

This warning is most urgent for the pregnant woman. The fetus's developing nervous system can metabolize only glucose for energy and can suffer irreparable damage if deprived of this fuel for even a short period of time.

Not only pregnant women, however, but all adults are warned not to diet this way. The diet raises blood uric acid, disposing the person to gout.[3] It lowers blood potassium, causing irregular heartbeats.[4] It causes sodium loss and consequent dehydration.[5] It causes fatigue and blood pressure abnormalities[6] and aggravates kidney problems.[7] It causes pronounced elevation of serum cholesterol concentration, a known risk factor for heart disease.[8]

Proponents of the low-carbohydrate diet have been extraordinarily irresponsible in ignoring these hazards. For example, R. C. Atkins is quoted as saying, "Of the thousands of people on my diet, *only 30 percent* . . . show any increase [in serum cholesterol]. . . . There's one other point that I'm sorry about. I recommended the diet during pregnancy. I now understand that ketosis in pregnancy could result in fetal damage."[9] (Emphasis added.)

In a diet that provides fewer than about 900 calories (for the average-size adult), it is pointless to supply any protein at all, because the protein will only be wasted to provide energy. Body protein is lost at the same rate in adults at that calorie level whether or not they are given any food protein.[10]

One conclusion to draw from all this is that a person who diets at the level of 900 calories a day might as well eat carbohydrate and fat alone, without protein. Carbohydrate-containing foods are less expensive than protein-rich foods, and both will serve the same purpose—supplying glucose. This is the choice made by the person on a juice fast, for juices contain only carbohydrate. But a wiser conclusion is that such a diet is unnecessarily low in calories, even dangerously so. The person who wishes to lose body *fat* will select a balanced diet of 1200 or more calories, one containing carbohydrate, fat, *and* protein. At this level, body protein will be spared, ketosis need not occur, vital lean tissues (including both muscle and brain) will not starve, and only the unwanted *fat* will be lost.

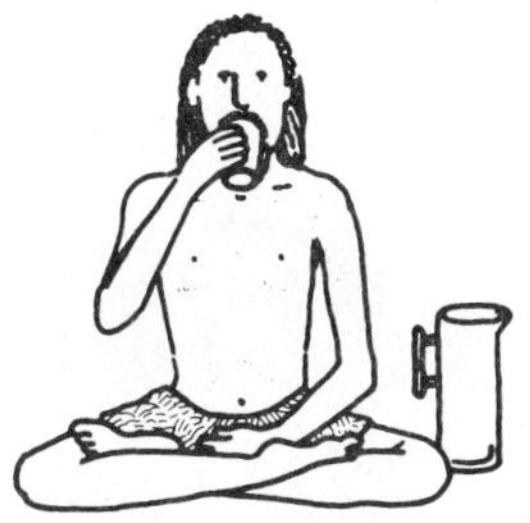

Juice fast = consuming carbohydrate to spare body protein.

People are attracted to the low-carbohydrate diet because of the dramatic weight loss it brings about within the first few days. They would be disillusioned if they realized that the major part of this weight loss is a loss of body protein with quantities of water and important minerals. A woman who boasts of losing seven pounds in two days on her diet may be unaware that at best she has lost a pound or two of fat and five or six of lean tissue, water, and minerals. When she goes "off" her diet, her body will avidly devour and retain these needed materials to restore its lean tissue, and her weight will zoom back to within a few pounds of where she started. The person willing to face the facts of nutrition and metabolism will learn to beware of those who promote quick-weight-loss schemes and to distinguish between loss of *fat* and loss of *weight*.

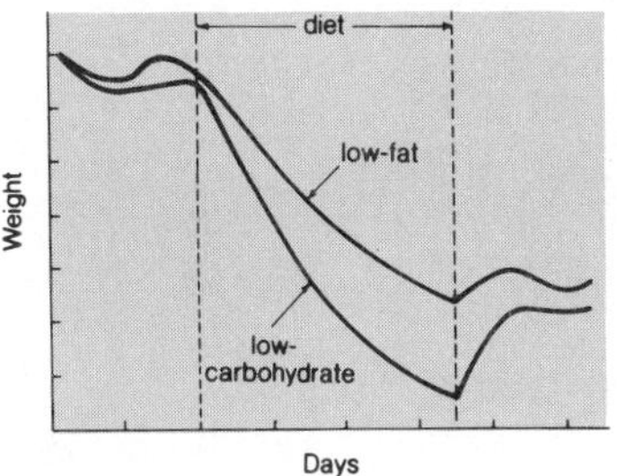

Weight loss during diets. The graph shows that some of the weight lost on a low-carbohydrate diet is "illusory" weight and is regained as soon as the diet is over. The amount of fat lost on both diets is virtually the same.

Adapted from S. B. Lewis, J. D. Wallin, J. P. Kane, and J. E. Gerich, *Effect of diet composition on metabolic adaptations to hypocaloric nutrition: Comparison of high carbohydrate and high fat isocaloric diets*, American Journal of Clinical Nutrition *30 (1977): 160-169.*

The protein-sparing fast. A variant on fasting is eating only protein. The hope is that the protein will spare lean tissue and that body fat will be broken down at a maximal rate to meet other energy needs. You may suspect that this is not so different from the low-calorie diet and will guess that this protein—together with the body's lean tissues—will be used to provide glucose. You are probably right. The idea sounded good when it was first advanced, but it has met with mixed results. It seems to become effective only after considerable lean tissue has already been lost, at which time the body may be conserving itself quite efficiently anyway; and the fast has not been shown more effective than a mixture of protein and carbohydrate. Furthermore, it doesn't seem to "stick" very well; most people regain the lost weight.[11] Thus the protein-sparing fast has to be judged at best a very moderate success and at worst a failure, for the ultimate criterion of success in any weight-loss program is maintenance of the new low weight.

Protein-sparing fast = eating only protein to spare body protein.
See Controversy 6 for the hazards of liquid protein diets.

The term *protein-sparing* has also been used in another connection. Malnourished hospital patients also lose body protein, and this is especially likely—and especially dangerous—if they are simultaneously fighting infection. The knowledgeable physician makes every effort to prevent the loss of vital lean tissue and supplies amino acids as well as glucose by some means—through a vein if the patient can't eat. No more than about 600 calories can be supplied in a day this way, so (as you would expect) the amino acids are used as glucose, not to build protein. But there is an advantage to using amino acids rather than glucose in this instance. The amino acids elicit less insulin secretion, and less insulin means that fat can come more easily out of storage. This helps to spare the patient's precious lean tissue. The main virtue of using protein-sparing therapy here, however, is that there is no better choicc. The doctor can't in any case provide more than a pitifully small ration; feeding 1200 calories is not an option.

The effort to provide protein-sparing *therapy* in these circumstances has met with notable success and has significantly reduced the death and disease rate in cases of severe hospital malnutrition. These praiseworthy efforts should not be confused with the profiteering efforts of faddists to sell the protein-sparing *fast.*

Moderate weight loss. The body's cells and the enzymes within them make it their task to convert the energy nutrients you eat into those you need. They are extraordinarily versatile and relieve you of having to compute exactly how much carbohydrate, fat, and protein to eat at each meal. As you have seen, they can convert either carbohydrate (glucose) or protein to fat. To some extent, they can convert protein to glucose. To a very limited extent, they can even convert fat (the glycerol portion) to glucose. But a grossly unbalanced diet or one that is severely limited in calories imposes hardships on the body. If calories are too low or if carbohydrate and protein calories are undersupplied, the body is forced to degrade its own lean tissue to meet its glucose need.

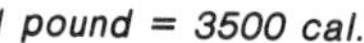
1 pound = 3500 cal.

People who want to lose body fat must reconcile themselves to a hard fact: There is a limit to the rate at which this fat tissue will break down. The maximum rate that can be sustained for more than a few weeks, except for a very large person, is one to two pounds a week. To achieve this kind of weight loss, the sensible course is to adopt a balanced low-calorie diet supplying all three energy nutrients in reasonable amounts and possibly to increase energy expenditure by getting more exercise. In effect, this means adjusting the energy budget so that intake is 500 to 1000 calories per day less than output. A person who wants to *gain* weight needs to make the opposite adjustment. It might seem that both efforts would require tedious counting of calories, but the following Food Feature shows that shortcuts are possible.

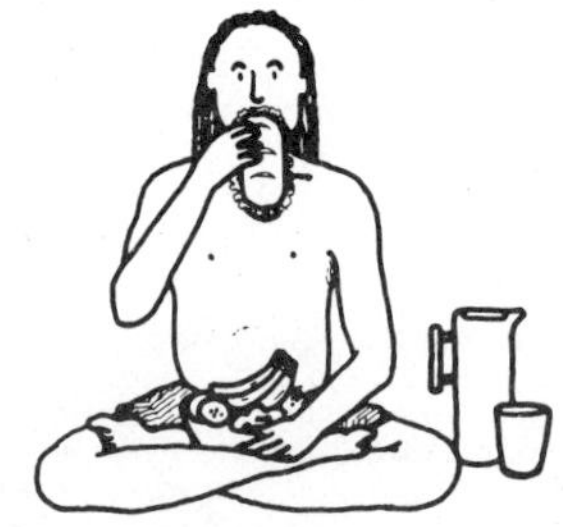
Balanced, low-calorie diet.

Food Feature: Counting Calories

Looking up every food in calorie charts is time consuming, and only the most motivated will persist at it for any prolonged period of time. For the rest of us who wish to keep track of calories, some acquaintance with the exchange system provides a simpler method. The foods depicted in the margin could be found one by one in Appendix H, but it's quicker to translate them into exchanges and add up the calorie values to get a rough idea. It is suggested that you do this and time yourself. With some practice, you can look at any plate of food and "sense" the number of calories it represents. The calorie amounts to remember are:

1 milk exchange—80 calories (for whole milk, add 2 fat exchanges).

1 vegetable exchange—25 calories.

1 fruit exchange—40 calories.

1 bread exchange—70 calories.

1 meat exchange—55 calories (for medium-fat meat, add ½ fat exchange; for high-fat meat, add 1 fat exchange).

1 fat exchange—45 calories.

So how many calories are in the meal in the margin? The answer is at the end of the chapter.

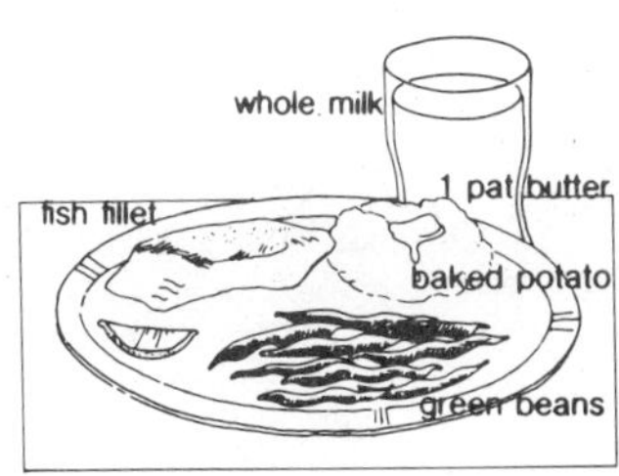

How many calories?

Energy Output

For every 3500 calories extra—above and beyond energy needs—that you eat, you can gain a pound of body fat; and for every 3500 calories that you *spend*—beyond your energy intake—you can lose a pound of fat. One of the questions people often ask is, "How many calories am I spending in my various activities?" The answer comes in three parts. Energy is spent for (1) basal metabolism, (2) muscular activity, and (3) assimilation of food.

(1) Basal metabolism. Most of the energy the average person spends goes to support the ongoing metabolic work of the body's cells, the **basal metabolism**. This is the work that goes on in the body all the time, without conscious awareness. The beating of the heart, the inhaling of oxygen and the exhaling of carbon dioxide, the maintenance of body temperature, and the sending of nerve and hormonal messages to direct these automatic activities are the basal processes that maintain life. The energy needs for these processes must be met before any calories can be used for physical activity or for the digestion of food.

Basal metabolic needs are surprisingly large. A woman whose total energy needs are 2000 calories a day spends as many as 1200 to 1400 of them maintaining her basal metabolic processes. Most people don't realize that so much of their energy is going to support the basic work of their bodies' cells, because they are unaware of all the work these cells do to maintain life.

The **basal metabolic rate** is influenced by a number of factors. In general, the younger a person is, the higher the basal metabolic rate. This seems to be due to the increased activity of cells undergoing division, because it is most pronounced during the growth spurts that take place during infancy, puberty, and pregnancy. After growth stops, the rate decreases by about 2 percent per decade throughout life.[12] Body surface area also influences metabolic rate. Research has shown that it is indeed surface area, not weight, that is crucial. The greater the amount of body surface area, the faster the metabolism. Thus, of two people with different shapes who weigh the same amount, the shorter, fatter person will have a slower metabolic rate than the taller, thinner person. The taller, thinner person has a greater skin surface from which heat is lost by radiation and so must have faster metabolism to generate heat to replace it.

Both weigh the same, but the tall, thin structure will lose more heat to the surroundings.

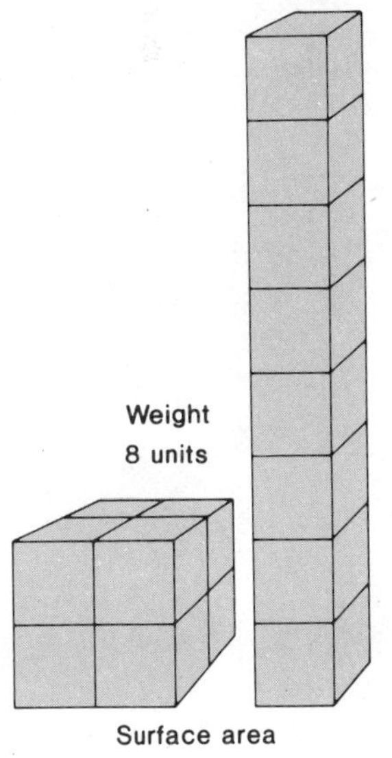

A third factor that influences metabolic rate is gender. Males generally have a faster metabolic rate than females. It is thought that this may be due to the greater percentage of lean tissue in the male body. Muscle tissue is highly active even when it is resting, whereas fat tissue is comparatively inactive.

Fever also increases the energy needs of cells. Their increased activities to fight off infection require more energy, and generate more heat, than normal.

Fasting and constant malnutrition lower the metabolic rate, partly due to the loss of lean tissues as well as to the shutdown of functions the body can't afford to support. This slowing of metabolism seems to be a protective mechanism to conserve energy when there is a shortage, and it hampers weight loss in a person who fasts or undertakes a too-strict diet.

Some glandular secretions influence metabolism. The adrenal glands secrete the hormone epinephrine into the blood in response to stress. The stress may be caused by as simple a situation as the command "Hurry, or you'll be late to work" or by as threatening a dilemma as the discovery of an intruder in the house. Whatever the cause, the body reacts by marshaling all its forces to meet the emergency. The increase in epinephrine increases the energy demands of every cell and thus temporarily raises the metabolic rate. This partly accounts for the weight loss you see in people experiencing extreme stress in their lives, although other factors also enter in (upset digestion causes loss of appetite).

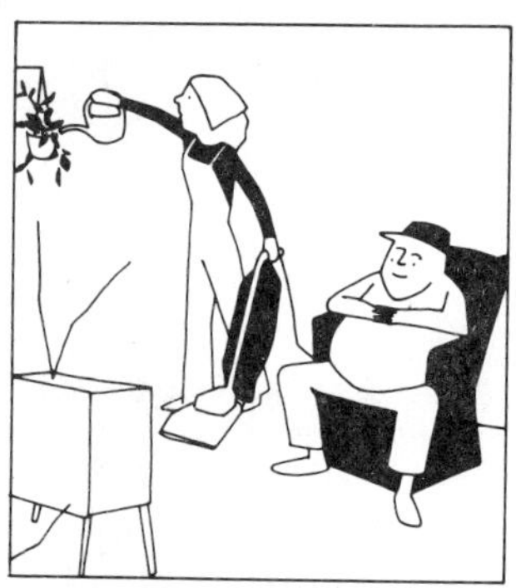

The metabolic rate influences behavior.

The activity of the thyroid gland has a direct influence on the basal metabolic rate. The less thyroxin secreted, the lower the energy requirement for maintenance of basal functions. Some persons move about their tasks in a slow, deliberate fashion, partly because of lower activity of their thyroid glands. Others race through the day, breaking dishes and becoming irritable, partly because of thyroid oversecretion. The difference in the two personalities, then, may reflect a difference in their basal metabolic rates.

To sum up, basal metabolic rate is higher in the young, in people with a large surface area, in males, in people with fever or under stress, and in people with high thyroid gland activity. It is lowered by increasing age, fasting, and malnutrition.

(2) Physical activity. Physical, muscular activity does not make such a big contribution to most people's energy output. It amounts to only about 30 percent of the total for most people. But unlike basal metabolism, which can't be changed, physical activity can be increased at will. If you want to tinker with your energy balance, this is the only component—on the output side—that you can alter significantly.

The energy spent on physical activity is the energy spent moving the body's skeletal muscles—the muscles of the arms, back, abdomen, legs, and so forth—and the extra energy spent to speed up the heartbeat and respiration rate as needed. Not all "active" people are active in this calorie-spending sense. The number of calories needed for an activity depends entirely on the involvement of the muscles. The greater the amount of muscular work, the heavier the weight being moved, and the longer the time the activity is engaged in, the more calories are spent. Table 1 shows the energy costs of various activities.

As disheartening as it may be for a college student to discover, mental activity requires very little energy, even though it may make you very tired. Studying for an exam may be hard work, but it won't burn off body fat. People who are very, very busy—writing letters, making phone calls, riding in their cars from place to place—may wonder why they tend to gain weight, because they think of themselves as active people. They may be socially active, or intellectually active, but this activity involves few muscles and therefore little energy expenditure.

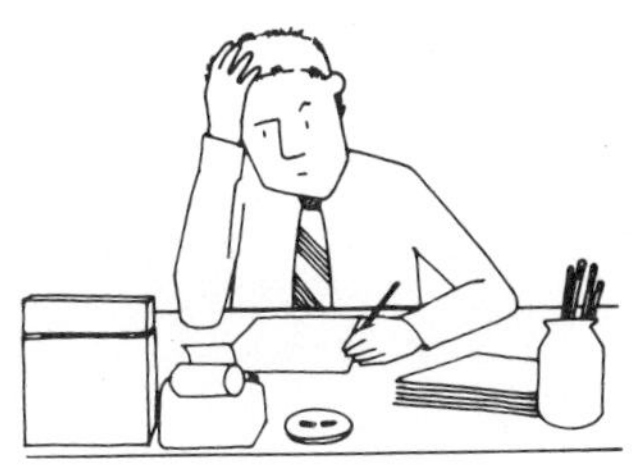

28 calories per hour.

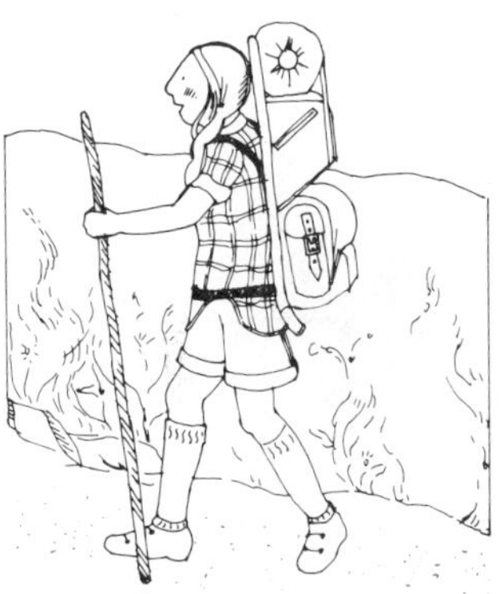

120 calories per hour.

As people age, their activities taper off somewhat. This slowing down varies greatly from one person to the next but averages out in such a way that people's total energy needs (including basal metabolic needs) probably decrease by about 5 percent per decade after the age of twenty.

(3) Assimilating food. The third component of energy expenditure has to do with managing food. When food is taken into the body, many cells that had been dormant begin to be active. The muscles that move the food through the intestinal tract speed up their rhythmic contractions; the cells that manufacture and secrete digestive juices begin their tasks. All these cells and others need extra energy as they "come alive" to participate in the digestion, absorption, and metabolism of food. In addition, the presence of food stimulates the general metabolism. This stimulation is the **specific dynamic effect (SDE)** of food, or the **specific dynamic activity (SDA)**, and is generally thought to represent about 6 to 10 percent of the total food energy taken in.

Food faddists make a big thing out of the specific dynamic effect, suggesting that a high-protein diet stimulates such tremendous energy losses that it will increase the rate of weight loss. Actually, high-protein and low-protein diets have the same effect.[13]

Total energy output. A typical breakdown of the total energy spent by a moderately active person (for example, a student who walks back and forth to classes) might look like this:

(1) Energy for basal metabolism:	1400 calories
(2) Energy for physical activity:	500 calories
(3) Energy spent assimilating 2000 calories of food:	200 calories
Total:	2100 calories

The first is the largest component—and you can't change it. The third is small and is affected little if at all by changes in diet. The second—physical activity—is the one you can change, and it is the subject of the last section of this chapter.

The most recent edition of the Recommended Dietary Allowances (RDA) for energy has abandoned the use of exact numbers of calories for each age-sex group. In 1978 it stated an energy allowance for "males, 23-50, 5 feet 9 inches tall, 154 pounds," as "2700 cal per day." In 1980 it changed the allowance to read "2700 cal—with a range of from 2300 to 3100 cal per day." This change acknowledges the immense differences in lifestyles and metabolism among people and leaves it to you to work out your energy balance knowing only the very wide range within which your output probably falls. There is an easy way to do this, though: Weigh yourself. Then comes the hard part. As stated in the *Dietary Guidelines*, if you are overweight "you must take in fewer calories than you burn. This means that you must either select foods containing fewer calories or you must increase your activity—or both."

The RDAs for energy are shown in Appendix I.

Increasing energy output. Table 1 shows the amount of energy a 150-pound person uses in an hour on various activities. Remembering that a pound of body fat stores 3500 calories, you may be impressed to see how small these numbers are. Even the most vigorous physical exertion, for a full hour, incurs an expense of only 900 calories. An hour of lawn mowing would consume less than a tenth of a pound of body fat. Obviously there is no way that you can go out and "work off" many pounds of excess body fat: You have to control the calorie input side, too. It is also obvious that only regular, frequent, and sustained exercise will make a difference in body weight. One hour of volleyball will have no detectable effect, but one hour of volleyball every other day for

Table 1. Approximate Energy Expenditure by a 150-Pound Person in Various Activities

Activity	Calories per Hour
Lying down or sleeping	80
Sitting	100
Driving an automobile	120
Standing	140
Domestic work	180
Walking, 2½ mph	210
Bicycling, 5½ mph	210
Gardening	220
Golf; lawn mowing, power mower	250
Bowling	270
Walking, 3¾ mph	300
Swimming, ¼ mph	300
Square dancing, volleyball, roller skating	350
Wood chopping or sawing	400
Tennis	420
Skiing, 10 mph	600
Squash and handball	600
Bicycling, 13 mph	660
Running, 10 mph	900

From the USDA/USDHHS Dietary Guidelines. Based on material prepared by Robert E. Johnson, M.D., Ph.D., and colleagues, University of Illinois.

three weeks will consume a pound of fat—and one hour of volleyball every other day for a year can make a fifteen- to twenty-pound difference.

When people realize that they want to make exercise a regular part of their lives, they become interested in their body structure, their muscles, and the contributions nutrition makes to athletics. Sometimes they fall in with trainers who know very little about nutrition or are influenced by faddists whose nutrition offerings are mostly misinformation. What athletes really need in the way of diet is the subject for Controversy 7.[1]

Answer to Food Feature Problem

We figure about 530 calories for the meal in the margin:

The milk (1 cup) is 1 milk exchange plus 2 fat exchanges	=	170 cal
The beans (½ cup) are a vegetable exchange	=	25 cal
The potato (one small) is a bread exchange	=	70 cal
The butter on it (one pat) is a fat exchange	=	45 cal
The fish (4 oz) is four lean-meat exchanges, assuming no fat is added	=	220 cal
The lemon wedge is negligible	=	0 cal
		530 cal

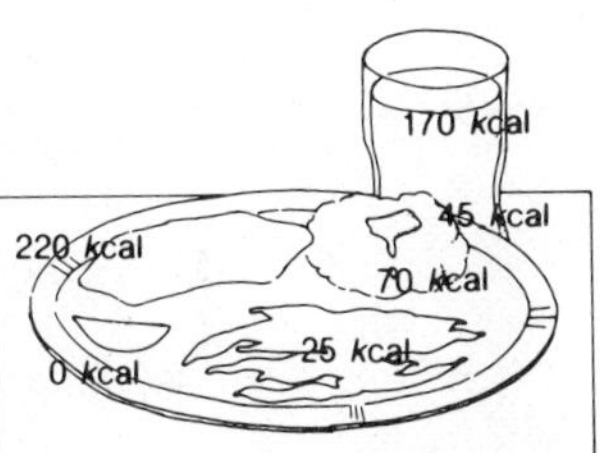

The answer: about 530 calories.

For Further Information

What happens when you fast is lucidly described in an article in *Scientific American:*

- Young, V. R., and Scrimshaw, N. S. The physiology of starvation. *Scientific American* 225 (1971): 14-21

The recommended references listed in Appendix J contain additional information on energy metabolism and nutritional imbalances associated with weight gains and losses.

[1] *Chapter Notes can be found at the end of the Appendixes.*

Controversy 7

Athletes

Do athletes need a special diet?

If you are serious about excelling in athletics you will do everything you can to promote your own success. And you will have many questions about diet. You have no doubt heard conflicting claims from different people—the coach, your fellow athletes, your nutrition-minded friends. One person will tell you to eat a high-protein diet because your muscles are made of protein. Another will tell you to eat a high-carbohydrate diet because muscles prefer carbohydrate as fuel. You may have had much advice about the use of protein powders, vitamin pills, and ergogenic foods. To prepare for an event, you may be urged to eat an enormous steak, or to drink only fruit juice and honey, or not to eat or drink at all. The subject of nutrition for athletes abounds with controversy and misinformation.

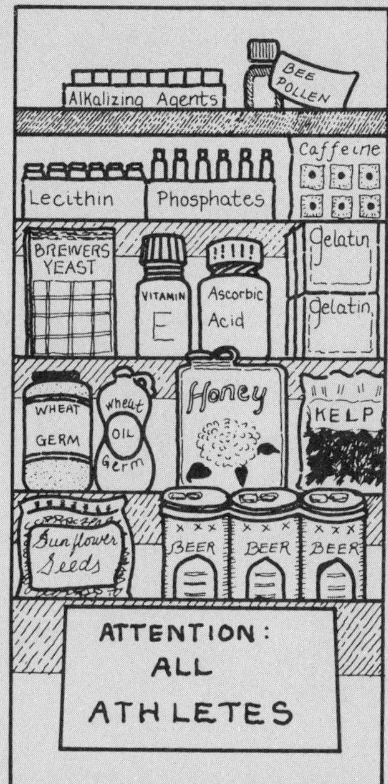

None of these foods or supplements is "ergogenic," no matter what the ads tell you.[1]

Much of what you may have heard about nutrition for athletes dates back so far that its origins are untraceable. As long ago as 500 B.C., trainers were advising athletes on what and when to eat and drink. Advice given to athletes today is a mixture of tradition, superstition, and scientific fact. Here, an attempt is made to sort the facts from the fantasies and give you some reliable references in case you would like to read further.

What builds muscles? Athletes have more muscles; exercise involves muscles; muscles are made of protein. It would seem, then, that athletes might need more protein than other people. This idea seems logical, but like so many ideas that seem logical, it doesn't stand up to scientific testing. The bodies of athletes contain more muscle than the bodies of nonathletes, and muscles do contain more protein than other tissues. But muscles are mostly (70 percent) water, and only half of the dry weight is protein, so there's less protein involved than you might think. To *maintain* muscle protein (that is, to replace the protein or nitrogen lost from it in a day) you need eat only as much total protein (nitrogen) as you lose, and an athlete loses only a little more than a nonathlete. This is probably not because of the greater muscle mass of the athlete, but because athletic events are stressful. Stress of any kind causes protein loss, but there is a stress factor built into the protein recommendations for all people, and they are high enough for the athlete.

To *build* muscle, you have to be in positive nitrogen balance (this was explained in Chapter 6), but even that doesn't mean you need to eat more protein. Unless you are very unusual, your diet already contains about twice as much protein as you can possibly use, and you are actually wasting about half of the protein you eat, in the sense that you are using it not to build body protein but rather for energy—a purpose any other energy nutrient could serve just as well, and less expensively.

There is no way that you can force extra protein into your muscles to make them grow just by eating more protein. Cells don't respond to what's given to them by helplessly accepting it. Actually, the way cells, including muscle cells, work is to respond to the demands put upon them and to select, from what is offered, what they need in order to perform. So the way to make muscle cells grow is to put a demand on them—that is, to make them work. They will respond by taking up nutrients, protein included, so that they can grow. In summary, don't *push* protein at them, but exercise them in order to demand that they *pull* protein in for themselves. Then make sure that protein is available by eating a diet that is adequate in protein. There's no need to make the diet "super-adequate" (whatever that might mean) and no advantage in doing so.[2]

A technique some athletes have used to try to increase muscle mass is to take hormone preparations designed to duplicate the hormones of puberty (androgens or anabolic steroids), which favor muscle development in growing boys. The evidence on their effectiveness has been reviewed, and the consensus seems to be that they are ineffective when used alone.[3] They may seem effective when used in conjunction with hard physical conditioning and increased food intake, but the effects seen under these circumstances are

Miniglossary

aerobic: Refers to processes requiring oxygen. Aerobic exercise is exercise performed at an intensity that causes oxygen intake and transport (breathing and heartbeat) to be speeded up (*aero* means "air, oxygen").

amenorrhea (ay-men-or-REE-uh): Failure to menstruate, reflecting a halted ovulatory cycle (*a* means "without"). *Athletic amenorrhea* refers to this problem in women athletes.

anaerobic: Refers to processes that do not require oxygen, like the first steps in the breakdown of glucose for energy (*an* means "without").

anabolic steroids: Hormones, produced normally in males during puberty, that bring about maturation; dangerous when used by athletes to try to promote muscular development (*anabole* means "building up"). Also known as *androgens* (*andro* means "man"; *gen* means "giving rise to").

ergogenic: A term used to refer to foods that are supposed to have unusual energy-producing power (*ergo* means "work"; *genic* means "gives rise to"). Actually, no foods are ergogenic.

lactic acid: An acid produced when oxygen is not available to oxidize pyruvic acid all the way to carbon dioxide and water. Lactic acid accumulates in hard-working muscles and makes them sore.

pyruvic acid (pye-ROO-vic): A breakdown product of glucose. Glucose can be oxidized to pyruvic acid without the help of oxygen, but pyruvic acid can be further oxidized only when oxygen is available and is shunted to lactic acid whenever oxygen is in short supply.

spermatogenesis (sperm-at-oh-JEN-uh-sis): The process of manufacturing sperm, a function that can be disturbed by the use of anabolic steroids.

testicular degeneration: Wasting of the testicles, a side effect of the use of anabolic steroids.

more probably due just to the increased exercise and food.[4]

Hormones have profound and far-reaching effects on many target tissues, and these hormones are no exceptions. Hazards associated with their use include disturbed spermatogenesis and testicular degeneration in older athletes. Younger athletes may never reach their full potential height, because the bones of the lower back fuse to terminate growth early in response to the large dose of the hormones of puberty.[5]

Gaining and losing weight. An athlete who wants to gain weight in a hurry, and who doesn't care whether it is muscle or fat, can add calories of any kind to the diet to achieve the desired gain. Because fat in foods is more calorie-dense than protein or carbohydrate, the athlete can most easily gain weight by eating a high-fat diet. This technique is said to be one of the most widespread nutrition-related abuses in sports; and it increases the risk of heart disease, to which athletes are not immune. The healthy way to gain weight is to build yourself up by patient and consistent training and to eat enough calories (of nutritious foods) to support the weight gain as you do so.

Don't forget, afterwards, to cut *down* on calories between or after training periods. Muscles respond to reduced demand by "growing" smaller. They lose mass. It would be magical thinking to believe that that mass simply disappears. In point of fact, the cells slowly break down, and the materials they are made of (mostly the familiar carbohydrate, fat, and protein) become available as potential fuel for other body cells. Of course this fuel will be stored as fat unless it is expended in activity. It should be no surprise, then, that a heavily muscled individual of twenty who stops working out but keeps on eating like a football player in training can become an oversized, flabby, and obese person at thirty. There's actually some truth in the notion that his muscle turned to fat, even though it's a slight oversimplification.

The athlete who wants to lose weight, like the one who wants to gain, can choose a wise or unwise course. To achieve ideal body composition —the optimum ratio of muscle strength to body mass—you must reduce only body fat, and you can't do this for more than a very few weeks at a rate faster than about two pounds a week. Hurry-up techniques, such as sauna bathing, exercising in a plastic suit (to sweat it off), using diuretics or cathartics, or inducing vomiting, achieve faster weight loss only by causing dehydration, and dehydration seriously impairs performance. The hazards of fasts and fad diets were described in Chapter 7, but a reminder should be repeated here: What is achieved by quick-weight-loss dieting is loss of lean tissue, glycogen, bone minerals, fluids—all materials vital to healthy body functioning. Abnormal heart rhythms have been seen in healthy adults after only ten days of fasting.[6]

Even if it is achieved by healthy methods, extreme weight loss can be hazardous to the athlete, as to any person. Occasionally one hears that an "elite runner"—in superb physical condition and at the peak of his career—has died suddenly at the end of an intensive exercise session. These deaths were a mystery until recently, but now a reason for them seems to be emerging. In each case, the person had been severely restricting calories and had reached a new, all-time low weight, while at the same time breaking his own previous records for distance or time. Exactly what causes the deaths is still not known, but severe calorie restriction and weight loss combined with hard training seem to be contributing factors.[7] Sometimes, however, an athlete obviously has heart disease, either hereditary or acquired. Diet can't always be blamed for sudden deaths in athletes.

Women athletes sometimes experience menstrual irregularity or even complete stoppage of the menstrual cycle. *Athletic amenorrhea*, as it is now termed, resembles the amenorrhea seen in women with anorexia nervosa (Chapter 14) or in the world's undernourished women, and has been thought to be due to loss of body fat. The theory is that a certain minimum amount of body fat is necessary to support the making and using of the female hormones, which are fat-like compounds themselves. However, low body fat may not be the only cause; a change in the brain's regulation of sex hormone output may be responsible in the case of athletic amenorrhea. In any case, the possibility serves as a reminder that all athletes should keep in mind the definition of ideal weight already mentioned: the optimum ratio of muscle strength to body mass. An optimum means having neither too much *nor too little* body mass.

What provides muscle fuel? The fuel of muscle work is not protein but carbohydrate and fat. Muscles normally use a mixture of the two; but during intensive exercise they require glucose, and they store it as glycogen within their cells so that it will be available when needed. Two-thirds of the body's glycogen is in the muscles, and only one-third is in the liver to serve the rest of the body's needs for blood glucose (Chapter 4). When a muscle uses glycogen, it first derives many glucose units from it, then breaks them down. The breakdown of glucose is a multi-step process that releases energy at several of its steps as Chapter 7 showed. (From other reading you may have learned that the energy from glucose isn't used directly but goes to make other compounds, ATP and CP.[8] The subsequent breakdown of these compounds provides the energy for the muscle to contract.) After glucose has released its energy, only carbon-dioxide gas and water are left—tiny waste products that can be excreted.

You may have noticed that if you exert yourself extremely vigorously without relaxing for a moment, you experience muscle fatigue or even exhaustion and can't work your muscles at all. This effect results from the buildup of lactic acid—and knowing where it comes from can help you to improve your endurance. The first few steps of glucose breakdown can be done without oxygen, until a compound called pyruvic acid has been produced.

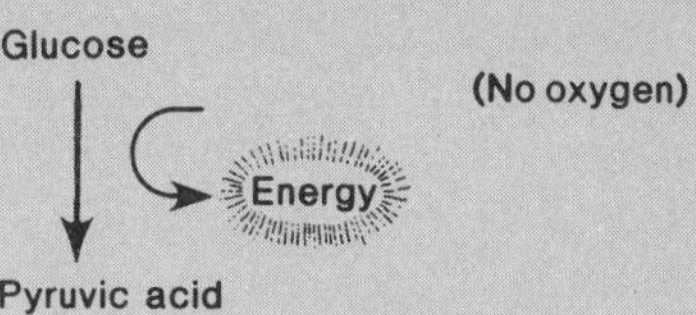

The anaerobic part of glucose breakdown.

The next few steps require oxygen and end with the complete breakdown of pyruvic acid to carbon dioxide and water.

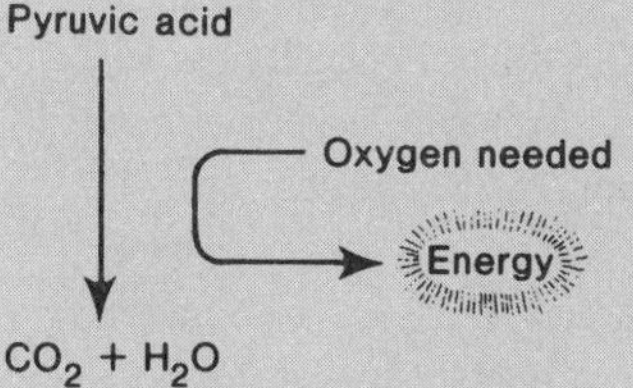

The aerobic part of glucose breakdown.

To break down glucose completely, then, and release the waste products, the muscle cells need abundant oxygen.

If the circulation can't bring them oxygen fast enough, the cells break glucose down as far as they can, to pyruvic acid, and then convert the pyruvic acid to a temporary waste product, lactic acid. That is all they can do without oxygen.

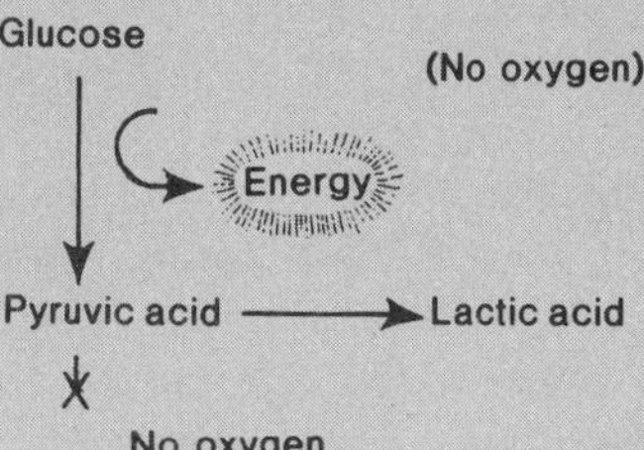

Pyruvic acid is shunted temporarily to lactic acid if oxygen isn't present to help oxidize it further.

This acid accumulates, changes the acid balance in the muscle, and causes fatigue.

You can prevent the accumulation of lactic acid in two ways. Breathing is most important. The more oxygen you can bring to the muscle, the longer it can work aerobically, getting all of the available energy from its stored glucose. (This is why to get in the best possible shape for an athletic event you have to condition your cardiovascular and respiratory system—that is, do aerobic exercise that requires speeded-up breathing and a rapid heartbeat, and not just weight-lifting or exercises that increase muscle strength only.) But during heavy physical exertion, the circulation can't keep up with the cells' need for oxygen, so lactic acid will accumulate. In this event, the strategy is to relax the muscles at any chance you have, so that the lactic acid and accumulated fluid can drain away. It can be relocated in the liver, if the circulation can carry it there, and be disposed of later, when oxygen again becomes available. (At the end of the event, too, you should shake and move your muscles to shift the fluid out of them so they won't become stiff.)

At the end of an event, you continue to breathe fast and your heart continues pounding for some time. What's happening is that oxygen is still being circulated to the tissues to help break down the accumulated lactic acid.

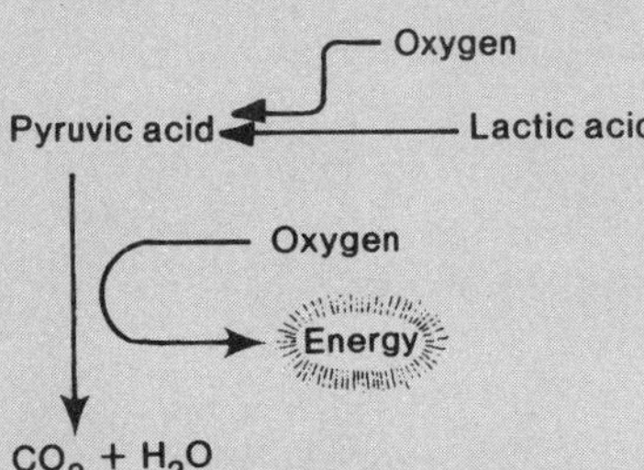

When oxygen is available again, lactic acid is reconverted to pyruvic acid and then completely oxidized.

The carbon dioxide that results stimulates the brain to make the heart and lungs stay speeded up until the waste products have been disposed of.

This description has shown what provides fuel for intense muscular activity: glycogen, that is, carbohydrate. The message for the athlete is that meals high in protein not only don't help build muscle but also don't help fuel its activity. Many experiments have shown that extra protein in the diet confers no advantage on the athlete in terms of strength, endurance, or speed.[9]

Fat is also used for fuel by muscles but can be broken down only as long as oxygen is available. Fat deposits therefore supply energy only for moderate muscular work. That's why long, slow, moderate intensity activity such as long walks can be very effective as an adjunct to a weight-loss effort. You don't need to exhaust yourself exercising; in fact it's better not to, for this reason. The best way to lose body fat is to have a moderate calorie deficit over many days' or weeks' time, so that the fat will gradually be used to meet the body's energy needs for daily (not strenuous) activity.

A great advantage to muscle conditioning is that it increases the muscles' ability to burn fat as fuel; they build up more fat-metabolizing machinery in response to demand. So if you train and get your muscles in good shape, you will find it easier to keep excess fat off. Conditioned muscles will burn fat longer during activity, or at a higher-intensity exercise level, than poorly-conditioned muscles. In competition, conditioned muscles will go much longer before starting to use glycogen. The point at which you start using glycogen is the beginning of the end, because glycogen stores are limited whereas fat stores are (in effect) unlimited.

When you are in training for an endurance activity such as long-distance running, cycling, or swimming, you may experience increasing fatigue as the days of training go on. One reason for this is that it takes forty-eight hours or even more to restore muscle carbohydrate to its pre-exercise level after it has been completely exhausted. To replace the used-up carbohydrate you have to eat a diet that is high in carbohydrate.[10] Two pointers for the athlete in training, then, are to take a periodic day's rest, if possible, during training, and to rest for a day or so before the event and eat a carbohydrate-rich diet.

What about glycogen loading? If you compete in a long-distance endurance event, you will naturally want to have as much stored energy in your muscles as you can. Glycogen loading is a technique of tricking the muscles into storing more glycogen than they normally have the capacity for. It involves first reducing carbohydrate intake for several days by eating meals high in protein and fat and simultaneously exercising heavily to deplete the muscle glycogen stores. The second step is to reduce exercise intensity and switch abruptly to a diet high in carbohydrate. Muscle glycogen stores rebound to about two to four times the normal level and thus provide fuel that will last longer in an endurance event. Marathon racers can tell when they've run out of glycogen (they "hit the wall" and suddenly slow down); those who have "loaded" can keep going longer and so have the edge in the competition.[11]

Until the mid-1970s, the hazards of this practice were unknown. Now, unfortunately, it is clear that there are hazards:

The use of this dietary regime is . . . not without possible risks. Glycogen retains water and both may be deposited in the muscle to such an extent that a feeling of heaviness and stiffness is experienced. The resulting weight increase due to water retention may reduce the ability of the athlete to take up oxygen maximally. Carbohydrate loading designed to increase endurance has also been reported to produce cardiac pain and electrocardiographic abnormalities in an older marathon runner. The effect of this practice on heart function is worrisome enough to caution all athletes against its use. . . .[12]

Many top athletes feel that the side effects of tampering with their diets, muscle and cardiac pain from the "stuffing," and weight gain cancel the benefits conferred by loaded glycogen. It is also strongly suggested that this not be done more than about three times a year, due to the effects on heart function. However, some athletes feel they can get away with it without ill effects; it may be an individual matter.

To maximize endurance, the athlete pays attention not only to fuel reserves in the muscle (that is, glycogen), but also to the muscle's ability to use that fuel. That means maximizing all of the following:

- Aerobic capacity (by heart-lung conditioning).
- Hemoglobin levels (by optimal iron and protein nutrition).
- Metabolic regulators (by optimal vitamin and mineral nutrition).
- Muscular fat-using ability (by muscular conditioning).[13]

What food is best before an event? There seems to be no special food that should be eaten before an athletic contest. A meal of steak may boost morale, but a meal so high in fat may also stay on the stomach long enough to hinder performance. There's no need to avoid milk; the idea that it causes "cotton mouth" is pure superstition. Olympic training tables are laden with carbohydrate foods such as fruit, and this is the best choice, for the reasons described in the previous section.

If you get very excited before competing, you may be unable to digest any food very well. For this reason, many athletes tolerate liquid meals best. But there is no magic ingredient in a liquid meal, even though advertisements may tell you there is. Whatever you eat, you should finish a good two or even three or four hours before the event, because digestion requires routing the blood supply to the GI tract. By the time you enter the contest, you want your circulating blood freed from the task of carrying newly arrived nutrients and available instead to carry oxygen and fuel to your muscles.[14]

The notion is widespread that it is smart to eat a candy bar or a few teaspoons of honey right before the event, for "quick energy." It may feel good to do this, but it probably confers a disadvantage physically, if it has any effect at all. The body's response is to secrete insulin, which retards fat use at a time when fat use should be maximal.

What liquids are best? During heavy exertion, you sweat, losing both water and salts from your body. There is no question that this can disable you more seriously than any other nutritional factor. Maintaining fluid balance is crucial to successful performance, because the first symptom of dehydration is fatigue. Sir Edmund Hilary is said to have attributed his success in the conquest of Mount Everest to the fact that he and his team took along fuel enough to melt about three quarts of water a day for each person during the final stages of the ascent.[15] A rapid water loss equal to 5 percent of the body weight can reduce muscular work capacity by 20 to 30 percent.[16] According to the Food and Nutrition Board, a person should begin replacing salt as well as water after having drunk more than four quarts of water to replace that lost in heavy sweating (see "Sodium" in Chapter 10), but according to recent research, the replacement need not be immediate and shouldn't be by way of salt tablets.[17] A person can sweat away as much as nine pounds of fluid and still perform well provided he or she drinks enough water, even without salt. When the event is over, eating regular food can make up the salt loss.[18] At that point, replacement of magnesium and potassium may be more important than the replacement of sodium.

You may be wondering how this statement can be made when the makers of Gatorade and other "sweat replacers" claim that their mixtures of water with glucose, sodium, chloride, potassium, magnesium, and calcium enter the system "faster than water" and help football players win games. Actually, although such mixtures do resemble sweat in composition (except for the glucose) and do satisfy thirst, they are probably absorbed less rapidly, not more rapidly, than water, because the glucose in them holds them back.[19] Moreover, the body of a trained athlete stores extra amounts of the minerals in question and can replenish them perfectly well—by eating and drinking ordinary food and fluids—after the competition is over.[20] Furthermore, a person who sweats heavily (say, two liters) during competition *cannot* replace the lost fluid even by drinking that much, because the stomach can't absorb more than one liter in an hour's time. The best fluid for a marathon event is *diluted* juice (for example, one part orange juice plus four parts water) or plain water in small quantities. However, there is probably no great harm in the moderate use of sweat replacers. The sugar in them provides a boost; they taste good; and most importantly, they bolster morale.

A note about adaptation. The body of a highly conditioned athlete is as perfectly adapted for its function as it can be. The muscles are developed specifically to perform the chosen sport, and the body's stores of glycogen and minerals are adjusted to meet the particular athlete's special needs. Other adaptations are also present. At one time, it was thought that there was a high incidence of anemia among athletes, and there was concern that this might be the result of nutritional deficiency. Now it seems that this anemia may be another of the body's adaptations. It may protect the blood from a tendency to form sludge when it is most concentrated, during periods of heavy exercise.[21] It is probable that the athlete only appears to be anemic and in fact has a greater number of red blood cells but an even greater plasma volume as a result of conditioning, so that the red blood cells are, in effect, diluted. This effect is enhanced when, during repeated days of heavy training, plasma volume may increase by almost a third because the kidney conserves sodium and water at these times.[22] (This is not to deny, however, that true anemia can occur in athletes, especially women athletes. Taking an iron supplement may be a good idea for them, as for all women).

No doubt other differences between the bodies of athletes and nonathletes will be discovered in the future, and the finger will be pointed at nutrition again: "You wouldn't be that way if you would eat right." But the athlete being told this should keep in mind that the body may be wiser than the accuser and that the reason the body is different may be because of the different tasks it is called upon to perform.

This note is intended to be a cautionary one. When new findings turn up in relation to nutrition and athletics, give them a chance to be responsibly investigated before jumping to conclusions, and especially before going to any extremes in terms of your food choices. In this field as in all fields of science, you can't find truth by a reasoning process, no matter how good the logic may be. It takes experimental testing before reliable conclusions can be drawn. Meanwhile, before the data are in and analyzed, be moderate in your nutritional practices.

Personal strategy. Unlike the subjects of previous Controversies, the subject of nutrition for the athlete turns out not to generate much disagreement among those who have researched it. The recommendations made here are simple, common-sense suggestions and have been summed up clearly this way:

A nutritious, normal diet should be adequate for extremely active athletes. The increased caloric intake of such individuals is likely to insure an adequate supply of all essential nutrients. The primary concern of athletes should be their water intake.[23]

But there *is* controversy between this view and that of the coaches, trainers, and others who promote the taking of a multitude of powders, syrups, granules, and pills to increase strength, endurance, speed, and skill. Food faddism, ignorance, and superstition are more widespread among athletes than among most other people interested in nutrition. To distinguish fact from fiction, when you hear nutritional claims made, ask the person making the claim where the facts came from. Generally speaking, you'll get the most valid information from an informant who has taken strong college or even graduate-school courses in the science of nutrition.

Meanwhile, it may be well to remember that one of the most effective things that food can do for you is to make you *feel* strong and swift. Contestants will go through extraordinary rituals to get into the winning frame of mind. If among these rituals is the taking of some unusual mixture of foods or nutrients, and if they do no harm, perhaps there is nothing to be said against them. In the final analysis, many athletes agree that what really wins athletic contests is the feeling of being "up for it" and the "will to win."

The Controversy Notes and For Further Information follow the Appendixes.

CHAPTER 8

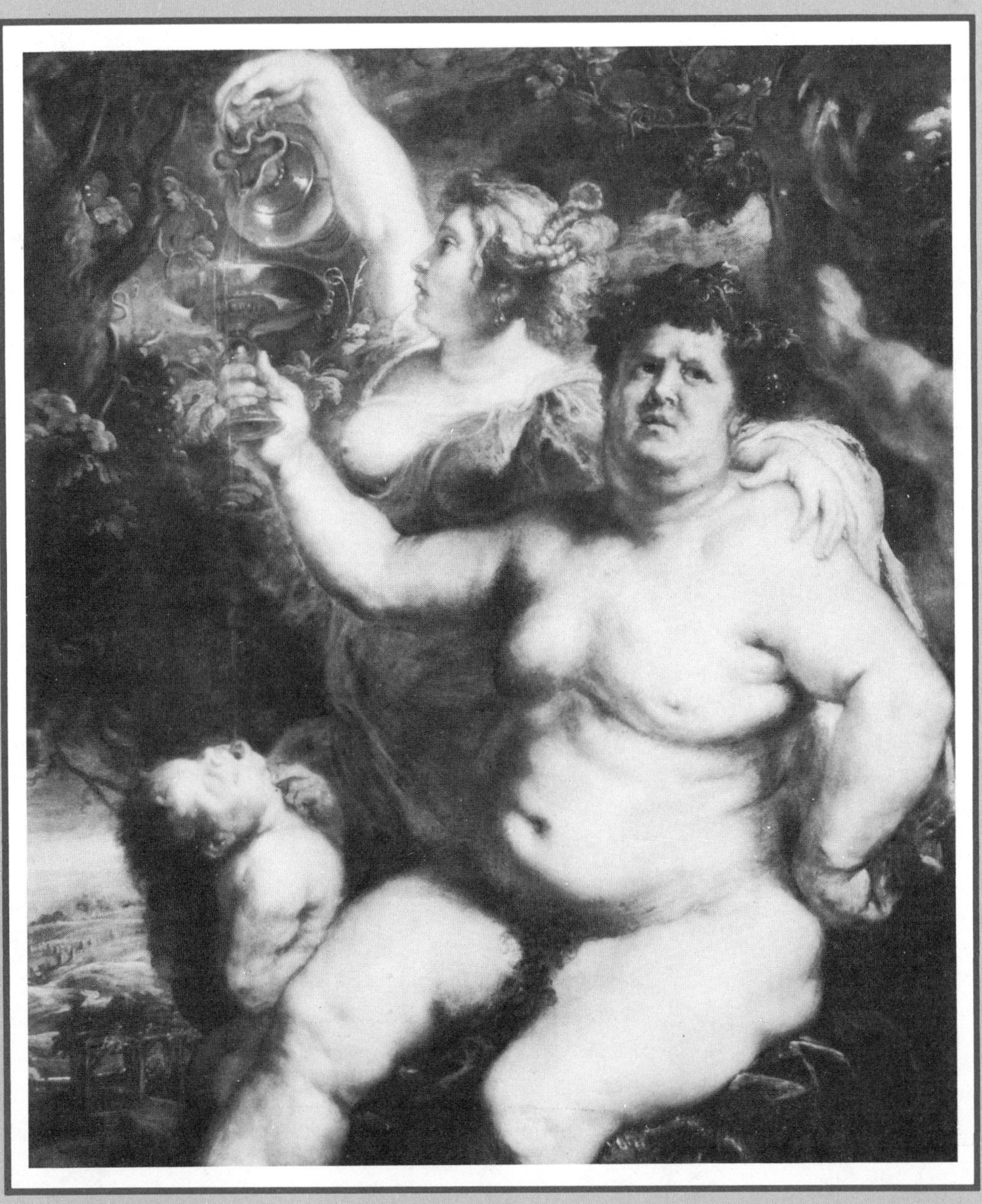

Energy Balance: Overweight and Underweight

Obesity is America's number-one malnutrition problem.[1] It is simultaneously one of the most important and least understood areas in the science of nutrition. Everyone knows roughly what it is: If you are too fat, you are obese. But why and how it occurs and what can be done about it are matters for much speculation, debate, and frustration. For the obese person who has earnestly tried every known means of losing weight—only to fail—frustration can turn to despair.

Less well recognized is the problem of underweight, which can be equally mysterious. A "skinny" person finds it as hard to gain a pound as a fat person does to lose one.

This chapter focuses on the problems of overweight and obesity, partly because they have been more intensively studied and partly because they are a more widespread health problem. This does not imply that the underweight person faces a less difficult problem. The concluding section shows that what we know about the one extreme sometimes applies equally well to the other.

It is appropriate to begin by defining terms. How fat is too fat, and how thin is too thin? The most important concept to understand is that obesity means being too fat but not necessarily being too heavy. This chapter therefore begins with a discussion of the relationship between body fat and body weight.

Opposite: Bacchus *by Peter Paul Rubens. Used with permission of The Hermitage Museum, Leningrad. Photograph (c) V. Terepenin.*

Body Weight and Body Composition

Body fat plays some important roles in maintaining health. It serves as an insulator from heat, cold, and mechanical shock and as an energy supply to be used when glycogen reserves are exhausted and refueling from food is delayed. Without a protective blanket of fat, as in the extreme of protein-calorie malnutrition, the human body is fragile and unable to withstand environmental stresses. Thus, some body fat is clearly desirable.

At the other extreme, however, excess body fat serves no useful function in a society where food is abundant and easily obtained. We need no large store of energy to carry us through periods of famine; in fact, the problem for some of us is that the famine never comes. The hazards of being obese are so numerous that they are treated in a separate section later in this chapter.

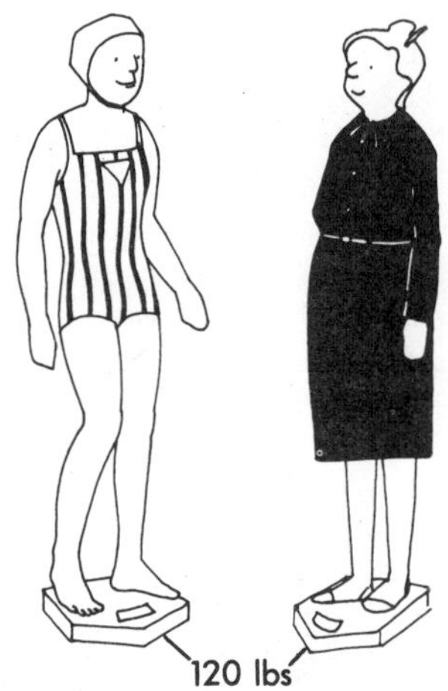

Both women weigh 120 pounds. One has more muscle and bone, the other more fat.

Body composition. Ideally, by a very rough approximation, fat will make up about 18 percent of a man's body weight and about 22 percent of a woman's, with the remainder being contributed by water (55 to 60 percent), muscle and other lean tissue (10 to 20 percent), and bone minerals (6 to 8 percent). The relative amounts of muscle and bone vary widely from one person to the next, and there is no easy way to estimate them.[2] Thus a dancer, an athlete, or a person doing heavy physical work, whose muscles are well developed and whose skeleton has become dense through constant stress on the bones, may have a slender figure with no excess fat tissue and still be heavier than another person of the same height, sex, age, and body shape. It follows that we cannot state an ideal weight for a person on the basis of height alone.

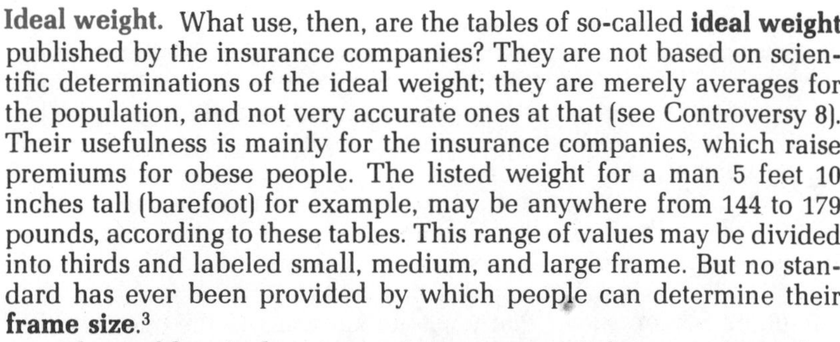

Ideal weight. What use, then, are the tables of so-called **ideal weight** published by the insurance companies? They are not based on scientific determinations of the ideal weight; they are merely averages for the population, and not very accurate ones at that (see Controversy 8). Their usefulness is mainly for the insurance companies, which raise premiums for obese people. The listed weight for a man 5 feet 10 inches tall (barefoot) for example, may be anywhere from 144 to 179 pounds, according to these tables. This range of values may be divided into thirds and labeled small, medium, and large frame. But no standard has ever been provided by which people can determine their **frame size.**[3]

The ideal-weight tables appear on the inside back cover. Average weights for U.S. citizens today are shown at the beginning of Controversy 8.

The problem is that you can't see a person's bones and muscles. Terms for **body types** have been developed in the attempt to make skeletal differences more meaningful. An ectomorph is supposed to be a person with a long and slender skeleton; an endomorph is one with a short, broad skeleton; and a mesomorph falls in between. But when a so-called endomorph (short and fat) starves, he may prove to have a very slight skeleton after all. The terms turn out to reflect body fatness, not skeletal type, and so have not proved useful.[4]

Body composition probably changes with age. People typically become less active as they get older. Their muscles get smaller, and their bones decrease in density. Thus a man who is lean at twenty-five may be fat at sixty-five without having gained a pound. Most of us should probably lose weight gradually after we have passed the age of thirty. The fact that it is "normal" for people to gain an average of twenty to thirty pounds during adulthood does not make it right.[5]

Choosing your own ideal weight is thus a matter of guesswork. To decide if you have "big bones," you can compare your wrist bone with those of several other people. Having decided on your frame size, you can decide whether you belong at the top, middle, or bottom of the range of suggested weights. But the matter is then complicated further by some additional considerations.

The notion that it is healthy to be thin has been changing recently, as new understanding of insurance company statistics has come to light. It was long thought that to be at the truly ideal body weight was to be 10 percent *under* the average weight on the charts, because statistics showed people at this weight to have the maximum life expectancy. We now know, however, that there was at least one wrong assumption underlying this view. Insured people are not typical of all people. Some overweight people buy life insurance because they already know that they have heart trouble or related problems that may shorten their lives. Others, who are "fat and happy" and unconcerned, may *not* buy life insurance. Thus the insurance company data are "skewed" as if fat people died younger.

According to insurance doctors, for every inch that your waist measurement exceeds that of your chest—not bust—your life expectancy decreases by two years.—J. Tragler: *The Bellybook*

In particular, people with high blood pressure have an increased risk of dying from heart attacks and strokes—the major killers of the developed countries—and it so happens that one condition obesity makes distinctly worse is high blood pressure. If you exclude individuals with this condition from the people being studied, the statistics then show a slight advantage (in terms of life expectancy) for people who are slightly *over*weight. This chapter's Controversy goes into the question of ideal weight in greater depth, but you can see that it may be a highly personal matter that depends on several factors including your familial health history and expectations.

Diagnosing overfatness: The fatfold test. With all their limitations, the ideal-weight tables are used to draw arbitrary lines between too much and too little body weight. A person who is more than 10 percent above the desirable weight on the tables is **overweight**; a person 20 percent or more above the desirable weight is **obese**. (Some authorities say obesity is 15 percent above the normal weight, some say 25.) Similarly, a person who is more than 10 percent below desirable weight is **underweight**. Obviously, for the reasons already given, these terms may be rejected in individual cases.

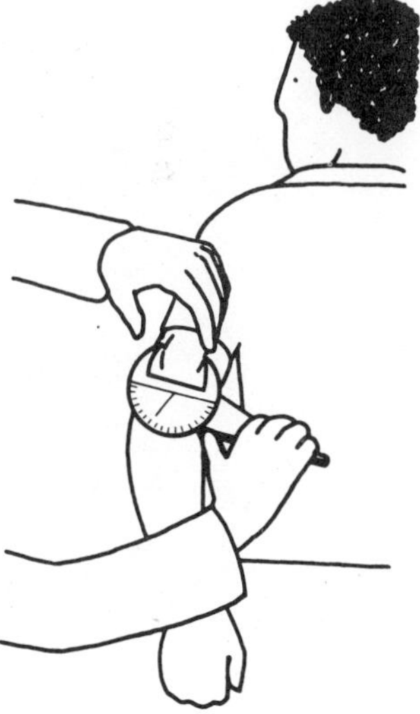

Fatfold test.

A direct measure of the amount of body fat can be obtained by means of the skinfold test—or, more accurately, the **fatfold test**. The clinician lifts a fold of skin from the back of the arm, from the back, or from other body surfaces and measures its thickness with a caliper that applies a fixed amount of pressure. Under these conditions, a fatfold over an inch thick indicates overfatness; under a half-inch reflects underweight. The fat attached to the skin in these regions is roughly proportional to total body fat. This technique is a practical diagnostic tool in the hands of trained people and is in increasingly wide use.

Finally, and most simply of all, one can use the mirror test: Undress and stand before a mirror. If you look too fat, you may be too

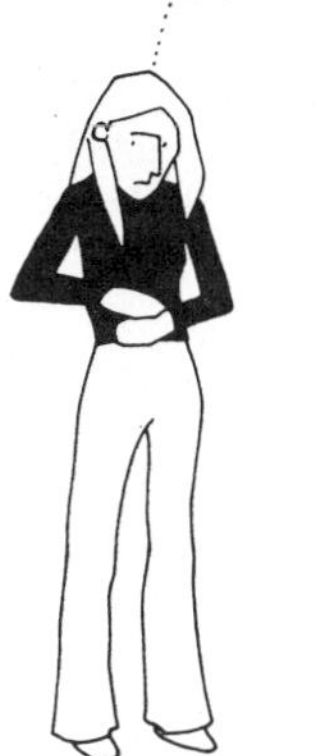

A notoriously poor judge of overfatness is the teenage girl.

fat. A notoriously poor judge of this test, however, is the teenage girl who thinks any amount of fat, no matter how small, is a serious blemish.

In women, a mild degree of obesity may be a desirable physiological state, according to some researchers. Teenage girls add more body fat than boys with the help of the hormones of adolescence.[6] The female hormones favor fat deposition.[7] Perhaps the tendency toward obesity (and a low basal metabolic rate) in females was an advantage during our evolution, when food was sometimes scarce. Those whose genes enabled them to store enough fat to survive and bear offspring passed on their successful genes and perpetuated the tendency in their descendants. (Those who didn't survive to maturity had no descendants!) Whether obesity now confers an advantage on women in the Western world, where food is plentiful, is questionable.

On the other hand, styles change, and our current image of the ideal—the leggy, fatless fashion model—may be unrealistically thin. Some girls who think they need to diet actually need to change their image of themselves.

Incidence and Onset of Obesity

Overweight or obesity is seen in more than 10 percent of the school-age children in the United States, in about 15 percent of the people under the age of thirty, and in 25 to 30 percent of the adults, according to most estimates; and its incidence is increasing. Among older people, a third of the men and half of the women are obese.[8] Certain subgroups of the population have a markedly higher incidence of obesity than others: the lower socioeconomic classes, blacks, Mexican Americans, Native Americans, and Eskimos. In some other countries, the poor are thin from lack of food and the wealthy are fat because it is stylish to be fat.

Juvenile- versus adult-onset obesity. Whatever the ideal may be, statistics show that some people become fat in childhood and others later on. Few of either type lose the excess weight. There is no specific age that divides **juvenile-onset obesity** from **adult-onset obesity**, but as the terms imply, there is a distinction between the two types.[9] Children who are obese will develop sturdy muscles and bones as they grow, to support their excess weight. Thus, as adults they will have both more lean body mass and more body fat than the average person and will likely always be stocky, even if they lose their excess fat.[10] People who become obese as children are also less likely to be able to reduce successfully than people who become obese as adults.

The fat-cell theory. Research on fat cells suggests a possible reason why early-onset obesity is especially resistant to treatment. Simply stated, early overfeeding stimulates fat cells to increase abnormally in *number*. The number of fat cells becomes fixed by adulthood. Thereafter, a gain in weight can take place only by increasing the *size* of the fat cells. The number of cells (the theory goes on) in some way regulates hunger: That is, the larger the number of fat cells, the more hungry the person will be. Thus, people with abnormally large numbers of fat cells will be abnormally hungry, no matter how thin they may be, and will always tend to overeat. On the other hand, people who gain weight in adulthood have normal numbers of fat cells and need only reduce their size; then they won't be abnormally hungry. The tyranny of a mass of fat cells is demonstrated by the fact that their number can be used as a predictor of success in weight loss efforts.[11] The idea that the number of fat cells is fixed in adulthood is being questioned, however, as animal experiments have revealed the possibility that the feeding of highly palatable foods may increase the number even after maturity has been reached.[12]

The best way to be thin when you are old is to have been thin when you were young.—paraphrased from J. Mayer

All we know about the subject seems to emphasize the fact that prevention is better than cure.—E. M. Widdowson and M. J. Dauncey

The fat-cell theory has been heavily criticized on several grounds.[13] But even the critics agree that there are certain periods in life when body fat increases more rapidly than lean tissue: during early infancy (up to about two years), again during preadolescence (and throughout adolescence in girls), and possibly again during the third trimester of pregnancy.[14] These are critical periods, in the sense that what happens at these times may be irreversible and crucial to the person's later physical fate. Prevention of obesity would thus be most important during these times. There is also agreement that, at whatever time fat is gained, it's hard to lose.

Prevention is the only road to true success in curing obesity.—B. B. Blouin

More on ways to avoid overstimulating fat development during critical periods—Chapters 12 and 13.

Hazards of Obesity

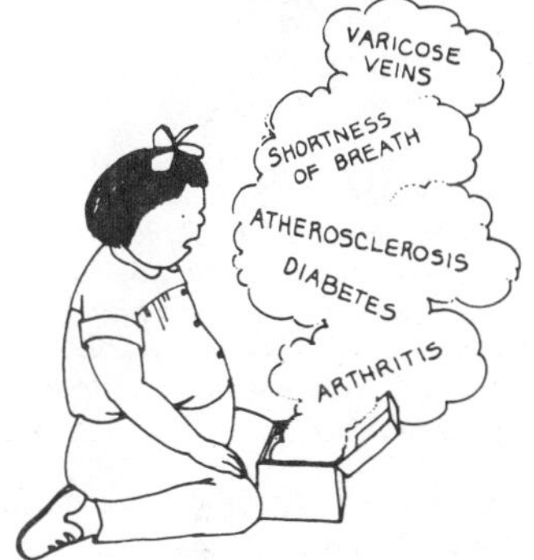

Hazards of obesity.

Insurance companies report that fat people die younger from a host of causes, and even while they have been wrong in defining how fat is too fat, they were observing accurately that overfatness can be a health disadvantage. Gaining weight often appears to precipitate diabetes.[15] Fat people more often suffer high levels of blood fat, hypertension, coronary heart disease, post-surgical complications, gynecological irregularities, and the toxemia of pregnancy.[16] The burden of extra fat strains the skeletal system, causing arthritis—especially in the knees, hips, and lower spine. The muscles that support the belly may give way, resulting in abdominal hernias. When the leg muscles are abnormally fatty, they fail to contract efficiently to help blood return from the leg veins to the heart; blood collects in the leg veins, which swell, harden, and become varicose.[17] Extra fat in and around the chest interferes with breathing.[18] Gout is more common and even the accident rate is greater for the severely obese.

As if this were not enough, there are also social and economic disadvantages. A fat person is less often sought after for marriage, pays higher insurance premiums, meets discrimination when applying for jobs, can't find attractive clothes so easily, and is limited in choice of sports.[19] Fat girls have only one-third the chance of being accepted into college that lean girls have.[20] The fat child often suffers ridicule from classmates and the unbearable humiliation of being left until last when the captains are choosing teams. The sailor who gains weight will be released from service.[21]

These many disadvantages justify our calling obesity a severe physical handicap. However, it is unlike other handicaps in two important ways. First, mortality risk is not linearly related to excess weight. Instead, there is a threshold at which risk dramatically increases. Being only a few pounds above this threshold weight may cause blood pres-

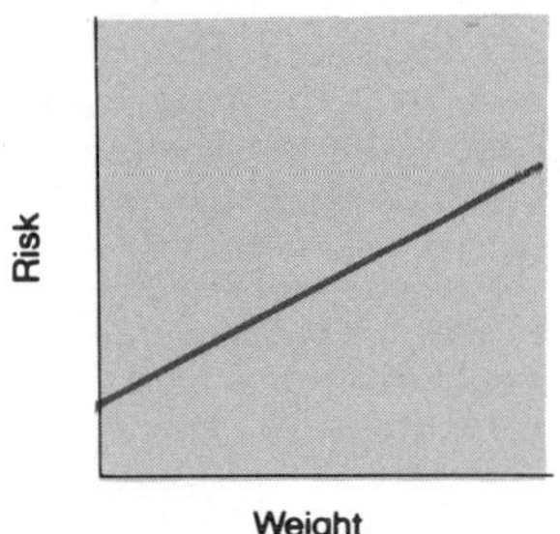

This would be a linear (straight-line) relationship.

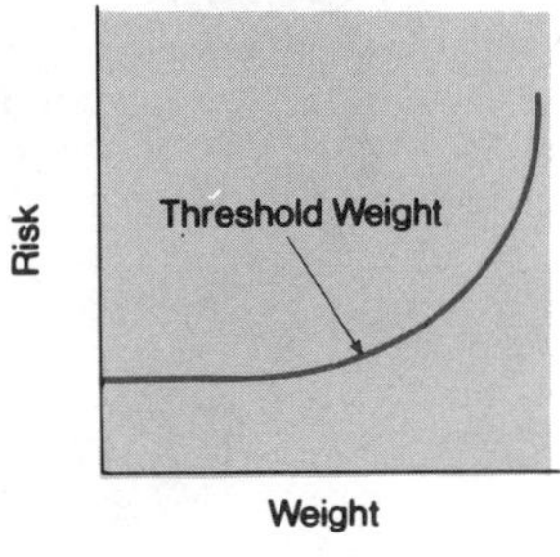

This is the actual relationship of risk to weight. The curve shows that beyond a certain point risk increases dramatically with weight gain. This is especially true for people with high blood pressure.

Adapted from C. C. Seltzer, Some re-evaluations of the Build and Blood Pressure Study, 1959, as related to ponderal index, somatotype and mortality, New England Journal of Medicine 274 (1966): 254-259, with the permission of the New England Journal of Medicine.

More about weight gain in pregnancy—Chapter 12.

Anyone who weighs more than he should has been eating more than he needs.—R. A. Seelig

sure, blood glucose, and blood lipids to zoom upwards. (The concept of a danger zone of weight is illustrated in the margin.) Second, obesity is reversible; and if it is corrected in time, some of its risks are, too.[22] Mortality rates (from insurance data) are not higher for the formerly obese than for the never obese.[23]

Ideally, a person would avoid having to struggle with the problem of obesity by never having become obese to begin with. Preventive efforts are needed, especially in vulnerable groups: infants, preadolescents, adolescents, and women before they are pregnant. (This is in no way meant to imply that a woman, once pregnant, should attempt to lose weight. Weight loss during pregnancy is even more hazardous than obesity.) Where prevention has failed, treatment is urgently needed. But how to treat? Before turning to the matters of diet, drugs, exercise, and other means of attacking the problem, it is necessary to try to figure out what causes obesity.

Causes of Obesity

The previous chapter made it clear that calories are not stored in fat until the body's other energy needs have been met. Excess body fat can accumulate only when the calories eaten exceed those needed for the day's metabolic, muscular, and digestive activities. To put it bluntly, obesity results from overeating.

This fact, however, neither explains the cause of obesity nor indicates the cure. Why do people overeat? Is it a hunger problem? An appetite problem? A satiety problem? Is it genetic? Metabolic? Environmental? Is it a matter of habits learned in early childhood? Is it psychological? Would you believe that all of these factors may play a role? To tell the truth, we do not know the cause. The following paragraphs only offer ideas that are presently being considered.

Hunger, appetite, and satiety. **Hunger** is said to be physiological—an inborn instinct—whereas **appetite** is supposed to be psychological—a learned response to food. **Satiety** is the sensation of fullness that follows a meal and is believed to have both physical and psychological characteristics. If all of these sensations worked in the ideal way, no one would have a problem with overeating. You would feel hunger and appetite simultaneously when your body needed food, and you would eat. When you had eaten enough to meet your body's need for food, you would experience satiety, and you would stop eating. But everyone knows it isn't always this simple. We have all experienced appetite without hunger: "I'm not hungry, but I'd love to have a piece." The too-thin person may often experience the reverse, hunger without appetite: "I know I'm hungry, but I don't feel like eating." And sometimes appetite and satiety occur together: "I'm really full, but I'll take just a little more." What goes on in your body to make you feel like eating or like stopping? Evidently the stomach and the brain both play a role.

A popular theory of hunger regulation is that the brain monitors blood glucose concentration and signals "eat" when glucose gets too low; but this theory, at best, accounts for only some of the facts. Sometimes eating that leads to a rise in blood glucose seems to satisfy hunger. But at other times—for example, when a person eats sweets late at night—the eating stimulates greater appetite, and more eating follows.[24] Insulin and other hormones are believed to be involved, and they don't always act consistently. Insulin secreted in response to the eating of complex carbohydrates including fiber may lead to satisfaction of the appetite, while insulin secreted in response to the eating of simple sugar may promote further eating. If you have noticed this, you may have described it by saying, "bread fills me up, but sugary foods stimulate my appetite." The key word—*appetite*—is so hard to define and explain that a monthly journal was started in 1980 devoted to articles about it.[25]

When you eat, you secrete not only insulin but also other hormones, and some of these act on the brain, perhaps affecting eating behavior.[26] Still others already circulating in your body—for example, the female hormone, estrogen—may influence the amount of hunger or appetite you experience. Women may find that this causes them to eat more during the days prior to their menstrual periods than during the days after.[27] And not only hormones but other factors respond to eating. Some fascinating research investigating these factors has shown that animals forced to overeat produce a factor that in other animals inhibits eating (a satiety factor).[28] Furthermore, eating has a calming effect, believed to be mediated by the making of a tranquilizing chemical in the brain. That is, when you eat, you make your own tranquilizer in response, and so you feel a comfort beyond that associated with the filling of your empty stomach.[29] This suggests that anything that causes arousal, and especially anxiety, may prompt eating behavior.[30]

Thus the brain seems to play a dominant part in the experiencing of hunger, appetite, and satiety. The stomach, on the other hand, has only a small part to play. It is responsible for sending messages to the brain when it is full,[31] but the brain has the task of receiving and interpreting the messages and altering eating behavior accordingly. Apparently the old idea that your stomach stretches when you overeat and shrinks when you diet is vastly oversimplified.

Some theorists think the key to obesity is a defective satiety center in the brain. A curious fact in favor of this notion is that infants born to undernourished mothers are more likely to become obese adults. This is especially likely if the malnutrition occurs during early or mid-pregnancy when that part of the brain believed to regulate satiety is developing.[32]

Not long ago, one of our patients with diabetes sat down to read a book with an open box of crackers by her side. At the end of an hour of absorbed reading, she noticed that the box was entirely empty. Thinking that someone else had emptied the box, she angrily accused her son and daughter of stealing the crackers. It was only with great difficulty that they persuaded her that they had seen her eat one cracker after another during the hour, until the whole box was consumed.—L. E. Hinkle

L. E. Hinkle, Customs, emotions, and behavior in the dietary treatment of diabetes, Journal of the American Dietetic Association 41 (1962): 341-343.

External cues. The person described in the margin is an unconscious eater; she seems to be eating merely because the food is there. Some obese people tend to do this. Rather than responding only to internal, visceral hunger cues, they respond helplessly to such external factors as the time of day ("It's time to eat") or the availability, sight, and taste of food. This is the basis of the **external cue theory**.

Of interest in this connection is the report of an experiment in which lean and fat people in a metabolic ward were offered their meals in monotonous liquid form from a feeding machine. The lean people ate enough to maintain their weight, but the fat people drastically reduced their food intake and lost weight. When calories were

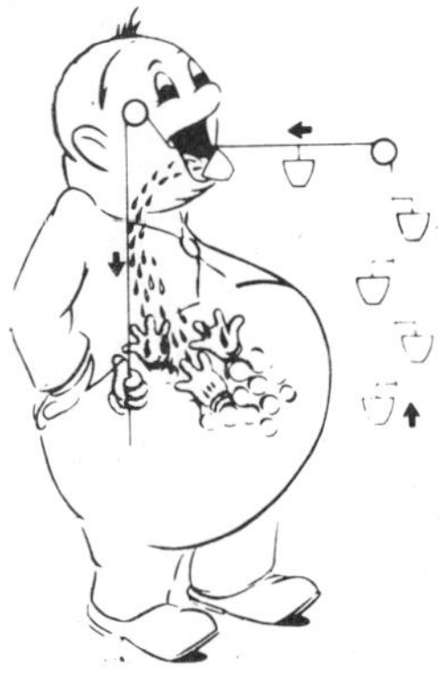

The "pull" theory of obesity proposes that a subtle metabolic disorder increases food intake either by affecting hunger-satiety signals transmitted to a "satiety center" or by altering the sensitivity of the satiety center to such signals.

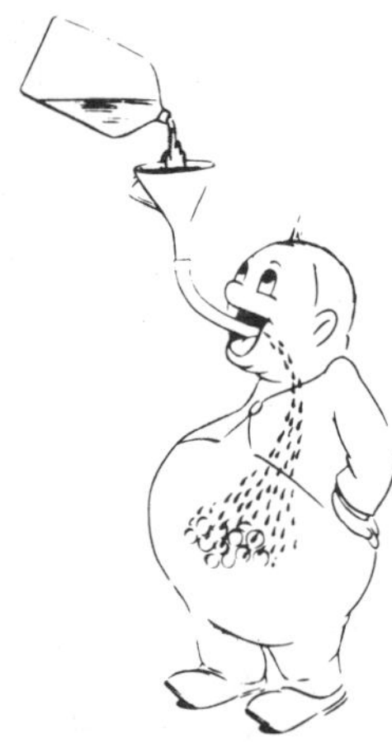

The "push" theory proposes that the obese person "force-feeds" himself, overeating for nonphysiological reasons.

From T. B. Van Itallie and R. G. Campbell, 1972, copyright The American Dietetic Association. Reprinted by permission from Journal of the American Dietetic Association 61 (1972): 386.

added to the formula, the lean people adjusted their intake to continue maintaining weight as if they had an internal, unconscious calorie counter. The obese people were insensitive to the change, continued drinking the same amount of formula as before, and stopped losing weight.[33]

For the person who eats in response to external cues, today's environment provides them in abundance. Restaurants, TV commercials, the abundance of food in our markets, vending machines in every office building and gas station—all prompt us to eat and drink high-calorie foods. There are no vegetable houses on our main streets, only steak houses. Kitchen appliances such as the hamburger cooker and donut maker make high-calorie foods easy to prepare and thus quickly available.

Psychology: Emotional needs. The psychiatrist Dr. Hilde Bruch, who has devoted as much attention to the human hunger drive as Freud did to the sex drive, states that both hunger and appetite are intimately connected to deep emotional needs. Two factors that she finds most important in this connection are the fear of starvation and "the universal experience in the early life of every individual that food intake requires the cooperation of another person." Feeding behavior is a response not only to hunger or appetite but also to more complex human sensations, such as "yearning, craving, addiction, or compulsion."[34]

Others agree that food is widely used for nonnutritive purposes, especially in a culture such as ours where food is abundant. An emotionally insecure person who feels unsure of acceptance by other people might eat as a substitute for seeking love or friendship. Eating is less threatening than calling a friend and risking rejection. Often, especially in adolescent girls, eating is used to relieve boredom. One researcher has found that eating helps ward off depression;[35] another, that it is used to get attention, to spite a spouse, to suppress assertiveness, to rebel against authority, to gain feelings of power by being "big," and for a host of other purposes.[36]

> The profound connection between emotion and food is a part of human nature that quacks often use to advantage. With their foods, pills, supplements, and diets, they offer an irresistible trinket in the package: love, beauty, youth, health, or long life. The victim cooperates by yielding to the child within, who wants to believe it is possible to have something for nothing. You can often identify quacks by their appeals to emotion and their promises of quick and painless results. We have labeled this trick *magical thinking* and suggest that you watch for it when evaluating what you hear and read about nutrition.

Obesity as a response to stress. Under conditions where there is a risk of physical harm, animals under stress have been observed to substitute one instinctive behavior for another. During a confrontation, for example, one animal may suddenly stop posturing and begin to groom itself intensively. It is possible that human beings also displace one behavior with another when they are threatened. Rather than fight or flight, the activity selected may be eating.

The hormones secreted in response to physical stress favor the rapid metabolism of energy nutrients to fragments that can be used to fuel the muscular activity of fight or flight. Under emotional stress, the same hormones are secreted, and if a person fails to use the fuel in violent physical exertion, the body has no alternative but to turn these fragments to fat.[37] If much blood glucose has been used up this way, then the lowered glucose level will signal hunger, and the person will eat again soon after. Stress eating may appear in different patterns: Some people eat excessively at night when feeling anxious, others characteristically go on an eating binge during an emotional crisis.[38] The overly thin often react in the opposite way. Stress causes them to reject food, thus becoming thinner.

Enzyme differences. It may be that some people have inherited a greater tendency to build body fat than others. Inheriting a metabolic trait like this means inheriting genes that code for enzymes that in turn work faster or move certain reactions along in preference to others. For example, when you need to oxidize a fuel to meet your energy needs, your body's cells can choose between glycogen and fat. Some people might tend to be glycogen users (because their glycogen-oxidizing enzymes are more active), while others might tend to be fat users. The glycogen users would experience lowered blood glucose more often and so would be hungry more often.[39] On eating, they would store both glycogen and fat, and then the fat would tend to stay in storage.

Insulin insensitivity. Once a person has become obese, the situation tends to perpetuate itself. The enlarged fat cells become resistant to insulin, the hormone that promotes glucose uptake into cells and its conversion to fat. The excess glucose remains in the bloodstream and stimulates the insulin-producing cells of the pancreas to multiply and secrete more insulin. This ultimately promotes more fat storage than in insulin-responsive people.[40] As if this were not enough, the enlarged fat cells are also less sensitive to other hormones that promote fat breakdown. Weight loss restores insulin levels to normal, but it first has to be achieved against these odds.

Heredity versus environment. Hormones and enzymes are under the control of genes, and genes are inherited. In some animal strains, obesity is inherited as predictably as hair or eye color. Is human obesity inherited? One way to test this possibility is to study identical twins raised in different families—one family fat and the other thin—because the twins have identical genes. If the genes determine fatness, then both twins will become equally fat or thin. But if the environment is responsible, the twins will resemble their respective families. Another approach is to study adopted children to see whether they resemble their natural or adoptive parents. Studies of both kinds suggest that the tendency to obesity is inherited.[41] But the environment is permissive; that is, it can enhance or inhibit the development of obesity when the potential is there.

An individual is probably endowed with a certain range of [numbers of fat cells] which can be modified by a variety of environmental influences.—J. L. Knittle

Inheritance of the tendency to obesity is probably very complex and governed by many different genes. To complicate the situation further, these genes probably occur with different frequencies in different populations.

Habits: Learned responses to food. Whatever a person inherits, the environment can doubtless promote overeating. Food-centered families encourage such behaviors as overeating at mealtimes, rapid eating, excessive snacking, and eating to meet needs other than hunger. Children readily imitate overeating parents and their behavior at the table persists outside the home. Obese children have been observed to take more bites of food per interval of time and to chew them less thoroughly than their nonobese schoolmates.[42]

People who eat small but frequent meals may tend to store less fat than those who eat large meals at irregular intervals.[43] Thus, families that allow their children to skip meals may be promoting obesity.

Inactivity. The many possible causes of obesity mentioned so far all relate to the input side of the energy equation. What about output? Obesity may be caused by eating too much, but it can also be caused by spending too little energy. It is probable that the most important single contributor to the obesity problem in our country is underactivity. The control of hunger and appetite actually works quite well in active people and only fails when activity falls below a certain minimum level.[44] Obese people, under close observation, are often seen to eat less than lean people;[45] but they are sometimes so extraordinarily inactive that they still manage to have a calorie surplus. If normal people actually swim thirty-five minutes during "an hour of swimming," obese people may only swim for seven minutes. Most of their time is spent sitting, standing, or lying in the sun.[46]

Individuality. No two people are alike either physically or psychologically, and no doubt the causes of obesity are as varied as the people who are obese. Many causes may contribute to the problem in a single person. Given this complexity, it is obvious that there will be no panacea. The treatment of obesity must involve a simultaneous attack on many fronts.

Treatment of Obesity

The only means of reducing body fat is to shift the energy budget so that energy-in is less than energy-out. This is most effectively done by eating less and exercising more. The concluding sections of this chapter address these strategies, but because rumors of other means fly about, they will first be dispensed with briefly.

Water pills. For the obese person, the idea that excess weight is due to water accumulation may be an attractive one. Indeed, temporary water retention, seen in many women around the time of the menstrual period, may make a difference of several pounds on the scale. Oral contraceptives may have the same effect. (They may also promote actual fat gain in some women. A woman who has this problem should consult her physician about switching brands.) In cases of severe swelling of the belly, as much as twenty pounds of excess body water may accumulate.[47]

If water retention is a problem, it can be diagnosed by a physician, who will prescribe a diuretic (water pill) and possibly a mild degree of salt restriction.[48] But the obese—that is, overfat—subject has a smaller percentage of body water than the person of normal weight.[49] Taking a self-prescribed diuretic does nothing to solve a fat problem, although it may make a person lose a few pounds on the scale for half a day and suffer from dehydration.

Diet pills. Some doctors will prescribe amphetamines ("speed") to help with weight loss (the best known are dexedrine and benzedrine). These reduce appetite—but only temporarily. Typically, after a week or two, the appetite returns to normal, the lost weight is regained, and the user then has the problem of trying to get off the drug without gaining more weight.[50] It is generally agreed that these drugs cause a dangerous dependency[51] and are of little or no usefulness in treating obesity.[52] No known drug is both safe and effective, and many are hazardous.[53] The only effective appetite-reducing agent to which tolerance does not develop in time is cigarette smoking, which of course entails hazards of its own too numerous to mention.[54]

These [amphetamine-type] drugs are central nervous system stimulants with serious abuse potential.—J. R. Crout, director of the Bureau of Drugs, FDA.

Health spas. One of the biggest weight-loss rip-offs is the health spa. Equipped with hot baths, massaging machines, health drinks, and the like, these places provide programs for the unsuspecting public to improve their figures while putting forth a minimum of effort. Health spas can be used to advantage. People who really exercise there benefit from the effort. But health spas can be extremely costly, and most of the gimmicks offer no real health advantage other than the psychological boost the consumer supplies. Hot baths do not speed up the basal metabolic rate so that pounds can be lost in hours. Steam and sauna baths do not melt the fat off the body, although they may dehydrate a person so that the weight on the scales changes dramatically. Machines intended to jiggle parts of the body while the person leans passively on them provide pleasant stimulation but no exercise and so no expenditure of calories.

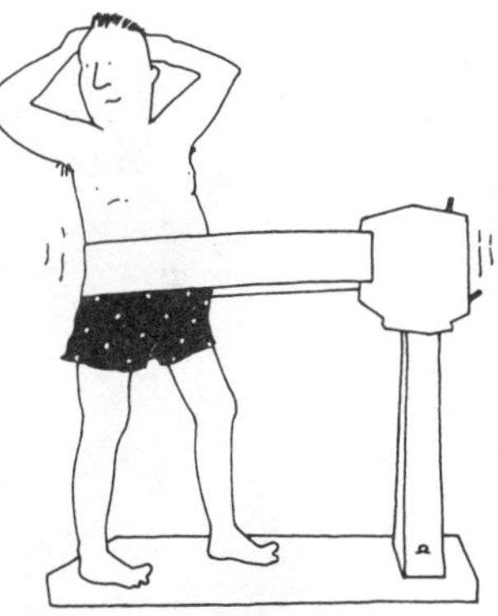

It feels good, but it isn't exercise.

Some people believe there are two kinds of body fat: regular fat and "cellulite." Cellulite is supposed to be a hard and lumpy fat that yields to being "burned up" only if it is first broken up by methods like the massage or the machine typical of the health spa. The notion that there is such a thing as cellulite received wide publicity with the publication of a book by a certain Madame R of Paris, which sold widely during the 1970s. The American Medical Association (AMA) reviewed the evidence on cellulite (there was none) and published a statement to the effect that cellulite was a hoax.[55] You are free to believe either Madame R or the AMA, of course, but it might

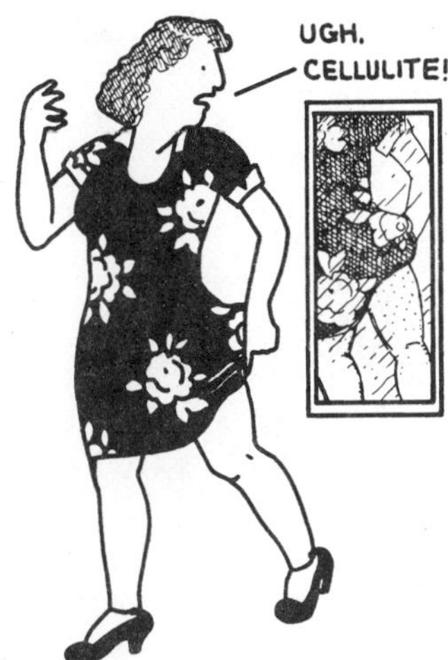

People believe in what they can see, and they think they can see "cellulite." Actually, this woman's connective tissue is pulling on, and puckering, her skin. Her fat is like anyone else's.

help to read the remarks made about books written for the public in Controversy 9 and to know that Madame R makes her living from sales of her book and the proceeds of her spa.

Hormones. Because hormones are powerful body chemicals and because many affect fat metabolism, it has long been hoped that a hormone might be found that would promote weight loss. Several have been tried. With testing, all have proven ineffective and often hazardous as well. Thyroid hormone, in particular, causes loss of lean body mass and heart problems except when medically prescribed for the correction of a thyroid deficiency—and thyroid deficiency is very seldom the cause of obesity.[56]

Among the hormones advertised as promoting weight loss is HCG (human chorionic gonadotropin), a hormone extracted from the urine of pregnant women. People have hoped that HCG would not only promote weight loss but also produce a more attractive body shape. But many controlled studies have shown that it has no effect on weight loss or shape and does not reduce hunger. A rash of "clinics" run by "doctors" that sprang up on the West Coast during 1976 and 1977 advertised tremendous success using HCG in the treatment of obesity. These outfits seem to have had one element in common: They prescribed an extremely rigid low-calorie diet, which accounted for their apparent effectiveness. The American Medical Association, the California Medical Association, and the Food and Drug Administration have concluded that the claims made for HCG are groundless and that the side effects are unknown and possibly dangerous.[57]

Surgery. Sheer desperation prompts some obese patients to request bypass surgery, an operation in which a portion of the small intestine is removed or disconnected. Then the patient can continue overeating but will absorb considerably fewer calories. Side effects from this procedure are many and highly undesirable; they include liver failure, massive and frequent diarrhea, urinary stones, intestinal infection, and malnutrition. Reports of mortality range from 2 to 10 percent,[58] and bypass surgery in particular has so many disadvantages that alternative surgical procedures are still being sought.[59] Still, surgery has been reported to be effective more than half the time for treating the massively obese where all other methods have failed.[60] It should be attempted only in otherwise healthy and cooperative patients under thirty who weigh more than 300 pounds and who have tried everything else.[61]

No matter how much you huff and puff, you can't just shake it off, rock it off, roll it off, knock it off or bake it off. . . . The only way is to eat less and exercise more.—American Medical Association

Desperation of the same kind leads some patients to request that their jaws be wired shut so that they will be forced to consume a liquid diet. This does bring about weight loss, but when the wires are removed, there is "relentless weight gain ... until the prewiring weight has been reached."[62]

The Successful Treatment of Obesity

It seems that the only realistic and sensible way for the obese person to achieve and maintain ideal weight is to cut calories, to increase activity, and to maintain this changed lifestyle for life. This is a tall order. Fewer than a third of those who lose weight manage to keep it off over the long run. To succeed means modifying all of the attitudes and behaviors that have contributed to the problem in the first place, sometimes against physiological pressures that can't be changed. Still, it can be and has been done successfully, as many former "fatties" can attest. A three-pronged approach usually accounts for their success: diet, exercise, and behavior modification.

The way a particular person loses weight is a highly individual matter. Two weight-loss plans may both be successful and yet have little or nothing in common. To heighten the sense of individuality, the following sections are written in terms of advice to "you." This is not intended to put you under pressure to take it personally, but to give you the illusion of listening in on a conversation in which an obese person (with, say, fifty pounds to lose) is being competently counseled by someone familiar with the techniques known to be effective. Notes in the margin highlight the principles involved.[63]

The *Dietary Guidelines* sound these warnings:

Do not try to lose weight too rapidly. Avoid crash diets that are severely restricted in the variety of foods they allow. Diets containing fewer than 800 calories may be hazardous. Some people have developed kidney stones, disturbing psychological changes, and other complications while following such diets. A few people have died suddenly and without warning. . . .

Do not attempt to reduce your weight below the acceptable range. Severe weight loss may be associated with nutrient deficiencies, menstrual irregularities, infertility, hair loss, skin changes, cold intolerance, severe constipation, psychiatric disturbances, and other complications.

If you lose weight suddenly or for unknown reasons, see a physician. Unexplained weight loss may be an early clue to an unsuspected underlying disorder.

Diet. No particular diet is magical, and no particular food must either be included or avoided. You are the one who will have to live with the diet, so you had better be involved in its planning. Don't think of it as a diet you are going "on"—because then you may be tempted to go "off." The diet can be called successful only if the pounds do not return. Think of it as an eating plan that you will adopt for life. It must consist of foods that you like, that are available to you, and that are within your means.

Do not—and this is hard advice to follow—allow yourself to get tempted into trying to follow a crash diet plan, and do not try to reduce your weight below the acceptable range. The risks of either of these courses are numerous and serious (see margin). Once you accept the fact that you will have to change your habits for a lifetime and lose the weight gradually to lose it permanently, you can put your energy into the positive effort of doing the job the way it has to be done.

Obese people have been administered every psychological battery devised and there is no correlation between psychological make-up and treatment outcome. What is important . . . is to . . . individualize the treatment.—H. A. Jordan

Choose a calorie level you can live with. If you maintain your weight on 2000 calories a day, then you can certainly lose at least a pound a week on a 1200-calorie diet. (A deficit of 500 calories a day for seven days is a 3500-calorie deficit—enough to lose a pound of body fat. But let's make a larger deficit, just to be sure.) There is no point in hurrying, because you will never go off the diet—and nutritional adequacy can't be achieved on fewer than about 1200 calories a day—1000 at the very least.

Involve the person.

Put diet adequacy high on your list of priorities. This is a way of putting yourself first. "I like me, and I'm going to take good care of me" is the attitude to adopt. This means including low-calorie foods that are rich in valuable nutrients—tasty vegetables and fruits, whole-grain breads and cereals, and a limited amount of lean protein-rich foods

Adopt a realistic plan.

Make the diet adequate.

Emphasize high nutrient density.

Individualize: Use foods you like.

Stress dos, not don'ts.

like poultry, fish, eggs, cottage cheese, and skim milk. Within these categories, learn what foods you like, and use them often. If you plan resolutely to include a certain number of servings of food from each of these groups each day, you may be so busy making sure you get what you need that you will have little time or appetite left for high-calorie or empty-calorie foods.

About a third of the calories in your diet should come from fat, to make your meals more satisfying. At least a third of the fat should be polyunsaturated fat—for example, from salad dressing or fish.[64] Read the label to be sure of the kind of fat. And measure your fat with extra caution: A slip of the butterknife adds even more calories than a slip of the sugar spoon. And speaking of empty calories—if you are willing, omit sugar, pure fat and oil, and alcohol altogether. Let your carbohydrate come from starchy foods and your fat from protein-rich foods.

Food Feature: Planning a Weight-Loss Diet

Two different distributions of energy nutrients are recommended for diets, depending on whether you are maintaining/gaining weight or losing weight. When you are *maintaining* weight (say, on 2400 calories a day), the following balance is suggested:

15 percent of calories from protein.

30 percent or less from fat.

55 percent or more from carbohydrate.

These calorie amounts translate into grams as follows:

Protein: 360 calories, or 90 grams.

Fat: 720 calories, or about 80 grams.

Carbohydrate: 1320 calories, or 330 grams.

Now suppose you want to *reduce* weight. You could cut your calorie amount in half, to 1200 calories per day. To avoid getting too hungry (for "satiety value") you must have ample protein and fat. But for health reasons, fat should not supply more than about a third of your calories. You must therefore cut the fat grams in half. For maximum satiety, then, leave the protein amount as is. (Protein, of course, should never be cut below two-thirds of the RDA.) So far, you have

Protein: 90 grams, or 360 calories.

Fat: 45 grams, or 405 calories.

This gives a total of 765 calories and therefore leaves only 435 to be supplied by carbohydrate. This means

Carbohydrate: 110 grams, or 440 calories.

You have had to cut your carbohydrate down to about a third of what it was formerly. This balance is typical of successful, nutritious weight-loss plans.[65] The protein may even be raised and the carbohydrate lowered a little more to deliver a nearly perfect ⅓-⅓-⅓ balance of calories from the three energy nutrients. In terms of exchanges, such a plan might be designed as follows:

Table 1. A Sample Balanced Weight-Loss Diet

Exchange Group	Number of Exchanges	Carbohydrate (g)	Protein (g)	Fat (g)
Milk (skim)	2	24	16	0
Vegetables	4	20	8	0
Fruit	3	30	0	0
Bread	2	30	4	0
Meat (lean)	11	0	77	33
Fat	2	0	0	10
Total		104	105	43

In this diet, carbohydrate supplies 34 percent of the calories, protein 34 percent, and fat 32 percent. The protein calories are higher than needed for maintenance. When the dieter returns to a maintenance plan by adding (mostly) carbohydrate foods, the ratio will resemble the recommended 15 percent protein, 35 percent fat, 50 percent carbohydrate. This diet is one of many that offers the needed balance. It could be higher in bread and fat and lower in meat exchanges.

The design of a weight-reduction diet—with all the protein, half the fat, and only a third the carbohydrate of a regular diet—may be responsible for many people's belief that cutting carbohydrate is necessary for weight loss. In a sound weight-loss diet, however, carbohydrate calories are not cut below about a third of the total. To eliminate carbohydrate altogether would be to invite a host of health hazards. Nor should you fast, except on a doctor's advice under very unusual medical circumstances.

More on low-carbohydrate diets and fasting in Chapter 7.

Eat regularly; and if at all possible, eat before you are very hungry. When you do decide to eat, eat the entire meal you have planned for yourself. Then don't eat again until the next meal. Save "free" or favorite foods or beverages for the end of the day, in case you are hungry once more.

Eat regular meals, no skipping—at least three a day.

You may have blamed yourself for eating compulsively in the past. That very character trait can work to your advantage: Compulsive people finish what they have started. So diet compulsively. Keep a record of what you have eaten each day for at least a week or two until your habits are beginning to be automatic.

Take a positive view of yourself.

It may seem at first as if you have to spend all your waking hours thinking about and planning your meals. Such a massive effort is always required when a new skill is being learned. (You spent hours practicing writing the alphabet when you were in the first grade.) But after about three weeks, it will be much easier. Your new eating pattern will become a habit. Many sound and helpful books and booklets are available to help you get started, some of which are listed in this chapter's references.

Visualize a changed future self.

Weigh yourself only once every week or two and always on the same scale, so that you can see clearly the progress you are making. Although 3500 calories roughly equals a pound of body fat, there is no simple relationship between calorie balance and weight loss over short intervals. Gains or losses of a pound or more in a matter of days reverse themselves quickly; the smoothed-out average is what is real. Don't expect to lose continuously as fast as you did at first. A sizable water loss is common in the first week, but it will not happen again.

Take well-spaced weighings to avoid discouragement.

If you see a gain in weight and you know you have strictly followed your diet, this probably represents a shift in water weight. Many dieters experience a temporary plateau after about three weeks—not because they are slipping but because they have gained water weight temporarily while they are still losing body fat.

You might be interested to know exactly how this happens. The fat you are hoping to lose must be combined with oxygen (oxidized) to make carbon dioxide and water if it is to leave the body. The oxygen you breathe in combines with the carbons of the fat to make carbon dioxide and with the hydrogens to make water. The carbon dioxide will be breathed out quickly. But the water takes awhile to leave the cell; it enters the spaces between the cells, then works its way into the lymph system, and finally enters the bloodstream. Only after the water arrives in the blood will the kidneys "see" it and send it to the bladder for excretion. While water is making its way into the blood, you have a weight gain, because the water weighs more than the fat that was oxidized.[66]

Anticipate a plateau (realistic expectations).

If you faithfully follow your diet plan, one day the plateau will break. You will know it by your frequent urination.

You may find it helpful to control your environment, to avoid situations that prompt you to eat. Begin at the grocery store. Shop when you aren't hungry, and buy only the foods you plan to use on your diet. Purge from your pantry all forbidden items. If you must keep them on hand for other members of your family, surrender them into someone else's possession and ask that they be kept out of your sight as much as possible. Have low-calorie foods ready to eat; prepare ahead. To help further with your motivation, mount a mirror on the refrigerator door.

Control external cues.

It is easier to exclude a food than to exercise away its calories. To remind yourself of the reality that calories eaten must be spent in physical activity, post the following table conspicuously in a place where you might otherwise be tempted to eat:

Discourage magical thinking.

Table 2. Activity Equivalents of Food Calorie Values

Food	Calories	Activity Equivalent to Work Off the Calories (minutes)		
		Walk[a]	Jog[b]	Wait[c]
Apple, large	101	19	5	78
Beer, 1 glass	114	22	6	88
Cookie, chocolate chip	51	10	3	39
Ice cream, 1/6 qt	193	37	10	148
Steak, T-bone	235	45	12	181

[a]Energy cost of walking at 3.5 mph, for a 70-kilogram person—5.2 calories per minute.

[b]Energy cost of running—19.4 calories per minute.

[c]Energy cost of reclining—1.3 calories per minute.

Data from M. V. Krause and M. A. Hunscher, Food, Nutrition and Diet Therapy, 5th ed. (Philadelphia: Saunders, 1972), p. 431.

After losing twenty or thirty pounds, expect to reach a stable plateau. Take this as a good sign. It means that you have lost so much weight that you now require fewer calories to maintain your weight. Take a deep breath (you knew this was coming, and you are courageous) and institute a change: Increase your activity, cut your calories further, or both.

Plateaus are absolutely inevitable. . . . It requires about 12 calories per pound to maintain body weight. When you lose 20 pounds, about 240 calories are no longer required . . . to maintain.—H. A. Jordan

If you slip, don't punish yourself. Positive reinforcement is very effective at changing behavior, but punishment seldom works. If you ate an extra 1000 calories yesterday, don't try to eat 1000 fewer calories today. Just go back to your diet. On the other hand, you can plan ahead and budget for binges. If you want to celebrate your birthday with cake and ice cream, cut the necessary calories from your bread and milk allowance for several days *beforehand*. Again, if you do this compulsively, your weight loss will be as smooth as if you had stayed with the daily plan.

Use positive reinforcement.

You may have to get tough with yourself if you stop losing weight or start gaining unexpectedly. You may be slipping on serving sizes. Many a dieter has in time begun to measure out meat exchanges too carelessly—and has added an extra 500 calories to the day's intake. Equally common is the "just this once" substitution of high-fat meat like steak for a fish fillet that was in the plan. You can get away with this only if you scrupulously omit the right amount of fat from other foods the same day. Ask yourself honestly (no one is listening in), "What am I doing wrong?" Very, very seldom does an unpredicted weight plateau of any duration have no explanation in the dieter's own choices.

Never blame, never punish.

Identify your problem and correct it.

Finally, if you stop losing weight or begin to gain, be aware that you may be choosing to stop. Your weight is under your control, and you are entirely free to change your mind about it. You may find you are choosing to take a break, to go into a holding pattern, and to get adjusted before going on. Rather than letting yourself suffer from guilt

Watch serving sizes.

Learn calorie values and fat contents of foods.

feelings and feelings of failure, hold your head high and take the attitude "This is me, and this is the way I am choosing to be right now."

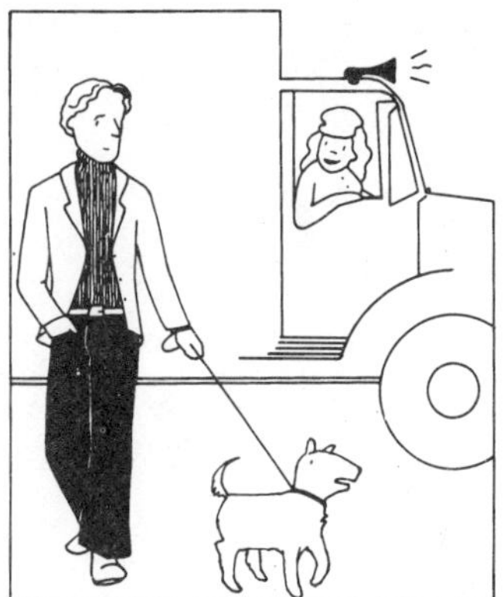

Moving your body becomes a pleasure, as does letting others see you move.

Exercise. Weight loss is possible without exercise. Obese people often —and very understandably—do not enjoy moving their bodies very much. They feel heavy, clumsy, even ridiculous. The choice of whether to exercise regularly, informally, or not at all is a strictly individual matter. But even if you choose not to alter your habits at first, let your mind be open to the possibility that you will want to take up sports, dancing, or another activity later on. As the pounds come off, moving your body becomes a pleasure, as does letting others see you move. And the health advantages of regular exercise are well documented. It can truly make you look, feel, and be healthier.

You must keep in mind that, if exercise is to help with weight loss, it must be active exercise—voluntary moving of muscles. Being moved passively, as by a machine at a health spa or by a massage, does not increase calorie expenditure. The more muscles you move, the more calories you spend.

Stress personal responsibility.

Honor the individual.

Pave the way for later changes.

More on exercise and its beneficial physiological effects in the adult years—Chapter 15.

If you are very inactive, you may eventually find yourself stuck at a plateau. At this point it may be time to come to terms with the fact that exercise will have to become a regular part of your life plan. One way to think of this is to realize that on a low-calorie diet, it is difficult to ensure nutritional adequacy. Exercise will increase your *need* for calories and so make it permissible to eat a little more nutritious food.

When you set about choosing an activity, don't feel obligated to choose one that you hate. Jogging is not for everybody. Let the activity be one that you can at least imagine learning to enjoy in time. What fits best with your self-image: Rapid walking? Bicycling? Running errands for friends? Many people find that after two or three weeks of effort, exercise becomes as habitual as binge eating was before: You can get addicted to it.

Behavior modification. Everybody is different, but people who overeat are often seen to behave in certain ways at the table. Hence the need for **behavior modification**. Most of us are only faintly aware of our eating behavior and can find it interesting, even funny, to observe ourselves. Notice your own table style and compare it to someone else's. How often do you put down your fork (if at all)? How often do you interrupt your eating to converse with a friend? How fast do you chew your food? Do you always clean your plate? Several good books and other resources (check the chapter references) can help you not only to observe yourself closely but also to set about systematically and effectively to retrain yourself to eat like a thin person.

For many people, learning to eat slowly is one of the most important behavior changes to adopt. The satiety signal indicating that you are full is sent after a twenty-minute lag. You may eat a great deal more than you need before the signal reaches your brain. Conversely, underweight people need to learn to eat more food within the first twenty minutes of a meal.

Some people seem to respond to sugar, specifically, as if they had a biochemically based addiction to it. If this is the case with you, you may have to kick the habit much as a drug addict has to do. Techniques developed for extinguishing drug addiction will be useful in this case.[67]

You may find it helpful to join a group such as TOPS (Take Off Pounds Sensibly) or Weight Watchers. A modest expenditure for your own health and well-being is certainly worthwhile (but avoid expensive, quick-weight-loss, "magical" ripoffs, of course). Many dieters find it helpful to form their own self-help groups structured around some of the resources already mentioned. Sometimes it also helps to enlist a family member's participation and cooperation. Correspondence groups are also available.[68]

In case you are a person who eats in response to external cues rather than internally felt hunger, you may need to keep a record for a while of all the circumstances surrounding your eating—the time, the place, the person you are with, the emotions you have at the time, the physical sensations, and other things. An example of such a record is shown below:

We make treatment contingent upon record keeping.—H. A. Jordan

Food Diary

Time	Place	Food	Amount	Reason Food Was Eaten	Mood
7 AM	kitchen	coffee	1 cup	to wake up	ok
11 AM	library	candy bar	2	hungry	ok
1:30 PM	kitchen	tuna sandwich	1	lunch	ok
4 PM	gas station	coke	12 oz	none	upset
4 PM	gas station	cookies	6	none	upset

In small step modification, it is important to ask the patient what he thinks would be the best approach . . . "Do you think you can do it?"—L. Haimes

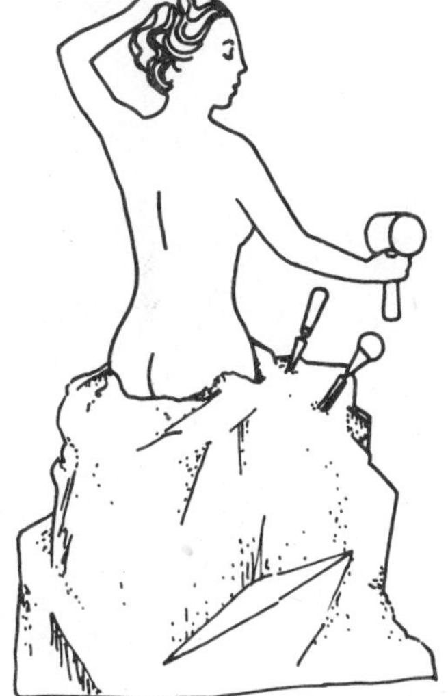

Inside of every fat person, a thin person waits to be freed.

Looking back, the writer can see what stimulates eating and can learn to control these stimuli. If you find that you are, indeed, eating for the "wrong" reasons—for example, boredom—this will pave the way for adopting behaviors that will better meet your needs than will compulsive eating.[69] You can begin to make rules for yourself, like "never eat when you're upset."

If you are especially sensitive to pressure from your family or friends or hosts (can't say no), it will help to have some assertiveness training. Learning not to clean your plate might be one of your first objectives.

From all the behavior changes available to you, you can choose the ones to begin with. Don't try to master them all at once. No one who attempts too many changes at one time is successful. Set your own priorities: Pick one trouble area that you think you can handle, start with that, and practice your strategy until it is habitual and automatic. Then you can select another trouble area to work on.

Enjoy your new, emerging self. Inside of every fat person, a thin person is struggling to be freed. Get in touch with—reach out your hand to—your thin self, and help that self to feel welcome in the light of day.

Deep inside there had always been a small child begging for my attention. . . . All I gave her was food. Now I give her love —E. Leshan

The Problems of Underweight

Much of what has been said about obesity applies to underweight as well, although its hazards are not as great. In fact, the only causes of death seen more often in thin people than in normal-weight people are infections such as tuberculosis. (Suicide is more common among underweight people, but the underweight is not thought to be a cause; rather, the severe depression that leads to suicide probably has caused **anorexia**, or lack of appetite.)

The causes of underweight may be as diverse as those of overeating. Hunger, appetite, and satiety irregularities may exist; there may be contributory psychological factors in some cases and metabolic ones in others. Clearly, there is a genetic component as well. Early underfeeding may limit the fat-cell number in the same way overfeeding may increase it. Habits learned early in childhood, especially food aversions, may perpetuate the problem. The demand for calories to support physical activity and growth often contributes: An extremely active boy during his adolescent growth spurt may need more than 4000 calories a day to maintain his weight. Such a boy may be too busy to take the time to eat that much. The underweight person states with justification that it is as hard for him to gain a pound as for an obese person to lose one. So much energy may be spent adapting to a higher food intake that it may take as many as 750 to 800 extra calories a day for the underweight person to gain a pound a week.[70]

Strategies recommended for weight gain mostly center on increasing food intake, using foods that provide as many calories in as small a volume as possible so as not to get uncomfortably full. Recommended are nutritious, high-calorie milkshakes; liberal servings of meat, bread, and starchy vegetables; and desserts. Where the weight loser is urged to select the lowest-calorie items from each food group, the gainer is encouraged to pick the highest-calorie items from those same groups. Often he or she may need to resort to systematic between-meal snacking in addition to regular meals. No known pill, shot, hormone, or surgical procedure will increase weight safely, and a reduction in activity is not recommended unless the condition is associated with illness or is so severe as to threaten overall health. As with weight loss, the person attempting a weight gain must anticipate a plateau, at which time a further increase in food intake will be necessary to continue the gain.[71]

An extreme underweight condition, **anorexia nervosa**, is sometimes seen, usually in young women who claim to be exercising self-denial in order to control their weight. They actually go to such an extreme that they become severely undernourished, finally achieving a body weight of seventy pounds or even less. The distinguishing feature of the anorexic, as opposed to other very thin people, is that she intentionally starves herself. Often there is a whole cluster of accompanying "typical" characteristics of the family and the girl's attitudes.

For more about anorexia nervosa, turn to Chapter 14.

Anorexia nervosa is a serious condition that demands treatment by an experienced doctor or clinic. Even if temporarily reversed by forced feeding, it can reappear. If the underlying cause is not successfully dealt with, this illness can result in permanent brain damage or death. Strategies for treatment are more effective than they have been in the past, and recovery can be hoped for.[1]

For Further Information

Recommended references on all nutrition topics are listed in Appendix J. In addition, we selected many to cite in this chapter's notes and Controversy.

A touching personal account by a woman who lost seventy pounds and recorded her thoughts and feelings throughout the experience:

- LeShan, E. *Winning the Losing Battle: Why I Will Never Be Fat Again.* New York: Bantam Books, 1981.

One of the most useful and well-written books we've seen to help with behavioral control of obesity is:

- Nash, J. D., and Long, L. O. *Taking Charge of Your Weight and Well-Being.* Palo Alto, Calif.: Bull Publishing Company, 1978.

It presents a complete program with step-by-step instructions and forms for eighteen weeks' worth of record-keeping.

Another excellent—and much smaller—book of the same kind advertises itself "for teenagers only" but is highly recommended for adults whose eating habits are the same as they were in the teen years:

- Ikeda, J. *Change Your Habits, Change Your Shape.* Palo Alto, Calif.: Bull Publishing Company, 1978.

A highly recommended weight-loss guide for young people is:

- Berg, F. *How to Lose Weight the Action Way.* Hettinger, N.D.: Flying Diamond Books, 1980.

A paper describing the ways in which a spouse can be helpful in the weight control efforts of an obese person is:

- Brownell, K. D., Heckerman, C. L., Westlake, R. J., Hayes, S. C., and Monti, P. M. The effect of couples training and partner cooperativeness in the behavioral treatment of obesity. *Behavioral Research and Therapy* 16 (1978): 323-333.

One of many recent popular books to help people learn to be more assertive is:

- Smith, M. J. *When I Say No, I Feel Guilty.* New York: Bantam Books, 1975 (paperback).

[1]*Chapter Notes can be found at the end of the Appendixes.*

The possibility that fiber and its interplay with insulin may have an important role to play in satisfying appetite and so controlling food intake is discussed in:

- Heaton, K. W., ed. *Dietary Fibre: Current Developments of Importance to Health.* Westport, Conn.: Food & Nutrition Press, 1979.

Weight Watchers, Inc., publishes several cookbooks, all based on the exchange system, that present a very sensible, nutritious, balanced diet for weight loss.

A diet book that uses the exchange system—and includes exchanges for fast foods—is Better Homes and Gardens' *Eat and Stay Slim*, 2d ed. Des Moines, Iowa: Meredith, 1979. The 1979 price was $3.95.

Consumer Guide put out a booklet in 1979 entitled *Diets '79*, which rated the Scarsdale Diet, the "Mayo Clinic" Diet, the Pritikin program, and many others as to whether they work, how safe they are, and how permanent their effects are. The booklet was so successful it will very likely be followed by another like it every now and then. Watch for these.

The entire issue of *Nutrition and the MD*, November 1979 (all six pages of it), was devoted to obesity: its causes, treatment, incidence in children, and so forth.

Controversy 8

Ideal Body Weight

What is it?

Svelte, lean, shapely, muscular, thin. These adjectives are often used to describe the healthy person. And it seems to be almost everyone's goal to fit these descriptions. Just think for a moment how many of your friends and acquaintances have just finished dieting, are on a diet, are planning to diet, or at least keep talking about how they "should lose a few pounds." This urge toward thinness is continually reinforced by advertisements, by television, by a continuing stream of diet and health books promoting the thin look. But is "thin" so "in"? What is the best weight for you, the weight that would really be ideal? Is there such a weight?

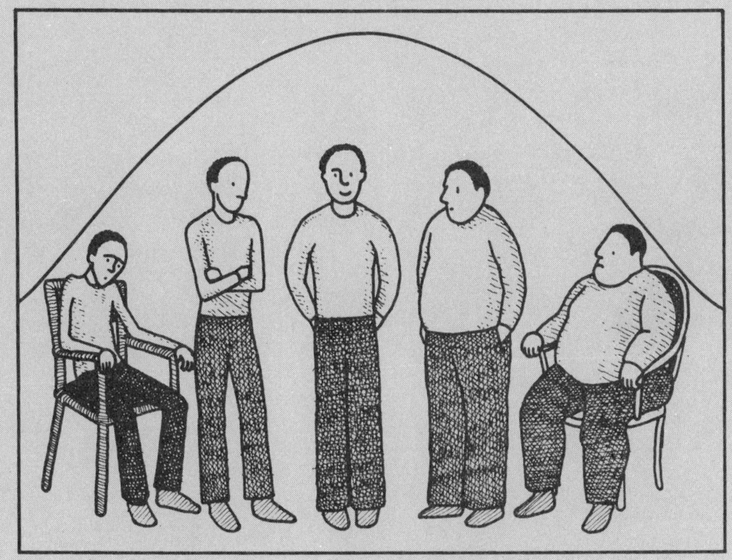

What's your ideal weight?

Marie is 5 feet 4 inches tall, 17 years old, and weighs 110 pounds. She is greatly disgusted with herself and is dieting strictly in the effort to lose 15 or more pounds. Emma is also 5 feet 4 inches tall but is 46 years old and weighs 130 pounds. She is facing surgery and is eating as much as she can in the effort to build herself up to at least 145 pounds before she goes into the hospital. If these women both reach their desired weight, Emma will be 25 pounds above the average weight for her height and Marie will be 25 pounds under. Who will be healthier?

Paul is 5 feet 10 inches tall, 24 years old, and weighs 155 pounds. He runs but is not as thin as some of the runners he admires. He isn't dieting, but

Average Weights of U.S. Citizens—HANES Survey, 1980[a]

Height (inches)	Age 18-24	Age 25-34	Age 35-44	Age 45-54	Age 55-64	Age 65-74
Men			Weight (pounds)			
62	130	141	143	147	143	143
63	135	145	148	152	147	147
64	140	150	153	156	153	151
65	145	156	158	160	158	156
66	150	160	163	164	163	160
67	154	165	169	169	168	164
68	159	170	174	173	173	169
69	164	174	179	177	178	173
70	168	179	184	182	183	177
71	173	184	190	187	189	182
72	178	189	194	191	193	186
73	183	194	200	196	197	190
74	188	199	205	200	203	194
Women						
57	114	118	125	129	132	130
58	117	121	129	133	136	134
59	120	125	133	136	140	137
60	123	128	137	140	143	140
61	126	132	141	143	147	144
62	129	136	144	147	150	147
63	132	139	148	150	153	151
64	135	142	152	154	157	154
65	138	146	156	158	160	158
66	141	150	159	161	164	161
67	144	153	163	165	167	165
68	147	157	167	168	171	169

[a]For comparison, look on the inside back cover at the tables of "ideal weight" published by the insurance companies.

he's holding back a little and increasing his daily mileage in preparation for a marathon event. At the time of the marathon he hopes to weigh 145 pounds. Meanwhile, Charlie, 51, the same height as Paul, is about to be married again after eight years of widowhood. At 185 pounds he is underweight compared to the husky, strong men of his family, and he is feeding himself liberally in hopes of weighing at least 195 pounds on his wedding day. If both of these men reach their goals, Charlie will be 50 pounds heavier than Paul. Who will be healthier?

Is it a surprise to learn that in the case of both the women and the men, the fatter one will probably be the healthier? There are severe risks to being too underweight. Marie has anorexia nervosa, and if she persists in her course she may end up with brain damage, hospitalized for life. (Chapter 14 describes this condition fully.) Paul is deluded in wanting to be as thin as possible; he hasn't heard of the sudden deaths of elite runners who lose too much weight (see Chapter 7).

But surely Emma and Charlie are facing severe health hazards in becoming so overweight? Not necessarily. The question is still being debated, but recent evidence suggests that—*unless they have high blood pressure*—these two people may not be risking any problems at all in letting their body weights exceed the average by up to 25 pounds.

Body weight and life expectancy in men. In 1900, life insurance companies were already insisting that people tell not only their ages but also their heights and weights when they applied for life insurance. Thinner people were then charged higher premiums—because if they contracted tuberculosis they would be the first to die, and tuberculosis was a major killer at the time. But much effort to cure tuberculosis was being expended, and it was rapidly being brought under control. Eventually the "thin" penalty premiums were eliminated.

Miniglossary

brown fat: A kind of fat found in hibernating mammals, and to some extent in humans, in which futile cycles take place so that energy nutrients are oxidized and generate heat without their energy being stored or used to do work.

futile cycle: A metabolic activity of the body's cells in which chemical reactions take place with a loss, and no storage, of energy. Futile cycles are believed to account for some people's "fast metabolism" and their ability to consume calories without the expected consequent weight gain.

set point: A term used to describe the point around which regulation takes place, as on a thermostat—the setting below which conservation measures are initiated and above which wasting measures take over. In body weight, the set point is considered to be the body's preferred weight, that to which it tends to return naturally after any disturbance.

Meanwhile, in 1912, a society of insurance people published a set of statistics showing that gross "overweight" also entailed a higher death rate than normal, and insurance premiums were raised for overweight applicants too. ("Overweight," here, means 25 to 30 percent above average weight.) Since that time, "thin" has been "in."

In 1980, Dr. Ancel Keys, professor emeritus of the School of Public Health at the University of Minnesota, presented a major lecture (the Atwater lecture) at a nutrition conference, reviewing the whole question of overweight and mortality.[1] He showed that the public has for years had several wrong impressions largely based on the insurance data and on the companies' use of the word *ideal*.

For one thing, Dr. Keys said, it was true that the overweight insured persons tended to die younger, but they were not a typical sample: They were people who were overweight *who knew they had an increased risk of early death* and so applied for life insurance. Certain conditions, especially high blood pressure, do entail an increased mortality risk; but for every 100 overweight men who applied and paid extra for life insurance, there were 200 other overweight men who didn't bother because they did not feel they needed that protection.

A second point made by Dr. Keys was that the so-called "ideal weight tables" published by the insurance companies were not only *not* ideal but were not even average weights for the population. "The fact is," he said, "the tables . . . are armchair concoctions starting with questionable assumptions and ending with three sets of standards for 'frame' types never measured or even defined." Actual average weights as determined by several other studies are about 15 percent higher than the table weights. For example, the insurance-company table weight for men 5 feet 10 inches tall is around 155 pounds, but the real average weight for these men is closer to 180 pounds (see table at start).

A great many analyses of a great mass of data were summed up by Dr. Keys, and his lecture is highly recommended reading. One other point he made that should be mentioned here is that a number of studies have shown that a slightly "overweight" condition may be advantageous in terms of life expectancy. To fully understand just what this means and doesn't mean, you have to understand the statistical methods used. Only data on men above 40 years of age were used. Those with high blood pressure were excluded. Then, Dr. Keys explained, you could look at the data in two ways. If you tried to see whether it was more advantageous to be overweight or underweight (the straight-line approach), overweight came out better. If you tried to see what weight was the very best (the curve approach), it turned out to be a weight "somewhat above the median," with the worst prospects for the most underweight *and* the most overweight men. This second approach, revealing both extremes as unhealthy, fit the data much better.

Finally, Dr. Keys offered an important caution. Remember, he said, that what was being measured was weight, not fatness. This means there may have been many heavily built, muscular men in the sample. Had only the overly *fat* men been studied, a greater connection between fatness and mortality risk might have been found. Scale weights, however, were the only available data. Fatfolds were not measured on the hundreds of men on whom these studies were made. Dr.

Keys' conclusion was succinctly stated:

We and other investigators find that in the absence of hypertension overweight is not a risk factor at all. But there is a tendency for persons with high blood pressure to be overweight. Such persons should be advised to reduce; the blood pressure often drops when weight is lost by the overweight person.

For the moment, then, it seems all right for men not to try to be thin.

For truly obese men there is a mortality risk, however, and it can be substantial. In very obese men of 25 to 34, the risk of death is twelve times greater than it is for men of normal weight.[2] But in the case of Charlie, whom we met earlier, at 195 pounds, he'll be only about 25 percent above the "ideal" weight for his height and only 5 to 10 percent above the average. This is probably fine, especially if he is of a muscular build.

What about women? Dr. Keys didn't have enough data to make any statements about women's weight and life expectancy, but others have attempted to make a start. The data from one of the studies Keys used (the Framingham study) revealed that minimal mortality for women occurred in those whose weight was 105 to 124 percent of "ideal."[3] To apply these numbers to Emma: At 5 feet 4 inches, her "ideal" weight is around 120 pounds; and 105 to 124 percent of this is about 125 to 150 pounds. Her goal weight of 145 pounds is within this range, and she can expect to lose some weight in the hospital; so maybe, for her, this is the best weight at which to approach surgery.

Not much more information is available on women's ideal weights, but other investigators who specialize in studies of energy balance have reached the conclusion that "mild obesity in women may well represent a desirable physiological state."[4] Very obese women, however, are advised to reduce because of a risk of breast cancer.[5]

The findings discussed above tend to point to the same conclusion: that it's all right to be fatter than we may have thought in the past. There is another line of thinking that seems to point in this direction, too: the body itself seems to know what weight it "wants" to be.

The body's own desired weight. In 1955, some investigators reported that they had put some genetically obese mice on a diet. When the mice had reached "normal" weight, they still had excess *fat* in their bodies. Their bodies had sacrificed lean tissue and held on to their fat.[6] Evidently their bodies were obeying a metabolic law that, for them, a high fat-to-lean ratio had to be maintained. That being so, weight loss was probably bad for them because it made them lose lean tissue. If there are some people like that, they too would probably be better off fat. Juvenile-onset obese people might fit into this category.

The body somehow seems to know how much fat it wants to store. Both animals and humans tend to regulate their body weight around some "set point" that is maintained with remarkable persistence, sometimes against heavy odds. For example, when subjects in an experiment are made to overeat so that they gain weight, they spontaneously lose weight back to whatever is normal for them as soon as the experiment is over. And when animals undergo surgical removal of fat tissue, they compensate afterwards by depositing more fat until they are back where they started from.[7] Most people can state, almost to the pound, their bodies' "natural" weight.

What accounts for the differences between different people's body weights? It is well known that people's energy needs vary widely. One reviewer puts it this way: "Some people, perhaps through some mechanism of adaptation, are able to be healthy and active on energy intakes which, by current standards, would be regarded as inadequate, [whereas] many fat people eat . . . less, than those who are not obese."[8] Another shows that most people of "normal" weight are "normal" because it's easy for them to be there. Even diabetics, who as a class are notorious for gaining weight uncontrollably, tend to maintain a normal weight if they happen to be of normal weight to begin with.[9]

And while it's easy for "normals" to be normal, it may be extremely hard for obese people not to be obese. One study shows, for example, that the fat cells of lean people resist taking up glucose, while the fat cells of obese people take it up eagerly and turn it into more fat. Not only that, but as they fill they become more and more "hungry" for glucose.[10]

How do different people's bodies regulate their weight so differently? Recently, much study has been invested in *futile cycles*—metabolic pathways in which energy nutrients are oxidized without their energy being captured and stored as fat.[11] Some people tend to store, others to "waste," energy, depending on the enzymes that happen to be active in their bodies. The fact that more weight is lost than one might predict under certain circumstances—with exercise and with stress—is partly attributable to an increase in futile cycling that occurs at these times.[12] In other words, some thin people can eat a lot of calories, but the enzymes in their bodies "burn" them up rather than storing them as fat. The difference may even be apparent in the type of body fat they tend to make: white versus brown.

It has been known for a while that some animals have two kinds of fat in their bodies: the regular kind (white), which stores energy for retrieval, and brown fat, which releases the energy as heat only, without using any of it to do cellular work. Brown fat is what hibernating animals use to keep themselves warm through the cold season: It burns like wood in a stove, dissipating heat and performing no other work. This is futile cycling. Some investigators speculate that humans, too, have brown fat that may "waste" energy (we know that babies are born with some). It remains to be seen whether this accounts for some of the differences between people.[13]

Whatever does account for the differences, however, they are real. The 1980 report of the Food and Nutrition Board, *Toward Healthful Diets*, acknowledges this in saying, "Energy expenditure among individuals doing similar amounts of work is variable, suggesting that different persons perform work with different efficiencies."[14] If you tend to be fat, then, it may be hard for you to lose, even if you exercise a lot. Moreover, if you decrease your calorie intake, you may use the calories with greater efficiency so that you tend to stay at the same weight. The same kind of thing in reverse may happen to a thin friend of yours who wants to gain weight. As she increases her calorie intake she may use calories more inefficiently (wastefully), so that she doesn't gain weight as you might expect.[15] Against these odds, it is as hard to gain as to lose from the point where the body "wants" to be. In view of this, should we try?

Personal strategy. If you weigh about 15 percent above the insurance tables' "ideal weight" for your height, should you try to reduce? From the standpoint of health, the effort may not be necessary. You may be at the average weight for the population, and there are no apparent health risks in staying where you are. Dieting is stressful, and stress itself can shorten life. It's been said this way:

Dieting is a stressor for many people who maintain a lower body weight than their set point. The constant physiological hunger may be a source of frustration and a drain on the ability to cope emotionally.[16]

Some people struggle so hard to control their weight that they are forced to conclude, in the end, that they are better off a little heavier than they might like to be, but without the constant anxiety incurred by dieting. The spouse, roommate, or other intimate of such a person may be grateful to see them give up dieting to free their energy for other, less self-involved interests.

If you have high blood pressure, however, and if this can be lowered by reducing your weight, you should definitely make the effort. And women whose breast cancer risk is high (if it runs in the family, and especially if it has already occurred and they are trying to avoid a recurrence) should be careful to avoid or correct obesity.

What about diabetics? Weight reduction normalizes a number of the metabolic abnormalities in the main form of diabetes (the non-insulin-dependent type), such as insulin resistance, high blood glucose, and high blood fat levels; and so it may be desirable from that standpoint. But while weight gain often precipitates diabetes, no one has yet shown that within that set of people who already have diabetes, the obese ones bear a greater mortality risk than the nonobese.[17]

Against these considerations one must balance the factors in favor of dieting. In our society, you can't ignore the cultural norms that dictate that, especially for women, slim is beautiful. A woman may have her self-esteem so tied to her body-image, and may be so firmly persuaded that only a very slim body is acceptable, that she may find it easier to maintain a strict diet than to change her mental attitude. Any person whose chief rewards, whether they be financial, emotional, social, or other, come from being very slim will find it worth the effort to fight the body's natural tendencies and maintain a fashionable figure. But such dieting should be done carefully and slowly to minimize stress on the body.

What about thin people who don't care so much about fashion but who care a great deal about their health? Should they make an effort to gain weight in order to reach the point on the curve where the statistical mortality risk is lowest? Probably not. Statistically, people's mortality risk is lowest at a weight slightly above average, but this doesn't mean a thin person can reduce his or her personal risk by gaining weight, especially by gaining body fat. Quite possibly, it's the other way around: People in the best health have the longest life expectancy, and their body weights may simply be a reflection (not a cause) of their good health.

This Controversy has tried to stay on the fence and not prescribe any particular course of action. Your body weight is a highly individual matter, and perhaps the most important new information offered here is that if there are risks to health in being different from the average, they exist at both extremes—overweight and underweight—and the area between the extremes may be broader than we have thought in the past. In addition, because stress influences health and dieting is stressful, and because the body itself exerts a force that tends to keep it at some preferred weight, there is something to be said for acceptance of reality. Within reason, perhaps the best course is to start by knowing yourself: Pick a weight you can comfortably maintain, and set about enjoying life in positive ways rather than struggling against what seems to be a powerful natural law.

An important caution has to be offered along with these ideas, however. Chapter 8 mentioned many health hazards of obesity and described the high incidence of obesity in the U.S. and Canada. Nothing that has been said here contradicts that information. Remember that obesity, as distinguished from overweight, is a condition to prevent and avoid. Add to this the fact that most authorities believe the primary cause of obesity is *underactivity*, and you have an element that should become part of anyone's self-prescription for good health: Be physically active. With abundant physical activity and a diet whose twin goals are nutritional excellence and enjoyment, you should be well on your way to a healthful and long life. Given these resolutions to start with, you can then maintain a weight that is comfortable and stop worrying about it.

The Controversy Notes and For Further Information follow the Appendixes.

CHAPTER 9

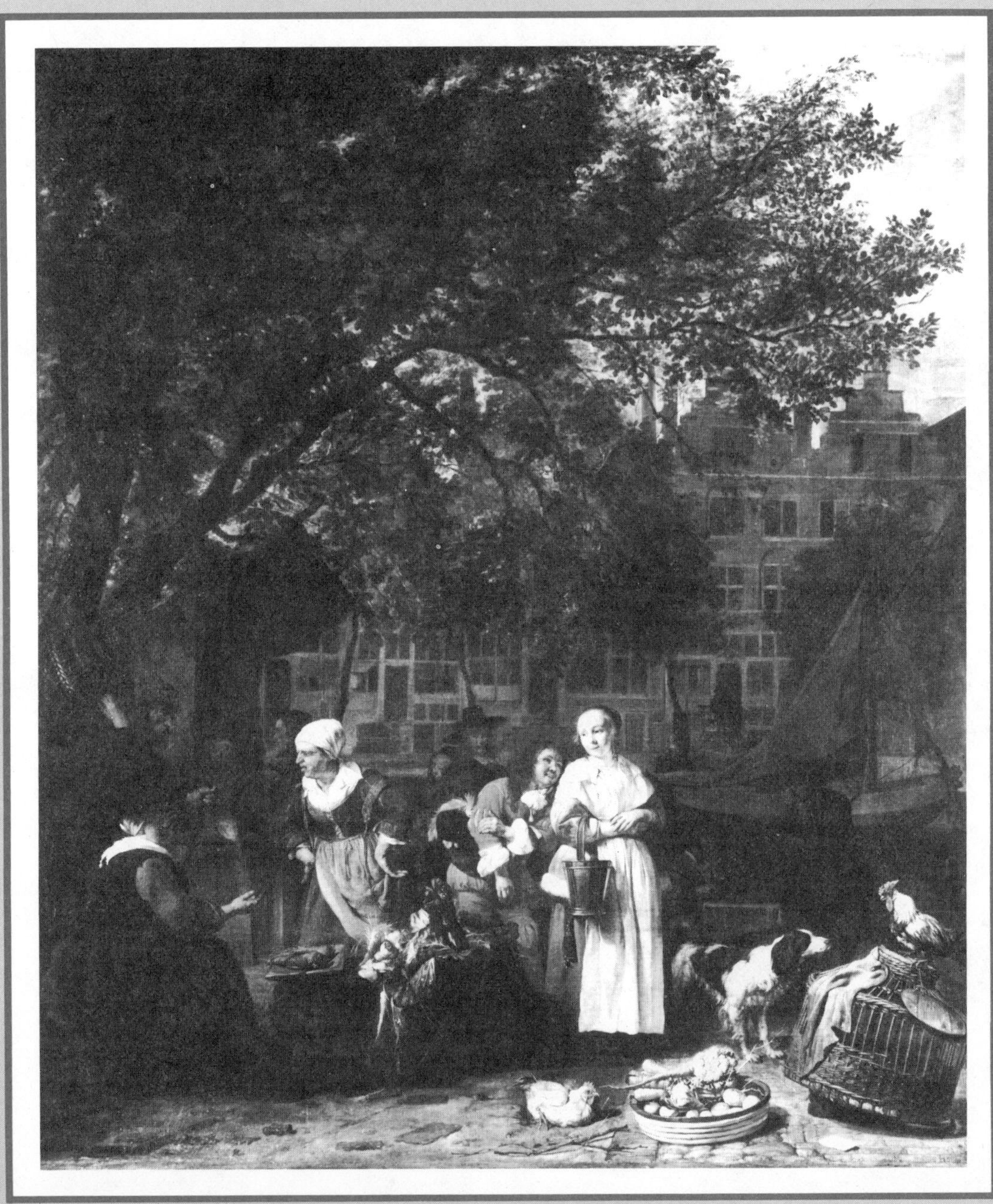

The Vitamins

The romance and excitement of nutrition is centered around the vitamins, especially in the minds of the general public. At the beginning of the twentieth century, the thrill of discovering the first vitamins captured the world's imagination, and out of the ensuing history has grown the multibillion-dollar vitamin supplement industry.

The story line was repeated over and over as each new vitamin was discovered: Whole groups of people were only half alive (or were going blind or were dying) until an alert scientist stumbled onto the substance missing in their diets. According to the plot, the scientist usually confirmed the discovery by feeding the vitamin-deficient food to chickens (or rats or guinea pigs). The animals responded to the diet just as the humans did, by becoming paralyzed (or going blind or bleeding profusely). Then, miraculously, they recovered when one missing ingredient was restored to the diet.

The only disease a vitamin will cure is the one caused by a deficiency of that vitamin.

Having read of dramatic events like these happening in real life, people continue to believe that a vitamin supplement will cure a wide variety of ailments. But the truth is that the only disease a vitamin will cure is the one caused by a deficiency of that vitamin. Vitamins, in general, are not cure-alls for such vague symptoms as tiredness. But if there is a deficiency of one of the vitamins essential to the release of energy from glucose, tiredness may be one of the symptoms. Restora-

Opposite: Vegetable Market at Amsterdam *by Gabriel Metsa at the Musées Nationaux de Louvre, Paris. Used with permission.*

tion of that vitamin to the diet, in that case, will alleviate the symptom.

The discovery of the vitamins is mostly a twentieth-century phenomenon. Ancient literature described diseases that we know today were vitamin deficiencies, and often the folk remedies for these were effective because they happened to replace the missing vitamins. However, it was not until 1897 that the vitamin era really began. In that year, Eijkman demonstrated that a diet of polished rice caused beriberi and that the addition of the rice polishings to the diet cured it. Since that time, each vitamin has become known as a specific chemical entity, indispensable to one or more body functions and purifiable from food.

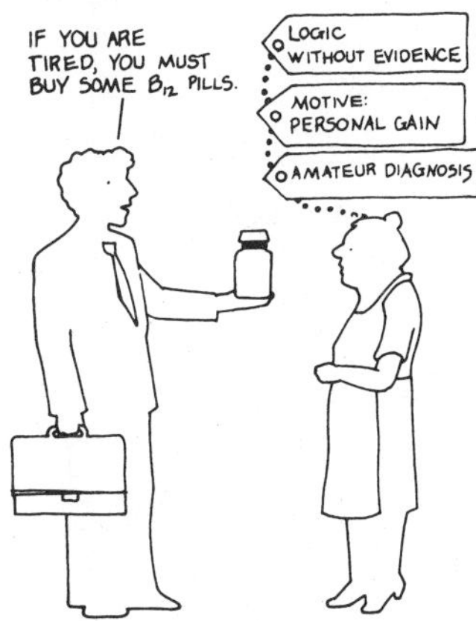
IF YOU ARE TIRED, YOU MUST BUY SOME B_{12} PILLS.
LOGIC WITHOUT EVIDENCE
MOTIVE: PERSONAL GAIN
AMATEUR DIAGNOSIS

Vitamins are frequently offered as cures for people's symptoms.

The term *vitamine* was given to these new dietary substances by Funk in 1912. He coined the word from *vita*, meaning "life," and *amine*, because the one he was working with contained a chemical structure called an amine. When it was later realized that most vitamins are not amines, the e on *vitamine* was dropped. At first, vitamins were given letters: vitamin A, vitamin B, vitamin C. Later, chemical analysis revealed that what had been thought to be one chemical was actually two or more, and sub-numerals were used to differentiate these: B_1, B_2, and so on. In addition, some vitamins received names to denote the diseases they cured, such as "antirachitic factor" for vitamin D, which cures rickets. This led to confusion that still exists today. Table 1 shows some of the common names and the correct names for the vitamins.

One reason why the discovery of vitamins came so late in the history of science was that they appear in foods and in the human body in such tiny amounts. It took a sophisticated knowledge of chemistry

Table 1. Common and Correct Names of the Vitamins

Original Name	Other Names	Current Names
Vitamin A	Anti-infective vitamin	Vitamin A (retinol)
Vitamin B	Antiberiberi vitamin	Vitamin B_1 (thamin)
	Antineuritic vitamin	
	Vitamin B_2 (G)	Vitamin B_2 (riboflavin)
	Vitamin B_3	Niacin (nicotinic acid, niacinamide, nicotinamide)
		Vitamin B_6 (pyridoxine)
		Vitamin B_{12} (cobalamin, cyanocobalamin)
	Vitamin M	Folacin (folic acid)
		Pantothenic acid
		Biotin
Vitamin C	Antiscorbutic vitamin	Vitamin C (ascorbic acid)
Vitamin D	Antirachitic vitamin	Vitamin D (calciferol)
Vitamin E	Antisterility vitamin	Vitamin E (alpha-tocopherol)
Vitamin K	Coagulation factor	Vitamin K (menaquinone, phylloquinone)

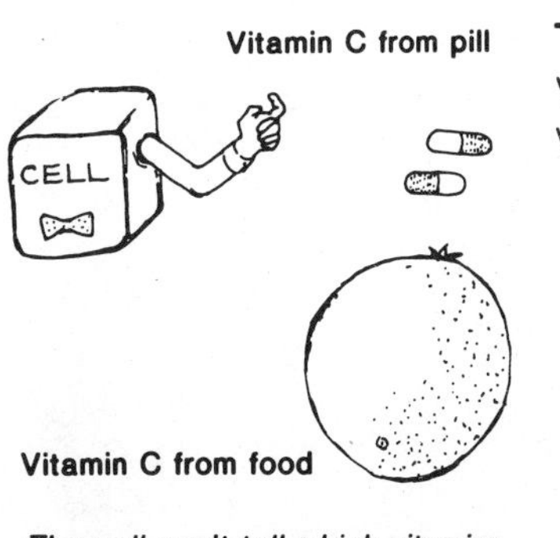

The cell can't tell which vitamins come from pills and which from foods.

and biology to isolate them and learn to distinguish them from one another. Today, chemists can synthesize most of them.

It should be repeated that the body's cells can't tell the difference between the synthesized vitamin and the "natural" vitamin, even though the marketers of "natural" vitamins would like you to believe otherwise. The word *synthetic* sometimes implies fake, as in a synthetic (fake) fur coat. To the chemist, however, to synthesize means to put together—and the product is not fake, it is identical to the real thing.

Vitamins sold as natural often have synthetics added anyway. For example, vitamin C pills made from rose hips would have to be as big as golf balls to contain significant amounts of the vitamin. The manufacturer therefore adds synthetic vitamin to the small amount of "natural" vitamin and sells the product for many times the original price.[1]

As we said earlier, a cell picking up vitamins from the bloodstream can't tell the difference between the vitamins from pills and those from foods. However, the digestive tract often does respond to the vehicle in which nutrients arrive. As you have seen, amino acids from whole proteins are better absorbed than purified amino acids. For some reason, synthetic vitamin C seems to be better retained than "natural" vitamin C when both are supplied in pill form.[2] But because the body evolved to utilize foods, not pills, we might guess that vitamin C would be retained even better if it came from foods. The lesson in this must be that it really is not natural to take any kind of pills.

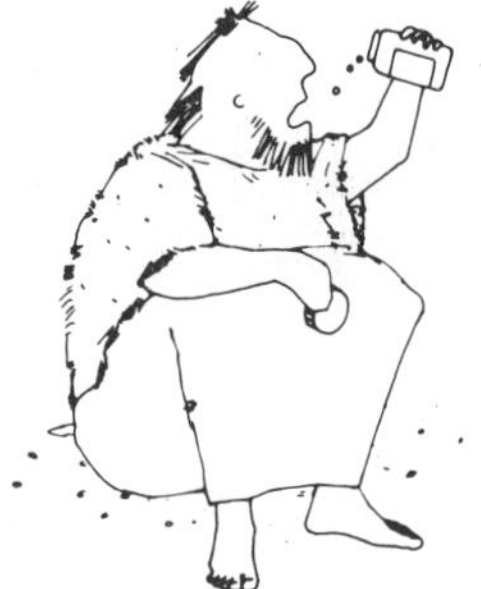

It really isn't natural to take any kind of pills.

Another stumbling block in the early work was in finding suitable animals for the investigations. A vitamin, it turns out, is not always a vitamin. One species may be able to synthesize a vital substance from other materials, whereas a second species, unable to synthesize it, will have to obtain it preformed in food. The substance, no matter how important to both species, is a vitamin only to the second. Human beings and guinea pigs must obtain vitamin C from their food, so for them it is a vitamin; rats, dogs, and cats, on the other hand, synthesize it from other elements taken in their food. Guinea pigs are therefore used for research on the effects of vitamin C deficiency; rats, dogs, and cats are of no use in this kind of research.

To learn when to take vitamin supplements, read Controversy 2.

Definition and Classification of Vitamins

A child once defined a vitamin as "what, if you don't eat, you get sick." Although his grammar left something to be desired, the definition was accurate and concise. Less imaginatively, the modern biochemist defines a **vitamin** as a potent, indispensable, noncaloric organic compound—needed in very small amounts in the diet—that performs specific and individual functions to promote growth or reproduction or to maintain health and life. This definition distinguishes the vitamins from the energy nutrients—protein, fat, and carbohydrate. Unlike these, the vitamins do not provide energy that the human body can use. The average adult may need several hundred grams of energy nutrients each day to maintain weight and support activity but may need only one-thousandth of a gram (a milligram) or one-millionth of a gram (a microgram) of each vitamin.

Many of the vitamins occur in foods in a form known as **precursors**, or **provitamins**. Once inside the body, these are changed chemically to one or more active forms, known as the active vitamins. Thus, in measuring the amount of a vitamin found in food, it is often most accurate to speak in terms of the total potential vitamin activity that the body will derive from the vitamin and its precursors.

One method of classifying the vitamins is to separate them on the basis of whether they are soluble in fats or in water. These are useful categories because they give an indication of the kinds of foods in which the vitamins can be found, the way the body can use them, and the way they should be handled during food preparation in order to preserve as much of their activity as possible.

Fat-soluble vitamins:
Vitamin A.
Vitamin D.
Vitamin E.
Vitamin K.

The fat-soluble vitamins—A, D, E, and K—are found in such foods as fish oils and plant oils. Just like the lipids, once they have been absorbed from the intestinal tract, they can't be excreted. Instead, they are stored in the liver and fatty tissues. They require the same special handling as other lipids. For example, they must have protein carriers to move them from one part of the body to another, because they are insoluble in water. Because excesses are stored, it is possible for them to reach toxic levels in the body. The only way they may be inadvertently lost is by being carried out of the body dissolved in fat. This can occur in a person whose fat absorption is poor or who uses mineral oil (which the body can't absorb) as a laxative.

All the other vitamins—the B vitamins and vitamin C—are water soluble. This indicates that they can be leached out of foods easily by incorrect preparation and that they can travel freely within the body in the blood and lymph. Some can be stored in the lean tissues for periods of a month or more; but these tissues are actively exchanging materials with the body fluids at all times, and so these vitamins are nowhere safe from being dissolved, carried away, and excreted by the kidneys. As a rule of thumb, it is recommended that you have daily, or nearly daily, intakes of the water-soluble vitamins.

Toxicity is unlikely if the sources of the water-soluble vitamins are foods. Only the large doses provided by vitamin supplements can reach toxic levels.

Although small in quantity, the vitamins accomplish mighty tasks. In some instances, their exact functions are still unknown. The most important facts will be discussed separately for each vitamin in the following sections.

The Fat-Soluble Vitamins

The fat-soluble vitamins are diverse, as you will see, but they have in common the fact that they are found only in complex animals and man and that they act somewhat like hormones in influencing events in the body. At least three of the four enter the body as precursors and then are converted to their active forms in one or more of the body's organs. A compound already mentioned that works in the same way is the essential fatty acid, linoleic acid; it may someday be classed as another fat-soluble vitamin.

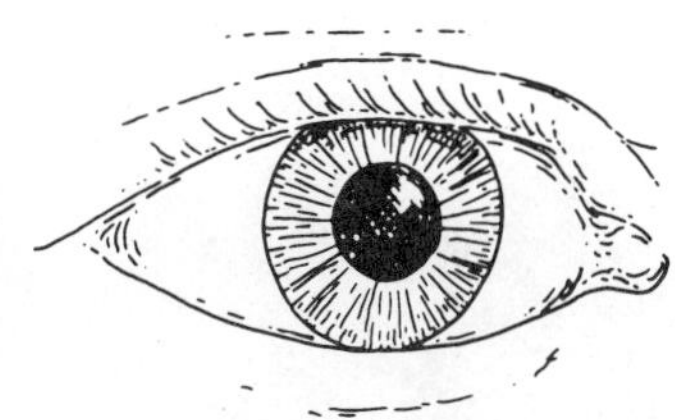

The cornea (outside covering) of the eye is maintained by vitamin A.

Vitamin A. Vitamin A has the distinction of being the first fat-soluble vitamin to be recognized. Its function of maintaining the **cornea**—the outside covering of the eye—was discovered early. In two laboratories simultaneously, rats being fed purified diets containing no fat failed to grow even though they were receiving sufficient calories. On this diet, the rats' eyes became red and inflamed. When butter or cod liver oil was added, growth resumed and the eye infection healed. Following this discovery, growth studies on English schoolboys showed that dramatic differences in height could be achieved by adding butter to the diet. It turned out, too, that **xerophthalmia** (inflammation of the eyes) could be prevented or cured by the addition of butter or cod liver oil to the diet.

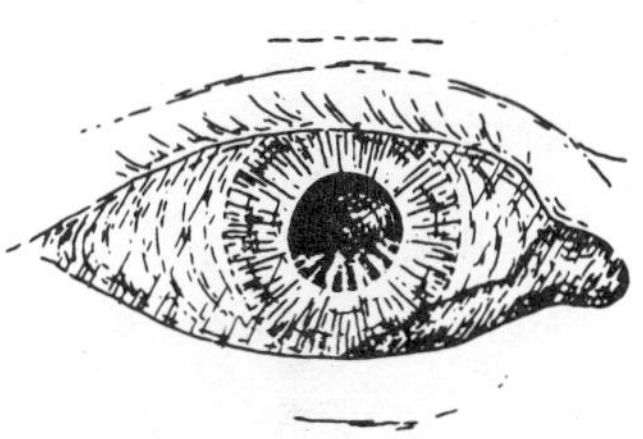

In advanced vitamin A deficiency, the cornea thickens and becomes opaque.

The term *vitamin A* continues to be used even though later research has shown that a number of compounds have vitamin A activity (one of the best known is **retinol**). These compounds are all of animal origin, except for a small amount found in spinach. The sources of the vitamin A precursors, however, are the dark green and yellow pigments in plants. These are the provitamins, which the animal liver converts to the active vitamins. The best-known provitamin is **carotene**, which occurs in squash, sweet potatoes, carrots, pumpkins, and other deep-orange vegetables.

Vitamin A, as stated earlier, plays a role in keeping the cornea of the eye healthy. In addition, all **epithelial tissue** (internal and external "skin") requires vitamin A to maintain its integrity (wholeness). Epithelial tissue includes the linings of the lungs, stomach, intestines, vagina, urinary tract, and bladder, as well as the eyes and skin. These cells secrete **mucus**, which protects them from infection. But if vitamin A is deficient, they secrete a protein (**keratin**) instead. Keratin is a normal body compound, the protein of hair and nails, but when it fills the epithelial cells, they become dry and hard (**keratinization**). The cells then cannot perform their job, and they die. Then they accumulate on the surface and become hosts to bacterial infection.

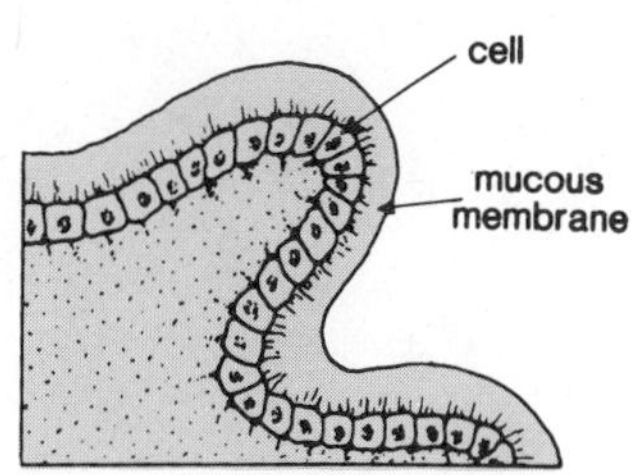

The cells of the intestinal lining secrete mucus, a function supported by vitamin A.

For a long while it was thought that vitamin A was an "anti-infection" vitamin because it promoted the healing of infected tissues in the respiratory tract, in the eyes, and on the skin. However, its role is now known to be maintenance of healthy epithelial cells, which can more effectively resist infection. The relationship of acne, an infection-like skin disorder, to vitamin A is not as simple, and acne cannot be cured by the taking of standard vitamin A supplements.

Controversy 14A discusses the causes of acne and the role of another form of vitamin A, retinoic acid.

Recent research has revealed another way in which vitamin A protects the epithelial tissue. Healthy skin and internal linings are able to interrupt the process by which cancers get started, but vitamin A deficiency handicaps this defense. Skin, lung, and bladder cancers and others become more likely when vitamin A is lacking.[3]

Vitamin A is involved in another eye function: restoring the ability

Foods containing vitamin A.

Table 2. Vitamin A Contents of Fifty Common Foods

Exchange Group[a]	Food	Serving Size[b]	Vitamin A (IU)
5M	Beef liver	3 oz	45,420
4	Pumpkin	¾ cup	10,943[c]
2	Dandelion greens	½ cup	10,530
2	Carrots	½ cup	7,610
2	Spinach	½ cup	7,200
2	Collard greens	½ cup	5,130[d]
4	Winter squash	½ cup	4,305
4	Sweet potatoes	¼ cup	4,250
2	Mustard greens	½ cup	4,060
3	Cantaloupe	¼	3,270
2	Broccoli	½ cup	2,363
3	Dried apricots	4 halves	1,635
3	Peach	1	1,320
2	Cooked tomatoes	½ cup	1,085
2	Tomato juice	½ cup	970
2	Asparagus	½ cup	605
5M	Egg	1	590
5L	Oysters	15; ¾ cup	555
3	Pink grapefruit	½	540
4	Green peas	½ cup	430
2	Summer squash	½ cup	410
2	Brussels sprouts	½ cup	405
1	Canned evaporated milk	½ cup	405
3	Tangerine	1	360
1	Whole milk	1 cup	350
1	Yogurt (made with whole milk)	1 cup	340
2	Green beans	½ cup	340
4	Corn on cob	1 small	310
3	Orange juice	½ cup	275
3	Orange	1	260
6	Cream, light	2 tbsp	260
4	Lima beans	½ cup	240
6	Cream, heavy	1 tbsp	230
4	Corn	⅓ cup	230
1	2% fat fortified milk	1 cup	200
5L	Sardines	3 oz	190
6	Soft margarine	1 tsp	156
3	Blackberries	½ cup	145
3	Banana	½ medium	115
5M	Creamed cottage cheese	¼ cup	105
4	Corn muffin	1	100
3	Raspberries	½ cup	80
5L	Chicken, meat only	3 oz	80
4	Yellow grits	½ cup	75
4	Pancake	1	70
5L	Canned tuna	3 oz	70
3	Blueberries	½ cup	70
3	Strawberries	¾ cup	68
5L	Canned salmon	3 oz	60
3	Pineapple	½ cup	50

These are not best food sources but are selected to show a range of vitamin A contents. Note how many 2s and 3s are at the top of the left-hand column, and how many 5s are at the bottom.

[a] The numbers refer to the exchange lists: 1 is milk; 2, vegetables; 3, fruit; 4, bread; 5L, lean meat; 5M, medium-fat meat; 6, fats and oils.

[b] Serving sizes are the sizes listed in the exchange lists, except for meat.

[c] Vitamin A activity reported in plants may be spuriously high. The actual amount of active vitamin A derived from plants depends on the body's conversion of the precursor, carotene, to the active vitamin.

[d] One serving of any of the first six foods contains the U. S. RDA of 5000 IU.

to see in dim light after the eyes have been "blinded" by strong light. There is a colored compound in the **retina** of the eye, **visual purple** (rhodopsin), that is bleached when light falls on it. The brain detects this bleaching and makes a judgment as to what it has "seen." Visual purple must then be regenerated before the eye can see again. Vitamin A is a part of the compound visual purple. It is broken off the protein part of the compound when bleaching occurs, changes its form, and then is restored to the compound again. A little vitamin A is destroyed each time this reaction takes place. The eye depends on an adequate supply of vitamin A in the blood to constantly regenerate the visual purple. If the supply is low, a lag occurs before the eye can see again. This lag in the recovery of night vision, termed **night blindness**, indicates a vitamin A deficiency.

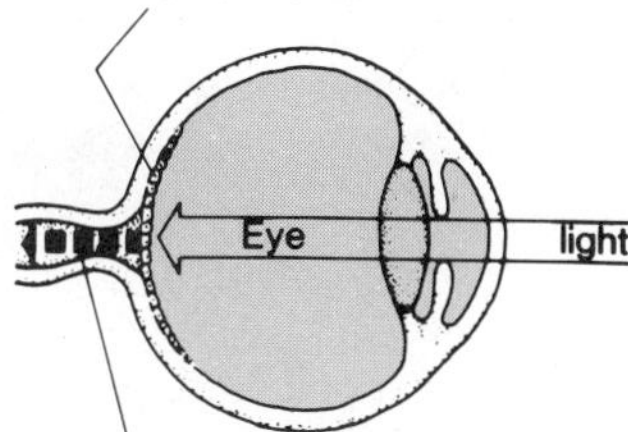

Light enters the eye.

The role that vitamin A plays in growth is not so clearly understood as its role in night vision. It is thought that the cessation of growth with a deficiency of vitamin A may be due to a loss of appetite. This, in turn, may be due to the deterioration of the epithelial cells of the intestinal tract or to keratinization of the cells of the tongue, which damages the taste buds. Failure of the bones to lengthen is one of the first symptoms to appear. Vitamin A seems to be involved in the remodeling of the ends of the bones, which is a prerequisite to the laying down of new bone. In the jawbone, vitamin A promotes normal tooth spacing. Crooked teeth and poor dental health can result from a deficiency.[4]

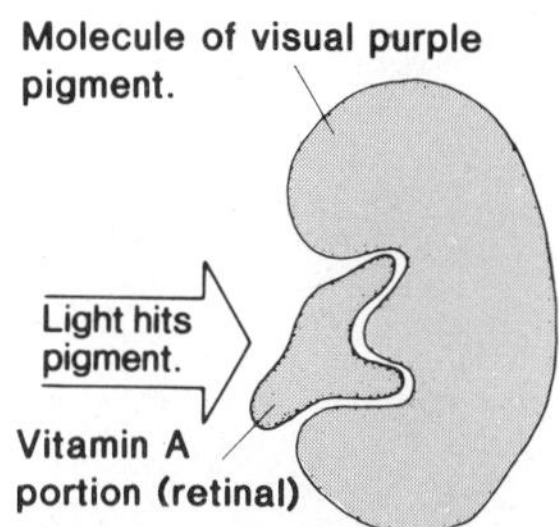

Vitamin A and the retina.

Vitamin A in food is fairly stable in light and heat but is easily destroyed by air (oxygen) and by sunlight (ultraviolet rays). Vitamin E helps prevent its oxidation by being oxidized in its place.

This point illustrates a by-now familiar principle: The nutrients depend on one another for their effectiveness. Vitamin A and vitamin E, both fat soluble, tend to occur together in foods, a naturally beneficial coincidence. People who try to outguess nature by taking single vitamins in pill form seldom hit on such winning combinations.

Foods containing high concentrations of vitamin A are fish oils like cod liver oil, liver, butter, fortified margarine, egg yolk, whole or fortified milk and cream, and cheeses made from whole milk or cream. Vegetables and fruits that contain the precursor carotene in abundance are collards, turnip greens, carrots, sweet potatoes, squash, apricots, peaches, and cantaloupe. Medium-green vegetables such as green beans or lettuce or yellow vegetables such as corn are not notable for their vitamin A content; hence the rule, familiar to most schoolchildren, that a person should include *dark* green or *deep* orange vegetables or fruits in the diet every other day. Other foods, such as meat, bread, and potatoes, are notoriously poor food sources of vitamin A; see Table 2.

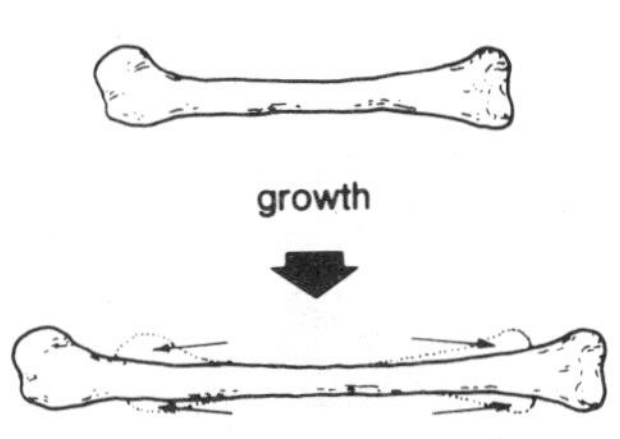

As bone lengthens, vitamin A helps remove old bone.

The amount of vitamin A needed is proportional to body weight.

Because it is stored, the vitamin does not need to be eaten every day, although the RDA states it as a daily amount. When an excess is eaten, it is stored mostly in the liver, where it is available constantly to the cells of the body. According to the RDA, to be assured of adequacy, the average man needs about 1000 **RE (retinol equivalents)** daily, and the average woman about 800 RE. Pregnancy increases the RDA for women to 1000 RE; and lactation, to 1200 RE. Children need from 400 to 700 RE up to about the age of thirteen years.

The RDA tables are on the inside front cover.

Vitamin A recommendations are expressed in RE as of 1980, but food contents of vitamin A are still expressed in the older style, with **IU (international units)**. Until this discrepancy is corrected in food tables, if you want to compare your vitamin A intakes with recommendations, you will have to convert from one to the other. A rule of thumb is that 1 RE = 5 IU. Thus, if you consumed 10,000 IU of vitamin A, that would convert to 2000 RE—more than enough by any standard.

1 RE = 5 IU, vitamin A.

Toxicity is a real danger for people who take vitamin A in capsule form. It can cause many symptoms, including joint pain, stunted growth and bone abnormalities, cessation of menstruation, nausea and gastrointestinal misery, rashes, and enlargement of the liver and spleen. Early symptoms of overdoses in children are loss of appetite, growth failure, and itching of the skin. The vitamin A precursor, carotene, is not so hazardous but has been known to turn people bright yellow if they take too much. Foods containing vitamin A can be eaten in large amounts without causing toxicity symptoms, with the possible exception of liver. Polar bears, because they eat fish whole (and thus fish livers), store very large amounts of the vitamin in *their* livers, which have therefore become notorious as a dangerous food source for arctic explorers.

Worldwide, vitamin A deficiency is second only to protein-calorie malnutrition as a world health problem. Infants and children are especially vulnerable. Once xerophthalmia has developed, it progresses more than half the time to blindness. The total number of new cases of blindness from this cause may be as many as 100,000 a year worldwide, placing a heavy burden on society.[5]

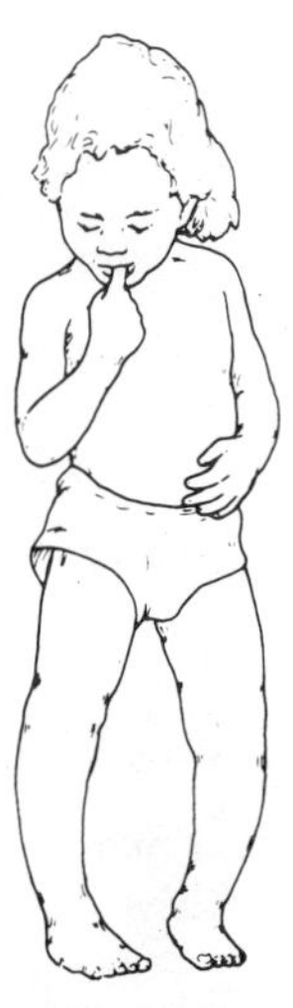

Rickets.

Vitamin D. Nearly a decade after vitamin A was discovered, it was learned that what had been considered one vitamin actually was two. The mixup was understandable. Both vitamins are fat soluble, and both are found in the same fatty foods. Any extraction of one would most likely contain the other. Finally, in 1922, McCollum separated the two and showed that only one, vitamin D, would correct the abnormal bone development called **rickets**.

Rickets had been recognized for several centuries, and it was even known in the 1700s that it could be cured with cod liver oil. However, not until the early 1900s was enough known about rickets for Mellanby to reproduce it in laboratory dogs. When the condition was reversed by the newly discovered fraction of vitamin A, the tragedy of rickets was largely eliminated. The bowed legs, knock-knees, and pigeon breast of rickets are no longer common sights.

Still another decade passed before it was learned, in 1936, that vitamin D can be formed in the body by the action of ultraviolet rays of the sun striking a cholesterol-like substance just under the skin. This makes vitamin D unique among the vitamins, because it can be obtained without the help of food. The vitamin D the body synthesizes is absorbed directly from the cells of the skin into the bloodstream; the vitamin D that enters the body with food is absorbed with fats.

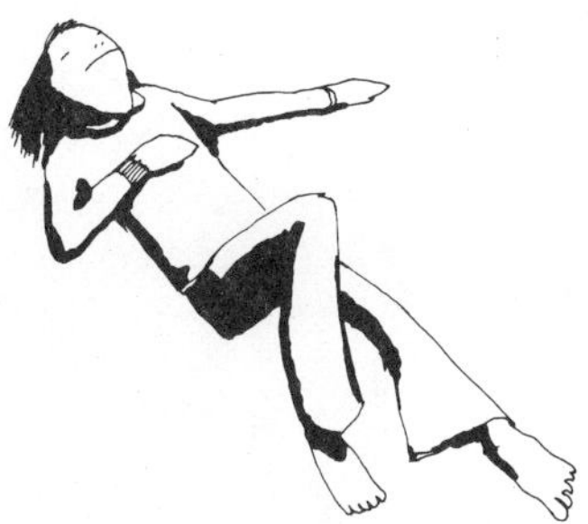
Sunlight promotes vitamin D formation in the skin.

The precise role vitamin D plays in the cells is still being investigated, but its importance and general functions are well known. The primary function of vitamin D is in the regulation of the body's handling of calcium and phosphorus. It promotes the absorption of these minerals by the intestine, their movement out of storage in the bones, their deposition in teeth, the prevention of their excretion, and the maintenance of their levels in the blood. This is why a vitamin D deficiency causes rickets; with the lack of vitamin D, calcium is poorly absorbed, and the bones are weak. The most noticeable deformity is the bowing of the leg bones under the weight of a child. In adults, the comparable deficiency disease is **osteomalacia**, in which calcium is withdrawn from the bones, making them brittle and easy to break.

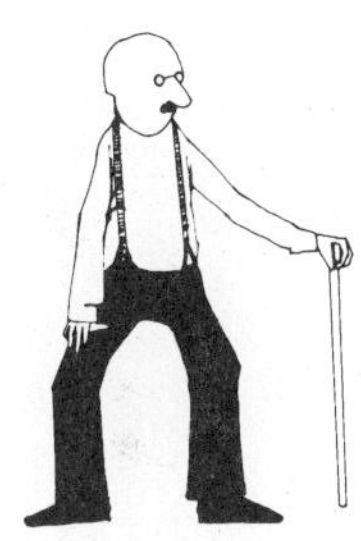
Osteomalacia.

There are no satisfactory tables of the vitamin D content of foods. The best natural food sources of vitamin D are fish oils (like cod liver oil), butter, cream, egg yolk, and liver. In the United States, milk, whether fluid, dried, or evaporated, is usually fortified with vitamin D. Milk is not naturally a rich source of vitamin D, because it contains only 4 to 5 percent cream, but it is an ideal vehicle for supplemental amounts because it is the main source of calcium for children. Breakfast cereals may also be fortified with vitamin D, as their labels indicate. The natural food sources of vitamin D vary with the seasons, with spring and summer contents being significantly higher. The amount of vitamin D received from sunlight is also higher in the summertime. The ultraviolet rays of the sun, the rays which promote vitamin D formation in the skin, are filtered out by clouds, smoke, smog, clothing, window glass, and even window screens.

Dark-skinned people make less vitamin D. The pigment in their skin which protects them from the sun in tropical countries may hinder their making enough of the vitamin in northern areas or smoggy cities, and it is in dark-skinned people that rickets most often appears. Anyone who gets into the sunlight much at all, however, should not have a problem with deficiency. The skin theoretically can make up to 10,000 IU a day of vitamin D.[6]

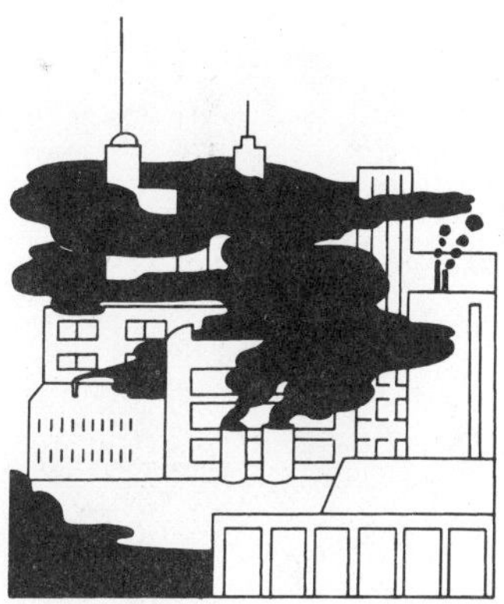
Smog filters out ultraviolet rays of the sun.

Children receive sufficient vitamin D if their milk is fortified, but rickets still occurs in children whose parents do not see the need to pay the cost of vitamin D-fortified milk.[7] Infants need formula that is fortified with vitamin D or supplements prescribed by the pediatrician if they are being fed breast milk.[8] There was a time when rickets seemed to have been almost completely eliminated from the developed countries, but in the 1970s it seemed to be creeping back, with cases being reported in inner-city children, especially blacks, in children breastfed for an exceptionally long time, and in vegetarian children.[9]

The RDA for vitamin D is 10 microgams per day for all individuals up to the age of eighteen, 7.5 micrograms per day to twenty-two, and 5 micrograms thereafter, with 5 micrograms extra recommended for women during pregnancy and lactation. Contrary to popular belief, people do need vitamin D in adulthood and can suffer from deficiencies, especially if they are housebound or in prison or if they work at night.[10] Milk is therefore a good food for adults as well as for children.

Daily intakes of vitamin D are not necessary, because excesses are stored. However, it is possible to receive an overdose with as little as four to five times the recommended daily intake.[11] Toxicity symptoms include diarrhea, headache, and nausea; if overdoses continue to occur, there will be calcium deposits in the soft tissues of the body as the vitamin mobilizes too much of the mineral from the bones. Obviously, this can happen most easily in infants whose overzealous mothers may go by the rule that if some is good for you, more is better. The health faddist, too, may easily overdose, not realizing that body tissues are building up a stockpile of the vitamin. Doctors don't always recognize the symptoms of vitamin D toxicity, and have sometimes performed unnecessary surgery or therapy.[12] The pathological conditions can be reversed by withdrawing the supplemental vitamin D, but if calcium deposits have formed in the heart's major artery, the aorta, the consequence of overdosing may be death.

Vitamin E. In a 1922 experiment, some investigators fed rats a purified diet, thinking that it contained all the needed nutrients, and found that the rats could not reproduce. Addition of wheat germ oil restored their fertility and provided the clue to a new vitamin. Vitamin E was later isolated from wheat germ oil and was named the antisterility vitamin, or **tocopherol** (*tokos* is a Greek word meaning "offspring").

The best-known function of vitamin E is as an **antioxidant**, protecting the polyunsaturated fats in the body from destruction by oxygen. It protects vitamin A in the same way, as already mentioned.

A deficiency of vitamin E produces a wide variety of symptoms in laboratory animals, but most of these symptoms have not been reproduced in human beings, despite many attempts. Two reasons given for this are (1) that the vitamin is so widespread in food that it is almost impossible to create a vitamin E-deficient diet and (2) that the body stores so much vitamin E in its fatty tissues that a person could not keep on eating a vitamin E-free diet for long enough to deplete these stores and produce a deficiency.

Many claims have been made for supplemental vitamin E for treatment of human complaints, ranging from trivial ones like body odor to serious ones like male impotence and heart problems. Most of these claims have been proved false, although it is not impossible that small supplemental amounts of the vitamin (up to 200 milligrams) may help prevent degenerative processes in elderly people.[13] The one proven vitamin E deficiency in humans is in premature babies, because there is little transfer of the vitamin from the mother to the infant until late in pregnancy. The mother's blood supply of the vitamin doesn't increase until the last trimester of pregnancy, in anticipation of lactation; a baby who is born early hasn't received the benefit of the rise in vitamin E supply. The deficiency symptom is breakage of the red blood cells. These cells' membranes contain large amounts of polyunsaturated fatty acids that need protection from oxidation when they are exposed to atmospheric oxygen in the lungs.

No one needs to take massive doses of vitamin E, and supplements are not given to infants except for premature babies. There seems to be some evidence that vitamin E provides a measure of protection for animals against lung damage from air pollutants such as nitrogen dioxide and ozone.[14] But there is absolutely no evidence that it is effective in the treatment of heart problems or muscular dystrophy, even though many well-designed experiments have been carried out to test these possibilities. Nor does it improve athletic prowess, prevent cancer,[15] or enhance sexual performance.[16] The muscular dystrophy seen in children is not even the same disease as the nutritional muscular dystrophy seen in animals deprived of vitamin E.

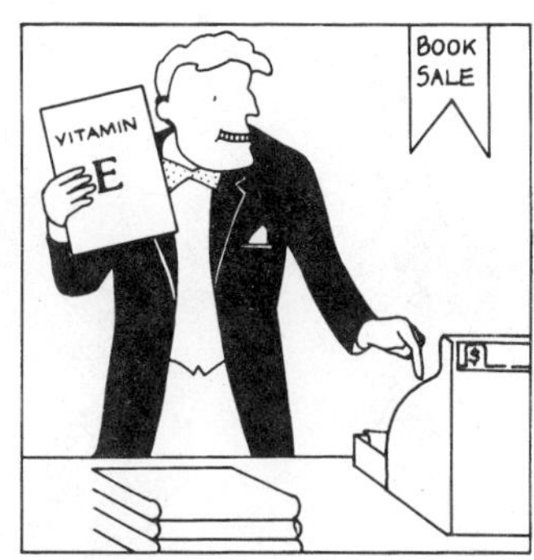

Vitamin E is said to have miraculous powers. There's more about vitamin E in Controversy 15.

The RDA for vitamin E is based on body size. For infants, it is about 3 to 4 milligrams; for females, 8 milligrams; for pregnant women and for males, 10 milligrams. The need for vitamin E increases with an increase of oils in the diet; but vitamin E is associated with the polyunsaturated fats in foods, so larger amounts automatically accompany added polyunsaturated fats.

Reports of vitamin E toxicity are rare. There are isolated reports in the medical literature of adverse effects on laboratory animals and of nausea, intestinal distress, and other vague complaints in human beings. However, the impression remains that "for most individuals daily doses below 300 IU are innocuous [harmless]."[17]

Vitamin E does not appear in standard food composition tables, although some information is available.[18] Most dietary vitamin E comes from vegetable oils, the richest being wheat germ oil. Cereal grains, green plants, egg yolk, milk fat, butter, liver, nuts, and vegetables are all good sources. Thus all four food groups provide generous amounts of vitamin E.

Vitamin K. Vitamin K is the fat-soluble vitamin necessary in at least two of the about fourteen steps in blood clotting. Protection against blood clots within the blood vessels is achieved by having all the ingredients for the formation of a clot present as precursors until the series of reactions is triggered by a rough surface such as a cut. Vitamin K participates by (1) helping to synthesize the protein **prothrombin**, which converts to thrombin in one of the first steps in the clotting process; and (2) changing the precursor protein fibrinogen into its active form, **fibrin**, which forms a net over the cut to trap the oncoming red blood cells.

Tables of the vitamin K content of foods are not available. Natural vitamin K is found in dark-green leafy vegetables. The only rich animal food source is liver. The vitamin is also synthesized by bacteria in the intestinal tract. Recent research shows that we obtain about half our daily needs from plants and about half through the courtesy of our intestinal inhabitants.[19] Newborn infants, whose intestinal tracts are not yet inhabited by bacteria, and people who have taken antibiotics that have killed the intestinal bacteria have a delayed clotting time. Vitamin K is often given to compensate. A newborn infant who suffers a wound can bleed to death without vitamin K.

A synthetic compound resembling vitamin K—**menadione**—is used widely in place of the natural vitamin. Several water-soluble substitutes for vitamin K have proved useful for people who have trouble absorbing fats and who therefore may fail to absorb the vitamin. Excesses of both the vitamin and its substitutes are toxic, so they are available only by prescription.

Water-soluble vitamins:
B vitamins.
Vitamin C.

In some heart patients, there is a need to prevent the formation of clots within the circulatory system. This is popularly referred to as "thinning" the blood. One of the best-known compounds for this purpose is Dicoumarol, which interferes with vitamin K in the synthesis of prothrombin. Vitamin K therapy is necessary in these cases if hemorrhaging occurs.

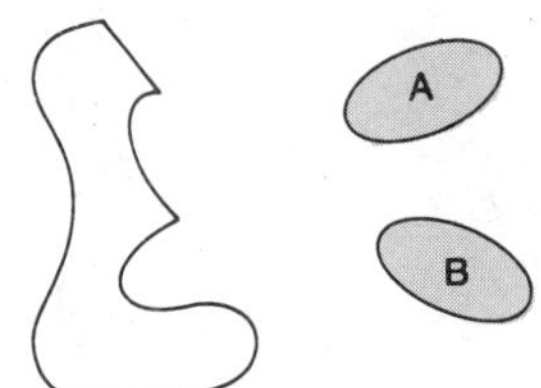

Coenzyme action. Without the coenzyme, compounds A and B don't respond to the enzyme.

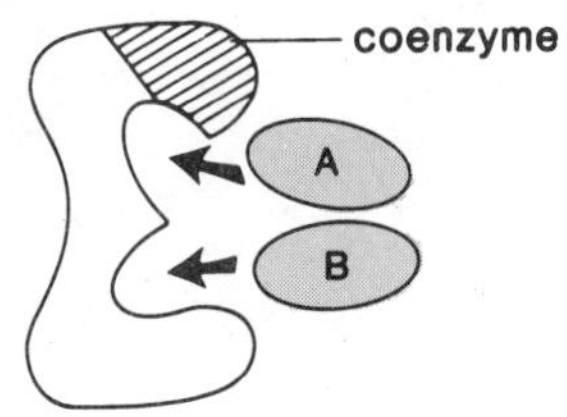

With the coenzyme in place, A and B are attracted to the active site on the enzyme, and they react.

The Water-Soluble Vitamins

The B vitamins, and possibly vitamin C, act as part of coenzymes. A **coenzyme** is a small molecule that can combine with an inactive protein to make it an active enzyme. It is thought that the vitamin part of the enzyme is the active site, where the chemical reaction takes place. The substance to be worked on is attracted to the active site and snaps into place, and the reaction proceeds instantaneously.

The architecture of each enzyme is designed to accomplish just one kind of job. Without its coenzyme, however, the enzyme is as useless as a typewriter without its ribbon. The vitamin is the part of the coenzyme that the body cannot make and so is an essential nutrient, needed daily in food.

The search for the roles of each of the vitamins has given rise to an enormous body of knowledge. About fifty years ago, the study of nutrition involved learning the symptoms associated with deficiency of each of the vitamins. Today, it is more concerned with vitamins' biochemical roles.

Thiamin. Some thirty years before the concept of vitamins began receiving attention, the medical director of the Japanese Navy showed that **beriberi** could be cured by requiring the seamen to eat more barley, vegetables, meat, and condensed milk, at the same time decreasing their intake of rice. His ideas were not widely accepted, and it took an observant Dutch physician in an East Indian prison to rediscover that beriberi could be cured with proper diet. This physician, Eijkman, noticed that the chickens at the prison developed a stiffness and weakness of their extremities similar to that of the prisoners who had beriberi. The chickens were being fed the polished rice left on the plates of prisoners. When the polishings, which had been discarded in the kitchen, were given to the chickens, their paralysis was cured. As might be expected, the doctor met resistance when he tried to feed the rice polishings—the "garbage"—to the prisoners. Later, in the Philippines, extracts of rice polishings were used to prevent infantile beriberi; still later, thiamin was synthesized.

Thiamin was at first named "water-soluble B" but then turned out to consist of two fractions. One fraction, vitamin B_1, was successful in treating beriberi and could be destroyed easily by heat; the other would cure pellagra and was more heat stable. Today these are called, respectively, **thiamin** and niacin.

Further research has revealed that a number of vitamins are closely related, and these are grouped together as the B-complex vitamins. They are found in the same groups of foods, and their work in the cells is largely related to releasing energy from food. In discussions of the individual vitamins, different deficiency symptoms are given for each member of the B-complex. Such clear-cut symptoms are found only in laboratory animals who have been fed diets lacking in just one ingredient. In real life, single B-vitamin deficiencies usually do not occur; further, their symptoms are not so easily distinguishable as textbook descriptions might lead us to believe. Because of the B-complex vitamins' interrelatedness, single-vitamin supplements are probably not useful.

The principal function of thiamin is to act as a coenzyme in the reactions that collect energy from carbohydrate (glucose) and trap the energy in a compound—ATP—that the cells can keep on hand. A thiamin deficiency produces nausea, severe exhaustion, emaciation, loss of appetite, tenderness in the calf muscles, and if continued, disabling paralysis of the extremities **(polyneuritis)** and abnormal heart action. These symptoms are thought to be largely due to the accumulation of substances that can't be dismantled without the aid of thiamin. It is as if thiamin is the signal that allows traffic to flow across a bridge. When the signal isn't working, a massive traffic jam results. The effects of this pileup are felt in every body cell and especially in those that are dependent on carbohydrate—the nerves and their responding tissues, the muscles. When thiamin is returned to the diet, the metabolic traffic flows again, and recovery can occur in a matter of a few hours. Exercise, carbohydrate foods, and alcoholic beverages hinder recovery because of the extra demand they place on the glucose-to-energy pathway in which thiamin is a crucial substance.

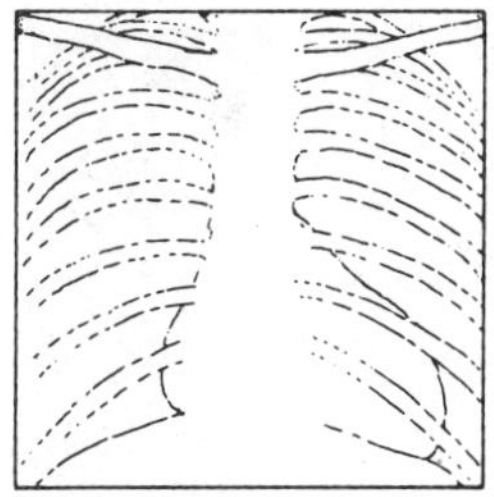

Effect of thiamin deficiency on the heart: enlargement.

If thiamin deficiency is prolonged enough and severe enough, however, recovery is not fully possible. The permanent brain damage seen in people who have abused alcohol for too long may result from their brain cells' having been unable to synthesize fatty acids and cholesterol because of the lack of the thiamin coenzyme.[20] Such people have a memory deficit, an inability to distinguish reality from fantasy, some problems with eye movement, and other traits well-known as characteristic of alcoholism. The alcohol itself hasn't caused the damage; what is responsible is the reduced food intake (and therefore thiamin intake) that goes with alcohol abuse, coupled with the increased need for thiamin incurred by the metabolism of alcohol.

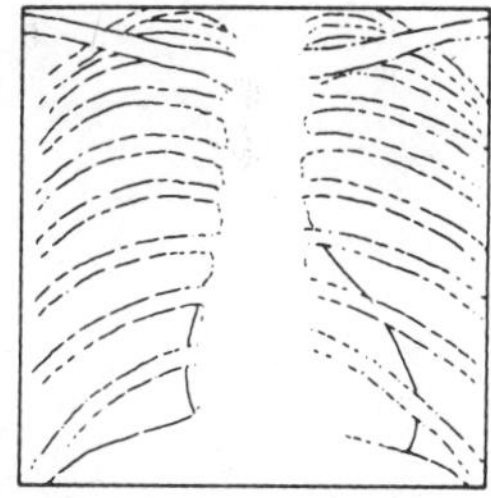

Decrease in size of heart after only one week of ample thiamin.

Lean pork is one of the richest sources of thiamin, and refined flour and polished rice (unenriched grains) are among the poorest. Other good sources are liver, yeast, legumes, and fresh green vegetables. Table 3 shows the thiamin contents of common foods.

Much thiamin is lost if the water used to cook green vegetables is discarded or if the drippings from cooked pork are not used. A common practice of a generation ago was to put a pinch of baking soda in the water to make green vegetables look brighter and fresher; this destroyed the thiamin. Fortunately, this practice is not in general use today. An acid medium does not harm thiamin, although temperatures higher than that of boiling water gradually inactivate it.

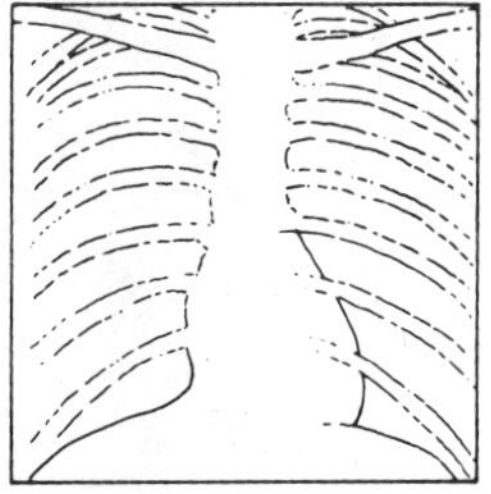

Heart back to normal with continued balanced diet.

Because it cannot be stored and is used up in the metabolism of food, thiamin should be included daily in the diet. Adult women need about 1 milligram a day; and men about 1.5 milligrams, because their energy output is greater. Infants require about half a milligram, and children about three-fourths. Because few foods other than pork sup-

Table 3. Thiamin Contents of Fifty Common Foods

Exchange Group[a]	Food	Serving Size[b]	Thiamin (mg)
5L	Ham	3 oz	0.40
5L	Oysters	¾ cup	0.25
5M	Liver, beef	3 oz	0.23
4	Green peas	½ cup	0.22
5M	Beef heart	3 oz	0.21
4	Lima beans	½ cup	0.16[c]
2	Collard greens	½ cup	0.14
3	Orange	1	0.13
4	Dried beans	½ cup	0.13
5L	Lamb, leg	3 oz	0.13
2	Dandelion greens	½ cup	0.12
4	Rice, enriched	½ cup	0.12
2	Asparagus	½ cup	0.12
3	Orange juice	½ cup	0.11
5L	Veal roast	3 oz	0.11
1	2% fat fortified milk	1 cup	0.10
4	Spaghetti, enriched	½ cup	0.10
4	Macaroni, enriched	½ cup	0.10
4	Cooked cereal	½ cup	0.10
4	Corn on cob	1 small	0.09
1	Skim milk	1 cup	0.09
4	Potato	1 small	0.08
4	Mashed potato	½ cup	0.08
1	Powdered skim milk	½ cup	0.08
1	Whole milk	1 cup	0.07
1	Yogurt (from whole milk)	1 cup	0.07
4	Corn muffin	1	0.07
4	Bran flakes	½ cup	0.07
4	Puffed rice	1 cup	0.07
4	Muffin	1	0.07
5M	Hamburger	3 oz	0.07
2	Cooked tomatoes	½ cup	0.06
2	Tomato juice	½ cup	0.06
2	Brussels sprouts	½ cup	0.06
3	Pineapple	½ cup	0.06
4	White bread	1 slice	0.06
4	Whole-wheat bread	1 slice	0.06
4	Hamburger bun	½	0.06
4	Potato chips	15 chips	0.06
4	French-fried potatoes	8	0.06
5L	Chipped beef	3 oz	0.06
2	Mustard greens	½ cup	0.06
2	Broccoli	½ cup	0.06
5M	Egg	1	0.05
3	Pink grapefruit	½	0.05
2	Summer squash	½ cup	0.05
1	Canned evaporated milk	½ cup	0.05
2	Green beans	½ cup	0.05
5L	Chicken, meat only	3 oz	0.05
5L	Lean roast beef	3 oz	0.05

These are not best food sources but are selected to show a range of thiamin contents. Note the presence of all food groups except fat as shown in the left-hand column.

[a] The numbers refer to the exchange lists: 1 is milk; 2, vegetables; 3, fruit; 4, bread; 5L, lean meat; 5M, medium-fat meat.

[b] Serving sizes are the sizes listed in the exchange lists, except for meat.

[c] One serving of any of the first six foods contains at least 10 percent of the U. S. RDA of 1.5 mg.

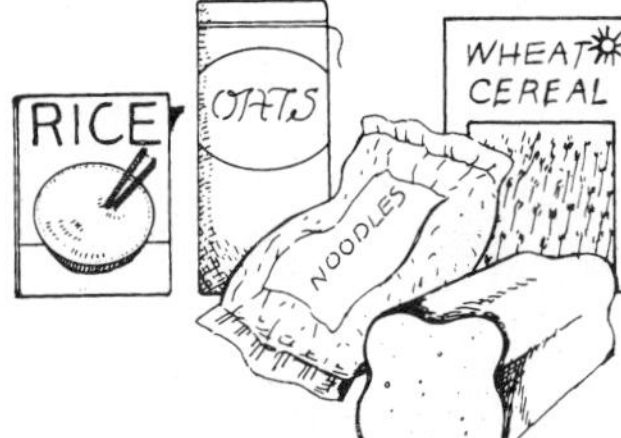

Foods containing thiamin.

ply thiamin in amounts higher than about a tenth of a milligram per serving, the most effective strategy for obtaining adequate amounts is to eliminate empty-calorie foods from the diet and to be sure to include whole-grain or enriched breads and cereals.

A rule of thumb for determining whether a diet is adequate with respect to thiamin is "ten servings a day of nutritious foods"—where "nutritious food" is defined as any food listed in the exchange system (Appendix L). In some persons who eat "junk foods" instead, signs of neurosis (mild mental illness) have been seen which cleared up with the administration of thiamin.[21]

The moral of this story would seem to be, "If you don't feel well (can't cope emotionally), check your diet. Be sure you're eating right before you go to the expense of having extensive checkups or therapy." One of the most intriguing things about the vitamins is the way in which deficiencies affect people's mental states. But watch out for charlatans who try to sell you the notion that your mental health can be improved by the taking of vitamin pills, special foods, supplements, and the like. While deficiencies do have effects on the mind and the emotions, overdoses from megavitamin supplements do nothing for people except to put money in the pockets of those selling them.

It is important in this connection to be aware that, if your calorie intake falls (for example, if you go on a diet or if your appetite is poor), your thiamin needs do not change. Even people who are fasting need as much thiamin every day as they did when they were eating a regular diet.[22] People on low-calorie diets—for whatever reason—should take vitamin-mineral pills (just the ordinary, daily supplement) until they can correct this situation. Thiamin doesn't give you energy, but it facilitates your getting energy, whether as the calories in food or as those in your body stores.

Surplus thiamin is excreted in the urine. Under ordinary circumstances, there need be no concern about taking an excess. However, as one person quipped, "If you take thiamin supplements, you may have the most expensive urine in town."

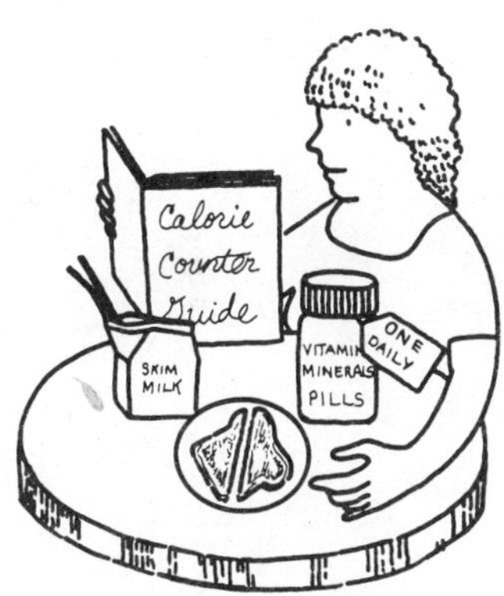

If you eat less than 1500 calories a day, you need a multivitamin-mineral supplement.

Riboflavin. Another member of the B-complex vitamins is **riboflavin**. It was first isolated from the greenish yellow, fluorescent pigment in milk.

The principal role of riboflavin is as a coenzyme-helper to the enzymes that transfer energy from one compound to another. Riboflavin also participates in the first step in the breakdown of the fatty acids for energy. Riboflavin plays a role in taking the nitrogen portion (the amine group) off amino acids when the amino acids are to be used for energy. Like thiamin, then, riboflavin is critical to the release of energy from food.

Table 4. Riboflavin Contents of Fifty Common Foods

Exchange Group[a]	Food	Serving Size[b]	Riboflavin (mg)
5M	Beef liver	3 oz	3.60
5M	Beef heart	3 oz	1.04
1	2% fat fortified milk	1 cup	0.52
1	Skim milk	1 cup	0.44
1	Canned evaporated milk	½ cup	0.43
1	Whole milk	1 cup	0.41
1	Dry skim milk	⅓ cup	0.40
1	Yogurt (whole milk)	1 cup	0.39
5L	Oysters	¾ cup	0.30
5L	Chipped beef	3 oz	0.30
5L	Veal roast	3 oz	0.26
5L	Leg of lamb	3 oz	0.23
5L	Lean roast beef	3 oz	0.19
2	Collard greens	½ cup	0.19
5M	Hamburger	3 oz	0.18[c]
5L	Sardines	3 oz	0.17
5L	Ham	3 oz	0.16
5L	Chicken, meat only	3 oz	0.16
5L	Canned salmon	3 oz	0.16
2	Dandelion greens	½ cup	0.15
5M	Egg	1	0.15
5M	Cheese, creamed cottage	¼ cup	0.15
4	Winter squash	½ cup	0.14
2	Asparagus	½ cup	0.13
2	Broccoli	½ cup	0.12
2	Brussels sprouts	½ cup	0.11
2	Spinach	½ cup	0.11
5L	Canned tuna	3 oz	0.10
2	Mustard greens	½ cup	0.10
4	Lima beans	½ cup	0.09
4	Green peas	½ cup	0.09
4	Pumpkin	¾ cup	0.09
4	Muffin	1	0.09
4	Corn muffin	1	0.08
3	Strawberries	¾ cup	0.08
2	Summer squash	½ cup	0.08
4	Corn on cob	1 small	0.08
4	Dried beans	½ cup	0.07
3	Pear	1	0.07
4	Spaghetti, enriched	½ cup	0.06
4	Macaroni, enriched	½ cup	0.06
3	Raspberries	½ cup	0.06
4	Pancake	1	0.06
2	Green beans	½ cup	0.06
4	White bread	1 slice	0.05
2	Cauliflower	½ cup	0.05
4	Mashed Potatoes	½ cup	0.05
3	Orange	1	0.05
3	Peach	1	0.05
4	Hamburger bun	½	0.04

These are not best food sources but are selected to show a range of riboflavin contents. Note, in the left-hand column, that the 1s and 5s cluster at the top; and 2s, 3s, and 4s, at the bottom.

[a] The numbers refer to the exchange lists: 1 is milk; 2, vegetables; 3, fruit; 4, bread; 5L, lean meat; 5M, medium-fat meat.

[b] Serving sizes are the sizes listed in the exchange lists, except for meat.

[c] One serving of any of the foods to this point contains at least 10 percent of the U. S. RDA of 1.7 mg.

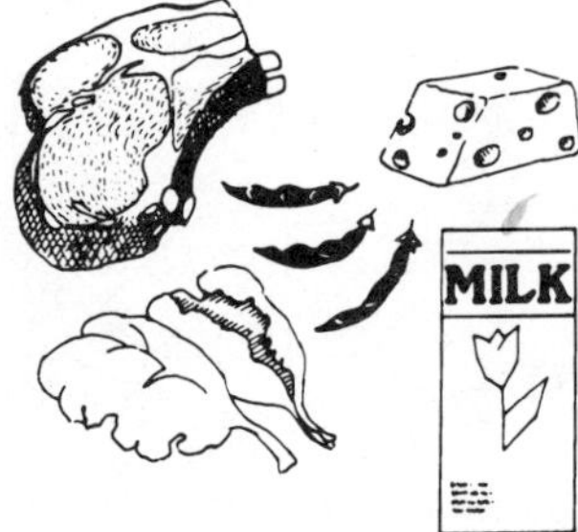

Foods containing riboflavin.

Clinically, deficiencies of riboflavin are rare except in alcohol abusers. Deficiencies can be recognized by severe skin problems including cracks in the corners of the mouth, a red, swollen tongue, teary eyes, or an invasion of blood into the corneas of the eyes. Laboratory animals on a riboflavin-deficient diet do not grow. Almost always, the symptoms of niacin deficiency are also present.

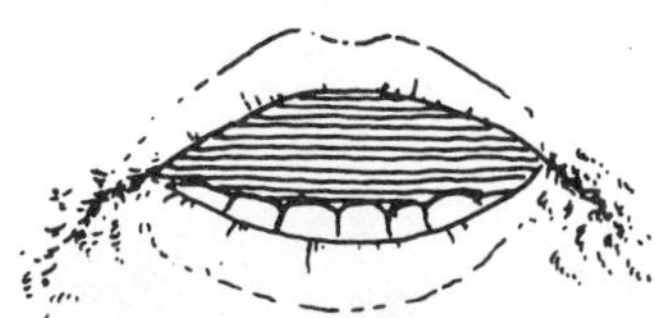

Adequate intake of riboflavin would have prevented the painful cracks at the corners of the mouth.

Riboflavin can be destroyed by ultraviolet rays—one reason why milk should not be delivered in transparent glass bottles. Cardboard cartons protect the riboflavin in milk from the ultraviolet rays of the sun. Fluorescent lights also destroy the riboflavin in milk; so it should be stored, as well as purchased, in opaque containers wherever these lights are used.[23] The same is true of enriched pasta products. As pretty as glass jars filled with noodles are to look at, the noodles will lose their riboflavin contents over time.

Although it is considered one of the water-soluble vitamins, riboflavin's solubility is slight; therefore, not much riboflavin is lost in washing vegetables or discarding cooking water. It is also stable in heat and acid but is destroyed by alkali such as baking soda.

Many foods contain riboflavin, but few are excellent sources. Milk and milk products like cottage cheese and yogurt contribute about half of the riboflavin most people consume, and meats about a fourth. Liver and heart are the best sources, but all lean meats, as well as eggs, provide some riboflavin. Leafy green vegetables and whole-grain or enriched bread and cereal products add smaller amounts to the total. Table 4 shows the riboflavin contents of common foods.

More about packaging and cooking of foods—Chapter 11.

The riboflavin RDA for women is about 1 to 1.5 milligrams, depending on age. The RDA for men is higher—1.5 to 2 milligrams—because they spend more energy daily.

Niacin. A confusing array of names is attached to the vitamin niacin. Any of these may be found on the labels of vitamin bottles. Some of the names are synonymous: **Niacin** and **nicotinic acid** refer to the same chemical structure. This chemical is easily converted in the body to the active form of the vitamin: **nicotinamide** or **niacinamide**. Technically it is not correct to say these are identical, but all of them do refer to the same vitamin. A similar word in common usage—**nicotine**, as in cigarettes—does not refer to the vitamin; it is a toxic drug.

Niacin is part of a coenzyme vital to obtaining energy from glucose. Without niacin to form this coenzyme, the glucose-to-energy reactions come to a screeching halt, and the result is **pellagra.** For over 200 years, this disease has been described in literature. In the United States, its devastating effects were seen in the South during the reconstruction period following the Civil War. Today, pellagra has been eradicated wherever enriched breads and cereals have been accepted, but it is still seen in poverty areas or where people eat predominantly corn and a low-protein diet.

Pellagra is characterized by disturbances of every body tissue, most marked in those that are most dependent on glucose for energy. Symptoms include weakness of the muscles, loss of appetite, lassitude, poor digestion, and digestive upsets such as diarrhea. In later stages, a typical skin rash of dark blotches appears on parts of the body exposed to the sun, and mental confusion develops with loss of memory, resembling insanity. Frequently these symptoms are referred to as the "three Ds" of pellagra: diarrhea, dementia, and dermatitis. There is a fourth D: death.

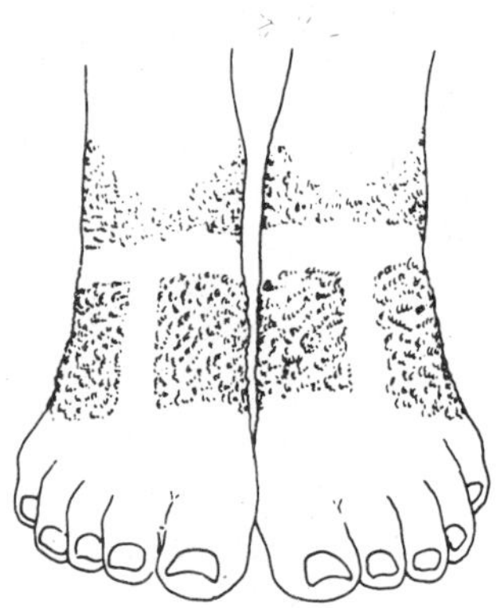

Typical dermatitis of pellagra develops on skin that is exposed to light.

In the early study of diets that produced pellagra it was found that some cultures that relied on corn for their staple grain did not develop the disease. The astonishing difference in the diets, it turned out, was in the dietary *protein*. **Tryptophan**, an amino acid present in the protein of lean meats but deficient in the protein of corn, is converted to niacin in the body. In fact, it is possible to cure pellagra by administering tryptophan alone. Thus a person eating adequate protein will rarely be deficient in niacin.

About 60 milligrams of tryptophan convert to 1 milligram of niacin in the body, and the average protein contains approximately 1 tryptophan among every 100 amino acids. However, tryptophan will first be used to build needed body proteins, and only the excess tryptophan is available for making niacin. Thus, calculating the amount of niacin available from the diet is a complicated matter. A means of obtaining a rough approximation is shown in the margin. However, the simplest assumption is that if the diet is adequate in complete protein, it will supply enough **niacin equivalents** to meet the daily need.

Rough approximation of niacin intake:

1. Calculate total protein consumed (g).

2. Subtract the protein RDA to obtain the "leftover" protein.

3. Divide by 100 to obtain the amount of tryptophan (g).

4. Multiply by 1000 to convert to milligrams (mg).

5. Divide by 60 to get niacin equivalents (mg).

6. Finally, add the amount of niacin obtained preformed in the diet (mg).

The association of niacin deficiency with "dementia" has led some people to reason, wrongly, that other forms of insanity might be curable by niacin. In particular, they have hoped that they could use niacin to cure the widespread and so-far unexplained mental disease of schizophrenia. This hope, together with others like it, underlies the schools of thought associated with "orthomolecular psychiatry" and "megavitamin therapy." Part of the appeal in the use of vitamins as opposed to drugs to treat mental illness is that vitamins are natural compounds found in the body (orthomolecular means "right molecules").

The claim is made that schizophrenic persons have an altered metabolism, with increased conversion of one hormone to another, which accounts for their symptoms. Niacin is thought to normalize this reaction. Schizophrenic people, then, are advised to dose themselves with up to 30 grams of niacin a day, 2000 times the RDA, with sizable vitamin C intakes on the side (to "protect" the niacin from oxidation). A 70 to 80 percent success rate in improvement of schizophrenic symptoms is reported.[24] When the evidence behind these claims is reviewed, however, many doubts arise.

A number of different biochemical abnormalities have been reported in schizophrenic persons, among them an altered level of epinephrine secretion. However, some people with schizophrenia do not exhibit this trait, and many nonschizophrenics do; so it is not specific to, or diagnostic for, schizophrenia. Even so, the niacin theory bears testing on the basis that it might alleviate a symptom, at least in some schizophrenic persons.

In 1973 a task force of the American Psychiatric Association reviewed the effectiveness of megavitamin therapy on schizophrenia and concluded that there was no solid evidence in its favor.[25] The reported "cures" have often been single case studies with poor follow-up. The persons "cured" may not have been accurately diagnosed as schizophrenic in the first place. Cures of mental illness seen in the early work with niacin were cures of the dementia of pellagra, not of schizophrenia. Nor is treatment low in cost, as its advocates have claimed; in instances where hospitalization is a part of treatment, it may be very costly.

When one person takes a vitamin and reports beneficial effects, it is never possible to conclude that the vitamin produced those effects. Faith also heals: Attention from the therapist plays a major role in improving a patient's state of mind. Only if two identical groups of people with schizophrenia are studied and all are treated in exactly the same way, except that one is given the vitamin, can sound conclusions be drawn. Both groups must receive similar pills, and neither group (nor their therapists) must know whether they are receiving the vitamin or a **placebo** (fake pill). The rating of success must be objective and must be performed by scorers who do not know which individuals received the vitamin. Such a study, which is called a controlled, double-blind study, has not been performed using niacin to treat people with schizophrenia. In fact, such studies are not feasible, because niacin is easy to recognize. In large doses, it produces a rush of blood to the skin surface with a flush and an associated tingling, painful sensation that is unmistakable.

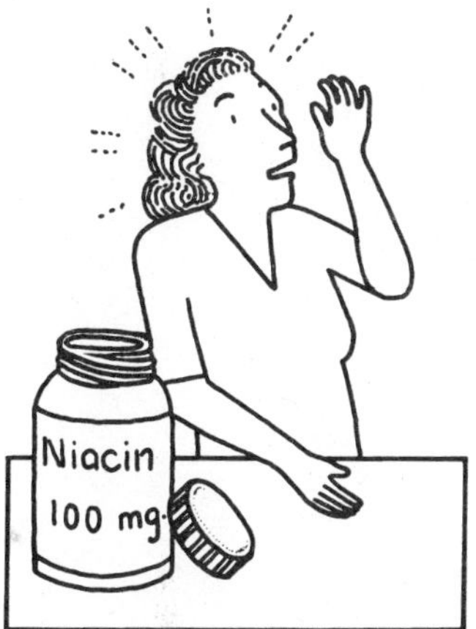

The niacin rush.

The task force members, reviewing the claims made for the use of niacin in schizophrenia, were unable to confirm that any success whatever had been achieved, much less a 70 to 80 percent cure rate. They gave full credit to the theory's proponents for caring about their patients and acknowledged that "the enthusiasm, dedication and personal investment of the megavitamin therapists may contribute to the well-being of their patients." They also acknowledged that valid theories are sometimes at first labeled as myths. It appears that the task force members were hopeful enough to have occasionally referred their own patients for megavitamin treatment. They expressed puzzlement and disappointment at their failure, after exhaustive searching, to find evidence in support of the theory.[26]

Possibly some good has come from introducing the orthomolecular idea to the public. It has supported the impression that mental disorders such as schizophrenia may be metabolic in origin. This relieves patients and their families of the destructive guilt and shame that often attend a "psychologically" caused disease. It is hoped that further investigations into the biochemistry of schizophrenia will yield more effective treatment strategies.

The use of megadoses of niacin in the attempt to treat schizophrenia and other such conditions has led to the discovery of toxic effects. This is a surprise, because niacin is a water-soluble vitamin, and it had been thought that excesses would be so promptly excreted that they would do no harm to the body. But with the increasingly widespread use of megadoses, niacin has been shown to cause liver damage with jaundice; skin rashes; elevated serum levels of glucose, uric acid, and enzymes; and peptic ulcers.[27]

Vitamin B_6. The term **vitamin B_6** refers to a group of B vitamins: **pyridoxine, pyridoxal,** and **pyridoxamine**. This group plays a vital role in many cellular reactions involving carbohydrate, fat, and protein. However, its most important roles involve proteins.

Vitamin B_6 helps to change one amino acid of which the cell has an abundance to another amino acid the cell needs; that is, it aids in the synthesis of nonessential amino acids. It also helps remove amine groups from amino acids that are fated to be used for energy. As a coenzyme, it acts in the conversion of the amino acid tryptophan to the vitamin niacin. It also helps convert the essential fatty acid, linoleic acid, to another important fatty acid, arachidonic acid. It plays a role in the synthesis of many other vital substances, such as hemoglobin and the secretions of the adrenal glands. B_6 also plays a role in maintaining the blood glucose level; it is part of the enzyme that releases glucose from glycogen stored in the liver.

Because the influence of vitamin B_6 is felt in so many areas, it is understandable that a deficiency should be expressed in generalized symptoms such as depression, nausea, and vomiting. Other symptoms include a greasy kind of skin disorder and some neuritis.

Pregnant women often show low blood concentrations of B_6 even though their diets are ample in the vitamin. It is thought that this is due to the high demand for B_6 by the fetus, whose blood normally has about five times more B_6 than the mother's. The vitamin is often prescribed for the relief of the nausea and vomiting of pregnancy as well as for the depression felt by women taking oral contraceptives, but it is not clear as yet whether it actually helps to relieve depression. Large doses should be avoided. For one thing, they have been shown to inhibit milk production in women breastfeeding their babies.[28]

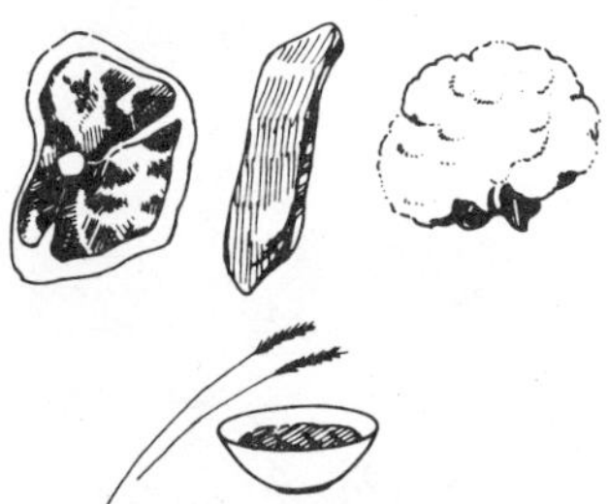

Foods containing vitamin B_6.

Vitamin B_6 is water soluble and, as a consequence, is not stored in the body. This means that foods containing it must be included in the diet daily. According to the RDA, the amount needed by adults is 2 milligrams a day; this is enough to handle 100 grams of protein. Pregnant and lactating women should receive 2.5 milligrams. Infants probably receive enough B_6 either from breast milk or from cow's-milk formula. There is some possibility that older people have a greater need for B_6 because of their slower synthesis of some key enzymes. Alcohol abuse makes B_6 deficiency likely.

No convenient reference tables showing B_6 contents of foods are available. However, the reader must by this time have realized that the B vitamins are found for the most part in the same groups of foods and that the only workable strategy for meeting B-vitamin needs is to eat a variety of nutritious foods. In the case of vitamin B_6, the richest food sources seem to be muscle meats, liver, vegetables, and whole-grain cereals.

Vitamin B_{12}. **Vitamin B_{12} (cobalamin)** was first identified as a factor necessary for the prevention and cure of **pernicious anemia**. Prior to 1926, pernicious anemia was a fatal disease; but in that year it was discovered that eating about three-fourths of a pound of nearly raw liver daily would control the condition. With this clue, research proceeded; today it is possible to control pernicious anemia with an injection of vitamin B_{12} about every three weeks.

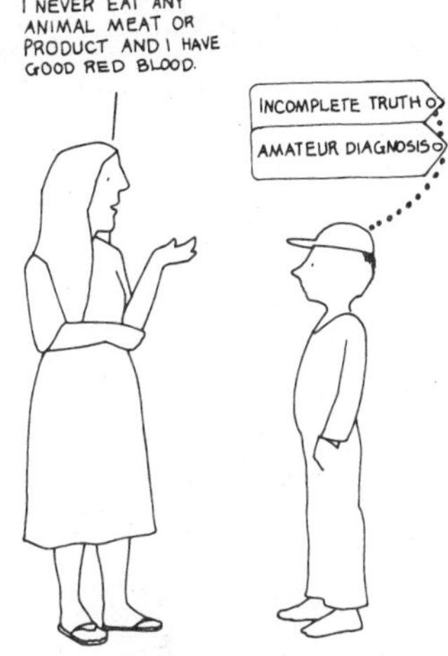
I NEVER EAT ANY ANIMAL MEAT OR PRODUCT AND I HAVE GOOD RED BLOOD.
INCOMPLETE TRUTH
AMATEUR DIAGNOSIS

The strict vegetarian may be incurring a vitamin B_{12} deficiency.

The formation of healthy red blood cells depends on an **extrinsic factor** (in foods, outside the body), now known to be vitamin B_{12}, and an **intrinsic factor** (inside the body), found in normal gastric secretion, that is necessary to help absorb the vitamin. Some persons do not inherit the ability to make the intrinsic factor and thus are unable to absorb the extrinsic factor (B_{12}). B_{12} is needed in very small amounts. The reason why the large amounts of liver were able to control pernicious anemia was probably because they provided such quantities of B_{12} that enough was absorbed, even without the help of the intrinsic factor, to keep the patient alive.

Absorption of vitamin B_{12} is affected by the levels of vitamin B_6 and iron in the body. It decreases with age and increases during pregnancy.

Vitamin B_{12} functions in maintaining the sheath surrounding and protecting nerve fibers and in promoting normal growth, as well as in producing mature red blood cells. A vitamin B_{12} deficiency, like iron deficiency, causes "tired blood" (anemia), but it shows up under the microscope as very large immature red blood cells (**megaloblastic anemia**). Other symptoms are intestinal injury and a swollen tongue. Early detection of a deficiency is necessary to avoid spinal injury and permanent nerve damage.

The vitamin is not present in plants but is produced by bacteria in the digestive tract of animals; thus the only sources are animal foods. Meats, poultry, fish, milk, cheeses, and eggs are all good sources; fortified cereal also includes B_{12}. The amount needed is very small (3 micrograms for adults is the RDA), so that almost everyone, except strict vegetarians (vegans), has an adequate intake. As for vegans, they may in some situations get enough B_{12} from their own intestinal bacteria.[29] When deficiency does develop in an animal-food eater, it is found to be a failure in absorption, and the cause is genetic rather than nutritional—a lack of the intrinsic factor. The cure for such a deficiency is to inject the vitamin, thus bypassing the intestinal failure to absorb it. Deficiency of B_{12} develops very slowly because up to three years' worth can be stored in the liver.

Folacin. **Folacin**, also known as **folic acid**, is probably more often deficient in the diets of people around the world than any other vitamin. It is essential for the formation and maturation of both white and red blood cells and for the making of all new cells by cell division.

Folacin deficiency may result from an inadequate intake, impaired absorption, or unusual metabolic need for the vitamin. A significant number of cases of anemia develop from these causes, especially among the poor and among pregnant women. The person with folacin-deficiency anemia, as with any anemia, is tired, weak, and apathetic, and may have headaches, irregular heartbeats, and labored breathing. The anemia of folacin deficiency is also characterized by a sore tongue, intestinal injury and diarrhea, lack of appetite, and weight loss and by behavioral symptoms such as irritability and forgetfulness. It is altogether a miserable condition.

Not only is folacin deficiency the most common vitamin deficiency in people, it is also the most likely to be caused by the taking of medication. Ten major groups of drugs have been shown to affect the body's use of folacin, including aspirin, anticonvulsants, and oral contraceptives.[30]

A reminder: Important as it is, folacin is not one of the nutrients found in the food composition tables (Appendix H) and is often not looked for when diets are evaluated for their adequacy. It is up to each individual, then, to make sure his or her diet includes foods that will supply generous amounts of this vitamin. The best way to do this, of course, is to balance the diet so that all food groups are included regularly and so that variety within each group is also a regular feature.

A high intake of folacin can mask the pernicious anemia caused by B_{12} deficiency. This tendency exposes the uninformed strict vegetarian to a special risk. Strict vegetarians are most apt to be deficient in vitamin B_{12}, because it is obtainable only from animal products. On the other hand, they are likely to be well supplied with folacin because, as its name—related to foliage—implies, folacin is found in vegetables and fruits. A deficiency of B_{12} needs to be detected early by the presence of very large immature red blood cells in order to prevent the nerve damage that otherwise will develop later, but the vegetarian's high intake of folacin helps the red blood cells to develop to normal size and maturity. This deceives the physician who examines a blood sample for signs of abnormality. However, the folacin can do nothing toward repairing the nerve damage caused by B_{12} deficiency, so this damage proceeds unchecked. Because of the danger of masking a lack of B_{12}, the amount of folacin in over-the-counter vitamin preparations is limited by law.

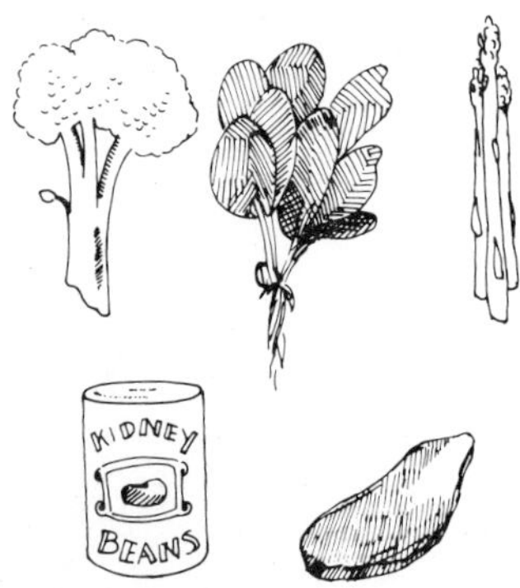

Foods containing folacin.

Folacin is widely distributed in foods. Tables of the folacin contents of foods are now being developed and probably soon will be incorporated into the standard table of food composition. The best sources are organ meats such as liver; kidney beans; green leafy vegetables like spinach, asparagus, and broccoli; beets; and members of the cabbage family. Among the fruits, oranges, orange juice, and cantaloupe are the best sources; among the starchy vegetables, corn, lima beans, parsnips, green peas, and sweet potatoes are good sources. Whole-wheat bread, wheat germ, and milk also supply folacin. It is absorbed easily from the digestive tract and is stored principally in the liver. Some is synthesized by bacteria in the intestines.

The presence of folacin in dark-green leafy vegetables is one reason for the Four Food Group Plan's recommendation that these vegetables be included in the diet at least every other day. Some forms of folacin are readily destroyed by cooking—hence the advisability of including raw vegetables like salad greens and fruits like citrus fruits in daily menus.

Other B vitamins. The six best-known B vitamins have been discussed already. Two other B vitamins needed for the synthesis of coenzymes active in a multitude of body systems are **pantothenic acid** and **biotin**. These are as important for normal body function as the vitamins to which many pages have been devoted in this chapter, but little is known about human requirements for them.[31] Both are widespread in foods, and there seems to be no danger that human beings who consume a variety of foods will suffer deficiencies. Claims that they are needed in pill form to prevent or cure disease conditions are, at best, unfounded and, at worst, intentionally misleading.

Another pair of compounds sometimes called B vitamins are inositol and choline. These are probably not essential nutrients for humans, although deficiencies can be induced in laboratory animals in order to study their functions. Like the B vitamins described above, they serve as coenzymes in metabolism. Even if they were needed for humans, supplements would be unnecessary, because they are abundant in foods. Choline has an interesting role with respect to a special kind of memory defect in the elderly, however, that is worth a moment of attention.

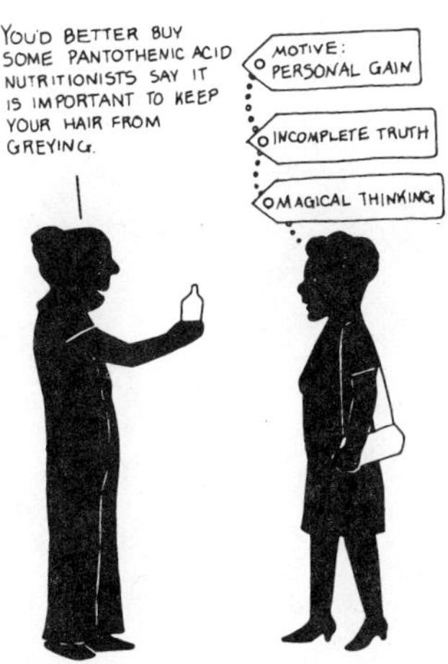
YOU'D BETTER BUY SOME PANTOTHENIC ACID NUTRITIONISTS SAY IT IS IMPORTANT TO KEEP YOUR HAIR FROM GREYING.
MOTIVE: PERSONAL GAIN
INCOMPLETE TRUTH
MAGICAL THINKING

The less the public knows about a vitamin, the more magical powers are attributed to it.

The nerves that are responsible for the storage and retrieval of information in the brain rely on a chemical known as acetylcholine to transmit their signals. Acetylcholine, in turn, is made from choline. Normally, the brain has to make all such substances for itself because it is shielded from the rest of the body by a protective barrier that won't allow changed concentrations of chemicals in the blood to affect the brain. The only exceptions are alcohol and a few powerful drugs such as narcotics. But choline is now known to be another exception to the rule. High doses given to animals raise the blood concentration, and then raise the brain concentration higher than normal—and the brain synthesizes more acetylcholine as a result.

Some elderly people develop Alzheimer's disease, a progressive impairment of memory which can lead over ten years' time to total incapacity to care for themselves. Some tentative work suggests that the progress of this disease may be slowed or halted by large doses of choline. The researchers working with it emphasize that this is not a deficiency disease but that "We are simply taking advantage of a curiosity of the brain to treat non-nutritional diseases." Poor memory caused by poor circulation, brain damage, social isolation, or other causes would not be helped by choline.[32]

Another specific use of choline is for mental patients who have been treated for a long time with the major anti-psychotic drugs. In reaction to the drugs they develop bizarre movements of the facial muscles, and this side effect seems to be countered by choline.[33] Both of these uses of choline are instances of non-nutritional therapies developed out of the discovery that large doses of a normal substance may sometimes have unexpected, beneficial drug-like effects. It is still too early to say, however, whether there may also be some risk or harm in these treatments.

A newcomer on the vitamin scene is "vitamin B_{15}," pangamic acid. First named in 1943, pangamic acid has had a mysterious and sleazy history which seems to be ending in disgrace (see Controversy 9). Whether or not it is a real compound, and whether or not it performs any necessary functions in the body, and whether or not a deficiency state will ever be observed, it is clear that the taking of pills or supplements given this name is not only unnecessary but in many instances—depending on what is really in them—may be hazardous. Their sale is illegal.

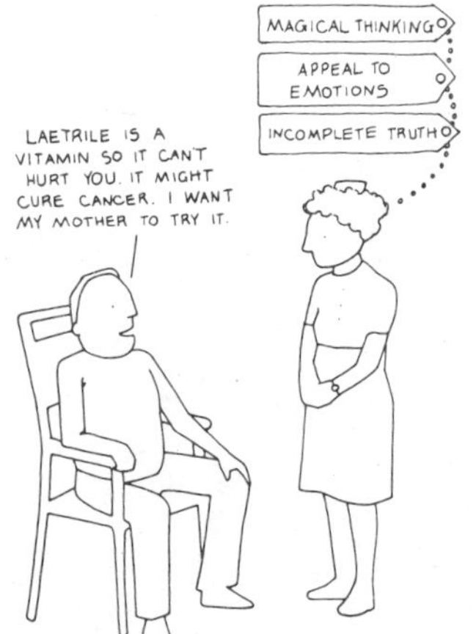

Victims of the laetrile fraud are cruelly deceived.

Two other compounds deserve mention here, if only to say that they are *not* vitamins: the bioflavonoids and laetrile. The bioflavonoids are natural body constituents to which vitaminlike characteristics have been attributed. Sold in some stores in purified form as "vitamin P," they have made much money for store owners. However, despite much work, no bioflavonoid deficiency has been induced in animals or discovered in humans, and there is, therefore, no need to make special efforts to include them in the diet. They were disqualified as vitamins by the American Institute of Nutrition and the American Society of Biological Chemists in 1950.[34] As for laetrile (also called amygdalin and dubbed "vitamin B_{17}" by its enthusiasts), it has been labeled a hoax by the FDA and proclaimed a cancer cure by the general public. Much of the success of products like vitamin P and vitamin B_{17} is due to their emotional appeal. The trick of inducing people to believe in miracle cures has been labeled magical thinking. In the case of laetrile, another kind of emotional appeal is also used: scare tactics. People fear cancer, perhaps more than they fear any other disease. Laetrile proponents have capitalized on this fear and added to it by scaring the public into believing that the medical establishment frowns on laetrile for dishonest reasons. "The doctors don't care if you die," they say, "so long as you pay huge sums for their services." Wanting to trust someone, wanting to hope that a cure is possible, victims of cancer and their friends and relatives can fall easy prey to this deception. The deception is the more cruel because the victims yield to it out of love of life, and their relatives go along because they are willing to try anything to help their loved ones get well.

Vitamin C. Vitamin C, or **ascorbic acid**, was first known as the factor that relieved the symptoms of **scurvy**; it was first isolated from lemon juice in 1932. The disease was the scourge of seagoing men of long ago, who carried cereals and live animals on long voyages but no fresh fruits or vegetables. Only ships that sailed on short voyages, especially around the Mediterranean Sea where fresh fruits and vegetables were available year-round in port, seemed free from the symptoms. On long voyages it was not unusual for two-thirds of the crew to die of scurvy.

The first nutrition experiment to be conducted on human beings was devised in 1747 to find a cure for scurvy. Dr. James Lind, a British physician, divided twelve sailors with scurvy into six pairs. Each pair received a different potential cure: vinegar, sulfuric acid, seawater, orange, or lemon. The ones receiving the citrus fruits were cured within a short time. Sadly, it was fifty years before the British Navy made use of Lind's experiment and required all navy vessels to carry sufficient limes for every sailor to have lime juice daily. The term *limey* was applied to the British sailors in mockery because of this requirement.

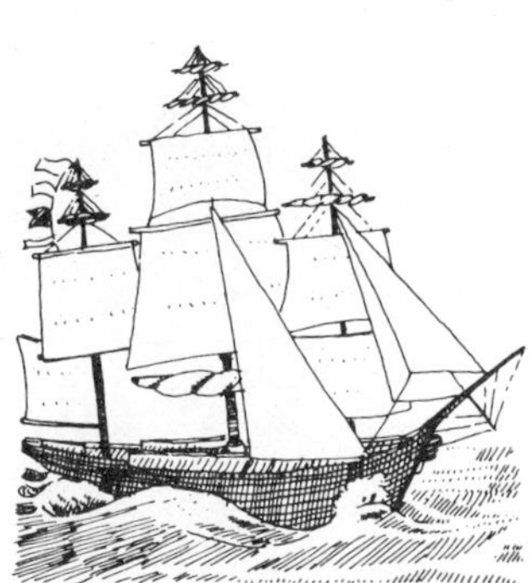

Long voyages without fresh fruits and vegetables spelled death by scurvy for the crew.

Vitamin C is required for the production and maintenance of **collagen**, a protein substance that forms the base for all connective tissues in the body—bones, teeth, skin, and tendons. Collagen is the scar tissue that heals wounds, the reinforcing structure that mends fractures, and the supporting material of capillaries that prevents bruises. Besides helping to produce and maintain collagen, vitamin C protects against infections, and promotes the absorption of iron. In times of stress, the supply of vitamin C is depleted because it is involved in the release of the stress hormones (epinephrine and norepinephrine) from the adrenal gland. The vitamin is also important to the production of thyroxin, the hormone that regulates basal metabolic rate and body temperature.

Most of the symptoms of scurvy can be attributed to the breakdown of collagen in the absence of vitamin C: loss of appetite and growth, anemia, tenderness to touch, weakness, bleeding gums, loose teeth, swollen ankles and wrists, and tiny hemorrhages in the skin.

In the United States, scurvy is seldom seen today except in infants. Breast milk supplies enough vitamin C, but the formula-fed infant must receive a supplement early. Orange juice is often added early to an infant's diet for this reason. By six months of age, a baby should be guaranteed enough vitamin C by also having some fruits and vegetables in the diet. Some subclinical evidence of vitamin C deficiency occurs in some groups, particularly male teenagers and elderly men who do not eat vegetables and salads. Smoking cigarettes seems to interfere with the use of vitamin C, but people's intakes are usually high enough to cover the needs incurred by smoking.

The RDA for vitamin C is 60 milligrams for adults, with an extra 20 to 40 milligrams recommended for pregnant and lactating women. This amount is midway between two extremes. At one extreme is the requirement, 10 milligrams per day, which is all you need to prevent the symptoms of scurvy from appearing. At the other extreme is the amount at which the body's pool of vitamin C would be full to overflowing: about 100 milligrams per day.[35] Other authorities have set different standards; for example, Canada recommends 30 milligrams

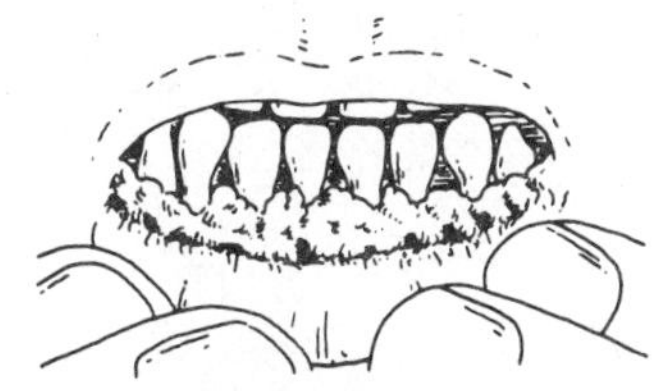

Vitamin C deficiency causes breakdown of collagen, which supports the teeth.

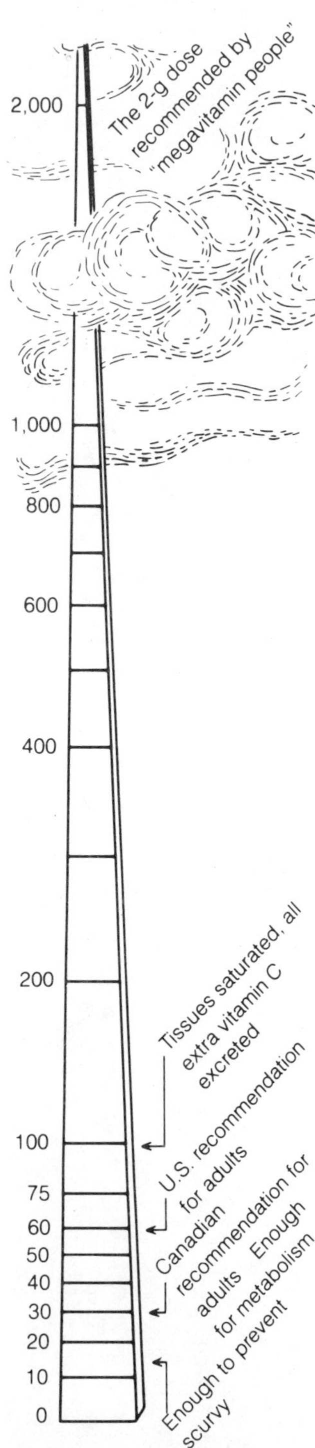

Recommendations for vitamin C intake (mg).

per day, and Germany 75. The differences between these recommendations may seem large, but when you consider that vitamin C intakes may vary from below 10 to over 1000 milligrams (a gram) a day, you can see that they are all within the same rather narrow range.

An advocate of the taking of large doses of vitamin C is Dr. Linus Pauling, whose book *Vitamin C and the Common Cold* first came out in 1970.[36] According to Pauling, much larger quantities than the RDA are necessary to enable the vitamin to perform functions other than preventing scurvy, like protecting cells from attack by cold-causing viruses. Pauling says that our ancestors evolved on a vegetarian diet which provided far more vitamin C than meat eaters consume at present. Because evolution takes place very slowly, our bodies doubtless have not changed since prehistoric times. Therefore, we still need large quantities of vitamin C today. Pauling advocates taking 1 or 2 grams (1000 to 2000 milligrams) of vitamin C per day, about twenty to forty times the RDA.

Many controlled, double-blind studies on vitamin C and colds have been performed since Pauling's controversial book first came out. A pooling of the data from eight of these showed that there was a difference of a tenth of a cold per year and an average difference in duration of a tenth of a day per cold in those subjects taking vitamin C over those taking the placebo.[37] These are enough data to support the tentative conclusion that the statistical effects of vitamin C, if any, are very small. This does not exclude the possibility that the effects on a few individuals might be considerable.

The difficulties of performing research of this kind were shown vividly in one study, in which a questionnaire given at the end revealed that a number of the subjects had guessed the contents of their capsules. A reanalysis of the results showed that those who received the placebo *who thought they were receiving vitamin C* had fewer colds than the group receiving vitamin C who thought they were receiving placebos![38] This demonstrated, as clearly as any research has ever done, the wonderful effect on your health of believing in the medicine you are taking (the **placebo effect**).

More recently, Pauling and others have suggested that vitamin C megadoses might be effective against cancer. A study reported by Pauling in which fifty cancer patients were given the vitamin tended to support this idea. However, the design of the study was flawed, the patients and researchers were not "blind," and the results therefore may have been due to faith, wishful thinking, or the like. A disciplined attempt was then made by way of follow-up: 150 patients with advanced cancer participated in a randomized, double-blind clinical trial using 10-gram-per-day doses of the vitamin, and no difference was seen in either symptoms or survival time.[39] The notion that vitamin C may cure cancer thus seems to be a false hope, although research will continue. No one questions the need for adequate amounts of vitamin C and all nutrients, however, to give the body its best defense against the onset of cancer and all other illnesses.

The widespread use of gram doses of vitamin C has enabled researchers to discover their toxic effects. They raise the uric acid level of urine and so can cause gout in people with that predisposition.[40] They cause hemolytic anemia in members of certain ethnic groups, including American blacks, Sephardic Jews, and Orientals.[41] They obscure the results of some medical tests, such as the urine test for sugar used by diabetics and the test for blood in stools used to diagnose colon cancer.[42] They impair the ability of white blood cells to kill bacteria, so that they can worsen infections rather than help clear them up.[43] And they may cause kidney stones and may affect fertility and the fetus.[44] These effects do not occur in all individuals, but there is no way of knowing in advance which individuals will be affected.

The ability of the body to cure itself is the mainstay of quacks and faddists.—**Unknown**

Infants born to mothers who take vitamin C megadoses during their pregnancies have been seen to develop scurvy shortly after birth.[45] Apparently, the infant's body adapts to high circulating levels of vitamin C by speeding up its destruction and excretion of the vitamin. Then, outside the womb on a normal intake, the infant destroys too much and suffers a severe deficiency. Known as "rebound scurvy," this withdrawal reaction may also occur in adults who stop taking megadoses, suggesting that the way to shift down to a normal intake would be to taper off rather than to quit "cold."[46]

There is a sensible argument against taking vitamin pills of any kind that seems relevant here. It goes like this: If you eat a balanced and adequate diet, you can meet all your nutrient needs within a reasonable calorie allowance. Having done this, you do not need to take supplements (pills). From another angle: If you eat an inadequate diet, you need to add vitamins, but how could you possibly know what vitamins to take? Doubtless you also need minerals—and these are often ignored.[47] Even a vitamin-mineral supplement is likely to include only five or six of the many minerals needed. The only way to be sure is to add or substitute *foods* to make your diet adequate.

When you have a cold, you are always advised to drink plenty of fluids to help your body rid itself of the metabolic wastes generated by fighting off the cold virus. A vitamin C pill has to be swallowed with fluid anyway; so why not forget the pill and just take a glass of water—or orange juice? Better yet, try the old Jewish remedy: a cup of hot chicken soup.[48]

Citrus fruits are among the best and most popular sources of vitamin C, and these can be fresh, canned, or frozen. Other vitamin C-rich fruits are strawberries and cantaloupe. The best vegetable sources

Table 5. Vitamin C Contents of Fifty Common Foods

Exchange Group[a]	Food	Serving Size[b]	Vitamin C (mg)
2	Brussels sprouts	½ cup	68
3	Strawberries	¾ cup	66
3	Orange	1	66
3	Orange juice	½ cup	60
2	Broccoli	½ cup	52
3	Grapefruit juice	½ cup	48
3	White grapefruit	½	44
3	Pink grapefruit	½	44
2	Collard greens	½ cup	44
2	Mustard greens	½ cup	34
2	Cauliflower	½ cup	33
3	Cantaloupe	¼	32[c]
3	Tangerine	1	27
2	Cabbage	½ cup	24
5M	Beef liver	3 oz	23
2	Cooked tomatoes	½ cup	21
2	Tomato juice	½ cup	20
2	Asparagus	½ cup	19
4	Green peas	½ cup	17
2	Turnips	½ cup	17
2	Dandelion greens	½ cup	16
3	Raspberries	½ cup	16
4	Potato	1 small	15
3	Blackberries	½ cup	15
4	Lima beans	½ cup	15
4	Winter squash	½ cup	14
3	Pineapple	½ cup	12
2	Spinach	½ cup	12
2	Summer squash	½ cup	11
4	French-fried potatoes	8	10
2	Radishes	4	10
4	Mashed potatoes	½ cup	10
3	Blueberries	½ cup	10
4	Pumpkin	¾ cup	9
2	Green beans	½ cup	8
4	Sweet potatoes	¼ cup	8
4	Corn on cob	1 small	7
3	Pear	1	7
3	Peach	1	7
2	Onions	½ cup	7
3	Pineapple juice	⅓ cup	7
3	Bananas	½ medium	6
4	Potato chips	15	5
2	Beets	½ cup	5
2	Carrots	½ cup	5
4	Corn	⅓ cup	4
1	2% fat fortified milk	1 cup	2
1	Skim milk	1 cup	2
1	Whole milk	1 cup	2
1	Yogurt	1 cup	2

These are not best food sources but are selected to show a range of vitamin C contents. Note, in the left-hand column, the clustering of 2s and 3s at the top and 1s and 4s at the bottom and the absence of 5s and 6s (fats).

[a] The numbers refer to the exchange lists: 1 is milk; 2, vegetables; 3, fruit; 4, bread; 5M, medium-fat meat.

[b] Serving sizes are the sizes listed in the exchange lists, except for meat.

[c] One serving of any of the foods to this point contains at least 50 percent of the U. S. RDA of 60 mg.

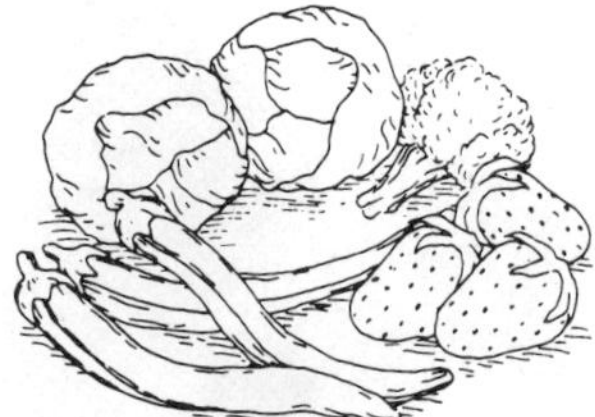

Foods containing vitamin C.

are broccoli and other members of the cabbage family and green leafy vegetables (see Table 5). Green peppers have a large amount of vitamin C but are not considered an excellent source because they are seldom eaten in quantity. Tomatoes and potatoes, if sufficient amounts are consumed, are considered good sources, although a single serving of either will not by itself meet the vitamin C RDA. Milk, meat, and eggs are very poor sources, as are breads and cereals. Thus the vegetable and fruit groups are the only ones providing ample amounts of vitamin C.

Food Feature: Cooking to Preserve Vitamins

Not only is it a healthy course of action to depend on foods, not pills, to obtain good vitamin nutrition, but also it is a sound practice to cook with the vitamins in mind. The problem of losing water-soluble vitamins when you expose them to heat or discard them in cooking water has been mentioned several times in this chapter. Understanding a few principles can help you avoid these losses. Because vitamin C is the most vulnerable of all the vitamins, it is emphasized here to illustrate these principles.

Vitamin C is an organic compound synthesized and broken down by enzymes found in the fruits and vegetables that contain it. The enzymes work best at the temperature at which the plants grow, normally about 70 degrees F (25 degrees C), which is also the room temperature of most homes. When a fruit has been picked, the enzymes that synthesize vitamin C stop working, because they require a continued input of energy from the sun to do their work. But the enzymes that break down vitamin C continue to work. Chilling the fruit stops the destructive work of these enzymes. To maximize and protect vitamin C contents, fruits and vegetables should be sun ripened, chilled immediately after picking, and kept cold until they are used.

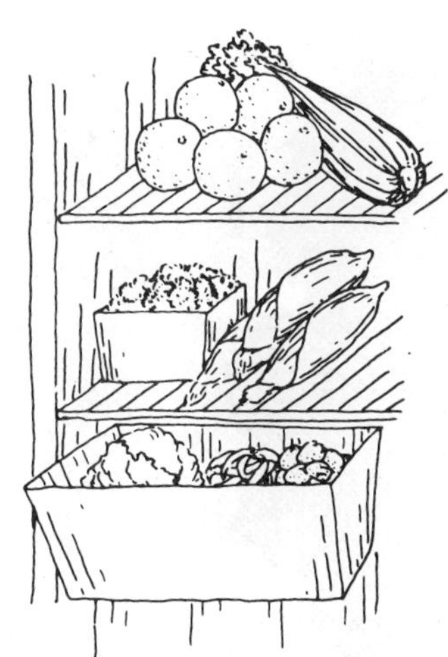

To preserve nutrients: refrigerate.

People sometimes wonder whether they should buy fresh vegetables instead of the canned or frozen varieties. Surprisingly, the rank order—in terms of vitamin content—often is (1) frozen, (2) fresh, and (3) canned. The reason for this is that freezing has very little effect on vitamin content, whereas standing at room temperature, as fresh vegetables sometimes do on their way to the market or in the store, does reduce the vitamin content. The canned vegetables come last because the high temperatures used in canning destroy some vitamins, and others leak out into the water, which is usually thrown away. Most nutritious of all, of course, are vegetables brought straight from the garden into the kitchen and cooked at once.

Because it is an acid, vitamin C is most stable in an acid solution; and because it can be destroyed by oxygen, it must be kept away from air. Citrus fruits, tomatoes, and many fruit beverages containing vitamin C are acid enough to favor its stability. As long as the skin is uncut or the can is unopened, the vitamin is protected from air. If you store a cut vegetable or fruit or an opened container of juice, you should cover it tightly with a wrapper that excludes air and store it in the refrigerator.

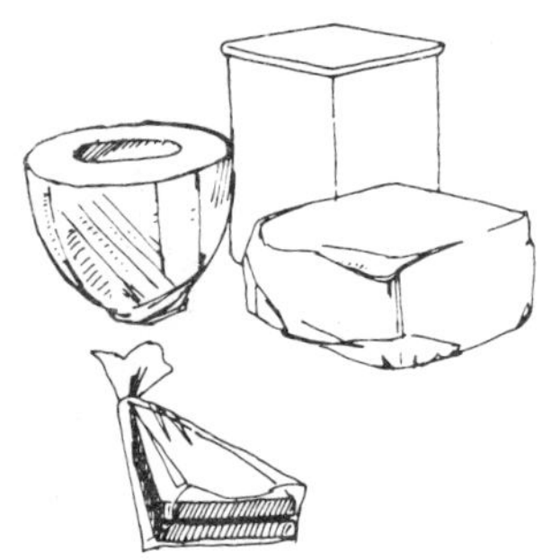

Wrap tightly.

On the subject of cutting, another pointer is not to pare or trim fruits and vegetables much when preparing them, because most of the nutrients are in the outer leaves or layers. Keep the skins on salad vegetables, and don't discard the broccoli leaves, for example. Cutting fruits and vegetables is only an advantage when it greatly shortens the needed cooking time.

Being water soluble, vitamin C readily dissolves into the water vegetables are washed in. Washing should be done quickly, in cold water, and the vegetables should not be allowed to soak. If cooking water is discarded, vitamins are poured down the drain with it. Cooking methods that minimize this kind of loss include steaming vegetables over water rather than in it, quick-frying them in a small amount of oil, or boiling them in a small volume of water. An amount of water equal to half the weight of the vegetable is probably best; more incurs vitamin losses, but less requires a longer cooking time. Of course, if the water is kept with the food, as in soups or casseroles, a larger volume of water can be used.

Overcooking is the greatest culprit causing vitamin losses; in fact, 100 percent of the vitamin C can be lost this way. Vegetables are most nutritious —and also most palatable—if they are cooked to the just-crisp point, not beyond. A pressure saucepan can be a great help for cooking vegetables; you can cut them up small because you are using little water, cooking time is very short, and you *can* open the saucepan to test for doneness midway in the process. Avoiding overcooking is a challenge for the user of a pressure saucepan, because it takes only a minute or two to bring most vegetables to the crisp state.

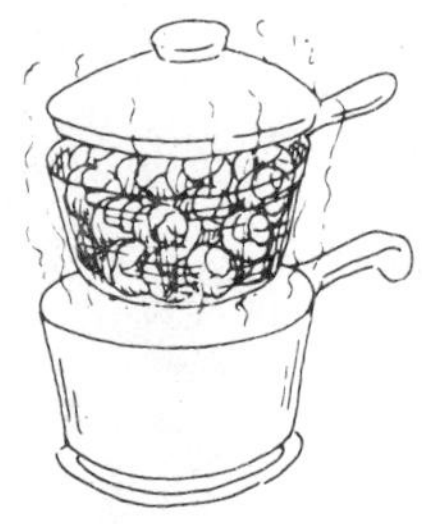

Cook over, not in, water.

Related to overcooking is the use of leftovers. Reheated leftover vegetables are usually seriously overcooked, and may be virtually valueless, nutritionally. A goal should be to cook only the amount of food, particularly vegetables, that can be consumed at one meal. Similarly, don't hold vegetables warm for long periods of time.

The composition of the cooking utensil has little or no effect on vitamin retention. Iron, like oxygen, destroys vitamin C by oxidizing it, but perhaps the benefits of cooking with iron utensils outweigh this disadvantage.

These are the main principles applying to the preservation of the water-soluble vitamin contents of foods. Other strategies can be adopted by the nutrition-conscious cook. You can keep a jar in the refrigerator for the surplus liquid from canned or cooked vegetables and the juice from cooked meats, then use this liquid for gravies or soups. Also, you can boil leftover bones to leach out the calcium and B vitamins and then use the resulting stock in the same ways.

A note of common sense might be appropriate to close this section. Considering the value of your time and energy, a law of diminishing returns probably operates in your kitchen. You have other things to do besides hovering over your foods, laboring to preserve every milligram of the vitamins they contain. If you adopt truly outrageous cooking methods—burning your meats, boiling your vegetables for hours, leaving foods out on your countertops to spoil—you can indeed suffer undesirably high losses of nutrients. But you can tolerate some losses if you make sure to start with foods containing surplus amounts of vitamins to begin with, and this takes no extra effort or time. Your time will be spent purchasing some kind of food, so it may as well be spent in purchasing the most vitamin-rich. For example, if you want broccoli but may not use it immediately, frozen rather than fresh may be the better buy. Remember that losses also occur under the following conditions:

When you buy more food than you can use.

When you buy packages of fruit and vegetables that contain more than you need, so that some of them spoil.

When you fail to read the labels, so that you buy sugar when you wanted to buy cereal.

When you buy the cheapest can and then discover that you have bought more water and sugar than food.

When you cook too much and have to throw away the leftovers.

When the way you cook is not appetizing, so that food is left uneaten.

And so forth.

Starting with a variety of nutritious foods and using reasonable precautions in their storage and preparation is enough to guarantee good nutrition without worry.

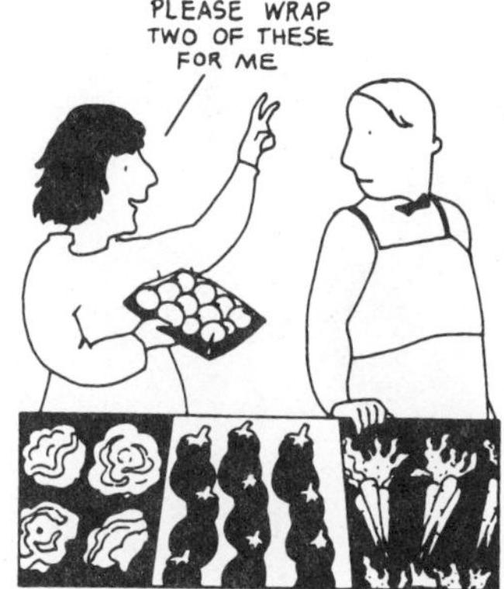
PLEASE WRAP
TWO OF THESE
FOR ME

Why should you buy food you can't use?

Putting It All Together

At this point, four of the six classes of nutrients have been considered: carbohydrates, fats, proteins, and the vitamins. Among these nutrients, linoleic acid, eight or nine amino acids, and all of the vitamins are essential nutrients; that is, they must be supplied by food. No single class of foods provides them all, but as Figure 1 shows, a balanced diet provides a virtual guarantee that all will be supplied. Only the "RDA vitamins" are included in the figure; food sources of the others are less well known. However, the variety of food selections suggested is so

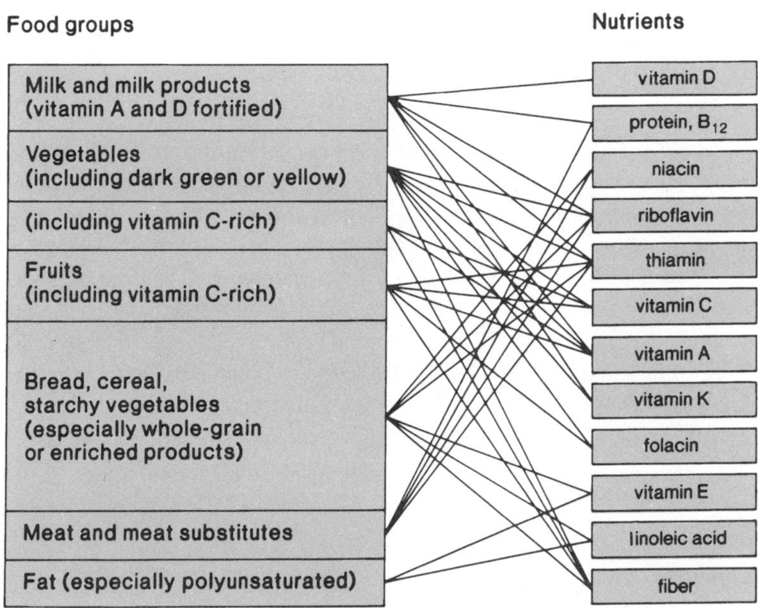

Figure 1. *The individual lines of the web may be of interest but the point of the figure is that it is a web. Different foods supply different assortments of nutrients, so a wide and varied selection is the best guarantee of adequacy.*

great that chances are good they will supply all the vitamins in amounts sufficient to meet the needs of virtually all members of a healthy population. This diagram will be repeated at the end of the next chapter, with modifications to show how to ensure adequacy for certain minerals.

The vegetarian has two special problems with respect to the vitamins. For one thing, the plant-food sources of vitamin D are unreliable, depending on how long and under what conditions the plant has been in the sun. Fortified milk is the only reliable source of vitamin D and is so important, especially for growing children, that all vegetarians should allow their children to drink milk even if they themselves do not.

The other problem is that there are no plant sources of vitamin B_{12}. The lacto-ovo-vegetarian can rely on milk or eggs, but the vegan needs to take a supplement (pill or shot) or use vitamin B_{12}-fortified soy milk. It may take as long as two or three years for the severe nerve damage of pernicious anemia to develop, but the damage can be extensive and irreversible before the victim is aware of it. This disease is seen periodically in adult vegans who fail to take vitamin B_{12} supplements and is especially likely in the breast-fed child of a vegan mother.

It must be abundantly evident by now why foods, not pills, are shown in Figure 1. Vitamin pills only contain the vitamins that human beings select to include in them. No pill or even combination of pills supplies all of the nutrients essential to life in the amounts in which they are needed. This point becomes even clearer when the minerals are considered.[1]

[1]*Chapter Notes can be found at the end of the Appendixes.*

For Further Information

Recommended references on all nutrition topics are listed in Appendix J. In addition, we recommend the following.

Some progress is being made in research on the possible therapeutic uses of large doses of vitamin E, although the results are not clear enough to report here as yet. The interested reader might want to refer to the Controversy 15 references and the following article:

- Horwitt, M. K. Therapeutic uses of vitamin E in medicine. *Nutrition Reviews* 38 (March 1980): 105-113.

Douglas Ramsey, who was captured by the Vietcong in 1966 during the Vietnamese War, personally experienced severe beriberi and scurvy and lived to tell the story in a moving account:

- Seven years in captivity as Douglas K. Ramsey tells it. *Nutrition Today*, May/June 1973, pp. 14-21.

A useful reference for the advanced student of nutrition is the review on choline, the lead article in *Nutrition Reviews* 36 (1978): 201-207.

L. Pauling's ingenious and thought-provoking arguments in favor of taking large doses of vitamin C are presented in:

- Pauling, L. Are recommended daily allowances for vitamin C adequate? *Proceedings of the National Academy of Sciences* 71 (1974): 4442-4446.

A fascinating story that we did not tell in this chapter is the story of Norman Cousins's "miracle cure" by vitamin C and laughter. Whether his recovery had anything to do with the vitamin itself is anyone's guess. The story is told in:

- Cousins, N. Anatomy of an illness (as perceived by the patient). *New England Journal of Medicine* 295 (1976): 1458-1463. Reprinted in *Nutrition Today*, May/June 1977, pp. 22-28.

A provocative sequel to this story is:

- Cousins, N. What I learned from 3,000 doctors. *Saturday Review*, February 18, 1978, pp. 12-16.

On cooking to conserve nutrients, see:

- Seelig, R. A. Conserving nutrients in fresh fruits and vegetables. United Fresh Fruit and Vegetable Association (address in Appendix J).

The American Dietetic Association makes available a cassette:

- Herbert, V. Megavitamin therapy. *CAM*, May 1977 (address in Appendix J).

Controversy 9

Vitamin B_{15}

Is it or is it not a vitamin?

Chapter 9 summed up what is known about each of the vitamins and briefly told a few of the more outrageous stories about frauds and fads connected with them. Hopefully, some of the rumors about their potency have been laid to rest. But knowing the falsity of these particular rumors won't provide a defense against others until you realize just how far a fraud can go. When you have learned to trust no source and no authority completely, then you will have learned to approach new claims made for vitamins (as for all nutrients) with the appropriate degree of wariness. The story of vitamin B_{15} is told here to illustrate this point.

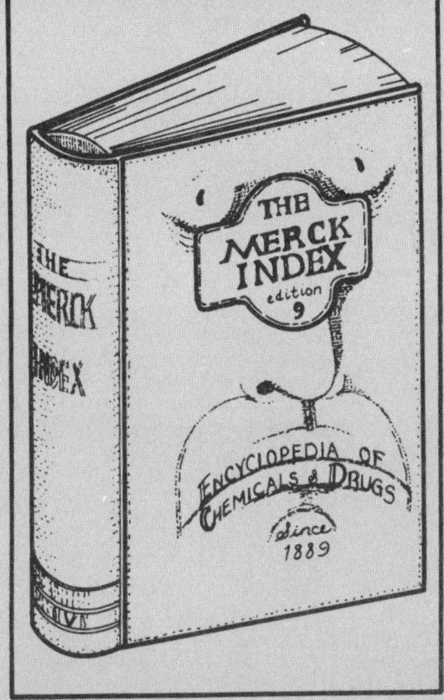

Even the Merck was fooled by this one.

Birth of B_{15}. According to a thoroughly researched review by Dr. Victor Herbert, professor of medicine at SUNY Downstate Medical Center in Brooklyn, New York, director of the Hematology and Nutrition Laboratory at the Bronx Veterans Administration Medical Center, and a highly respected, long-time scholar and researcher of vitamin facts and fallacies, it was in 1943 that this controversial entity first appeared on the scene. In that year, two researchers, Ernst Krebs, Sr., and Ernst Krebs, Jr., applied for a patent for a substance they claimed to have isolated from apricot kernels, which they called pangamic acid. They patented a trade-name for it: vitamin B_{15}.[1]

Immediately, the first moral of this story can be drawn: Naming a compound a vitamin doesn't make it a vitamin. In the same way, Krebs, Jr., gave the name vitamin B_{17} to another chemical, laetrile, also isolated from apricot pits. Similarly, if you wished, you could name your next baby "Doctor" instead of Rachel or Nzingha or Cromwell, and the child could then be known by this name all its life without ever having earned an M.D. degree. As an adult, if the child decided to publish a diet, it could be called "Doctor So-and-

So's" diet. (But to pursue this reasoning further would be to tell another story.)

B_{15} into the 1980s. The *World Review of Nutrition and Dietetics* published in 1977 a review, "Pangamic acid," which was "supported in part by a grant from the McNaughton Foundation" and which claimed that a similar review would soon be published in the *American Journal of Clinical Nutrition* with over 125 references, most of them clinical. The *Merck Index*, 9th edition, 1976, also published the structure of pangamic acid.

To the experienced reader of nutrition literature, these appear to be impressive evidence of legitimacy. But a closer look shatters the claims for pangamic acid based on them. First, the author of the review in the *World Review* is Krebs' son-in-law—not that a family relationship immediately proves a bias, but it does suggest the possibility. Second, the "McNaughton Foundation" is a front name for Andrew McNaughton, the owner of a factory manufacturing laetrile. The "foundation's" previous publications were booklets promoting pangamic acid and laetrile as if they were vitamins. The review "to be published in the *American Journal of Clinical Nutrition*" was indeed submitted to the journal but was refused because it included:

- No quotation marks on the word "vitamin" as applied to pangamate, implying falsely that pangamate was already officially accepted as a vitamin.
- No mention of the Canadian and U.S. food and drug authorities' positions that evidence for pangamate as a vitamin was nonexistent and that its safety and benefit were not proven.
- No data on the chemical reactions in which pangamate might participate in the body.
- No data on absorption, blood levels, and other factors normally studied for vitamins.
- No foundation for the claims made or citation of conflicting evidence or claims.

In short, the review was not a scientific review and critique of all the available evidence but rather an uncritical collection of stories and uncontrolled studies from which no positive information could conclusively be drawn.[2] Hence it was rejected for publication.

A second moral is perhaps apparent in this tale by now. "To be published" does not mean "published"; it may be a statement of wishful thinking. And the fact that someone claims he or she has "clinical" evidence of a vitamin's effectiveness is not to say that such evidence actually exists. In other words, people sometimes lie.

One strong fact stands out in favor of the reality of pangamic acid as a substance, however: its publication in the *Merck Index*. Every chemist uses "the Merck" as a reference for the structure and properties of chemical compounds. The Merck is the standard for chemical identity; in short, the chemist's dictionary. So in spite of the lack of evidence and reliable publications on pangamate at present, the substance does exist and research in the future will show us exactly what it does. Right?

Wrong. Amazingly, the Merck slipped up—not once, but twice—when it came to pangamic acid. According to Dr. Herbert,

The Merck Index, 8th edition, 1968, notes pangamic acid as a mixture of sodium gluconate,

Miniglossary

laetrile (LAY-uh-trill): A substance isolated from apricot pits, advertised as a cancer cure and sold under the trade-name "vitamin B_{17}" but actually not a vitamin and never shown to be either safe or effective as a cancer cure. See Controversy 11A for the details.

pangamic acid/pangamate: A name used for a substance supposed to be isolated from apricot pits. Actually, pangamate has no particular chemical identity. See also vitamin B_{15}.

refereed journal: A journal that refuses to publish research or review articles submitted to it until they have been approved by two or more referees, experts in the specific subject area of the articles and in the research methods used.

vitamin B_{15}: Trade-name for pangamic acid. The term *vitamin* in this name does not signify that B_{15} is an essential nutrient.

vitamin B_{17}: See *laetrile*.

glycine, and diisopropylamine chloroacetate. The 9th edition of the Merck Index gives the structure as D-gluconic acid 6-bis (1-methylethyl) amino acetate. The editor of the Merck Index indicated to this reviewer that "pangamic acid" and "vitamin B_{15}" will be deleted from the 10th edition, since they were deceived into listing it. Products marketed as B_{15} or pangamic acid, or calcium pangamate could contain any or all of the above materials, plus other materials, since there is no standard of identity for the product.[3]

Dr. Herbert, for all of the above and many more reasons, has concluded that vitamin B_{15} *alias* pangamic acid is "a label and not a substance." Its creator, he says, is a twice-convicted criminal who is a "doctor" only because he was given an honorary doctorate in science by a small Bible college in Oklahoma which had "no science department and no authority from Oklahoma to award the degree."[4] (That was a short story about "doctors.") The college itself no longer exists. (Here we could draw a moral about institutions of higher learning.)

When bottles labeled "pangamic acid" are bought and analyzed they are found to contain a variety of ingredients, not always the same but always identifiable as other compounds, not as pangamic acid. One of these is a chemical which produces blood vessel dilation and a drop in blood pressure so that the user experiences a "high" very shortly after taking it. The reaction of the uninformed: "Wow, this is really a powerful vitamin. I feel great already!" The promoters, who also sell laetrile, have become multimillionnaires.[5] By now we have gleaned a multitude of morals, but there are still more to come.

The FDA and the *American Journal of Clinical Nutrition* have soundly condemned pangamic acid. *Nutrition and the MD* dubbed it the "quack nutrient of the year" in 1978. More recently it has been shown that one of the ingredients sometimes in the bottle is a compound that not only is not a vitamin but is a cancer-causing agent.[6] The sale of pangamate as a food, dietary supplement, or drug is illegal.[7] Canada has prohibited the sale of pangamate altogether for over ten years.

Still, as this book goes to press, thousands of bottles of these compounds are being sold each week in health food stores, bearing the label "vitamin B_{15}" or "pangamic acid." The FDA has made a number of seizures of these products but has not stemmed the flow of them to the ever-believing public. No doctor can legally use or prescribe the material without first securing permission from a committee composed of doctors authorized to make decisions about the ethics of experiments using human beings as subjects. Nor can a doctor proceed until after obtaining informed consent from the patient—*informed*, meaning that the patient reads a statement that the item has no known value in the treatment of any disease, is not known to be safe, and may be dangerous. However, doctors and self-titled doctors are as enthusiastic, impulsive, and ill-informed in many cases as the customers who hope to buy miraculous cures in pill form under this name.[8]

Personal strategy. Suppose that you want *not* to be misled into believing false information about vitamins. How can you see through such convincing claims as those made for pangamic acid?

There are many elements of skill involved in assessing the validity of nutrition (or any) information. Some of them have been suggested in previous chapters. In this case the profit motive was clearly in evidence: Score one against the sellers of B_{15}. Their credentials don't stand up to close examination, either: Score two. Their "evidence" was of the anecdotal, "case-history" kind which is never acceptable as sound scientific evidence of the safety or efficacy of a nutrient or drug in therapy for any condition. They had no controlled clinical studies of large samples of people with unbiased, double-blind scoring of results: Score three. But what this story illustrates, perhaps better than any other told so far, is that any authority, no matter how credible and reputable, can make an error on occasion, as the *Merck Index* did in this case. Seeing a statement on the pages of a book in black and white—

no matter what the book—is no guarantee that it is a fact.

If you earnestly want to find out whether new nutrition information is valid, you have some effective strategies at your disposal, but you have to be willing to expend the time and energy to use them. To check on the credentials of a speaker, an inquiry by telephone to the institution where he or she claims to have gotten a degree is likely to be informative. To find out about the reality or reputation of an institution of higher learning, you can go to any good library and ask for a directory of colleges and universities or, in the case of organizations, for the *Encyclopedia of Associations*.[9]

In reading published nutrition information, seekers after truth can glean much information by simply asking themselves why it was published. Was it a newspaper article, a book written for the public, a textbook, or a report in a scientific journal? Newspapers pride themselves on keeping the public informed, and they try to print the truth as they perceive it. But they also welcome the opportunity to break sensational stories, sometimes before they have been confirmed. They stand to gain by being the first to report new findings, and they have little to lose by publishing misinformation. A newspaper article may lead you to some interesting further reading, but by itself it will support nothing but conversation.

As for books, those written for the public are often written to make money, and they vary widely in reliability. Again, seeing a statement in black and white on the pages of a book is no guarantee that it is a fact. Book writers cannot be punished by law for publishing misinformation unless a court case shows that they have caused bodily harm. "Because of the protection afforded by the First Amendment (Freedom of the Press), those who prey on the public do so not with products, but with books."[10]

The public is not generally aware that many books on nutrition are so unreliable that most professional organizations have had to form committees to combat the misinformation in them. An example is the Committee on Nutritional Misinformation of the Food and Nutrition Board, National Academy of Sciences/National Research Council. The statement about books quoted above was made by the chairperson of that committee.[11] If there is a reward for working on these committees, it is not a dollar reward. On the contrary, it costs time and energy for people to serve on them and money to the organizations to publish their statements.

What about textbooks? Perhaps we, the authors, stand too close to the subject to speak without bias. However, it is our impression that factual and reliable textbooks are more widely used, so writers strive to make their textbooks factual and reliable. We also stand close enough to know that those who write textbooks welcome, even seek, criticism from others in the field. One of the sources of our motivation is plain curiosity, which drives us to keep reading and studying in the hope of getting satisfactory answers to our own and our students' questions.

By far the most reliable of all publications on nutrition, however, are the scientific journals. Those that you can rely on are what we call reputable journals. They are the publications of such organizations as the American Medical Association and the American Dietetic Association, which require confirmed credentials and training for membership. The general reader may find journal articles unspeakably dull, but the motivated reader finds them a gold mine of information. Once the purposes and methods are understood, a journal article can be more exciting than a detective story.

Whether or not we find them exciting, however, we can rely on the reputable journals because, unlike other publications in which information appears, they are usually *refereed.* (You can find out from the *Encyclopedia of Associations* whether an association's journal is refereed.) This means that the articles submitted for publication are not automatically accepted. Each article is sent to at least two experts in the field who can judge the validity of each article and who are encouraged to be critical and careful in making their judgments. Only when these referees, or reviewers, have passed on an article is it allowed into print. That the *American Journal of Clinical Nutrition* was alert enough to stop the misinformation about pangamic acid from going any further testifies to the critical judgment of its reviewers and shows how the screening of information for publication makes these journals far more trustworthy than most leaflets, pamphlets, and books you may pick up in the local food store or bookstore.

This section has perhaps told you more than you wanted to know about the publication of science facts. But there was an excuse, remember? Today's pangamic acid will disappear from the scene tomorrow, as surely as the snake-oil medicines of the 1920s have disappeared today. What you need to arm you against the next massive fraud of this kind is not the knowledge, specifically, of the history of pangamic acid, but the techniques to be able to determine—for *any* news—whether or not you should believe it.

The Controversy Notes and For Further Information follow the Appendixes.

CHAPTER 10

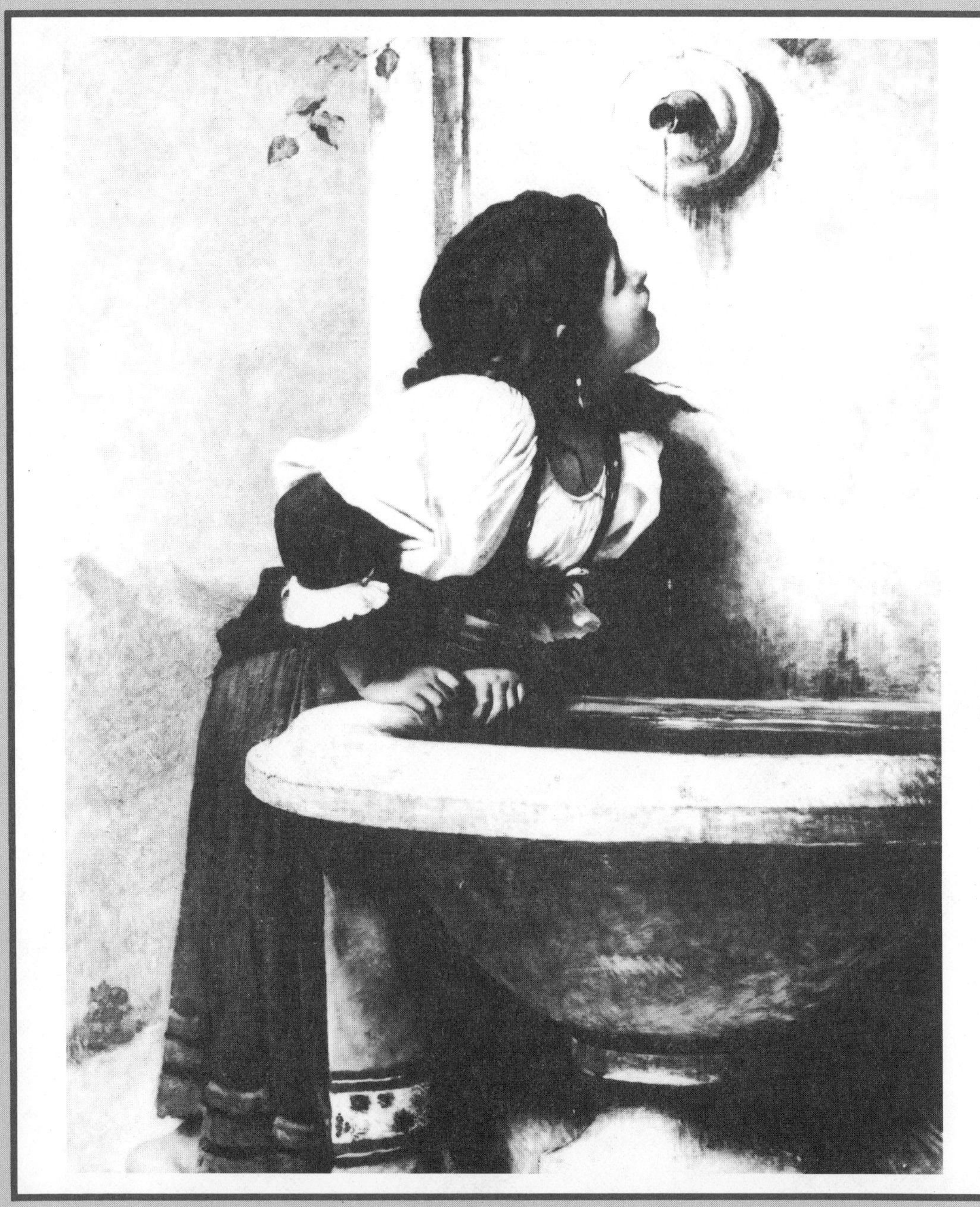

Minerals and Water

"Ashes to ashes and dust to dust." This familiar quotation is used often to remind us of our mortality. Perhaps we need this reminder to put our own importance into perspective, but it is not quite accurate. For one thing, a person does not spring like a phoenix from the ashes. A living person begins when two living cells merge into one; and when the life force leaves the body, what is left behind is at first more than a small pile of ashes. Carbohydrates, proteins, fats, vitamins, and water are also present, but these soon disappear.

The carbon atoms in all the carbohydrate, fat, protein, and vitamins combine with oxygen to produce carbon dioxide, which vanishes into the air; the hydrogens and oxygens of those compounds unite to form water; and this water, along with the water that was a large part of the body weight, evaporates. Then only the minerals are left behind as ashes. The small pile of ashes, about five pounds, is not impressive in size, but when you consider the tasks these minerals performed, you may realize their great importance in living tissue.

Consider the calcium and phosphorus. If you could separate these two minerals from the rest of the pile, you would take away about three-fourths of the total. Crystals made of these two minerals, plus a few others, form the structure of the bones and so provide the architecture of the skeleton.

Run a magnet through the fourth of the pile that remains and pick up the iron. It would not fill a teaspoon, but it is billions of billions of iron atoms. As part of the protein hemoglobin, each iron atom has the

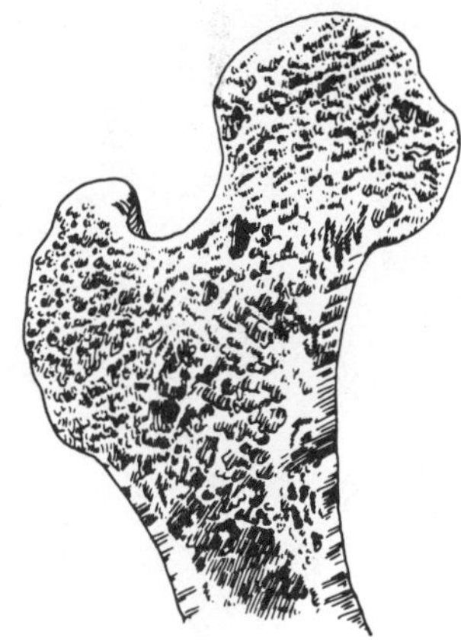

Most of the body's major minerals are found in the crystals of the bones.

Opposite: A detail from Roman Girl at a Fountain *by Leon Joseph Florentin Bonnât. Used with the permission of the Metropolitan Museum of Art, Bequest of Cathrine Lorillard Wolfe, 1887.*

Only twenty-five chemical elements are essential to life:
Carbon.
Hydrogen.
Oxygen.
Nitrogen.
Major minerals:
Calcium.
Phosphorus.
Chlorine.
Potassium.
Sulfur.
Sodium.
Magnesium.
Trace minerals:
Fluorine.
Silicon.
Vanadium.
Chromium.
Manganese.
Iron.
Cobalt.
Nickel.
Copper.
Zinc.
Selenium.
Molybdenum.
Tin.
Iodine.

special property of being able to attach to atmospheric oxygen and deliver it to the billions of cells deep inside the body.

If you were able to extract all the other minerals except for copper and iodine from the pile of ashes, you would want to close the windows before you did it. A slight breeze would blow these remaining bits of dust away. Yet the copper in the dust is the catalyst necessary for iron to hold and release oxygen; and iodine is the critical mineral in the hormone thyroxin, which controls the speed with which the body carries on its metabolic activities.

Figure 1 shows the amounts of minerals in the human body. A line separates the **major minerals** from the **trace minerals**. The major minerals are those present in amounts larger than 5 grams (a teaspoon); they are also called macrominerals or macronutrient elements. The trace minerals (microminerals or micronutrient elements) number a dozen or more; only four are shown. A pound is about 454 grams; thus only calcium and phosphorus appear in amounts larger than a pound.

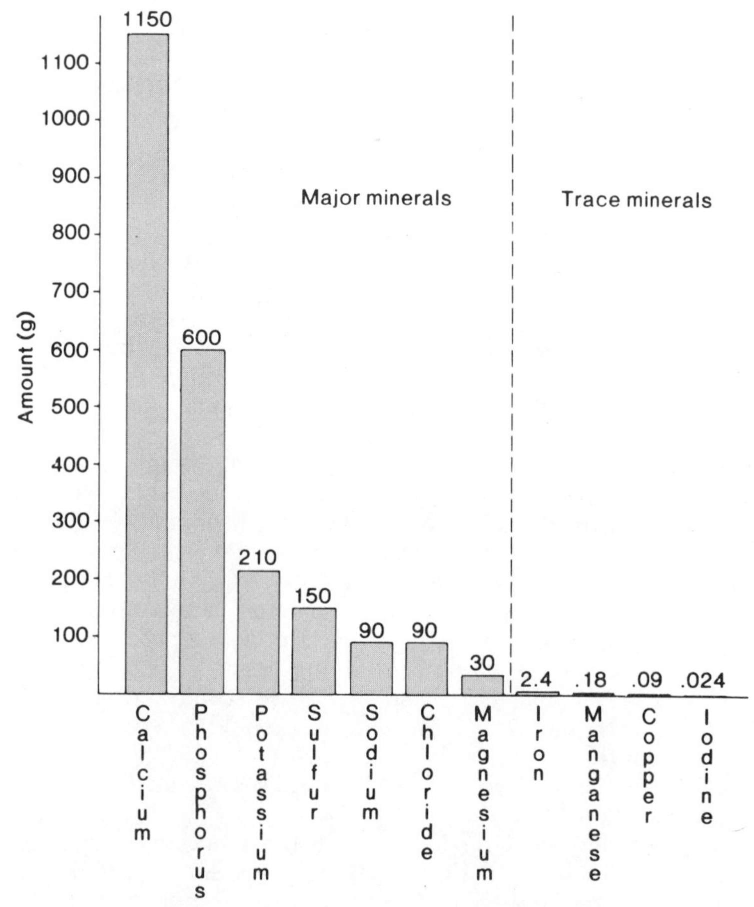

Figure 1. Minerals in a 60-kilogram person.

The distinction between the major and the trace minerals doesn't mean that one group is more important than the other. A deficiency of the few micrograms of iodine needed daily by the body is just as serious as a deficiency of the several hundred milligrams of calcium. However, because the major minerals occur in larger total quantities in the body fluids, they have certain effects on the characteristics of those fluids.

This chapter begins with a discussion of the characteristics of water—the most indispensable nutrient of all—and then goes on to show how certain minerals affect it. Lastly, the minerals that play other specialized roles in the body will be discussed one by one.

Water

Water is such an integral part of us that we seldom are conscious of its importance—unless we are deprived of it. Our bodies can survive a deficiency of all the other nutrients for long periods of time, some of them even for months or years, but they can survive only a few days without water. You began life as a single cell bathed in a soupy medium, getting all your nourishment from that fluid. Even after you became a beautifully organized body of billions of cells breathing air, each individual cell had to remain next to water in order to remain alive. That water brings to each cell the exact ingredients it requires and carries away the end products of the life-sustaining reactions that take place within its boundaries. Water makes up about 60 percent of the body weight.

Characteristics of water. Water in the body is not simply a river coursing through the arteries, capillaries, and veins, carrying the heavy traffic of nutrients and waste products. Some of the water is a component of compounds, literally a part of the chemical structure of compounds that form the cells, tissues, and organs of the body. For example, protein holds water molecules within its structure. This water is locked in and is not readily available for any other use.

We, too, live in water. See the discussion of lymph in Appendix A.

> The water held by protein molecules often discourages the very obese person who has dieted to the point of starvation and lost lean body mass. Eating a small amount of food restores some of this lean body mass, and restoring even one pound of protein tissue brings with it the retention of four pounds of water. Small wonder the obese person thinks that any tiny amount of food causes enormous weight gains. As a result, many such persons conclude that, for them, dieting is futile.

Water also participates actively in many chemical reactions, instead of being merely the medium in which they take place. A good example of this is the splitting of a disaccharide into two glucose units. Water participates by being split, with a hydrogen going to one glucose and an oxygen and hydrogen going to the other. By this action, the two glucose units are made complete.

Boasting scientist: *I'm working on discovering the Universal Solvent.*
Skeptical backwoodsman: *Is that so? Well, when you've got it, what are going to keep it in?*

As the medium for the body's chemical traffic, water is very nearly a universal solvent. Luckily for our bodily integrity, this is not quite the case, but water does dissolve amino acids, glucose, minerals, and many other substances needed by the cells. Fatty substances are specially wrapped in water-soluble protein so that they too can travel freely in the blood and lymph. Water thus makes an ideal transportation medium.

Another characteristic of water, important in its service to the body, is its incompressibility: Its molecules resist being crowded together. Thanks to this characteristic, water can act as a lubricant around joints. For the same reason, it can protect a sensitive tissue such as the spinal cord from shock. The fluid that fills the eye serves in a similar way to keep optimal pressure on the retina and lens. The unborn infant is cushioned against blows by the bag of water it develops in. Water also lubricates the digestive tract and all tissues moistened with mucus.

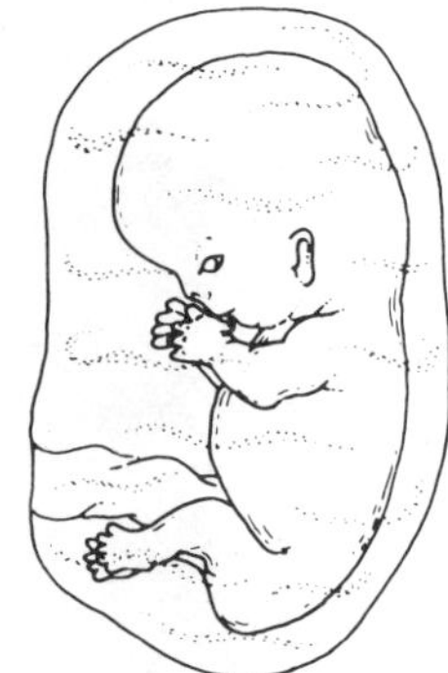

Life begins in water.

Still another of water's special features is its heat-holding capacity. This characteristic of water is familiar to coastal dwellers, who know that land surrounded by water is protected from rapid and wide variations in temperature from day to night. Water itself changes temperature slowly; at night, when the land cools, the water holds its heat and gives it up gradually to the air, moderating the coolness of the night. In contrast, the desert has a wide variation in temperature from day to night because of the lack of water on the land and in the air. In our bodies, water helps to maintain our temperature at a constant 98.6° F (37° C) by resisting fluctuations in temperature.

Related to this characteristic is the fact that a great deal of heat is required to change water from a liquid to a gas. This serves the body when cooling is needed. In a very hot environment, we sweat: Water is brought to the body surface through the sweat glands. When the sweat evaporates, it carries off all the absorbed heat and so cools the body.

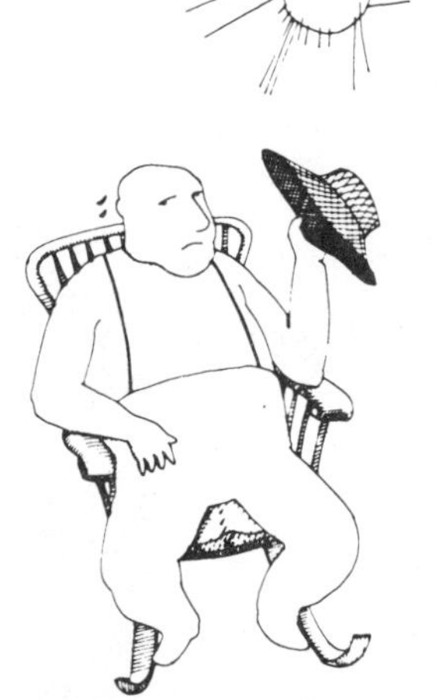

Water evaporates and helps cool the body.

A fascinating characteristic of water that makes life possible on earth is the fact that although it contracts as it gets colder like other substances, it abandons this behavior at 4° C and then expands as it freezes. (It is most dense at 4° C.) Ice is therefore lighter than cold water and so floats instead of sinking. This protects the water beneath from the coldness of the air. Thus pond water below a protective sheet of ice can remain unfrozen, and living things in a pond can survive through hard winters, even when the temperature of the air goes many degrees below freezing. If it were not for this characteristic of water, ponds and lakes would freeze from the bottom up, they would become solid and colder than ice, and all living things in them would die.

The expansion of water during freezing explains why the packages of frozen foods tell you "Do not refreeze." As it freezes, the water disrupts the structure of the food and so changes its texture. People sometimes wonder if there is any danger in eating a twice-frozen food. Provided that they haven't let it spoil while it was thawed, the only problem is that the food may be less appealing. Its nutrient content is not affected by refreezing.

Hard versus soft water. Water can contribute significant amounts of minerals to the diet. The chief mineral in **soft water** is sodium; in **hard water** the chief minerals are calcium and magnesium. Soft water makes more suds with less soap and is considered desirable for many other reasons, such as the ease with which it can be rinsed away. People in hard-water areas sometimes choose to install water softeners in their homes to obtain this advantage. Depending on the type they select, however, they may be trading calcium and magnesium for sodium. Persons who need to control their sodium intakes should be aware of this.

The major minerals in body water. About 40 percent of the body's water weight is found inside the cells, and about 15 percent bathes the outsides of the cells. The remainder is in the blood vessels. Special conditions are needed to regulate the amounts of water inside and outside the cells so that the cells do not collapse from water leaving them or swell up under the stress of too much water entering them. The cells cannot manage this by pumping water across their membranes, because they are freely permeable to water. However, they can pump minerals across their membranes, and these minerals can attract the water to come along with them. This is how the cells maintain water balance. The special form in which minerals are used for this purpose is as **ions**. In this form, as single, electrically charged particles, the minerals act to maintain not only water balance but also acid-base balance, and to play many special roles in the body. Examples are the calcium ions in the fluid that bathes the cells and the sodium ions that help send electrical impulses along nerves.

Diffusion and Osmotic Pressure

All matter is in constant motion; that is, the atoms and molecules of a substance are in constant motion. This motion is not visible to the eye but is no less real. Because of it, the molecules of two adjacent substances diffuse into each other. The direction of the **diffusion** is toward the place where there is less of the substance. For example, a person far from the kitchen can detect the frying of breakfast bacon. The molecules of the odor diffuse from the kitchen (the place of high concentration) to the bedroom (a place of lower concentration). Eventually, the bacon smell will be the same in both rooms, and although diffusion will continue, there will be no net direction.

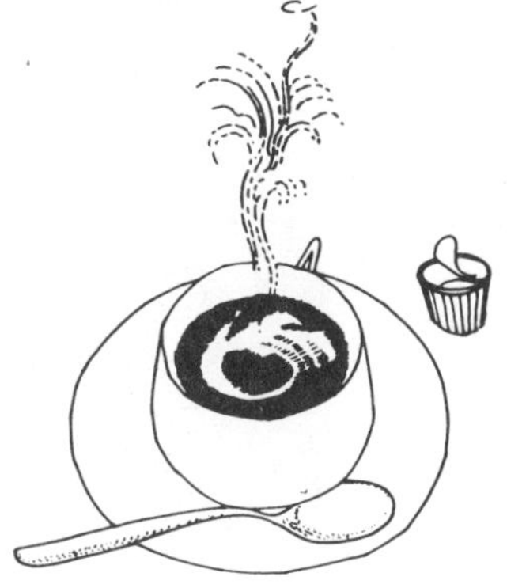

This movement of an odor in air is an example of a gas diffusing in a gas. You have seen a liquid diffuse into a liquid when you poured cream into a cup of coffee. Even without stirring, you could watch the cream molecules diffuse into the coffee. Two substances separated by a membrane can even diffuse through the membrane until their concentrations on both sides are equal.

When you read that a particular nutrient can diffuse out of the intestinal tract, you need to understand that the molecules of the nutrient are small enough to go through the membranes of the cells lining the intestinal tract

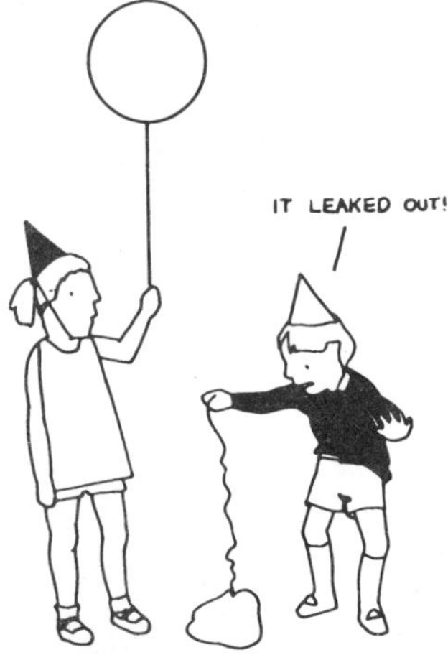

and that they do not have to be helped across. Because of their constant motion, they bombard the cell membranes and find their way through to the other side. Oxygen in the lungs will diffuse through the membranes into the bloodstream if the concentration of oxygen in the bloodstream is lower (in other words, if the blood "needs" the oxygen).

Suppose the membrane would not permit certain particles to go through. Then a force would be created.

The force created by fluids and particles on two sides of a membrane that will let only certain particles through is **osmotic pressure**. In the body, the pressure of fluids on the two sides of a cell membrane must remain equal, or there will be movement of fluid across the membrane. The pressure is caused by the bombardment of particles against the membrane and is, therefore, in direct proportion to the concentration of particles in the cell fluid. If the pressure outside a cell is greater than inside, water will flow out of the cell to dilute the concentration and thus reduce the pressure. The simplest way to state what it is about osmotic pressure that moves water from one side of a membrane to the other is to say that "water follows salt."

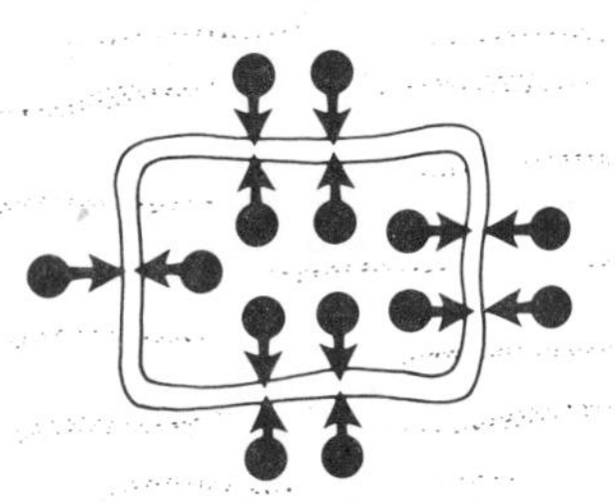

Equal bombardment of particles on both sides of cell membrane —no net direction of flow of water.

Say that on one side of a membrane there is a very concentrated solution of particles in water and that on the other side there is a weak solution. Say, too, that the membrane lets the water through easily and makes it difficult or impossible for the particles to go through. The water will move from the dilute solution to the strong solution until the *concentration* of particles is the same on both sides. There will then be more water where there are more particles and less water where there are fewer particles.

You have seen this phenomenon if you have ever salted a lettuce salad and let it set a half hour before eating it. When you returned to it, the lettuce was wilted and the salad bowl had water in it. The concentrated salt solution on the outside of the lettuce cells had a higher osmotic pressure than the fluid inside the cells. Therefore, the water flowed out of the cells toward the higher concentration of salt to bring the solutions to equal concentrations (and equal osmotic pressures). The walls of the lettuce cells collapsed when their fluid was withdrawn.

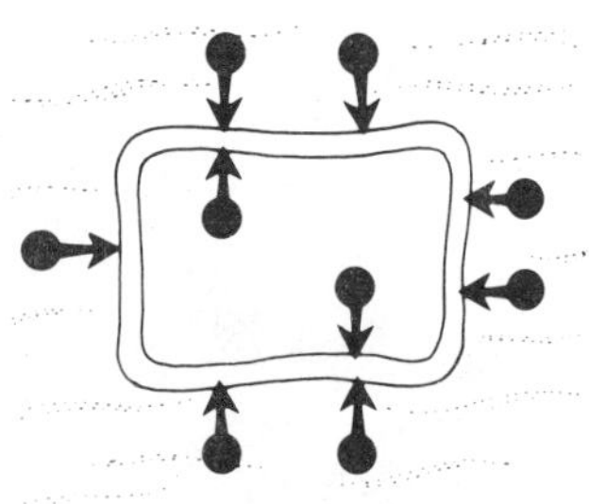

Greater bombardment of particles against outside of cell membrane —net direction of flow of water is toward the greater pressure to equalize the concentration and thus the pressure.

Water can flow freely across the membranes of most cells inside the body, so the body uses minerals to keep the water in the needed amounts in different places. The sodium ion is the special mineral used outside cells, and the potassium ion is inside cells. Proteins in the cell membranes act as pumps to keep each ion in its proper compartment. As long as the body stays healthy, the water balance will be maintained by the mineral ions. To say this another way, the osmotic pressure will be equal inside and outside the cells as long as the concentrations of the ions remain correct.

If, however, something happens to overwhelm the system, severe illness can result quickly. For example, in vomiting or diarrhea, the shift of water out of the intestinal tract pulls water from between the cells in every part of the body. This leaves a high concentration of sodium outside the cells, so water will leave the inside of the cells to equalize the concentration. Meanwhile, the kidney will detect the water loss and will attempt to retrieve water by retaining sodium, driving the concentration outside the cells even higher and bringing more water out of them. When this happens, the very serious condition of **dehydration** occurs. The water lost in vomiting or diarrhea comes from every body cell.

Among the major minerals, the calcium, potassium, sodium, and magnesium ions are positively charged (plus), and the chloride, phosphate, and sulfate ions are negatively charged (minus). The total number of plus and minus charges in the body fluids must remain balanced within narrow limits to allow the cells to do their work. For example, if some of the calcium were to be lost from the blood, the body would suffer not only from the loss of calcium's special functions but also from the loss of the plus charges contributed by calcium.

Base formers:
Calcium.
Magnesium.
Sodium.
Potassium.

Acid formers:
Chloride.
Phosphate.
Sulfate.

A very few of the atoms of water (H_2O or H-O-H) also exist as ions: H^+ (hydrogen ion) and OH^- (hydroxyl ion). Excess hydrogen ions in a solution make it an **acid**; excess hydroxyl ions make it a **base**. The positive mineral ions, such as calcium, occur in association with negative hydroxyl ions, which make a solution basic; thus they are called base formers. The negative mineral ions are called acid formers.

The ability of minerals to form acids or bases is one of their most important characteristics. It enables them to aid the tissues by maintaining the acidity (or alkalinity) at which the enzymes there work best. For example, the blood must be maintained in a very narrow acid-base range—between pH 7.2 and 7.4. (A **pH** between 0 and 7 is acid, 7 to 14 is alkaline, and 7 is neutral.) If the body's pH should vary more than 0.2 of a point, many of the reactions that take place in the blood would cease.

The body protects itself against changes in the acid-base balance of its fluids by providing **buffers**—large molecules, mostly protein, that can accommodate excess plus or minus charges (ions). The action of a buffer is shown in Figure 2.

Cereals and grains contain the acid-forming minerals; fruits and vegetables contain base formers. This comes as a surprise to people who think that citrus fruits, for instance, are acid. You may have heard someone say, "I can't eat oranges or tomatoes; they're too acid for me." In truth, although citrus and tomatoes may taste sour, or acid, in the mouth, their ash is composed of base-forming minerals. After the organic acids in the fruit have been digested and metabolized, they are excreted as carbon dioxide and water, leaving only the minerals. Therefore, fruits and vegetables ultimately form bases in the body.

Meat, eggs, poultry, and fish contain the acid-forming minerals. Milk and milk products contain both acid- and base-forming

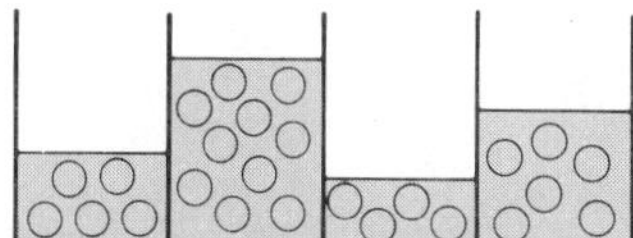

Normally, the ratio of particles of minerals to particles of water (the concentration) is the same on both sides of cell membrane.

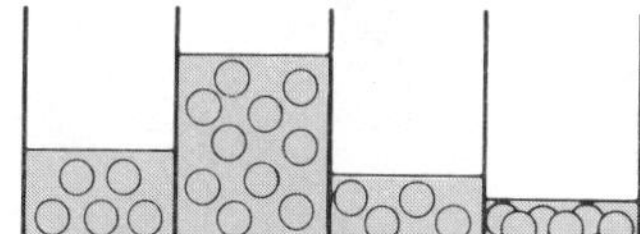

If diarrhea occurs, water will flow from the intestinal wall cell in an attempt to equalize the concentration.

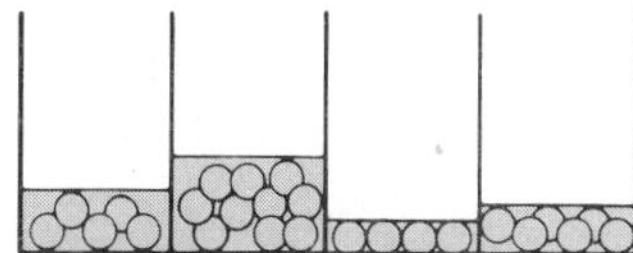

Eventually, the water must flow out of every cell. This is dehydration.

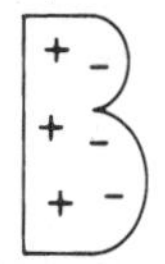

A buffer can be neutral (an equal number of plus and minus charges).

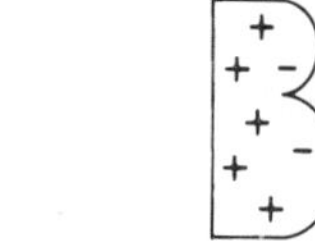

A buffer can be acidic (an excess of plus charges).

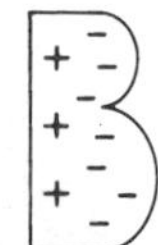

A buffer can be alkaline, or basic (an excess of minus charges).

In a solution, a buffer helps the solution keep its acid-base balance by soaking up excess plus or minus charges or giving them up to the solution.

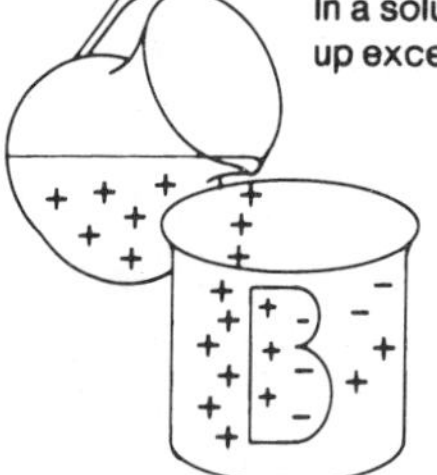

If the solution receives excess plus charges, tending to make it acidic,

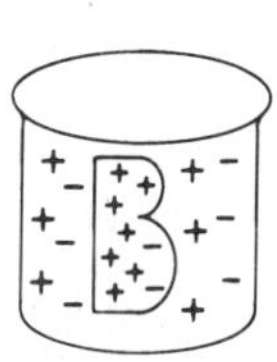

the buffer will pick these up. The solution keeps its acid-base balance.

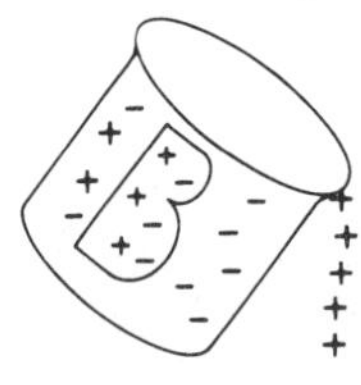

If the solution loses plus charges, tending to make it alkaline (basic),

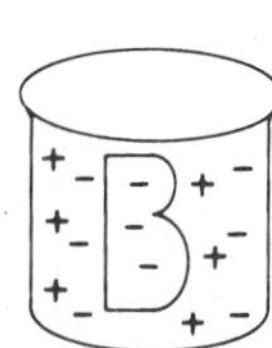

the buffer will give up its plus charges. The solution keeps its acid-base balance.

Figure 2. *A buffer is a large molecule, usually protein, that can accommodate plus or minus charges (ions).*

substances. The breakdown of the protein in milk does produce some acid; but the large amounts of calcium in milk cause milk to be classified as a base former in the body.

The Major Minerals

While all of the major minerals help maintain water balance and acid-base balance in the body, each also plays some special roles of its own. These roles are described in the following sections. The order does not imply that the first are the most important.

Calcium. Many people have the idea that calcium and phosphorus, once deposited in bone, stay there forever—that once a bone is built, it is inert, like a rock. Not so. Bones are in a state of constant flux, with formation and dissolution taking place every minute of the day and night.

Calcium is essential to the formation of bone. Calcium forms phosphate and carbonate salts which, with some other minerals, particularly fluoride, crystallize on a foundation material composed of the protein collagen. Vitamin D helps in this process. In the infant, these crystals invade the collagen and gradually lend more and more rigidity to the maturing bones, until they are able to support the weight they will have to carry. Thus, the long leg bones of a child can support its weight by the time it has learned to walk.

The increase in length of the long bones involves a dismantling of the crystals near the ends of the bone to allow for the growth of the collagen and the subsequent reinvasion by mineral crystals. This lengthening does not take place continuously throughout the growing years but occurs in spurts, the last great surge taking place during puberty.

The formation of teeth follows very much the same pattern, with the same calcium compounds forming crystals to give strength to the teeth. Calcification occurs during the latter half of the infant's time in the womb and is fairly complete for the "baby" teeth by the time of their eruption. The calcification of the permanent teeth takes place during early childhood, up to about the age of three; that of the "wisdom" teeth begins at about the age of ten. There is not such a rapid turnover of calcium in teeth as there is in bone, but some withdrawal and redepositing does take place throughout life. Fluoride plays an important role in the hardening of teeth by retarding the withdrawal of calcium for use in other parts of the body.

About 99 percent of the calcium in the body is in the bones and teeth; less than 1 percent is found in the fluid that bathes the body's cells; and an even smaller amount is inside the cells. These minute amounts play major roles, however, in the health of the body. Calcium

Regulates the transport of ions across cell membranes and is particularly important in nerve transmission.

Is required for muscle contraction and therefore for the maintenance of the heartbeat.

Plays a role in the clotting of blood.

Maintains the collagen, which is the "glue" that holds cells together.

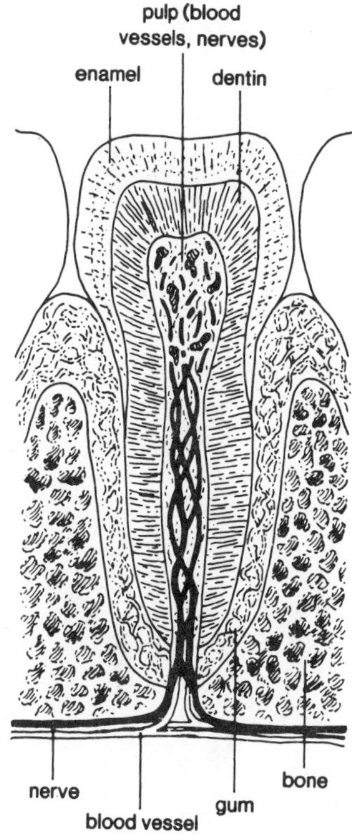

The outer two layers of the teeth are composed largely of calcium compounds.

With such major roles to play in the body fluids, calcium must be furnished to the cells on demand. This is accomplished by maintaining a constant, carefully regulated concentration of 10 milligrams of calcium per 100 milliliters of plasma at all times. To this end, the bones serve as banks where calcium can be deposited and withdrawn as needed. Calcium in the fluids surrounding the bone cartilage is deposited as crystals of calcium phosphate and calcium carbonate. If the blood level of calcium falls, these crystals are redissolved from the bone structure. Withdrawal or deposition of calcium in the bones is not at the mercy of the amount taken in food but is regulated by hormones sensitive to blood levels of calcium.[1]

The writer of a popular nutrition book made extravagant claims for calcium.[2] For example, she suggested taking calcium tablets for pain before going to the dentist or when giving birth to a baby—because calcium helps regulate nerve activity. The fact she ignored was that blood calcium is not influenced by the amount ingested; if there is a sudden need for calcium, a mineral bank is available in the bones for instant withdrawal of any amount needed. Taking a few tablets of calcium has no effect on blood levels. Similarly, calcium spurs or calcium deposits in joints are not related to dietary intakes but to hormone imbalances.

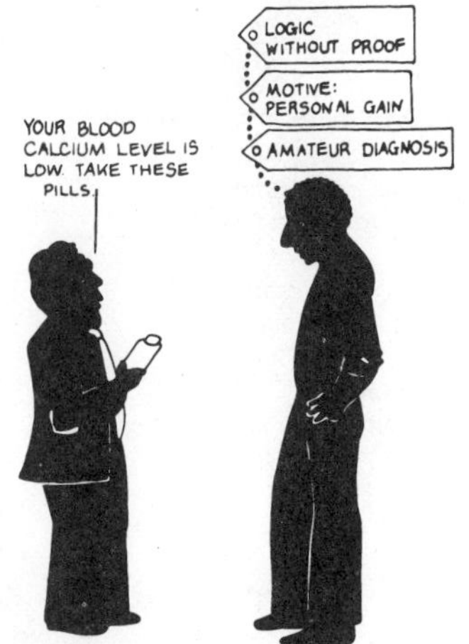
YOUR BLOOD CALCIUM LEVEL IS LOW. TAKE THESE PILLS.
LOGIC WITHOUT PROOF
MOTIVE: PERSONAL GAIN
AMATEUR DIAGNOSIS

People don't regulate their bodies' calcium concentrations. Hormones do.

The guarantee that blood calcium levels are always maintained might seem to imply that you need make no effort to obtain calcium in your daily diet. However, if your diet lacks calcium, you will pay a price—perhaps not today, but years from now—in the weakening of your bones caused by withdrawal of calcium to meet the body's constant demands. Between the ages of twenty and fifty you can lose up to a third of the total calcium in your skeleton without even being aware of it. It is important to know not only good food sources of calcium but also how calcium is absorbed, because absorption is tricky and is influenced by many factors.

The absorption of calcium from food varies with each individual and with various times in life. During periods of growth and during pregnancy and lactation, absorption increases. Infants and children absorb up to 60 percent of ingested calcium, pregnant women about 50 percent, and other adults about 30 percent.

During a prolonged period of very low calcium intake, the body adjusts by absorbing as much as 60 percent of that consumed. When supplied for years with abundant calcium, the body may absorb only 10 percent. It takes time to adjust to changing intakes. Thus in diet planning it is important to keep the calcium intake constant. A well-fed person from the United States going to a country where there is no milk may not be able to adapt in time to avoid incurring a calcium deficiency that will have a profound impact on his or her bones. In contrast, the people of that other country, whose bodies have been adapted to a low intake for a lifetime, may never suffer bone abnormalities. Vitamin D is indispensable for the absorption of calcium across the intestinal cell membranes, so it is important to include foods containing vitamin D with calcium sources.

Calcium must be soluble if it is to be absorbed. Acid, such as the hydrochloric acid in the stomach, increases solubility, as do vitamin C (ascorbic acid) and some of the amino acids. But a high-fat diet may inhibit the absorption of calcium by forming insoluble calcium soaps, which are then excreted in the feces. This may be the case in any of the diseases that affect the absorption of fat, leaving a high fat content in the intestine to combine with calcium.

Aids to calcium absorption:
Body's increased need.
Acid environment:
Hydrochloric acid in stomach.
Ascorbic acid.
Some amino acids.
Lactose in milk.
Vitamin D.
Phosphorus in 1:1 ratio.

The lactose in milk forms a soluble compound with calcium. This enhances the value of milk as one of the best food sources of calcium. (Remember, too, that milk is chosen as the vehicle for fortification with vitamin D.) Calcium is lower in human milk than in cow's milk, but babies absorb it better, probably because of the higher lactose and vitamin C (acid) contents of human milk.

An important relationship exists between calcium and phosphorus. Each is better absorbed if they are ingested together. Authorities differ on the ratio that might best favor health, but it seems probable that most would agree on a one-to-one ratio; perhaps any ratio from three-to-one to one-to-three is all right. However, a too-high phosphorus intake can promote the excretion of calcium. (The body has to excrete the excess phosphorus and it excretes calcium along with it, as if the phosphorus were pulling calcium out of the body.) This may create a problem for people who, for example, not only don't drink milk but make heavy use of phosphate-containing beverages like diet sodas in its place. They may be asking for trouble in the form of osteoporosis in later life.

Most of the calcium taken with food, about 50 to 70 percent, never enters the body but is excreted in the feces. This amount varies with intake. Excretion of calcium by way of the urine remains constant at about 100 to 150 milligrams a day. Some is lost in perspiration; this becomes significant only if unusually hard physical labor is performed in an extremely dry, hot climate.

Calcium deficiency in children leads to bone malformation and the disease known as **rickets**. In adults, the corresponding disease is **osteomalacia**. The cause of the calcium deficiency is most likely a lack of vitamin D. (There may be ample calcium in the diet, but it cannot be absorbed without the vitamin.) In **osteoporosis**, a disease of older persons in which there is a decline in the total amount of bone, a prolonged deficiency of calcium probably is the cause. Hormone imbalances or conditions, like diarrhea, that speed the passage of foods through the digestive system interfere with absorption and cause a deficiency of calcium.

People do not always realize that hip fractures in the elderly, which result from osteoporosis, can cause death or permanent disability.[3] One in six women who suffer a hip fracture by age 90 will die within three months of her injury—as a direct result of the weakened bone. And in case this sounds like something that "can't happen to you": one-fourth of all postmenopausal women in the United States develop an unhealthy degree of bone loss.[4] Adults, who do not sense the gradual weakening of their bones by mineral loss, are often unaware that milk may be even more important for them than it is for young adults. Even late in life, adequate intakes of calcium can retard or reverse bone loss. A public service announcement first broadcast on television in 1978 shows a young girl saying, "Grandma and I need three cups of milk a day." Take heed, Grandma!

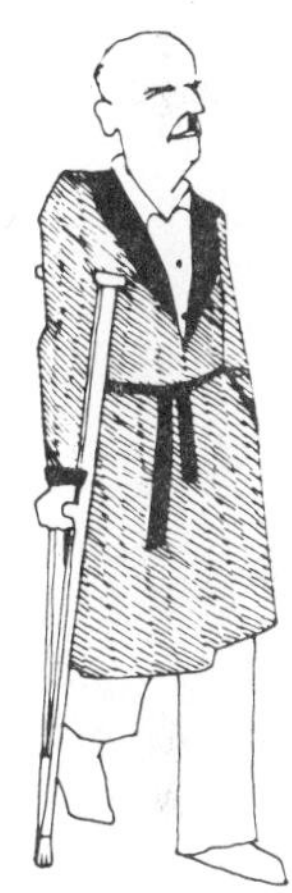

Hip fractures in the elderly can cause death or permanent disability. Ample calcium intakes may help prevent them.

Human beings can adjust to very low intakes of calcium. In some countries people achieve balance on only 200 milligrams a day.[5] This makes setting recommended intakes for calcium difficult. The RDA for calcium has been set at 800 milligrams daily for U.S. adults, but women's intakes should perhaps be even higher. More (1200 milligrams) is recommended for pregnant and lactating women, because they are supplying calcium to another growing person. Of course, during pregnancy and lactation, the absorption of calcium is probably increased. The extra 400 milligrams is recommended for the protection of the mother's bones, not the infant's, because the mother's bones will supply the calcium for the fetus or nursing infant if her diet is low in calcium.

The U.S. and Canadian recommendations for calcium intake are high compared to those of other countries, but are rightly so because most adults consume large quantities of meat and other protein foods. Both the protein and the phosphorus in these foods enhance the excretion of calcium, making the need higher than it would otherwise be. Around the time of the menopause, women are advised to increase their calcium intakes still further, to around 1200 milligrams a day, to be sure of avoiding bone loss.[6]

The main food source of calcium is milk. Other dairy products, such as yogurt, cheese, and ice cream, are good sources. Butter and cream contain negligible calcium, because this mineral is not soluble in fat. The calcium of milk is unusually well absorbed because of the lactose, protein, and, if the milk is fortified, vitamin D content. Canned fishes with edible bones, such as sardines and canned salmon, are another good source. Dark green vegetables contain calcium but in a form that is not so well absorbed. Vegetarians may rely on these and on soymilk and bean curd (tofu) for their calcium. Cereal grains contain only small amounts; but if the diet is composed mainly of cereal, it may be a major contributor. The calcium contents of some common foods are shown in Table 1.

Phosphorus. Phosphorus is the mineral in second largest quantity in the body. About 85 percent of it is found combined with calcium in the crystals of the bones. Its concentration in blood plasma is less than half that of calcium: 3.5 milligrams per 100 milliliters of plasma. But as part of one of the body's major acids (phosphoric acid), it is a part of the structure of all body cells.

The average person hears very little about phosphorus, even through it plays a critical part in all cell functions. This lack of publicity in popular nutrition writing is probably due to the fact that deficiencies are unknown. Phosphorus is widespread in foods in association with calcium and protein; if these nutrients are adequate in the diet, then phosphorus is too.

Phosphorus is intimately associated with the calcium in bones and teeth as calcium phosphate, one of the compounds in the crystals that give strength and rigidity to the structures. (The suffix *ate* in *phosphate* indicates that oxygen is bound to the phosphorus.) It is also a part of the nucleic acids, which are components of DNA and RNA, the genetic code material present in every cell. Thus phosphorus is necessary for all growth, because DNA and RNA provide the instructions for new cells to be formed.

Phosphorus plays many key roles in the cells' transfers of energy. Many enzymes and the B vitamins become active only when a phosphate group is attached. The B vitamins, you will recall, play major roles in energy metabolism. Again, phosphorus is critical in energy exchange. ATP itself, the energy carrier of the cells, uses phosphate groups to do its work.

Some lipids contain phosphorus as part of their structure. These phospholipids help to transport other lipids in the blood; they also form a part of the structure of cell membranes, where they affect transport of nutrients into and out of the cells.

Phosphorus in the plasma is one of the most important buffers. An earlier diagram showed how a buffer works in a solution such as blood to maintain the required acid-base balance.

Animal protein is the best source of phosphorus, because phosphorus is so abundant in the energetic cells of animals. People who eat large quantities of animal protein have high phosphorus intakes. This circumstance accounts for the recommendation that people in the

Table 1. Calcium Contents of Fifty Common Foods

Exchange Group[a]	Food	Serving Size[b]	Calcium (mg)
5L	Sardines with bones	3 oz	372
1	2% fat fortified milk	1 cup	352
1	Canned evaporated milk	½ cup	318
1	Skim milk	1 cup	296
1	Dry skim milk	⅓ cup	293
1	Whole milk	1 cup	288
1	Yogurt	1 cup	272
5L	Oysters	¾ cup	170
5L	Canned salmon with bones	3 oz	167
2	Collard greens	½ cup	145
2	Dandelion greens	½ cup	126
2	Spinach	½ cup	106[c]
2	Mustard greens	½ cup	97
4	Corn muffin	1	96
5M	Creamed cottage cheese	¼ cup	58
4	Pancake	1	58
3	Orange	1	54
2	Broccoli	½ cup	49
4	Dried beans	½ cup	45
4	Pumpkin	¾ cup	43
4	Muffin	1	42
4	Lima beans	½ cup	40
3	Tangerine	1	34
2	Cabbage	½ cup	32
2	Green beans	½ cup	32
6	Cream, light	2 tbsp	30
4	Winter squash	½ cup	29
2	Turnips	½ cup	27
5M	Egg	1	27
2	Summer squash	½ cup	26
3	Dried fig	1	26
2	Onions	½ cup	25
4	Whole-wheat bread	1 slice	25
2	Brussels sprouts	½ cup	25
4	Mashed potato	½ cup	24
2	Carrots	½ cup	24
3	Blackberries	½ cup	23
4	White bread	1 slice	21
3	Pink grapefruit	½	20
3	White grapefruit	½	19
4	Rye bread	1 slice	19
4	Green peas	½ cup	19
5M	Peanut butter	2 tbsp	18
3	Strawberries	¾ cup	17
5L	Chipped beef	3 oz	17
2	Asparagus	½ cup	15
4	Hamburger bun	½	15
3	Raspberries	½ cup	14
3	Cantaloupe	¼	14
4	Sweet potatoes	¼ cup	14

These are not best food sources but are selected to show a range of calcium contents. Study of the left-hand column will help you to generalize about which foods contribute calcium.

[a]The numbers refer to the exchange lists: 1 is milk; 2, vegetables; 3, fruit; 4, bread; 5L, lean meat; 5M, medium-fat meat; 6, fats and oils.

[b]Serving sizes are those in the exchange lists, except for meat.

[c]To this point, all foods supply at least 10 percent of the U.S. RDA of 1 g.

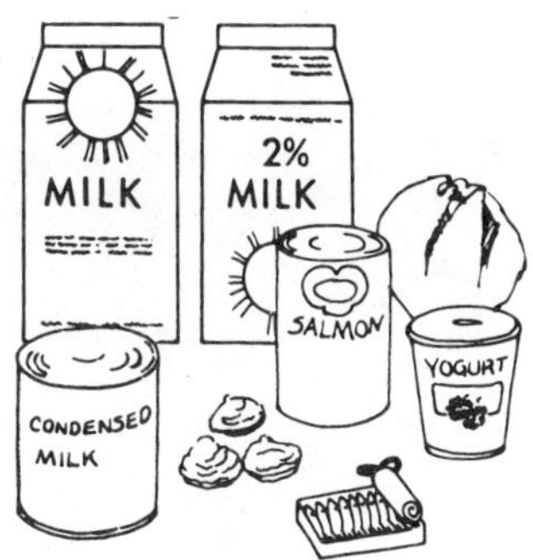

Foods containing calcium.

United States and Canada take in more calcium than other peoples. The recommended intakes of phosphorus are the same as those for calcium to maintain a one-to-one ratio.

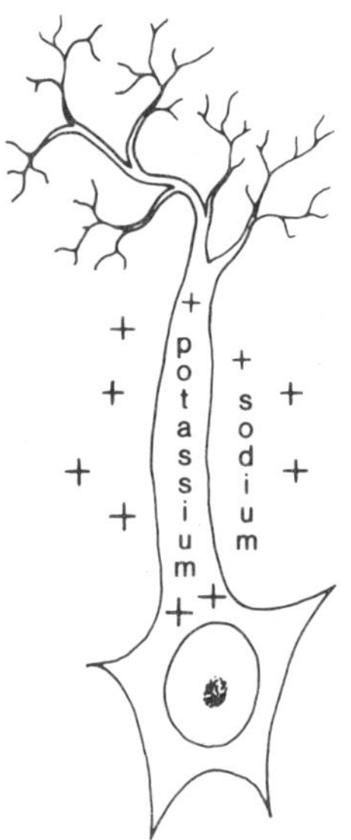

Nerve cell with ions.

Sodium. Sodium is the positive ion in the compound sodium chloride, ordinary table salt.[7] Salt has been known throughout recorded history. The Bible's saying "You are the salt of the earth" means that a person is valuable. If, on the other hand, "you are not worth your salt," you are worthless. Even the word *salary* comes from the word *salt.* Carnivores generally do not travel to find salt, because they get it from eating other animals, but a grazing animal will travel many miles to a salt lick, driven by its body's need for sodium.

There is seldom a sodium shortage in the diet. Foods usually include more salt than is needed, and it enters the body fluids freely. The kidneys filter the surplus out of the blood into the urine. They can also sensitively conserve salt and return it to the blood in the event of a deficiency, which might occur during heavy sweating or starvation. Intakes vary widely, especially because of cultural differences in diets. Orientals, who use a great deal of soy sauce and monosodium glutamate (MSG or Accent) for flavoring, consume about 30 to 40 grams of salt per day; most people in the United States average about 6 to 18 grams of salt per day.[8] Vegetarians probably consume much less than this.

The total amount of fluid in the body depends primarily on the sodium and potassium ions present. Cells can move these ions across their membranes, and they work constantly to keep sodium on the outside and potassium on the inside. Nerve transmission and muscle contraction depend on the cells' permitting a temporary exchange of sodium and potassium ions across their membranes. About 30 to 45 percent of the body's sodium is thought to be stored on the surface of the bone crystals, where it is easy to recover if the blood level drops.

The activity of the kidney in regulating the body's sodium level is remarkable.[9] Sodium is absorbed easily from the intestinal tract, then travels in the blood, where it ultimately passes through the kidney. The kidney filters all the sodium out, then with great precision returns to the bloodstream the exact amount needed. Normally, the amount excreted equals the amount ingested that day.

If the blood level of sodium rises, as it will after a person eats heavily salted foods, the thirst receptors in the brain will be stimulated. The fluid intake will increase, to make the sodium-to-water ratio constant. Then the extra fluid will be excreted by the kidneys along with the extra sodium.

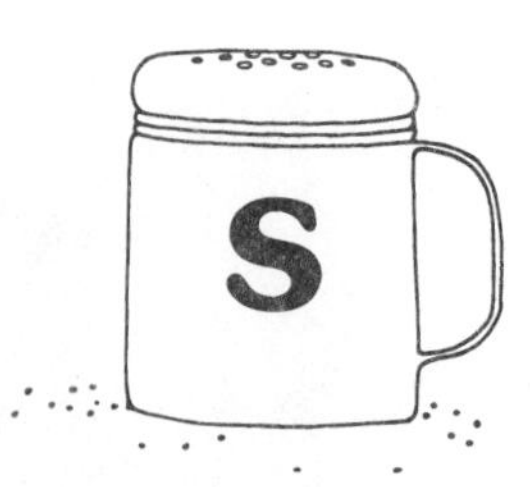

Sodium chloride.

Dieters sometimes think that eating too much salt or drinking too much water will make them gain weight, but this is not the case. Excess water is excreted immediately. Excess salt is excreted as soon as enough water is drunk to carry the salt out of the body. From this perspective, then, the way to keep body salt (and "water weight") under control is to drink more, not less, water.

If the blood level of sodium drops, as it does during vomiting, diarrhea, or heavy sweating, both water and sodium must be replenished. If only water is replaced, the blood concentration of sodium will drop and water will migrate into the cells. This will result in symptoms of water intoxication: headache, muscular weakness, lack of concentration, poor memory, and loss of appetite. Times when such a condition might exist are during heavy physical work in the heat, after extensive burns, or following accidents or surgery that involve loss of blood. Overly strict use of low-sodium diets in the treatment of kidney or heart disease may also deplete the body of needed sodium. The symptoms quickly vanish with the return of both sodium and water.

No recommendation needs to be made for daily sodium intake, because of the sensitive controls operating in the body. Just remember that salt is more abundant in animal foods than in plants. Furthermore, cooks add salt generously in food preparation, and diners add more from the salt shaker on the table. The highest concentrations in foods are in cured ham, bacon, salted peanuts, pickles, potato chips, pretzels, and cold cuts, where the salt acts as a preservative. Pregnant women should normally not restrict their salt intake.

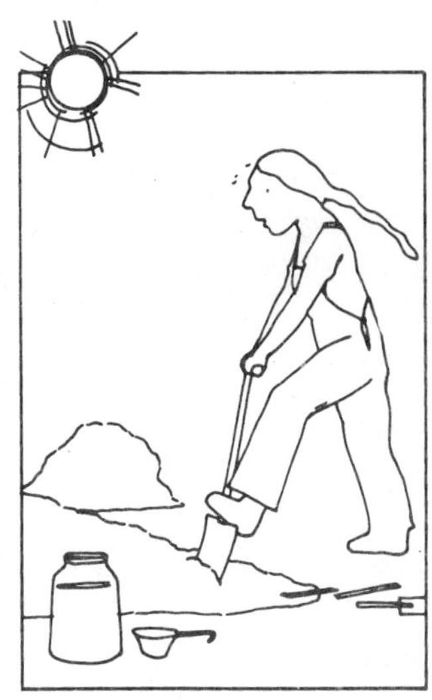

Rule of thumb: If you have drunk more than four quarts of water in a day to replace water lost in sweat, you should take a gram of sodium chloride with each additional quart.

1 g sodium chloride = ⅕ tsp salt.

Salt tablets are usually 1 g each.

Athletes, however, should probably wait until after competition and then replenish their sodium by eating food. See Controversy 7.

The use of highly salted foods may contribute to high blood pressure (**hypertension**). This may be true only for those who have a genetic tendency to develop high blood pressure—about 17 percent of U.S. adults. Black Americans are especially at risk in this respect. With a high sodium level in the blood, the blood pressure rises until it is high enough to cause excretion of the excess sodium.[10] With a greater volume of blood coursing through the arteries, the heart has to work harder to pump the extra fluid around. Added weight (obesity) raises the pressure further, and added fat means miles of extra capillaries through which the blood must be pumped. The ultimate danger of high blood pressure is damage to the heart from overwork or closing off of arteries from hardening or clot formation (heart attack or stroke).

The *Dietary Guidelines* recommend that we avoid too much sodium. This advice would be particularly important for people who have high blood pressure or who have reason to think they may have inherited the tendency to it. But it is possible that as many as three out of four people have high blood pressure by the time they are sixty-five, so perhaps everyone should pay attention to these guidelines.[11] Table 2 shows a sampling of the sodium contents of commonly eaten foods, and the notes in the margin provide general suggestions for avoiding sodium in foods.

The old idea that salt excess may cause hypertension gains additional support almost daily. It is now clear that there is a strong genetic factor in this association. Thus, many people lack genetic susceptibility and are immune to the effects of salt excess, while others . . . are susceptible.—Nutrition and the MD

Persons who wish to avoid salt need to know that what they pour from the salt shaker may be only a third of the total salt they consume. One-fourth to one-half comes from processed food, to which it is added as a preservative and flavoring agent. Not only salt but also other common additives contain sodium. This makes eating something of a guessing game because (as of 1981) labels are not required to declare the sodium contents of foods. The serious sodium-avoider must stay away from fast-food places and Oriental restaurants and stop using many canned, frozen, and instant foods at home.[12]

"High blood pressure" is defined differently for different purposes. Here, if the higher of the two numbers is over 140 or if the lower is over 90, it is considered to be too high.

Processed foods don't always taste salty. Most people are surprised to learn that a serving of cornflakes contains more sodium than a serving of cocktail peanuts—and that a serving of chocolate pudding contains still more.[13] A perusal of the sodium contents of foods in

To avoid too much sodium:

Learn to enjoy the unsalted flavors of foods.

Cook with only small amounts of added salt.

Add little or no salt to food at the table.

Cut down on:

Foods prepared in brine, such as pickles, olives, and sauerkraut.

Salty or smoked meat, such as bologna, corned or chipped beef, frankfurters, ham, luncheon meats, salt pork, sausage, smoked tongue.

Salty or smoked fish, such as anchovies, caviar, salted and dried cod, herring, sardines, smoked salmon.

Snack items such as potato chips, pretzels, salted popcorn, and salted nuts and crackers.

Bouillon cubes; seasoned salts (including sea salt); soy, Worcestershire, and barbecue sauces.

Cheeses, especially processed types.

Canned and instant soups.

Prepared horseradish, catsup, and mustard.

Read labels. You may be surprised to learn that some processed foods which contain no table salt and don't taste salty have lots of sodium. Look for the word soda or sodium or the symbol "Na" on labels. Examples are sodium bicarbonate (baking soda), monosodium glutamate, most baking powders, disodium phosphate, sodium alginate, sodium benzoate, sodium hydroxide, sodium propionate, sodium sulfite, and sodium saccharin.—USDA

Table 2. Representative Sodium Contents of Foods

Food	Serving Size	Sodium (mg)
Meat, fish, poultry, cooked without added salt (average)	3 oz	100
Ham, cured	3 oz	860
Bacon	3 oz	1077
Egg, whole	1	61
Milk, whole	1 cup	120
Vegetables (average)	½ cup	40
Potato, boiled	3 oz	2
Peanut butter	1 tbsp	91
Cola beverage	12 oz	15
Salt	1 tsp	2000
Soy sauce	1 tbsp	912

If you want to limit sodium, try not to have more than 3 g (3000 mg) sodium (equals 7½ g salt) in a day. See Appendix E for more details on sodium in foods.

Appendix E and other references is well worth while for anyone wishing to prevent or reduce high blood pressure.

Avoiding sodium is not only tricky but also hard to do because foods are far less attractive and tasty without salt. With practice, however, people can learn to enjoy the flavors of many unsalted foods and, where spices are needed, to make liberal use of sodium-free spices like those listed in the margin.

As already mentioned, public water (if it is soft water) can contribute significant sodium to people's intakes. In some areas, where the water supply contains more than 100 milligrams of sodium per liter, some people's blood pressure is affected. Where highways are salted in winter to melt the snow, the runoff may contribute to this problem by adding more salt to the underground water. A sodium standard for public water, of perhaps 20 milligrams per liter, might need to be adopted in these areas.[14]

Chloride. The element chlorine occurs naturally as a poisonous gas; but when it combines with sodium in salt, it is not poisonous but is part of a life-giving compound. It occurs in salt as the negative chloride ion. The chloride ion is the major negative ion of the fluids outside the cells, where it is found mostly in association with sodium. Chloride can move freely across membranes and so is also found inside the cells in combination with potassium.

In the stomach, the chloride ion is part of the hydrochloric acid that maintains the strong acidity of the stomach. The cells that line the stomach continuously expend energy to push chloride into the stomach fluid. One of the most serious consequences of vomiting is the loss of chloride ions from the stomach, which upsets the acid-base balance of the body.

Chloride deficiency is uncommon because of the abundance of salt, but has been seen in infants given a formula that was mistakenly too low in chloride. Their acid-base balance was upset, and they failed to grow, but recovered when the error was corrected.[15]

A chlorine compound is added to public water to sterilize it before it flows through pipes into people's homes. (Remember that chlorine is a deadly poisonous gas.) The chlorine gas kills dangerous microorganisms that might otherwise spread disease and then evaporates, leaving the water safe for human consumption. The addition of chlorine to public water is one of the most important public health measures ever introduced in the developed countries and has eliminated such waterborne diseases as typhoid fever, which once ravaged vast areas, killing thousands of people.

Sodium-free spices and flavorings include:

Allspice.
Almond extract.
Bay leaves.
Caraway seeds.
Cinnamon.
Curry powder.
Garlic.
Ginger.
Lemon extract.
Mace.
Maple extract.
Marjoram.
Mustard powder.
Nutmeg.
Paprika.
Parsley.
Pepper.
Peppermint extract.
Pimiento.
Rosemary.
Sage.
Sesame seeds.
Thyme.
Turmeric.
Vanilla extract.
Vinegar.
Walnut extract.

In many instances, an essential nutrient has a limited range of concentrations within which it is safe. At higher concentrations it may have adverse effects and may even be a deadly poison. Nutrients especially noteworthy in this respect are vitamins A and D and many of the minerals, but it is not an exaggeration to say that the same principle applies to all nutrients and all substances, even water. Understanding this principle alerts the consumer to be wary of taking the naive view that "if some is good for you, more is better" or its opposite, "If a high dose is bad for you, then even a low dose must be bad."

It is easy to fall into this naive reasoning. Consider the reasoning implied in the following statements:

Some fiber is beneficial, so we should eat all the fiber we can.

Too much sugar may be bad for us, so we should eat no sugar at all.

Protein is a vital nutrient, so we should eat a high-protein diet.

Iodine is a poison, so we should avoid it altogether.

Additives may be harmful, so we should avoid them altogether.

It is tempting to go along with these statements, perhaps partly because it is easier to make distinctions between black and white than between shades of gray. However, they are as misleading as the obviously wrong conclusion drawn from this sort of reasoning:

(1) A match is useful because you can light little fires with it.

(2) Fires are useful because they keep you warm.

(3) Therefore, it would be ideal if we could ignite the earth.

There is no law that says that a correlation has to hold true to either extreme.

Chlorine can combine with water pollutants, however, to form highly toxic chemicals, an unexpected effect. See Controversy 10B.

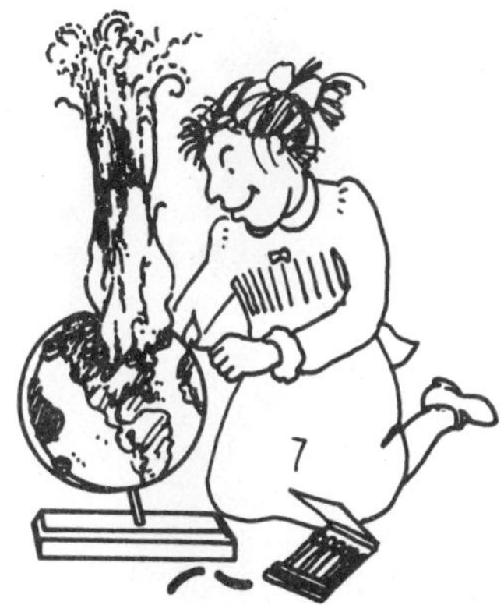

There's a fallacy in mindless extrapolation.

On the other hand—and this is important—there is no law that says that a correlation will not hold true to either extreme. An example of a correlation that does not hold relates to vitamin C: At a low concentration, it acts as an essential nutrient, but at a high concentration, it acts as a drug. An example of a correlation that may hold (we don't know yet) relates to certain additives, which are known to cause cancer at high concentrations and which may continue to do their deadly work even at concentrations below the level at which they can be detected. The assumption that small amounts of cancer-causing agents do, in fact, cause cancer at a low but predictable rate is the basis for a part of the law (the Delaney Clause) that says they may not be permitted in foods at any level whatsoever.

To avoid being misled by nutrition quacks, watch out for oversimplified reasoning. At the same time, when assessing new information about benefits and harms associated with nutrients and additives, keep an open mind and think in shades of gray.

Potassium. Potassium is critical to maintaining the heartbeat. The sudden deaths that occur during fasting or severe diarrhea and in kwashiorkor children are often due to heart failure caused by potassium loss. As the principal positively charged ion inside body cells, it plays a major role in maintaining water balance and cell integrity.

During nerve transmission and muscle contraction, potassium and sodium briefly exchange places. Nerve and muscle cells, then, are especially rich in potassium, but all cells must contain some. Potassium is also known to play a catalytic role in carbohydrate and protein metabolism, but the exact nature of this role is not known.

When sodium is lost in water loss from the body, the ultimate damage comes when potassium is pulled out of the cells and excreted. Dehydration is especially dangerous, because potassium deficiency affects the brain cells early, making the victim unaware of the need for water. Water loss can therefore be a grave danger, and adults are warned not to take **diuretics** (water pills) except under the direction of a physician. When a person uses diuretics and consults another physician for a different health problem, that physician should be alerted to the fact that a diuretic is in use. Any physician prescribing diuretics will tell the patient to eat potassium-rich foods to compensate for the losses.

For potassium-rich foods, see Appendix E.

Gradual potassium depletion of the body can occur when a person sweats profusely day after day and fails to replenish his potassium stores. A study of this effect shows that up to about 3 milligrams of potassium can be lost in a day. The average diet in this country supplies about 1.5 to 2.5 milligrams. If a person sweats heavily and often, the authors of this study recommend that he eat about five to eight servings of potassium-rich food each day.[16]

It has been pointed out several times previously that there are advantages to eating food instead of taking supplements. Salt tablets contain sodium and chloride, but foods contain a multitude of minerals. The body evolved in dependence on foods, not supplements. Body builders who think fruit is only for delicate people might take note that because of the potassium it contains, fruit may do more for their muscles than meat.

For an alternative view, that the body adapts and stores more potassium, see Controversy 7: Athletes.

A borderline food is the liquid "sweat replacer," like Gatorade, designed especially for such athletes as football players. In choosing one of these, the buyer should look for potassium on the label.

The principal sources of potassium among foods commonly eaten are orange juice, bananas, dried fruits, and potatoes. Potassium supplements are not advisable except when prescribed, because too much potassium is as dangerous as too little. Even salt substitutes containing potassium should be avoided, especially by heart patients, except as recommended by a physician. The story of a woman who killed her baby by giving it potassium supplements was told in Controversy 2.

Sulfur. Sulfur is present in all proteins and plays its most important role in determining the contour of protein molecules. Sulfur helps the strands of protein to assume a particular shape and hold it—and so do their specific jobs, such as enzyme work. Some of the amino acids contain sulfur in their side chains; once built into a protein strand, these amino acids can link to each other by way of sulfur-sulfur bridges. The bridges stabilize the protein structure. Skin, hair, and nails contain some of the body's more rigid proteins, and these have a high sulfur content. The sketch in the margin shows parts of a protein strand linked by sulfur bridges.

There is no RDA for sulfur, and no deficiencies are known. Only a person who lacks protein to the point of severe deficiency will lack the sulfur-containing amino acids.

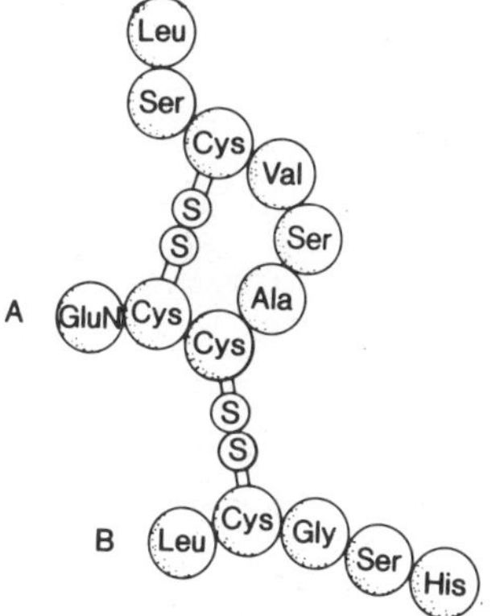

A portion of the insulin molecule.

Magnesium. Magnesium barely qualifies as a major mineral: Only about 1¾ ounces are present in the body of a 130-pound person. Most of this is in the bones. Bone magnesium seems to be a storage reservoir to ensure that some will be on hand for vital reactions regardless of recent dietary intake.

Magnesium also acts in all the cells of the soft tissues, where it forms part of the protein-making machinery and where it is necessary for the release of energy. Its major role seems to be as a catalyst in the reaction that adds the key high-energy phosphate bond to the cells' energy-carrier, ATP. Magnesium also helps relax muscles after contraction and promotes resistance to tooth decay by helping to hold calcium in tooth enamel.

Deficiency of magnesium may occur as a result of vomiting, diarrhea, alcoholism, or protein malnutrition; in postsurgical patients who have been fed incomplete fluids into a vein for too long; or in persons using diuretics. Deficiency causes weakness, confusion, and if extreme, bizarre muscle movements, especially of the eye and facial muscles, and difficulty in swallowing.[17] It is not known to what extent magnesium deficiencies exist in the general population.

It is interesting to note that, in areas that have a high magnesium content in their water supply, there is a lower incidence of sudden death from heart failure.[18] It seems likely that magnesium deficiency makes the heart unable to stop itself from going into spasms once it starts.[19] A severe deficiency causes tetany, an extreme and prolonged contraction of the muscles very much like the reaction of the muscles when calcium levels fall. Magnesium deficit is also thought to cause the hallucinations experienced by alcoholics during withdrawal from alcohol.

The magnesium RDA is 350 milligrams a day for adult males, 300 milligrams for females. The amounts in foods have not been thoroughly studied as yet, but good food sources include nuts, legumes, cereal grains, dark green vegetables, seafoods, chocolate, and cocoa. The kidney acts to conserve magnesium; that not absorbed is excreted in the feces.

The Trace Minerals

Laboratory techniques developed in the last two decades have enabled scientists to detect minerals in smaller and smaller quantities in living cells. Knowledge of the "new" trace elements is coming out of this research. Those trace minerals identified as essential nutrients include silicon, vanadium, nickel, and tin. Arsenic and cadmium are still being studied. An obstacle to determining their precise roles lies in the nearly impossible task of providing an experimental diet lacking in the one element under study. Thus, research in this area is limited to study of laboratory animals, which can be fed highly refined, purified diets in environments that are free of all contamination.

Not all of the trace minerals will be discussed here. Three for which RDAs were established and published as of 1974 were iodine, iron, and zinc. Others on which research is active and the findings are of special interest are copper, fluoride, cobalt, selenium, and chromium. Whole books have been published on the trace minerals alone.[20].

Iodine. Iodine occurs in the body in an infinitesimally small quantity, but its principal role in human nutrition is well known, and the amount needed is well established. Iodine is a part of **thyroxin**, a hormone secreted by the thyroid gland. Thyroxin is responsible for the basal metabolic rate—the rate at which the body uses energy from food. The hormone enters every cell of the body to control the rate at which the cells use oxygen. This is the same as saying that thyroxin controls the rate at which energy is released.

Iodine must be available for thyroxin to be synthesized. The amount in the diet is variable and generally reflects the soil in which plants are grown or on which animals graze. Iodine is plentiful in the ocean, so seafood is a completely dependable source. In the United States, in areas where the soil is iodine-poor (most notably the Plains states) the use of iodized salt has largely wiped out the iodine deficiency that once was widespread.

People sometimes wonder whether sea salt, made by drying ocean water, is preferable to purified sodium chloride for use in the salt shaker. Sea salt does contain trace minerals, but its iodine flies off as a gas during the drying process. Thus, in a region where goiter is a risk, iodized sodium chloride is the salt to choose.

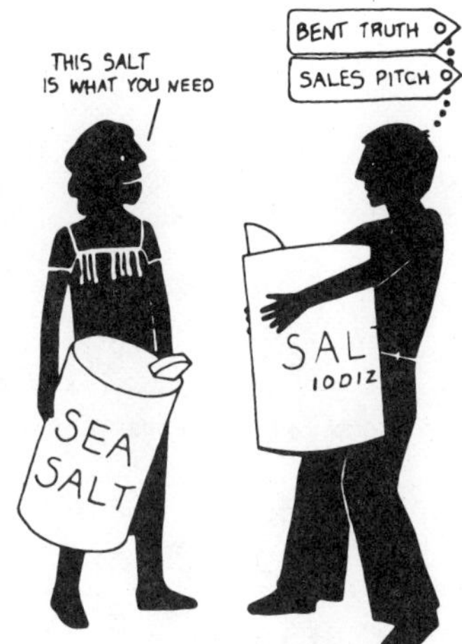

Ironically, sea salt contains less iodine.

When the iodine level of the blood is low, the cells of the thyroid glands enlarge in an attempt to trap as many particles of iodine as possible. If the gland enlarges until it is visible, it is called a simple **goiter**.[21] In addition to causing sluggishness and weight gain, a thyroid deficiency may have serious effects on the development of an infant in the uterus. Severe thyroid undersecretion during pregnancy causes the extreme and irreversible mental and physical retardation known as **cretinism**. A cretin has an IQ as low as 20 and a face and body with abnormalities like those shown in the margin. Much of the mental retardation can be averted by early diagnosis and treatment during pregnancy.

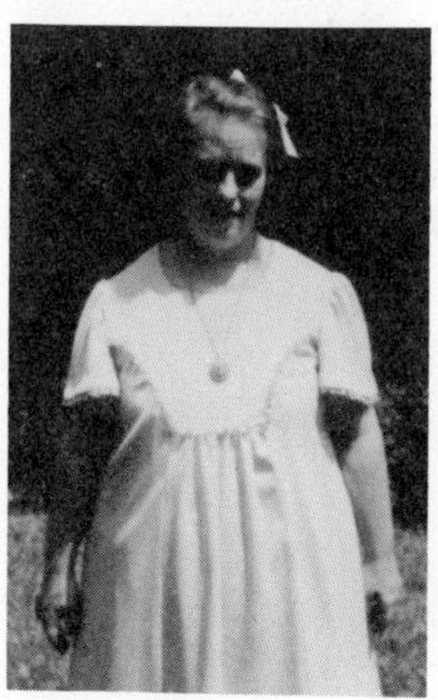

Laura Drake, a cretin, shown at the age of thirty-eight.

The iodization of salt in the Plains states eliminated the widespread misery caused by goiter and cretinism in the local people during the 1930s. Once these scourges had disappeared a new generation of children grew up who never saw the problem and so had no appreciation of its importance. Rejecting iodized salt out of ignorance, they allowed the problem to creep back into their lives. Hopefully, now, education is keeping them informed on the need to continue the measure.

The RDA for iodine for adults is 100 to 140 micrograms a day, a miniscule amount. Like chlorine and fluorine, iodine is a deadly poison in large amounts, but traces of it are indispensable to life. The RDA is easily met by consuming seafood, vegetables grown in iodine-rich soil, and (in iodine-poor areas) iodized salt.

Goiter . . . is being rediscovered by the grandchildren of those who suffered from it.
—L. M. Henderson

Iron. Iron is an essential trace element, probably the best known of all the minerals to the layperson. Television viewers, particularly, know that the wife who "takes good care of herself" takes iron supplements every day and that "you should, too."

Most of the iron in the body is a component of the proteins **hemoglobin** and **myoglobin**. Both these compounds carry oxygen and release it; iron is their crucial element because of its ability to have either a +2 or a +3 charge. As circumstances in the cells change, ionized iron can change from one to the other charge, thereby releasing or holding on to oxygen, which has a −2 charge.

Hemoglobin is the oxygen carrier in the blood, and its iron can have either charge. Myoglobin is found in the cells, especially the skeletal and heart muscle cells, and can have only a +2 charge. Myoglobin has a greater holding capacity for oxygen than hemoglobin

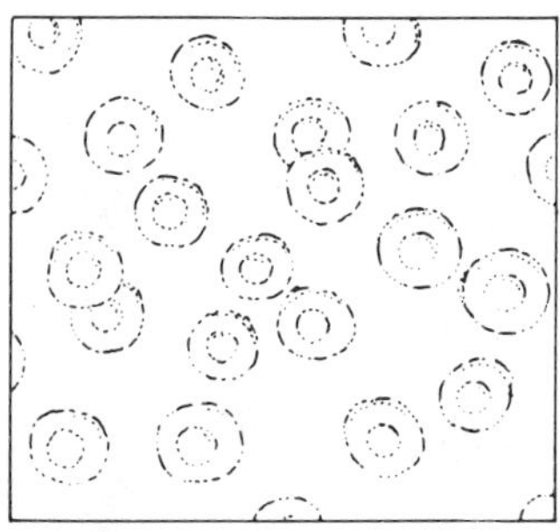
Blood cells in anemia.

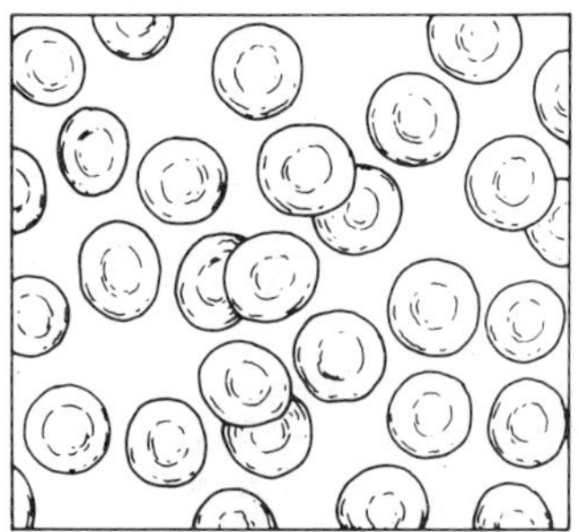
Normal blood cells.

and because of this serves as a reservoir for oxygen in the cells. The presence of myoglobin seems to draw oxygen into the cells.

In **iron-deficiency anemia** (which is only one of several nutritional anemias), the red blood cells contain less hemoglobin and lose their ability to hold oxygen. Therefore, less oxygen is delivered to the body. The cells of the body then operate with lowered energy. The symptoms of iron deficiency are those you would expect—tiredness and apathy. A sample of iron-deficient blood examined under the microscope shows smaller cells that are a lighter red than normal cells.[22] To diagnose iron deficiency, the physician usually measures the blood hemoglobin level.

Long before the mass of the red blood cells is affected, however, a developing iron deficiency may affect other body tissues, including the brain. As researchers have become better acquainted with iron, they have learned that it plays roles in the body, including the brain, not earlier appreciated. For example, iron works with an enzyme that helps to make neurotransmitters, the substances that carry messages from one nerve cell to another. Children deprived of iron show some psychological disturbances, such as hyperactivity, decreased attentiveness, and even reduced IQ. These symptoms are among the first to appear when the body's iron level begins to fall and among the first to disappear when iron intake is increased again.[23]

A curious side effect seen in some iron-deficient subjects is an appetite for ice, clay, starch, and other nonnutritious substances. People have been known to eat as many as eight trays of ice in a day, for example. This behavior has been observed for years, especially in women and children of low-income groups, and has been given the name **pica**. Pica clears up dramatically within days after iron is given, long before the red blood cells respond.[24]

Iron-deficiency anemia is a major health problem in both the United States and Canada and even more so in the rest of the world. It is especially common in older infants, children, women of childbearing age, and people in low-income and minority groups. The incidence of iron deficiency in these groups ranges from 10 to over 50 percent.[25] It tends to cluster with other indicators of low socioeconomic status, such as family instability, little money spent on food, little attention given to children.[26] But no segment of society is free of iron-deficiency anemia, and these groups are not the only ones affected. For example, one out of every twenty Canadian men is at moderate risk (hemoglobin 12 to 14), and one out of every hundred is at high risk (hemoglobin below 12).[27] Among college women, one-fourth may have depleted iron stores.[28]

Iron-deficiency anemia can be caused by a low-grade constant blood loss such as might occur from a bleeding stomach ulcer, bleeding hemorrhoids, parasites, or cancer. In any of these conditions, iron supplements might temporarily improve the anemia but delay its discovery and correction. In such cases, over-the-counter medicines that promise to cure iron-deficiency anemia might be very dangerous.

Iron-deficiency anemia may also be caused by an iron-poor diet or poor absorption of iron from food. A normal, healthy person absorbs only about 10 percent of the iron he or she consumes, about 2 to 10 percent from vegetables and about 10 to 30 percent from red meats. Increased absorption occurs in the presence of need and also when vitamin C and certain amino acids are taken with the iron-rich food.

In foods, iron is generally found with a +3 charge. However, it is absorbed better when it has a +2 charge. The body provides for this change by means of the stomach acid, which reduces the +3 ion to a +2 ion. The presence of vitamin C (because it is an acid—ascorbic acid) favors iron absorption in the same way. For this reason, a prescription for supplemental iron often includes vitamin C to help the taker to absorb the iron.

The facts about iron absorption underscore the foolishness of taking self-prescribed antacid preparations. You are already aware that the stomach must be acid to do its work; putting alkaline tablets into the stomach not only alters the acidity but also hinders the absorption of iron and counteracts the work of vitamin C. In fact, ulcer patients who have to take antacids easily develop iron-deficiency anemia. There are special instances when these tablets are needed, but they should be prescribed by a doctor, not by a huckster on television.

Periods of growth—infancy, childhood, adolescence, and pregnancy—involve enlargement of the blood volume to feed the new tissue. During such periods, the body accomplishes increased absorption of iron by synthesizing extra carrier proteins to pick up iron from the digestive tract. Often, however, this still does not meet the demands of new red blood cells for iron. Increased emphasis on iron-containing foods is necessary at these times, along with adequate vitamin C and protein.

Once iron is absorbed, the only normal route of excretion is menstruation in women. Otherwise, iron is carefully conserved. Red blood cells are manufactured in bone marrow and sent into the blood, where they live about three to four months. When they die and are broken down, the liver retrieves their iron and recycles it to the bone marrow for reuse. Only minute losses occur in the clipping of nails, the cutting of hair, and the shedding of skin cells.

For women only: You are often told that you need more iron, yet you may often have had your blood cell count or hemoglobin level pronounced normal. Does this mean that you don't need more iron? Not necessarily. The difference between you and the men you know is a difference in your body stores of iron, which doesn't show up in these tests. Most men eat more food than women do, because they are bigger; and so their iron intakes are higher. Besides, women menstruate, and so their iron losses are greater. These two factors—lower intakes and higher losses—put you much closer to the borderline of deficiency. Even though you may never have been diagnosed as iron deficient, you are likely to be deficiency-prone. Should you lose blood for any reason (even by giving a blood donation) or become

Table 3. Iron Contents of Fifty Common Foods

Exchange Group[a]	Food	Serving Size[b]	Iron (mg)
5L	Oysters	¾ cup	10
5M	Beef liver	3 oz	8
4	Bran flakes, enriched	½ cup	6.2
5M	Beef heart	3 oz	5
5L	Chipped beef	3 oz	4
5L	Lean roast beef	3 oz	3
5L	Veal roast	3 oz	2.9
5M	Hamburger	3 oz	2.7
3	Prune juice	¼ cup	2.6
5L	Sardines	3 oz	2.5
4	Dried beans	½ cup	2.5
2	Spinach	½ cup	2.4
4	Lima beans	½ cup	2.2
5L	Ham	3 oz	2.2[c]
5L	Canned tuna	3 oz	1.6
2	Dandelion greens	½ cup	1.6
4	Green peas	½ cup	1.5
5L	Leg of lamb	3 oz	1.4
5L	Chicken, meat only	3 oz	1.4
2	Mustard greens	½ cup	1.3
3	Strawberries	¾ cup	1.1
5M	Egg	1	1.1
2	Tomato juice	½ cup	1.1
4	Rice, enriched	½ cup	0.9
2	Brussels sprouts	½ cup	0.9
3	Dried apricots	4 halves	0.8
4	Winter squash	½ cup	0.8
4	Whole-wheat bread	1 slice	0.8
3	Blackberries	½ cup	0.7
4	Pumpkin	¾ cup	0.7
5L	Canned salmon	3 oz	0.7
4	Cooked cereal	½ cup	0.7
3	Blueberries	½ cup	0.7
4	Spaghetti, enriched	½ cup	0.7
4	Macaroni, enriched	½ cup	0.7
2	Broccoli	½ cup	0.7
4	Potato chips	15	0.6
3	Raspberries	½ cup	0.6
5M	Peanut butter	2 tbsp	0.6
4	White bread	1 slice	0.6
3	Dried fig	1	0.6
4	Muffin	1	0.6
4	Corn muffin	1	0.6
3	Applesauce	½ cup	0.6
2	Cooked tomatoes	½ cup	0.6
4	French-fried potatoes	8	0.6
4	Popcorn, no fat	3 cup	0.6
3	Pear	1	0.5
4	Potato	1 small	0.5
4	Corn on cob	1 small	0.5

These are not best food sources but are selected to show a range of iron contents. Note the preponderance of 5s at the top of the left column and the total absence of 1s in this table.

[a]The numbers refer to the exchange lists: 2 is vegetables; 3, fruit; 4, bread; 5L, lean meat; 5M, medium-fat meat.

[b]Serving sizes are those in the exchange lists, except for meat.

[c]To this point, all foods supply at least 10 percent of the U.S. RDA of 18 mg.

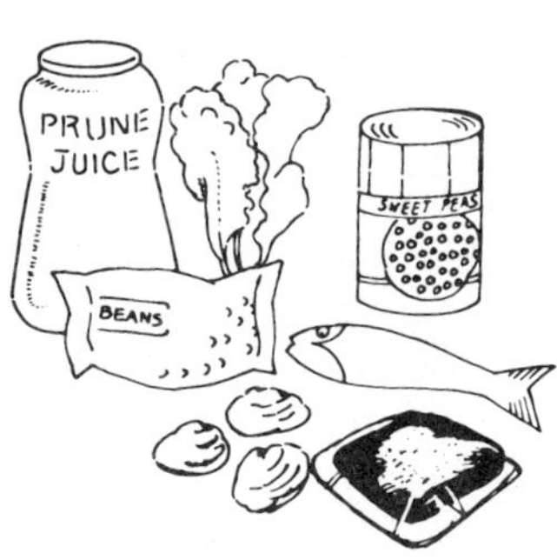

Foods containing iron.

pregnant (so that your blood volume would need to increase), you would need to pay special attention to your diet in an effort to maintain your iron stores. The information about iron in foods, which appears later in this chapter, is especially important to you.

The RDA is 10 milligrams a day for adult males and older women. For women of childbearing age, the RDA is 18 milligrams. This amount is necessary to replace menstrual losses and to provide the extra iron needed during pregnancy. Because of the television advertising of iron compounds, there is a general misunderstanding that only females need be concerned about their iron intakes. As a matter of fact, teen-age males need the same 18 milligrams as females. This need stems from the enormous growth spurt that males experience during their teen years. On the other hand, grown men experience iron-deficiency anemia rarely but may occasionally exhibit the toxicity condition, **iron overload**. When a man has a low hemoglobin, this alerts his physician to examine him for a blood-loss site.

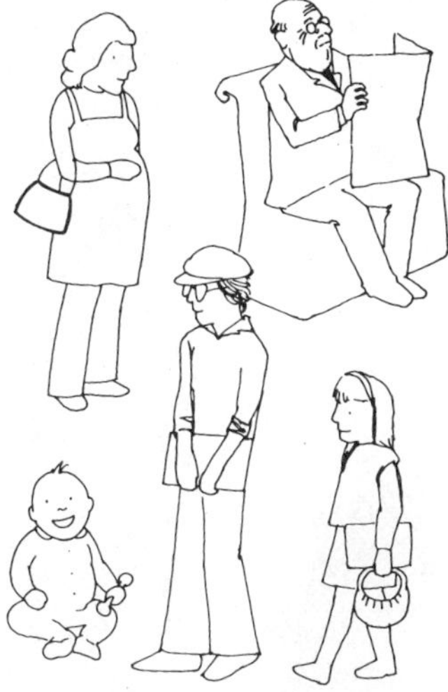

These people may need more iron. The people missing from this picture are adult males and adult women after menopause. The very elderly are included because they frequently have lowered stomach acidity, which interferes with absorption.

The normal hemoglobin value for male adults is 14 to 15 grams of hemoglobin per 100 milliliters of blood. For females, the normal value is 13 to 14 grams per 100 milliliters. Blacks are generally found to have lower average values than these, and it is not yet known whether this is a racial characteristic or is due to insufficient iron intakes.

The iron contents of common foods are shown in Table 3. Notable among them are liver and other organ meats, beef, dried fruits, dried peas and beans (legumes), nuts, green leafy vegetables, molasses, and whole-grain breads and cereals. Besides eating some of these foods daily, many females and teenage males may need iron supplements (the doctor should decide). The possibility that more iron should be added to enriched foods has been much debated. As of 1978, however, it had been decided that enrichment was to remain at its present level. This leaves it up to the consumer to meet her iron needs as best she can from foods. Enough strategies can be adopted to make this a relatively easy task.

Food Feature: Meeting Iron Needs from Foods

Iron from supplements is poorly absorbed, even though they may contain as many as 50 milligrams per dose. To be assured of meeting your iron needs, it is best to rely on foods. It will help you to learn to think in terms of nutrient density. The usual Western mixed diet provides only about 5 to 6 milligrams of iron in each 1000 calories. Thus an adult man, whose RDA is 10 milligrams and who eats upwards of 2500 calories a day, has no trouble meeting his RDA. A woman, whose RDA is 18 milligrams, and who may eat fewer than 2000 calories a day, understandably does have trouble. She must increase the iron-to-calorie ratio of her diet so that she will receive about double the average amount of iron, at least 10 milligrams per 1000 calories. It can be done by following the guidelines long familiar to nutrition-minded consumers. From each food group select those foods that are notable for their high iron content:

Milk and cheese. Milk and cheese have negligible iron content, so don't overdo (but don't omit these foods either; you need them for calcium). Drink skim milk, to free up calories to be invested in iron-rich foods.

Meat. Use liver and other organ meats frequently, perhaps every week or two. Meats, fish, and eggs are second-best iron sources.

Meat substitutes. Don't forget legumes: A cup of peas or beans can supply up to 5 milligrams of iron. For vegetarians, legumes are an indispensable part of the diet.

Breads and cereals. Use only whole-grain, enriched, and fortified products.

Vegetables. The dark-green leafy vegetables are richest in iron.

Fruits. Dried fruits like raisins, apricots, peaches, and prunes are high in iron.

Knowledgeable cooking and menu planning can enhance the amount of iron delivered by the diet. The iron content of 100 grams of spaghetti sauce simmered in a glass dish is 3 milligrams, but it's 87 milligrams when the sauce is cooked in an unenameled iron skillet. Even in the short time it takes to scramble eggs, their iron content can be tripled by cooking them in an iron pan. Foods containing 25 milligrams or more of vitamin C can more than double the amount of iron absorbed from iron sources eaten at the same meal.[29] Therefore, two additional suggestions are:

Cook with iron skillets whenever possible.

Serve vitamin C-containing foods at every meal.

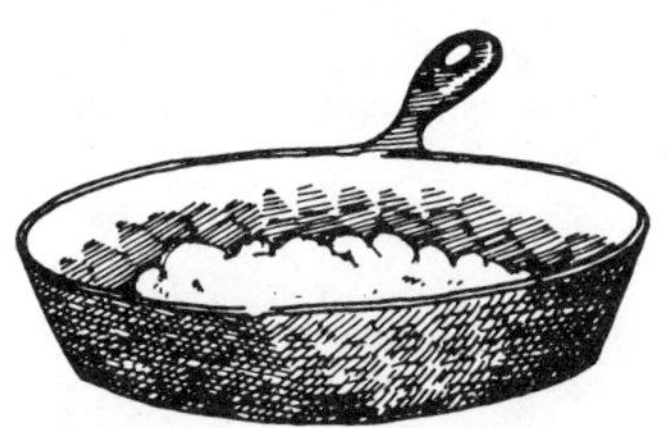

The old-fashioned iron skillet adds a much needed nutrient to the diet.

The use of fortified foods is another option. Some breakfast cereals boast that they contain 100 percent of the recommended daily intake of iron. The use of these may indeed boost the day's iron intakes, even though absorption of the iron used in them is poor. A number of proposals have been made for further fortification. Canada is considering adding iron to milk;[30] other ideas are to add it to coffee, to junk foods, even to salt. At present, 25 percent of all the iron consumed in the United States derives from fortified foods. A proposal to increase further the iron level in enriched bread has been defeated. Ultimately, it is up to consumers themselves to see that they get enough iron.

Zinc. Zinc occurs in a very small quantity in the body (about 2 grams) but is a helper for some twenty enzymes and forms part of the structure of bone. High concentrations of zinc appear in the eye, liver, muscles, and male reproductive organs. It is involved in DNA and protein synthesis, the action of insulin, the immune reactions, and the utilization of vitamin A. With all of these vital roles, it is not surprising that zinc is necessary for the healing of wounds; a deficiency can seriously retard this process. Zinc is also required for a normal sense of taste. The impressive accumulation of new information about zinc in recent years has led to the conclusion that this mineral is as important as protein in the normal processes of growth and the maintenance of body tissues.

A deficiency of zinc was first observed in humans in the 1960s in the Middle East, where a high-cereal, low-animal-protein diet was common. It was marked by dwarfism and poor male sexual development, which responded to the administration of zinc. Since then, zinc deficiency has also been seen in some children in the United States, suggesting that the problem may be more widespread than has been thought in the past. Zinc deficiencies are now suspected to exist among preschoolers, older people, hospital patients, and other populations whose protein intakes may be limited (vegetarians).

Animal foods are good sources of zinc, with the richest being oysters, herring, milk, and egg yolks. Among plant foods, whole grains are richest in zinc, but it is not so well absorbed from them as from meat. The RDA of 15 milligrams per day for adults is probably easily met by the diet of the average person. As a rule of thumb, a person who eats enough food protein probably gets enough zinc; vegetarians should emphasize whole grains.

Teenagers and college students who are concerned about acne may learn that zinc has been effective in its treatment in cases where vitamin A has not been.[31] However, self-dosing with zinc can cause toxicity with severe consequences: muscle incoordination, dizziness, drowsiness, lethargy, renal failure, anemia, and others.[32] As with all the nutrients, and especially the trace minerals, overdoses of zinc are dangerous. Besides, acne can have so many different causes that it would be foolhardy to self-diagnose. The person who wants to consider the use of zinc for acne should ask first for the help of a dietitian or nutritionist to see if it is reasonable to suspect a zinc deficiency and then for the help of a dermatologist to work out the details of therapy.

By the same token, people who are experiencing altered taste sensations should not jump to the conclusion that zinc deficiency is the cause. The sense of taste is affected by many things—including such serious conditions as early cancer. Loss of taste does not respond to the administration of zinc if it is caused by something else.

Copper. Copper, too, is an essential trace mineral for humans. About 75 to 100 milligrams of copper appear in the entire body.

Copper performs a vital role as a catalyst in the formation of hemoglobin and as a component in some of the compounds necessary to the release of energy. It has a possible role in the formation of collagen. Also, it helps to maintain the sheath around nerve fibers. Most of what is known about copper is from animal research, which has provided clues as to its possible roles in humans. The critical roles of copper seem to have to do with helping iron shift back and forth between its +2 and +3 states. This means that copper is needed in many of the reactions having to do with respiration and the release of energy.

A copper deficiency is rare but not unknown. It has been seen in children with kwashiorkor and with iron-deficiency anemia. Low intakes of copper, on the other hand, appear to be quite common, but it is not known what the health implications may be.[33]

Best food sources of copper include grains, shellfish, organ meats, legumes, dried fruits, fresh fruits and vegetables—a long list showing that copper is available from almost all foods. About a third of that taken in food is absorbed, and the rest is eliminated in the feces.

Fluoride is the bone-seeker par excellence.—H. C. Hodge

Fluoride. Only a trace of fluoride occurs in the human body, but studies have demonstrated that, where the fluoride content of the diet is high, the crystalline deposits in bones and teeth are larger and more perfectly formed.

Drinking water is the usual source of fluoride. In communities where the water contains 2 to 8 parts per million (ppm), mottling of the teeth may occur; where fluoride is lacking, the incidence of dental decay is very high. Fluoridation of water where needed, to raise its fluoride concentration to 1 ppm, is recommended as an important public health measure. Not only does fluoride protect children's teeth from decay, but it makes the bone crystals of older people more resistant to the degeneration of osteoporosis. Despite fluoride's value, violent disagreement often surrounds the introduction of fluoridation in many communities at first.

Arguments for and against fluoridation appear in Controversy 10B.

Cobalt. Cobalt is another essential trace mineral for humans, needed in minute amounts but absolutely necessary for optimum health. One of the first trace minerals to be studied, it is known to form a crucial part of the large vitamin B_{12} molecule, a catalyst in reactions involved in the manufacture of red blood cells. Thus this mineral, like iodine in thyroxin, functions by being part of a large organic complex that has a unique place in human physiology. It seems to be an emerging generalization that many of the minerals work this way. Cobalt confers on vitamin B_{12} its alternative name, cobalamin.

More on vitamin B_{12}—Chapter 9.

Selenium. Selenium, too, is a trace element that functions as part of large molecules, especially certain enzymes. It also acts alone as an antioxidant and can substitute for vitamin E in some of the vitamin's antioxidant activities. Deficiencies are unknown, and food sources are abundant.

Chromium. The element chromium is now known to be essential in human nutrition. Experiments on animals have shown that chromium works closely with the hormone insulin, facilitating the uptake of glucose into cells and then the breakdown of that glucose with the release of energy. When the mineral is lacking, the effectiveness of insulin is thus severely impaired. The concentration of chromium in human tissues declines as people age, and apparently the resulting deficiency accounts for the onset of what looks like diabetes in some cases.[34] There is some concern that chromium deficiency may be becoming a serious public health problem because of the increased refinement of foods and the resulting loss of their trace minerals.[35]

Like iron, chromium can have two different charges: The +3 ion seems to be the most effective in living systems. It also occurs in association with several different complexes in foods. The one that is best absorbed and most active is a small organic compound named the **glucose tolerance factor (GTF)**. This compound has been purified from brewer's yeast and pork kidney and is believed to be present in many other foods. It may be that, when more is known, the GTF, rather than chromium, will be dubbed an essential nutrient and will be classed among the vitamins.

Depleted tissue concentrations of chromium in human beings have been linked to adult-onset diabetes and growth failure in children with protein-calorie malnutrition.

Just twenty years ago I wrote: "For the overwhelming bulk of mankind a diet well-balanced and adequate in other respects is likely . . . to provide the normal individual with an abundance of all the trace elements." . . . Today, such a definite statement could not be made. . . . Marginal or overt deficiencies of iron, zinc and chromium have been recognized widely. . . . These have been shown to be related mainly . . . to changes in dietary patterns, particularly to increases in the consumption of refined, processed, and prepared foods . . .—E. J. Underwood

Putting It All Together

This chapter has treated fifteen different minerals essential in human nutrition and has pointed out that many more may be needed. The end of Chapter 9 presented a scheme whereby the nutrients so far discussed could be obtained in food. Now, with the addition of all these minerals, is it still possible to achieve an adequate diet without exten-

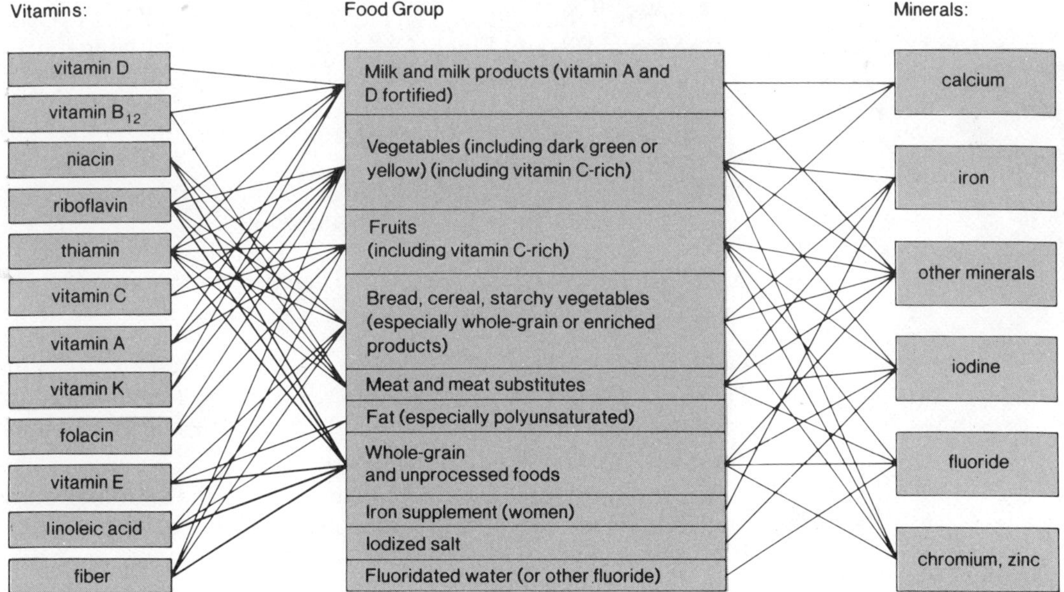

Figure 3. Chapter 9, Figure 1, with modifications. *Although the figure looks complex, it still presents a small number of food groups to meet the body's needs for a large number of nutrients.*

sive planning? Evidently, some modifications of the figure at the end of Chapter 9 are now needed.

The mineral element iron may be too sparsely provided by the diet to meet the needs of women and adolescent boys, and some authorities recommend that these groups take a supplement. In the case of two other mineral elements—iodine and fluoride—food sources are unreliable enough in some geographical locations to necessitate the inclusion of iodized salt and fluoridated water for protection against deficiencies. Some trace elements, such as chromium, are lost during the refining of foods, so there is some basis for believing that unrefined foods should be used in preference to "enriched" foods. To cover these needs, some additions must be made to the diagram presented at the end of Chapter 9 (see Figure 3).[1]

For Further Information

Recommended references on all nutrition topics are listed in Appendix J.

"The Sodium Content of Your Food," by A. C. Marsh, R. N. Klippstein, and S. D. Kaplan, published by the USDA (Booklet No. 233 in the Home and Garden Bulletin Series) is available for $2 from the U.S. Government Printing Office (address in Appendix J). Mention stock number 001-000-04179-7 when ordering.

A technical reference which tells how to estimate the amount of iron you actually get from your foods, taking the vitamin C and meat effects into consideration, is:

- Monsen, R. R., Hallberg, L., Layrisse, M., Hegsted, D. M., Cook, J. D., Mentz, W., and Finch, C. A. Estimation of available dietary iron. *American Journal of Clinical Nutrition* 31 (1978) 134-141.

On diet and oral health, an excellent review is:

- DePaola, D. P., and Alfano, M. C. Diet and oral health. *Nutrition Today*, May/June 1977, pp. 6-11, 29-32.

Nutrition Today and the American Dietetic Association make several teaching aids available:

- Fletcher, D. Trace elements in nutrition. *Cassette-a-Month*, February 1975. This and the White reference that follows are cassettes with lecture notes, available from the American Dietetic Association (address in Appendix J).
- Robinson, J. Nutrient metabolism—water, the essential nutrient (slide set with lecture notes). Nutrition Today Society (address in Appendix J).
- White, H. S. Iron nutrition—an update. *Cassette-a-Month*, September 1977.

[1]*Chapter Notes can be found at the end of the Appendixes.*

Controversy 10A

Iron Superenrichment

Should we superenrich breads to prevent iron deficiency?

In 1971 the FDA proposed an increase in the levels at which iron should be added to enriched grain products. Until that time, enrichment had restored iron in refined products to the concentrations normally found in the original whole-grain products before refinement. The FDA proposed raising the iron content of these products about threefold. A lively debate ensued, with well-informed expert opinions expressed along all points of the spectrum. The major arguments follow.

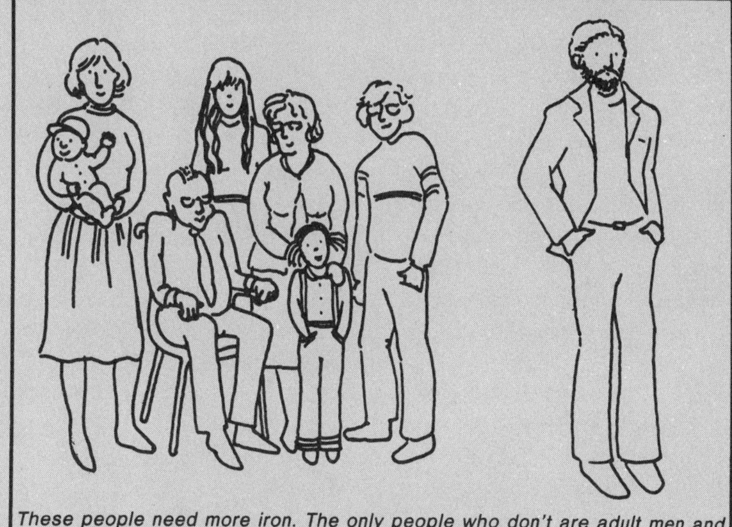

These people need more iron. The only people who don't are adult men and post-menopausal women.

Arguments pro. The FDA based its proposal on the data that show low hemoglobin levels in extensive segments of our population—especially in women, infants, children, the elderly, and low-income and minority groups. The rationale for superenrichment is the same as that underlying the original Enrichment Act: Wheat products are widely consumed in the United States, accounting for about a fourth of the total calorie intake, and two-thirds of these products are now enriched. Higher proportions of wheat products are consumed by low-income groups, in whom iron deficiency is also more common. Thus superenrichment of these products is a practical means of delivering needed iron to the target population.[1]

The American Medical Association Council on Foods and Nutrition, as well as the Food and Nutrition Board[2] and the American Association of Pediatrics, supported the proposal. The council observed that a diet that would provide 20 milligrams of daily iron intake for women would result in men's having about 50 milligrams a day (because men consume more calories). The council was of the opinion that this intake would be "well tolerated." It found the increase "consistent with the principles of preventive medicine and with a conservative approach." By way of illustration, it reasoned as follows: The absorption of iron from meat is about 20 percent, and that from bread is about 5 percent. Under the new regulations, the average boy would get about 4 more milligrams of iron from bread than he does now; this would be the equivalent of 1 milligram from meat. Thus the effect on his iron status would be the same as if he ate an additional ounce of cooked hamburger each day.

The advocates of superenrichment argued further that iron-deficiency anemia is "the end stage of iron deficiency."[3] In developing an iron deficit, the body goes through several earlier stages of negative iron balance, with symptoms not normally seen because they are not looked for. These include fatigue, impaired work performance, and reduced mental ability. If we improve the iron nutriture of our people enough to raise the lowered hemoglobin levels of a few people to normal, countless other people will benefit by remediation of these less obvious symptoms.

Arguments con. But wait a minute, say the opponents: Consider the risks. It may be true that the average male might not suffer an iron overload, but what about those with abnormally high iron stores? Inevitably, increased iron intakes will precipitate severe toxicity symptoms in some.[4] Besides, there are causes of low blood hemoglobin other than iron-deficient diets; consider the case of bowel cancer. It is an accepted fact that "a *man* who is iron deficient is bleeding; the cause of his blood loss is a problem far more important than his iron deficiency."[5] It would be inexcusable to endorse a measure such as superenrichment to solve one public health problem only to cause another—the masking of bleeding that demands prompt diagnosis.[6] Enrichment, which is directed at 2 percent of the population, would put 100 percent at risk.[7]

Moreover, the benefits of superenrichment are only theoretical. It has not been demonstrated that raising our low hemoglobin levels would relieve fatigue and other such symptoms. One authority draws a line at a hemoglobin score of 10 (10 grams of hemoglobin per 100 milliliters of blood) to indicate deficiency in women (12 in men), but symptoms seldom appear until a person's hemoglobin level falls to 7 or 8. We must base our definition of deficiency on real harm to health, and this is not seen in subjects with low hemoglobin levels. Contrary to expectations, according to this authority, adding iron does not always relieve anemia.[8] It may be, too, that blacks are supposed to have lower hemoglobin levels than whites by virtue of their different genetic heritage.[9]

Superenrichment would be a mistake from another point of view as well: It would give consumers a false sense of nutritional security.[10] If iron deficiency reflects poor nutrition in our country, then we had better correct the causes of poor nutrition. A spokesman emphatically states the case:

> *Admittedly, it is much easier to add more iron to flour than it is to improve the economic status of our population, to reduce unemployment, to lower food prices, and to improve sanitation and health education. However, in the long run, these logical, corrective steps are far more likely to be effective in relieving nutritional iron deficiency, not to speak of their other, far-reaching beneficial effects, than to cover our eyes, shut our minds, triple the dietary iron and hope for the best.*[11]

It seems that for every voice crying "Fortify!"[12] there is another answering "Educate!"[13]

All of the above arguments are based on logic. To test their validity, experiments have been done, and some of the relevant questions have been answered.

What are the actual effects of iron deficiency? In 1970, Elwood reported the results of increasing iron stores in thousands of women in Wales.[14] At the outset, many were anemic and exhibited such symptoms as easy fatigue and dizziness. After a year of corrective iron treatment, their average hemoglobin levels had increased considerably, but their symptoms had not changed. Elwood was forced to conclude that it was not until the level of hemoglobin fell to the 8-gram range that disability resulted from iron deficiency.[15] These findings converted him to the opinion that no significant "harm to health" is caused by the great majority of low hemoglobin levels seen in the United States. A careful review by Elwood of the evidence available at the time also showed inconclusive evidence from other studies regarding the effect of iron deficiency on work capacity, fatigue, mental ability, and psychomotor function.[16]

Elwood also observed that there might be a correlation between low-to-normal hemoglobin levels and a lowered risk of heart disease. Iron-deficient subjects, he said, have lower serum cholesterol and more artery branches that have grown to feed tissues if major arteries become blocked. He expressed surprise that more attention had not been focused on these correlations.[17]

As often happens, heat generated by the controversy has prompted some researchers to undertake studies. Among the reports is one that clearly shows effects of mild to moderate iron-deficiency anemia that qualify as "harm to health." This study demonstrates that iron-deficiency anemia markedly reduces women's ability to perform physical work and concludes that "a strong case for its correction and prevention can be made on a basis of economics, as well as of health."[18]

A recent review of the evidence linking iron deficiency to behavioral problems in human beings shows that there are connections. For example, "motivation to persist in intellectually challenging tasks may be lowered, attention span shortened, and over-all intellectual performance diminished." However, it is impossible to tell whether these problems are a consequence of iron deficiency alone or of "a general nutritional inadequacy of which iron deficiency was only a readily identifiable component."[19] Another review reports additional symptoms, such as hyperactivity, reduced attentiveness, and lowered IQ. At least sometimes, iron therapy provides a remedy before anemia becomes established. The authors of this article support the view that iron-deficiency anemia is the end stage of iron deficiency and state that "storage, transport . . . and even enzyme . . . iron may be exhausted before the circulating mass of red cells is affected."[20] It is thus a real possibility that iron deficiency so mild that it does not even cause anemia does cause "harm to health" and needs to be identified and corrected. In reporting to the President in 1977, the Biomedical Research Panel accepted the view that iron deficiency is associated with learning disability.[21]

But what about the risks of superenrichment? One opportunity to study the risks of superenrichment is provided by Sweden, where legislation has increased dietary iron by 42 percent. A careful look at 197 men in one community there revealed nine new cases of abnormally raised hemoglobin levels and at least four of iron overload.[22] When a U.S. agency was asked to assess the risk in this country, however, it demonstrated that iron overload was too rare and that any such study would require the examination of too many individuals and would cost too much to be feasible.[23] For the present, at least, the question has not been satisfactorily answered.

By 1978 the FDA had yielded to the counterarguments, and the idea of superenrichment was abandoned.[24] Enrichment will remain at its present levels. This leaves it up to the individual consumer to identify and solve the problem of iron deficiency where it exists.

Personal strategy. If you are concerned about meeting your own iron needs, the suggestions in Chapter 10's Food Feature will be helpful. Learn to think in terms of nutrient density, select the most iron-rich foods from each food group, cook with iron utensils, and serve foods containing vitamin C at every meal.

We had better be informed in the realm of public policy, too. It may help to get the original FDA proposal in perspective if we realize that wholesale addition of iron to all grain products was never the intention, only to such enriched products as flour, bread, buns, and rolls. Whole-wheat, rye, and raisin bread would not have been affected.[25] If and when the proposal is revised, it should be accompanied by a means of labeling to enable consumers (for example, men versus women) to make an educated choice between superenriched and whole-grain products. The effectiveness of the measure should be monitored by sampling segments of the target population at intervals for changes in the incidence of iron-deficiency anemia or other iron-deficiency symptoms.

You are urged not to assume that the evidence presented here is a balanced representation of the available information (although we have tried to make it one). New and important publications on the iron controversy are still appearing. The consumer and consumer advocate who seek to be truly well informed will read not only the references cited here but the others to which they refer and those not yet in print.

The Controversy Notes and For Further Information follow the Appendixes.

Controversy 10B

Fluoridation

Should fluoride be added to community water supplies?

Wherever fluoride concentrations in the water supply are higher than one part per million (ppm), tooth decay is less prevalent—and tooth decay is a major public health problem in this country, contributing to a host of other ills. Fluoridation of water supplies that lack natural fluoride is an obvious, safe, and cost-effective measure to reduce this problem. So say the fluoridation advocates.

The opponents disagree. They argue that altering the community water supply is "unnatural" and deprives its consumers of their freedom of choice. Those who want fluoride can get it by way of drops, tablets, toothpaste, or dental treatments, leaving those who do not want it free to choose. Some people are opposed to fluoridation on religious grounds: "If God had intended to have fluoride in the water supply, He would have put it there." Others fear accidental overdoses: Fluorine is a highly volatile chemical and is deadly in excess. Still others claim that fluoridated communities have an increased cancer rate.

These arguments have raged in one community after another since the first controlled experiments in 1945. By the 1970s, about 100 million people in the United States were drinking fluoridated water in more than 5000 communities. The map shows the extent to which fluoridation had been adopted before 1980.

Evidence pro. The first experiments in fluoridation, now famous, were performed in the 1940s in the paired communities of Kingston and Newburgh, New York, and in Grand Rapids and Muskegon, Michigan. In each instance, one of the two communities treated its water supply with fluoride, and the other did not. At the end of ten years, the dental records showed a reduction in the number of decayed, missing, and filled teeth of the Newburgh children (whose water was fluoridated) as compared with the children of Kingston. The youngest children (ages six to nine) showed the greatest improvement—57.9 percent reduction—but even those aged sixteen had benefited, with a 40.9 percent reduction. The medical team reported no significant differences in other aspects of the children's health and concluded that the fluoride had had no adverse side effects.[1] Similar results emerged from the Michigan studies and from others conducted thereafter. It seems from these experiments that fluoride stabilizes the developing tooth

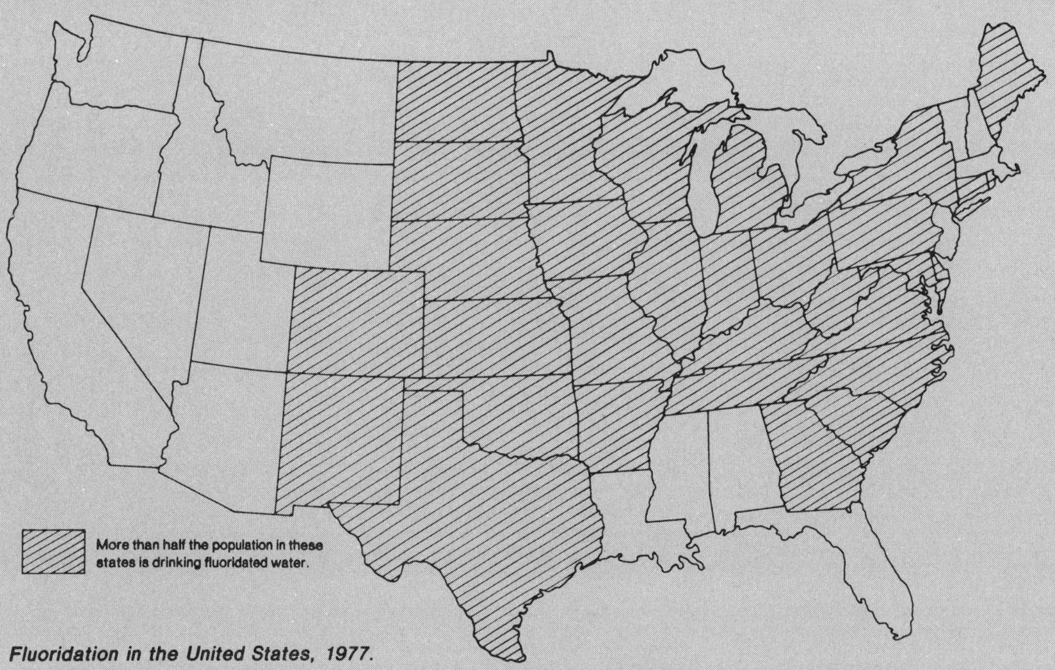
More than half the population in these states is drinking fluoridated water.

Fluoridation in the United States, 1977.

Adapted from D. P. DePaola and M. C. Alfano, Diet and oral health, Nutrition Today, *May/June 1977, pp. 6-11, 29-32, and presented with the permission of the authors and of* Nutrition Today *magazine, 703 Giddings Avenue, Suite 6, Annapolis MD 21401, May/June 1977.*

structure, making it resistant to decay.

More recently, accumulating evidence has suggested that fluoride may protect bone structure, in a similar way, against the gradual leaching out of minerals known as osteoporosis, or adult bone loss. The causes of osteoporosis are probably many, but one of the nutritional factors affecting it seems to be fluoride. A typical research report, comparing two North Dakota communities, found a significantly higher incidence of osteoporosis in the community with the lower fluoride concentration in its public water.[2] The researchers ruled out differing calcium intakes as an explanation of the difference, noting that milk and cheese consumption in both communities was the same. As a result of studies of this kind, there is general agreement that "fluoridation of city water supplies is beneficial in ways other than in the prevention of [tooth decay]."[3]

The Committee on RDA states that fluoride is found in all normal diets, is required for growth in animals, and is an essential nutrient for humans. The committee acknowledges that fluoride is toxic in excess but points out that chronic intakes, for years, of 20 to 80 milligrams a day are required to produce toxicity symptoms. The amount consumed from fluoridated water is typically about 1 milligram a day. "The first identifiable indication of an excess [is] slight mottling of the [tooth] enamel," and this, although unsightly, is not harmful to health.[4]

On the basis of the accumulated evidence of its beneficial effects, fluoridation has been endorsed by the National Institute of Dental Health, the American Medical Association, the National Cancer Institute, and the National Nutrition Consortium.[5]The allegation that it causes cancer has no identifiable basis in fact and has been refuted by the National Cancer Institute, the American Cancer Society, and the National Institute of Dental Research.[6]

Evidence cannot be cited

for or against the emotional arguments against fluoridation, because they cannot be tested by experiments. The issues of human freedom and religion often clash with public health measures, and they have with this one. Perhaps it is relevant to note, however, that fluoride's close relative, chlorine, is routinely added to city water supplies. The benefits of this measure so far outweigh the risks that it has been gratefully accepted.

Arguments con. In spite of the manifest benefits of fluoridation, the debate continues, and some responsible scientists are raising important questions.[7] No evidence has been collected that bears on these questions as yet, but they should be kept in mind for the future. For example, now that fluoride has been added to many water supplies, the amounts in foods processed in plants supplied by that water are increasing, so that the total fluoride consumed by certain populations may be greater than expected. There is no indication, as yet, that these effects extend into the area where any hazard is likely, but it is important to be aware of the possibility.

Another basis for concern relates to the possible interaction of fluoride with other elements and pollutants in the environment that could give rise to harmful combinations. The unquestionably beneficial addition of chlorine to city water supplies has had an unexpected side effect of this kind. Where water is heavily polluted with organic waste materials, they can combine with the chlorine to make materials that in some instances cause cancer. This effect can't be blamed on chlorine, of course, but shows that the addition of any element into the environment—no matter how harmless that element may be by itself—has to be viewed in the light of all possible interactions and combinations, and not as a simple matter. This makes monitoring and testing of the water supply increasingly important.

Personal strategy. In communities where fluoride in the water supply falls short of 1 ppm, individual consumers who want the protection provided by fluoride have several options. (One is, of course, to fight for fluoridation.) They can use fluoride toothpaste or tablets and can made sure their children do the same. During pregnancy, women can request a fluoride-containing supplement from their doctors and a similar one for their newborn infants. During their early years—up to sixteen—children should receive twice-yearly fluoride applications directly on their teeth as part of dental care.

The Controversy Notes and For Further Information follow the Appendixes.

PART THREE

APPLICATIONS

This one-chapter section offers an opportunity to put together the information about nutrients presented in the last seven chapters. Nutrients, after all, reach people by way of the foods they eat, and the problem of acquiring good nutritional status therefore becomes a problem of combining foods into balanced diets. Once this section has addressed the questions adults most often ask about foods and diets today, Part IV turns to the special concerns of people in other life stages from infancy to old age.

CHAPTER 11

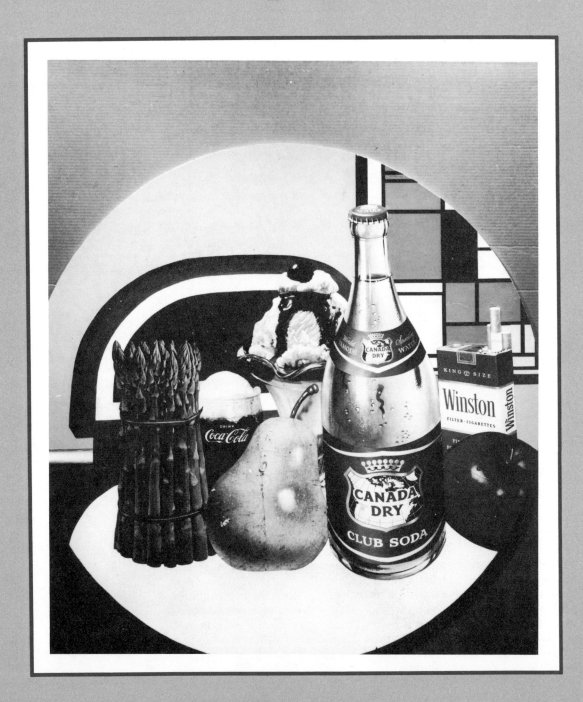
DRINK
Coca-Cola
CANADA DRY
CANADA DRY
CLUB SODA
KING SIZE
Winston
FILTER · CIGARETTES
Winston

Foods, Food Labels, and Additives

The last seven chapters have been devoted to the nutrients and energy in foods. It is time again to focus on the foods themselves. Which ones are the "best"—the most nutrient-dense, the most desirable to use in menu-planning? Which are the ones to avoid? Questions many people these days are especially concerned about are: What is in the processed foods? Are the additives in foods safe?

It is suggested that you review the personal strategy section at the end of Controversy 1, and Figure 1 in Chapter 2, before you begin reading this chapter. The review will help you to remember the main classes of foods and the generalization that whole, farm-grown foods are usually more nutritious than refined, processed foods. This chapter begins by paying special attention to the processed, convenience, and fast foods of today's popular marketplace. It explains how you can tell from a food label what is in the food and what may be missing. Then it turns to the matter of the additives in foods and tries to provide a perspective that will help you make intelligent food choices.

The New Foods

The nutrition scene in the United States and Canada is changing fast. New in the picture since the 1940s are all kinds of foods: fast foods, convenience foods, fabricated foods, engineered foods. All of these are

Opposite: Mondrian Still-Life #18 *by Tom Wesselmann. Used with the permission of the Sidney Janis Gallery, New York.*

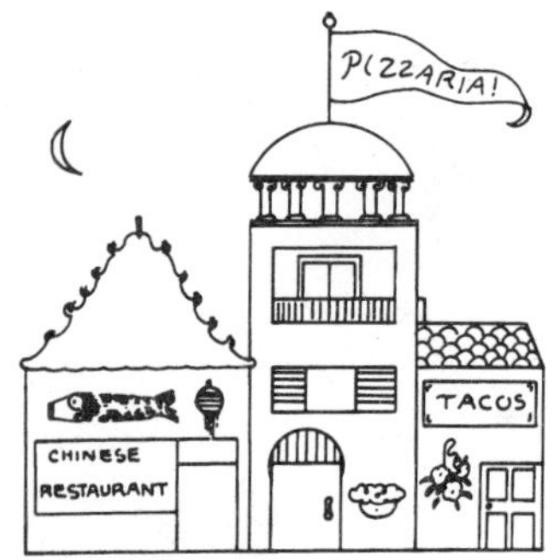

Fast foods come in all nationalities.

prepared by people other than ourselves, and there are more of them all the time.

According to one estimate, 40 percent of all meals, whether consumed in restaurants, fast-food places, or at home, are now prepared outside the home; in ten years, 70 percent will be.[1] Among the trends creating the demand for these foods is the recruitment of women into the work force. The number of working mothers has more than doubled in the past two decades. Only 10 percent of all people in this country eat lunch at home even once a week, except on weekends.[2] Thus reliance on the new foods, which are easy to store and carry along and quick to prepare, is greater than it has ever been before. But people who use these foods daily may be inclined to wonder what sort of nutrient contributions they make.

Those who oppose and fear this trend say that the new foods are "empty calorie foods," "junk foods," and that often—because their labels claim large amounts of vitamins and minerals—they are fraudulently called nutritious. Others applaud the new technology, which represents the achievements of thousands of laboratory-trained food scientists. The two opposing views have been expressed like this:

> Food is now not only nutritious, but it is safe, convenient, of high quality, flavorful, and presented to the consumer at a cost, relative to earnings, which is competitive with any other country in the world at any other time in history, or the present. It is a gross injustice for consumers to have their confidence in the safety and nutritive value of their food supply destroyed. . . .[3]

> Manufacturers . . . make whatever junk they like and add some vitamins and minerals to make that high-sugar, high-fat food look extremely nutritious. . . .[4]

Before getting into the pros and cons of this issue, it will be helpful to define some of the terms.

The **fast foods** are those prepared in quick-order restaurants, such as the hamburger stands and fried-chicken places that line our nation's main streets and highways. **Convenience foods** are those prepared at home from foods that have already been cooked or otherwise processed before reaching the market. They include:

Cold breakfast cereals, to which you add milk and sugar.

Powdered drinks, to which you add water and ice.

Preprepared meals and desserts, to which you add water or milk and then stir, cook, and serve hot or cold.

Canned foods that you open, heat if desired, and serve.

Frozen foods such as frozen vegetables, concentrated juices, and TV dinners.

All of these convenience foods are **processed foods**—cooked, frozen, freeze-dried, or the like. Some are **natural foods** in the sense that they are prepared from farm-grown animal or plant foods (for example, concentrated orange juice, frozen vegetables, bread made from whole-wheat flour). Others are **engineered foods**, or **fabricated foods**, made entirely from ingredients purified and mixed in laboratories (for example, drinks composed of sugar, additives, colors, and vitamins). Fabricated foods may be called **imitation foods**, a term whose use on labels now has precise legal limits.

The complete nutrient contents of typical fast foods are shown in Appendix G.

The terms **junk food** and **empty calorie food** may be applied to any food by a person who feels that it has little or no nutritional value. Snack foods found in convenience stores are most often deemed junk, especially if they contain large amounts of sugar, fat, or salt. *Empty calorie food* is a less emotion-laden term, referring to foods of low nutrient density. The user of these terms often contrasts them with their opposites—*health foods* and *organic foods*—but these terms may also be misleading.

More about "health foods" and "organic foods"—Controversy 1.

Finally, there are enriched and fortified foods. **Enriched** traditionally refers to four nutrients (iron, thiamin, riboflavin, and niacin) added back to refined grain, from which they have been lost in processing, and added in the approximate amounts in which they were originally present (double, in the case of riboflavin). **Fortified** refers to the addition of any nutrient to a food, even one that may not have been there originally, and may involve adding nutrients in amounts well above those found naturally in a food. A fortified breakfast cereal may have such large quantities of nutrients added that one serving provides 100 percent of the U.S. RDA for all of them. Other examples of fortified foods are

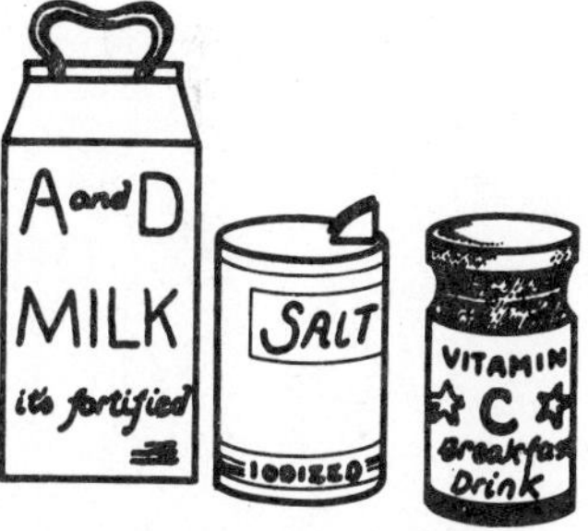

Salt to which iodine is added.

Milk to which vitamins A and D are added.

An orange-colored drink composed mostly of sugar to which vitamin C is added.

The canny consumer will realize that the word *fortified* sometimes conveys an emptiness of other nutrients: Fruit *juice* is more nutritious than fortified fruit *drink*, even though the drink may be higher in vitamin C content.

For the exact definitions of enriched and fortified, turn to the glossary.

It is the food scientist, not the nutritionist, who is concerned with the technology underlying all these different foods. A complete discussion of this subject is beyond the scope of this book; but since all these foods are controversial, you need some information about them in order to make informed choices. It helps to know how to read labels and to understand the debate surrounding additives.

Food Labels

Three sections of the labeling laws of the 1970s deal with nutrition. One has to do with how the label itself should appear. The second sets standards for foods—especially convenience foods—that bear certain names on their labels. The third requires that certain foods be labeled "imitation." These aspects of the labeling laws are discussed in the three sections that follow.

Claims and information on labels. The original authority for the government to move into the field of nutrition labeling came from the

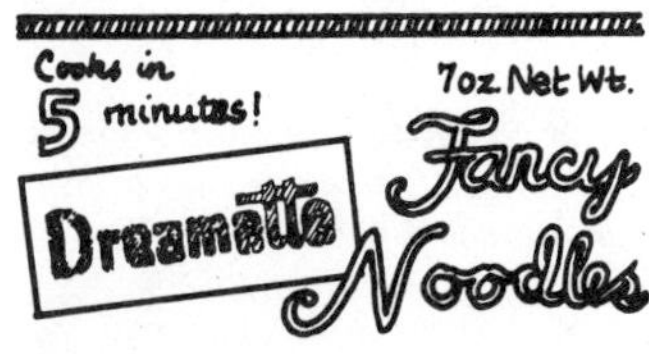

For forty years, labels have had to give this much information.

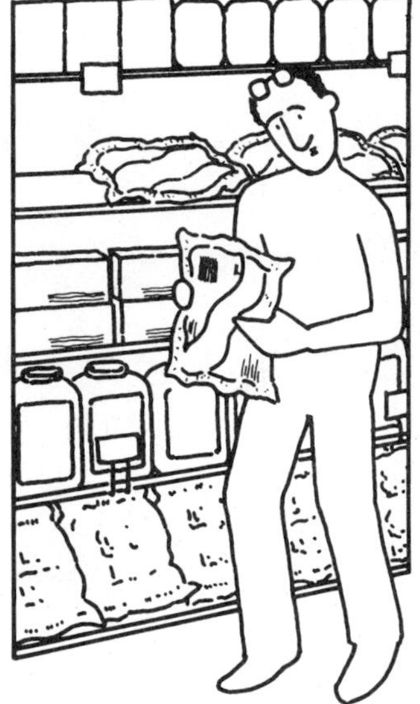

Now, the buyer wants to know more.

Food, Drug, and Cosmetic Act of 1938. Regulations under this act require that labels state:

The common name of the product.

The name and address of the manufacturer, packer, or distributor.

The net contents in terms of weight, measure, or count.

The ingredients listed in order of descending predominance.

These requirements, however, were not sufficient to make labels informative to consumers. Manufacturers often printed the information in type too small to be read and placed it on an inconspicuous part of the label. In 1966, therefore, Congress passed the Fair Packaging Labeling Act, which required, in part, that information for the consumer's use be put in a prominent place on the label and that words used to convey this information be those ordinarily used. For instance, adjectives such as *economy* or *giant* could not be used to describe the size of the package, because they do not ordinarily have a size connotation. With these new regulations, labels began to be much more informative than they had been in the past.

Still, as consumers began to learn more about nutrition, many of them realized that the food labels still lacked important information. They were buying new products on the basis of advertising claims and then continuing to use them if the taste, appearance, convenience, or price was right. But they began to wonder if the foods were of high quality nutritionally, and so they demanded still more information. The consumer had learned to read the fine print that listed the ingredients and knew that they were listed in order of predominance. Seeing sugar in first place on a label, for example, told the consumer there was more sugar than anything else in the package. But now the buyer wanted to know more: "How much protein does it contain? How much thiamin?"

Consumer demand for nutrition information on labels led, during the 1960s, to the formulation of the labeling laws in effect today, which deal specifically with the nutrient contents of foods. According to the laws, the manufacturers of food products are free to add or not to add nutrients to their products and to advertise or not to advertise the nutritional superiority of their products. If nothing is added and no claim is made, no nutritional information need appear on the package other than the statements already mentioned. But if manufacturers decide to add a nutrient (for example, vitamin D to a breakfast drink), or if they decide to make an advertising claim (like saying that orange juice is a good source of vitamin C), then they must comply *fully* with the nutrition labeling requirements. Without a complete information panel, nutrition claims could deceive the consumer about the true nutritional value of a food.

Several types of claims on labels are forbidden. It cannot be claimed:

(1) That a food is effective as a treatment for a disease.

(2) That a balanced diet of ordinary foods cannot supply adequate amounts of nutrients (excepting the iron requirements of infants, children, and pregnant or lactating women).

(3) That the soil on which food is grown may be responsible for deficiencies in quality.

(4) That storage, transportation, processing, or cooking of a food may be responsible for deficiencies in its quality.

(5) That a food has particular dietary qualities when such qualities have not been shown to be significant in human nutrition.

(6) That a natural vitamin is superior to a synthetic vitamin.[5]

The nutrition labeling section of the law then states that, if any nutrition information or claim is made on the label of a food package, it must conform to the following format under the heading "Nutrition Information":

Serving or portion size.

Servings or portions per container.

Calorie content per serving.

Protein grams per serving.

Carbohydrate grams per serving.

Fat grams per serving. (When fatty acid composition is declared, the information must be placed on the label immediately adjacent to the statement on fat content; when cholesterol content is declared, the information must immediately follow the statement on fat content—and fatty acid content, if stated.)

Protein, vitamins, and minerals as percentages of the U.S. RDAs. (No claim may be made that a food is a significant source of a nutrient unless it provides at least 10 percent of the U.S. RDA of that nutrient in a serving. No claim may be made that a food is nutritionally superior to another food unless it contains at least 10 percent more of the U.S. RDA of the claimed nutrient per serving.)

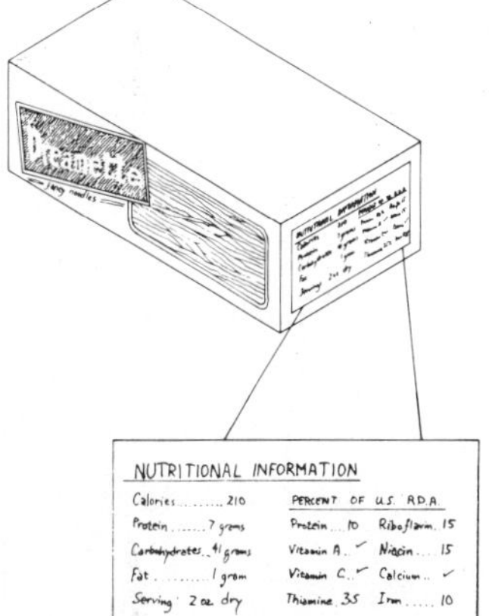

The nutrition information panel must always be on the right side from the front of the package.

Knowing these labeling laws can help you, the buyer, to "see" the inside of the packages you pick up in the store. If the package simply says "breaded fish sticks" or "lima beans," you can read the ingredients on the panel and glean a lot of information. Looking up the ingredients (fish, enriched bread crumbs, and so on) in a table of food composition like the one in this book (Appendix H) will tell you what nutrients are present.

If a nutritional claim is made on the label, or if something has been added to the food, then the full nutrition information panel must appear and you can find out exactly how many calories and what amounts of the nutrients are present. To fully understand the meaning, you must be able to interpret statements about vitamins and minerals made in terms of the U.S. RDA, which are not quite the same as the RDA.

The U.S. RDAs, as explained in an earlier chapter, were designed from the RDA tables of 1968 for the purpose of labeling. The RDA tables have different recommendations for each age group. But for the U.S. RDA, it was decided to use one recommended amount for each nutrient: whichever was the highest in the RDA tables (not counting those for pregnant and lactating women, whose needs are too high to use as a general standard). Thus, in picking a U.S. RDA for iron, the decision makers chose the woman's RDA of 18 milligrams, which is higher than that for any other group. In setting a U.S. RDA for magnesium, they chose 400 milligrams—the RDA of males aged fifteen to eighteen—because it is the highest RDA for any age group. The only exceptions were for calcium and phosphorus—set a little lower than the very highest because needs vary so widely—and for four nutrients that did not appear in the RDA tables of 1968: biotin, pantothenic acid, copper, and zinc. These were already known to be essential for human beings, and so tentative amounts were set for them in order to enable manufacturers to list them if they wished. RDAs have since been set for these four nutrients; they are not different enough from the 1968 estimates to cause concern, and so they have not been changed.

The U.S. RDAs include two values for protein. If the protein is of high quality, less is needed, and the U.S. RDA is 45 grams. If it is of lower quality, then the U.S. RDA is 65 grams. This rule enables the consumer to "buy protein" in appropriate amounts, without having to understand how protein quality is evaluated.

The table of U.S. RDA shows that there are actually four different U.S. RDAs. The set of figures in the third column is the one used on most labels. This set expresses the nutrient contents of foods in terms of the allowances for adults and children four years of age and older. The other three are for products intended for special categories of people: infants under one year of age, children under four, and pregnant or lactating women.

The four sets of U.S. RDAs have survived much court litigation in which many other labeling proposals have fallen by the wayside. The U.S. RDA for adults promises to be the standard on nutrition labels for years to come and is the single set of figures best understood by the public. The more varied and specific RDA figures will continue to be used for research.

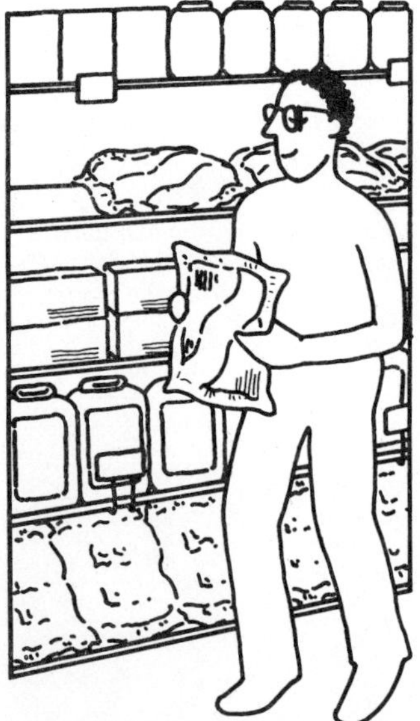

The U.S. RDAs make labels more understandable. The table of the U.S. RDA is on the inside back cover.

In the years since 1968, when the U.S. RDAs were designed, the RDA tables have been revised three times, and the values for most of the nutrients have changed somewhat in accordance with new information emerging from research. However, the U.S. RDAs have not been revised, for several reasons.

For one thing, the 1968 RDAs are generally higher than the later versions, but they are safe to consume. The most likely mistake the public will make is to think of them as maximum amounts ("I must get *up to* 100 percent of the U.S. RDA")—so it's better to let them be a little high than a little low. For another thing, it would cost the industry a lot of money to relabel all the food packages now ready for distribution. A third reason is the confusion that would result for foods labeled as either "enriched" or "fortified." Nutrients inserted in a food at levels higher than 50 percent of the U.S. RDA have to be labeled as "supplements." If the U.S. RDAs were lowered to agree with the 1980 RDAs, some "enriched" and "fortified" foods would end up as "supplements" and then would have to comply with further regulations and definitions. Whenever new regulations are costly to industry, the cost is borne ultimately by the consumer. The FDA did not believe that changing the U.S. RDA would result in a benefit that was worth the rise in price.

With this understanding of the U.S. RDA you can extract a lot of information from a nutrition label. If you just want to know generally what amounts of nutrients are in the package, the percent-of-U.S.-RDA will tell you that without your having to do any calculating. If you read, for example, that a serving of breakfast cereal provides "Vitamin A—25 percent," then you can be sure it provides at least a quarter of *your* vitamin A allowance for a day (unless you are pregnant or lactating). If you want to know exactly how many units of vitamin A are in a serving, you can look at the U.S. RDA table (inside back cover), find out that the U.S. RDA is 5000 IU, and figure 25 percent (a quarter) of that is 1250 IU.[6] For the nutrients included in the RDA tables, then, all the information that most consumers might want is available on a nutrition label.

U.S. RDA—inside back cover.

Labeling laws also require that any food claiming to be "low in calories" must state the absolute number of calories per serving. Any food calling itself a "reduced calorie" food must be at least a third lower in calories than the food it most closely resembles and must carry a nutrition label. Furthermore, wherever additives are listed on labels, their functions must be stated.

The information just presented helps you with ordinary foods labeled "fish" or "beans" and with foods that present information panels, like breakfast cereals. But what about foods that simply say "TV dinner" or "macaroni and cheese"?

Nutrients in convenience foods. The FDA has devised guidelines for the nutrient contents of many kinds of convenience foods: frozen dinners, breakfast cereals, meal replacements, noncarbonated vitamin C-fortified fruit- or vegetable-type beverages, and main dishes such as macaroni and cheese or pizza. If a product complies with the nutritional quality guidelines, it may carry on its label the statement that it "provides nutrients in amounts appropriate for this class of food as determined by the U.S. government." For example, frozen dinners must contain one or more sources of protein from meat, poultry, fish, cheese, or eggs, and these must make up at least 70 percent of the total protein; they must include one or more vegetables or vegetable mixtures other than potatoes, rice, or cereal-based products; and they must have a certain minimum nutrient level for each 100 calories, as shown in the accompanying table. Thus, the important concept of nutrient density (nutrients per calorie cost) is beginning to be conveyed on labels.

Required Nutrient Content of Highly Processed Foods, Such as Frozen Dinners

Nutrient	For Each 100 Calories	Total Nutrient in Package[a]
Protein (g)	4.60	16.0
Vitamin A (IU)	150.00	520.0
Thiamin (mg)	0.05	0.2
Riboflavin (mg)	0.06	0.2
Niacin (mg)	0.99	3.4
Pantothenic acid (mg)	0.32	1.1
Vitamin B_6 (mg)	0.15	0.5
Vitamin B_{12} (μg)	0.33	1.1
Iron (mg)	0.62	2.2

The package must contain these minimum amounts of nutrients regardless of the number of calories.

What if the label says nothing more than a name, such as *mayonnaise*? The Food, Drug, and Cosmetic Act of 1938 gave some items **Standards of Identity** and excused them from the requirement to list ingredients. Standards of Identity exist for such foods as bread and mayonnaise—common foods that at that time were often prepared at home, so that the basic recipe was understood by almost everyone. Certain ingredients must be present in a specific percentage before the food may use the standard name. Any product like mayonnaise, for example, may use that name on the label only if it contains 65 percent by weight of vegetable oil, either vinegar or lemon juice, and egg yolk. The FDA does not have the authority to require that ingredients be listed for these foods, but it urges manufacturers to give the consumer more detailed information, and many manufacturers do so voluntarily.

Imitation foods. Still another class of foods that concerns consumers includes foods developed in imitation of, and as substitutes for, familiar foods. A section of the original Food, Drug, and Cosmetic Act of 1938 required that, if a food is an imitation of a traditional food, this fact must be stated on its label. With the new food technology, however, many imitation food products on the market may very well be superior to traditional foods; it is misleading to the consumer to imply that they are inferior. For this reason, the regulation now requires that the word *imitation* must be used on the label only if the product is "a substitute for and resembles another food but is nutritionally inferior to the food imitated. . . . Nutritional inferiority is defined as a reduction in the content of an essential vitamin or mineral or of protein that amounts to 10 percent or more of the U.S. RDA."

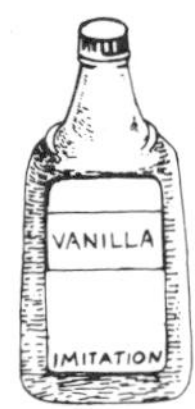

If a food is nutritionally inferior to the food it imitates, it must say "imitation."

Thus, if you read *imitation* on a food label, you may conclude that it is a poor imitation nutritionally. This may be of no consequence when the food is an incidental item in your diet, like vanilla, because you do not depend on vanilla for any nutrients. But if—for example—it's a fruit drink that you use daily, and if you usually include no other items from the fruit and vegetable group in your diet, then the label may alert you to a needed change.

Coping with the new foods. The understandings won from learning to read labels can help you to mix and match new and traditional foods to your advantage. "You are not a bad mother if you use a cake mix!" So says the American Council on Science and Health.[7] Less humorously, Dr. Howard Appledorf, professor of nutrition at the University of Florida, says, "Franchise fast-food meals can be an acceptable source of nutrition."[8] And Dr. Daniel Rosenfield, director of Nutrition Affairs, Miles Laboratories, says that even an imitation food, while inferior to conventional foods by a legal definition, might have desirably lower levels of some compounds and might be nutritionally superior.[9]

Many people fear that the new foods are inferior, however. Some are so put off by them that they try to avoid them altogether. Most use them with mixed feelings; the pleasure of the really delightful taste sensations sometimes offered is tainted with anxiety and guilt. (Some don't even think about it, of course.) Whatever your feelings on the subject, the chances are that you can't escape the new foods altogether. They are part of modern life, and in many ways a very desirable part. They are easy to store and prepare, they save a tremendous amount of time and energy, and they are often tasty to eat. Formulated foods used in school lunches are acceptable to children, who waste less of them, and they are lower in cost than conventional foods.[10] They have won wide acceptance in institutional settings as well as by homemakers and individual consumers, and their use is on the rise.[11] Rather than trying to avoid them altogether, it makes sense to learn to use them to your advantage.

In 1940, there were 1,000 food products on the market in North America. By 1965, the number had risen to 6,000, and in 1975 the figure was probably 12,000.
—P. R. Lee

Not all are of equal value, of course. A substitute for hamburger made from textured soy protein, soy flour, wheat germ, and artificial flavors and colors may be lower in fat, higher in fiber, and equal in protein quality to a hamburger—that is, superior for some purposes. On the other hand, a TV dinner may cost twice as much as, and provide fewer nutrients than, the same meal prepared from the raw materials at home; and a fast-food meal may be three times as expensive as its home-made equivalent. The habitual use of a fortified breakfast cereal may prevent iron deficiency in a woman whose calorie intake is low, while the use of toasted, jam-filled, unenriched pastries for breakfast by her children may dilute the nutrients in their day's menus.

A strategy for dealing with the new foods is based on several principles. First, ask yourself how often you eat the food in question. The more often you use a food product, the more impact it will have on your diet, and the more important it is to be aware of the contributions it is, or isn't, making. Second, when you consider its nutrient contributions you must do so in the context of the other foods in your diet. For example, the lack of vitamin C in the potato chips you eat is of no concern to you if you drink plenty of fruit juice, especially citrus juice, every day. But if you are relying on a food as a staple, to provide the nutrients usually contributed by a class of similar foods—for example, if you are regularly using a meat substitute in place of meat or soy milk instead of milk—then you owe it to yourself to be sure that the substitute is nutritionally similar to the missing food and is of high quality. Third, you should keep the calories in mind. No matter how attractive, if a food you often use donates more calories than you can afford to consume, you have a hard fact to face up to.

Finally, put the spotlight on yourself. No matter how nutritious the food you eat, it cannot compensate for other flaws in your lifestyle. A balanced, health-oriented approach to life including adequate rest, some exercise, and adequate time for appropriately timed meals will pay off in dividends no selection of foods by itself can offer you. Within such a context, common sense should help you to avoid unnecessary extremes. It is possibly true that you should try to include foods that contribute vitamin C in every day's meals. On the other hand, the idea that you should always eat farm-fresh foods, sitting down, with a placemat under your plate, may reflect a set of values that you may or may not wish to call your own. Drinking your breakfast or bringing home your family's dinner in a bucket can be part of a satisfactory nutrition picture and of a lifestyle that you find comfortable and acceptable. For ourselves, it seems appropriate to draw the line where adequate, balanced, and safe nutrition is achieved and to be open-minded about all other options.

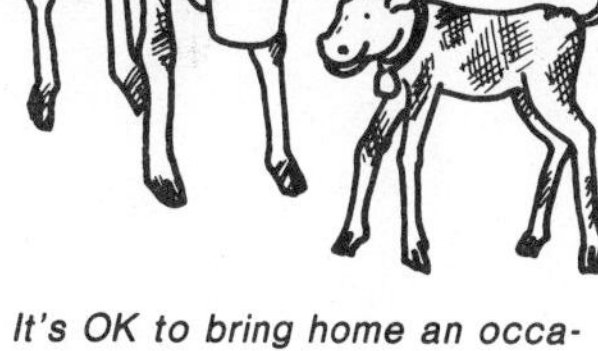

It's OK to bring home an occasional dinner in a bucket.

Present Concerns about Labeling

Up to this point you have learned you can tell from a food label:

What the ingredients are.

Whether anything has been added.

The number of calories.

Often you can also tell:

> The amount of protein, fat, and carbohydrate and of the vitamins and minerals listed in the RDA tables.

You also have a feel for the nutrient contributions that are made by processed and convenience foods and by imitation foods. But the discerning reader may still ask, "Is this enough information? What else do I need to know?" The question is worthwhile, because nutrition-minded people are still concerned about several aspects of food labeling. For one thing, despite all the regulations forbidding false claims, labels can still be misleading. For another, foods labeled "fortified" may not be as nutritious as they appear to be. A third concern has to do with the sugar and salt in processed foods.

Misleading labels. As they presently appear, food labels provide useful information. The listing of calories alone serves as a stimulus to better weight control by people who need to watch their weight. The listing of ingredients, nutrients, and additives helps educate the public in nutrition and provides motivation to food producers to make their products not only tasty, attractive, convenient, and low in cost but also nutritious. But labels still can be improved. The need is not to add more in-depth nutrient analysis (this would be expensive and most people don't use all the information on the label anyway), but to make nutrition information still more clear and easy to understand.

A survey of the membership of the Society for Nutrition Education found widespread agreement that food advertising can give consumers useful nutrition information and that advertisers should be permitted to make their claims on labels. The people who responded to the survey felt, furthermore, that the claims should continue to be stated in terms of the U.S. RDA. But most of them also were of the opinion that consumers must be well informed if they are not to be taken in.[12]

According to the survey, the law still allows loopholes through which can slip certain kinds of true but misleading claims. You might be interested in trying your own skill at selecting from the following the two claims that are misleading even though true (all three claims are true):

(1) A label says one serving of the food in the package provides thirty-five times as much iron as an 8-ounce glass of whole milk.

(2) A label says a fortified fruit drink contains "more vitamin C than fresh orange juice."

(3) A label says that a brand of instant nonfat dry milk has "all the calcium, protein, B vitamins of whole milk."

Check this chapter's Notes for the answers.[13] Two other ways a consumer might be led off the track are when:

(4) A label claims that an artificially constituted food or dietary supplement contains all of the vitamins and minerals known to be essential in human nutrition, in amounts equal to the U.S. RDA wherever this has been established. This implies a completeness that may be overestimated. A critic points out that "it is often not appreciated that we really do not know everything that should be included in artificially constituted foods."[14]

(5) A breakfast bar or snack food label gives nutrition information showing that the protein, fat, carbohydrate, and certain vitamin and mineral contents are the same as those found in a milk, egg, and toast breakfast with orange juice. This fails to mention that the carbohydrate is sugar (versus the complex carbohydrate in toast), that the fat is saturated fat (versus the oil the egg might have been fried in), or that there is considerable salt in the food. Proposals under consideration for new labeling laws would require listing added sugar and salt in a prominent place on the label.

Consumers are putting pressure on legislatures to provide labeling laws that will make such misleading claims illegal.

Of particular concern to us, with the advent of nutrition labeling, is that the average consumer may be led to feel that all he needs to do is consume something that provides "100 percent of his daily requirements" and he can forget about nutrition.—D. M. Hegsted

"Fortified" versus "nutritious" foods. Another area of concern has to do with the addition of nutrients to foods. Earlier, this chapter quoted the accusation that "nutrition labeling is an inducement for manufacturers to make whatever junk they like and add some vitamins and minerals to make [it] look extremely nutritious." Debate centers around this accusation and around the question of how nutrition labeling should be regulated to prevent this kind of hoax.

To understand the issue, recall that the nutrients that have to be listed on labels that make nutritional claims are only a few of the essential nutrients and are in no way more important than the unlisted nutrients. It is as if the state of your wardrobe were measured by counting the number of items of jewelry you own, and ignoring all your clothes and shoes. Another person who had nothing at all in his clothes closet could make himself appear to be better equipped than you simply by displaying more jewels. This problem has been a theme throughout this book, from the first comparison made between an orange and a vitamin C pill. Many authorities have expressed concern about it in many ways. Some of them are quoted in the margin.

The regulations do not require the listing of the remaining 12 nutrients for which U.S. RDAs have been established or the many other nutrients essential to man . . . fortification can give consumers a false sense of nutritional security.—H. A. Dymsza

A desirable solution may be to relieve consumers of the burden of reading details on labels by allowing certain foods to state that they are nutritious. To accomplish this, the designers of the legislation will have to define the term *nutritious* very carefully. As you might expect, proposals make use of the concept of **nutrient density**.

It is naive to think that processors fortify foods mainly in order to deliver nutrients to the consumer. They fortify them because they can label and advertise them as fortified—and fortification sells.—E. N. Whitney

The object is to distinguish between nourishing foods—those that provide some nutrients besides calories—and *nutritious foods*, a term which requires a very precise definition. To identify a **nutritious food**, you have to consider two questions:

> How much of the nutrients does a serving of this food supply in relation to my need?
>
> How many calories does a serving supply in relation to my need?

Fortification of a food with one vitamin or mineral does not redeem a food that contains excessive amounts of sugar or fat or a potentially harmful food additive.—H. A. Guthrie

If the food supplies half of your daily allowance for a vitamin and at the same time only one-tenth of your daily allowance for calories, then it is a very good source of that vitamin. You could obtain a substantial quantity of the vitamin from it, at a low "calorie cost."

You can actually attach numbers to foods to express their nutritional quality, by scoring each nutrient against the calories in the foods. For example, if a serving of a food provides 30 percent of the RDA for vitamin C and 10 percent of the RDA for calories, then it gets a 30/10 score—or a 3—for vitamin C. A nutritious food could then be defined as a food that had a score of 1 or more for several nutrients or a score of 2 or more for, say, two nutrients.[15] Or, thinking of each nutrient separately, the food could be called a "poor" source of a nutrient if it had a score of less than 0.5 for that nutrient, "fair" if its score was between 0.5 and 0.9, and "adequate" if it had a score of 1 or above for the nutrient.[16]

Food labels of the future will be permitted to carry words like "good source of iron" or "nutritious food" if the legal definitions of these terms can be worked out. An important consideration, though, is that foods with nutrients *added* to them by fortification may appear to be more nutritious than they are. One proposal for the definition of the term *nutritious* carefully rules out the possibility:

> Such a term can be applied "only to foods derived directly or indirectly from animal or vegetable products which can be expected to supply small but important amounts of many other naturally occurring essential nutrients and which have not been fortified to levels more than 15 percent above those of their unprocessed forms."[17]

A nutritious food must provide more than just energy.—H. A. Guthrie

This proposal illustrates the kind of guidelines by which labels of the future may be simplified and by which you may measure the nutritional value of the foods you select for yourself. The scores to be given foods have been called the **NCBR (nutrient-calorie benefit ratio)** or **INQ (index of nutritional quality)**, and the details of how they will be calculated are still being worked out. But they all have the same objective: to help you distinguish between truly nutritious foods and those whose stated value is inflated. Recognizing nutrient density, you will be able to choose foods with greater sophistication than if you were simply to reject all processed foods and embrace all natural, unprocessed foods. An exercise in the use of this concept is presented in this chapter's Self-Study.

Sugar and salt. Another problem still to be resolved in nutrition labeling has to do with the amounts of sugar and salt in foods. Consumers want, and are entitled to, this information, but food producers are concerned that the labels not put them at an unfair disadvantage; so the exact requirements for labeling still have to be worked out. What should be called "sugar," for example: all monosaccharides and disaccharides, including those found naturally in the food; or all added sugars, including honey, corn syrup, and the like; or only added sucrose (see Controversy 4A)? How should sugar contents be listed: if in grams per serving, then the amount of sugar in a cola beverage will be seen to be more than that in a serving of sugar-coated cereal; but if sugar is stated in percent, then the amount in the cereal will appear very high because it isn't diluted by water. As for salt, should it be listed as salt or as sodium? Should just the added salt or sodium be listed, or should that occurring naturally in the food be included?

Whatever decisions are finally made, the labels that include this information will benefit consumers who wish to limit their intakes of these additives. It isn't enough to stop using the sugar bowl and the salt shaker, because only about one-third of your total intake of these items is self-selected that way. The other two-thirds are added to foods during processing. When you eat processed foods, your intake of these items is involuntary. That's why they were called *additives* above.

With the information so far presented, you are in a position to make some quite accurate judgments about what's in the foods you choose to use. But if you are very skeptical or anxious about foods you buy in the grocery store, you may still have questions:

> How do I know how many nutrients have been lost during the processing of this food?
>
> How do I know what harm may come to me from the additives and preservatives listed on the package?

These questions are addressed in the following sections.

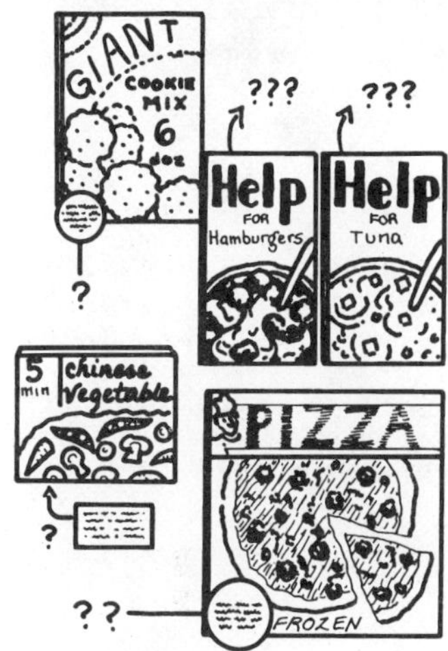

What's been lost from these foods? What's been added to them?

Nutrient Losses from Foods

If you are concerned about the effect processing has on food, you are not alone. The food industry has been responding to people's concern in recent years by paying increased attention to the nutritional quality of its products. This is a desirable trend in view of the fact that nearly two thirds of the foods we consume have been processed in some way.

People often wonder about the effects of the different kinds of processing. The question most often asked is "Which is most nutritious: fresh, canned, or frozen food?" Understanding the effects of food processing can help you buy and store foods so as to maximize their nutrient value. Some of the answers may surprise you. In general, food processing is a tradeoff, in the sense that it makes food safer and gives it a longer usable lifetime than fresh food, but at the cost of some vitamin and mineral losses. In some instances, however, processed food has the edge over its unprocessed counterpart, even in terms of nutritional quality.

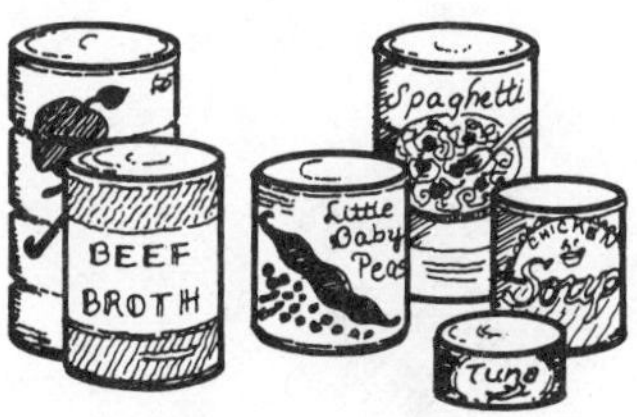

Canned foods are likely to be thiamin-poor.

Canning is one of the better methods for preserving food against the microbes (bacteria, fungi, and yeasts) that might otherwise spoil it, but canning unfortunately does diminish nutrient retention. Like other heat treatments, the canning process is based on time and temperature. Each small increase in temperature has a major killing effect on microbes with only a minor effect on nutrients. By contrast, long treatment times are costly in terms of nutrient losses. Therefore high-temperature-short-time (HTST) treatments are best for nutrient retention.

To answer the question how much of a food's nutritional value is lost in canning, food scientists have performed many experiments. They have paid particular attention to the three very vulnerable water-soluble vitamins, thiamin, riboflavin, and vitamin C. Acid stabilizes thiamin but heat rapidly destroys it; therefore the foods that lose the most thiamin during canning are the low acid (alkaline) foods like lima beans, corn, and meat. Appendix H shows that up to half, or even more, of the thiamin in these foods can be lost during canning.

To see the effect of canning on thiamin in foods, look at Appendix H, items 134 and 135 (3 ounces of raw claims vs 3 ounces of canned clams). Or check the thiamin in items 215 and 216 (1 cup green peas vs 1 cup canned green peas). While you're looking, what other effects of canning on thiamin do you see?

Unlike thamin, riboflavin is stable to heat, but is sensitive to light, so it is glass-packed, not canned, foods that are most likely to lose riboflavin. Vitamin C's special enemy is an enzyme (ascorbic acid oxidase) present in fruits and vegetables as well as in microorganisms. By destroying this enzyme, HTST processes such as canning actually aid in preserving vitamin C. As for the fat-soluble vitamins, they are relatively stable and are not affected much by canning.

Compare the riboflavin, vitamin C, and other vitamin contents of the items you just checked for thiamin. What's the greatest difference you find between the fresh and canned products? What's the average effect of canning on these nutrients (estimate), according to Appendix H?

Minerals are unaffected by heat processing because they can't be destroyed as vitamins can be, but they can of course be lost by leaking into water which is then thrown away. Losses are closely related to the extent to which tissues have been broken, cut, or chopped, and to the length of time the food is in water.

> The nutrient contents of canned foods are usually shown as "solids and liquids." If you throw away the liquid from a canned food, you are throwing away all the nutrients that have leaked into it. A bit of southern folk wisdom related to the cooking of "greens" (dark green vegetables) is to pour off the liquid and drink it rather than throwing it away; this is known as drinking the "pot liquor." The user of canned vegetables who can think of a way to use the "liquor"—for example by saving it to make soups, cook rice, or moisten casseroles—is displaying similar wisdom.

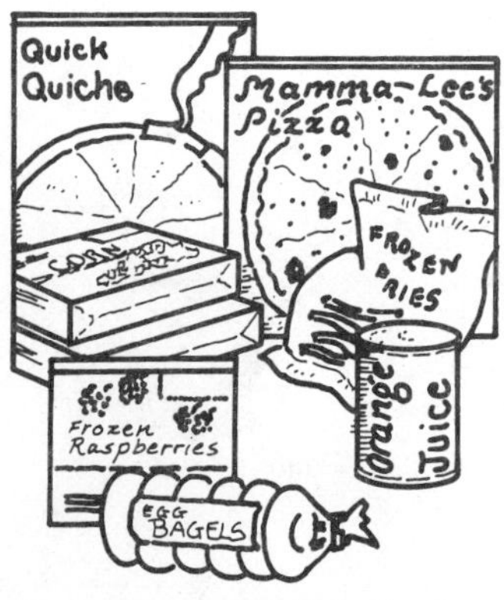

Frozen foods may lack vitamin C.

An alternative to canning, as a means of preserving food, is freezing. The freezing process itself does not destroy nutrients, but losses may occur during the steps taken in preparation for freezing such as blanching, washing, trimming, or grinding. Vitamin C losses are especially likely, because they occur whenever tissues are broken and exposed to air (oxygen destroys vitamin C). Uncut fruits, especially if they are acid, don't lose their vitamin C; strawberries, for example, may be kept frozen for over a year without losing any vitamin C.

An important point to remember in connection with freezing, however, is that to be really frozen, a food has to be kept at a temperature colder than 18°C or 0°F. Conversion of vitamin C to its inactive forms occurs rapidly at warmer temperatures. Food may seem frozen at 2°C, but much of it is actually unfrozen and enzyme-mediated changes can occur. Under these conditions, the vitamin C in a frozen food can be completely lost in as short a time as two months.

In general, for frozen foods, the lower the temperature the longer the storage life and the greater the nutrient retention. If you want to maximize the nutritive value of the foods you store at home, invest in a freezer thermometer and monitor the temperature of your frozen-food storage place. Freezing is an excellent way to preserve nutrients, and if foods are frozen and stored under proper conditions, they will often contain more nutrients when served at the table than fresh fruits and vegetables that have stayed in the produce department of the grocery store even for a day.

Canning and freezing are the most familiar, but not the only, processing methods common today; another is drying or dehydration. Advantages of these methods are that they eliminate microbial spoilage (microbes need water to grow) and greatly reduce the weight and volume of foods (because foods are mostly water). Furthermore, these processes don't incur major nutrient losses. Special types of drying, such as vacuum puff drying or freeze drying, are especially good for nutrient retention, as they allow the use of cold temperatures.

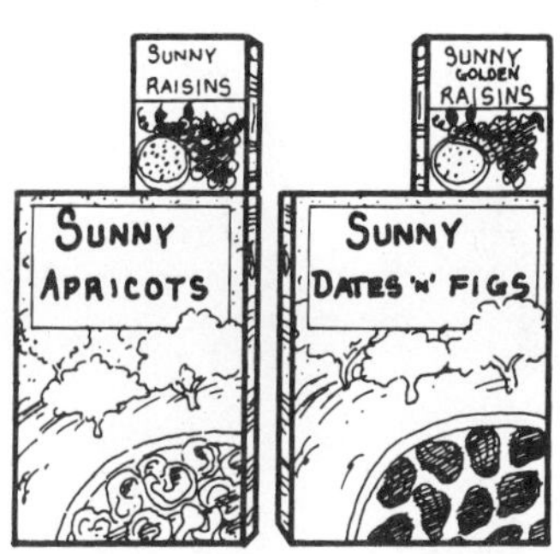

Dried fruits don't lose their original nutrients.

During the drying of fruits such as peaches, grapes (raisins), and plums (prunes), sulfur dioxide is added to prevent browning. Sulfur dioxide happens to help preserve vitamin C as well, but it is highly destructive of thiamin. The overall effect of its addition is probably beneficial, because most sulfured, dehydrated products are not major sources of thiamin anyway.

Some food products, particularly snack foods, have undergone a process known as extrusion. In this process, the food is heated, ground, and pushed through various kinds of screens to yield different shapes, usually bite-size or smaller, like the "bits" you sprinkle on salad. Considerable nutrient losses occur during extrusion processes, and nutrients are usually added to compensate. But foods this far removed from the original fresh state may still be lacking significant nutrients, and should not be relied on as major components of the diet (staples). A better way to make use of them is to enjoy them in moderation as snacks and to add them to foods to enhance the appearance, taste, and variety of meals.

These pointers have answered the specific questions people most often ask about processed foods. There is also a generalization you may find useful in selecting and preparing foods. As food quality (appearance, taste, and texture) deteriorates, there is often a corresponding deterioration in nutrient content. For example, when a food smells bad, the odor reveals that oxidative or enzymatic changes have occurred—the same kinds of reactions as those that have adverse effects on nutrients. Thus, some of the "natural" or unprocessed food sold in health food stores may be a poor choice in spite of the claims made for it. If it has lost its freshness, it may well have lost its vitamins too, because no processing means no measures have been taken to prevent oxidative and enzymatic changes. Thus your "sixth sense," which tells you that a food "doesn't look quite right" can be trusted to give you true information.

In modern commercial processing, losses of vitamins seldom exceed 25 percent. In contrast, losses in food preparation at home can be 100 percent, and it is not unusual to see losses in the 60-75 percent range. These facts put the matter of food processing into perspective and reveal that what you buy, in the way of food, makes a difference, but what you do with it in your kitchen makes considerably more difference. The Food Feature in Chapter 9 was devoted to the home preparation of nutritious foods.

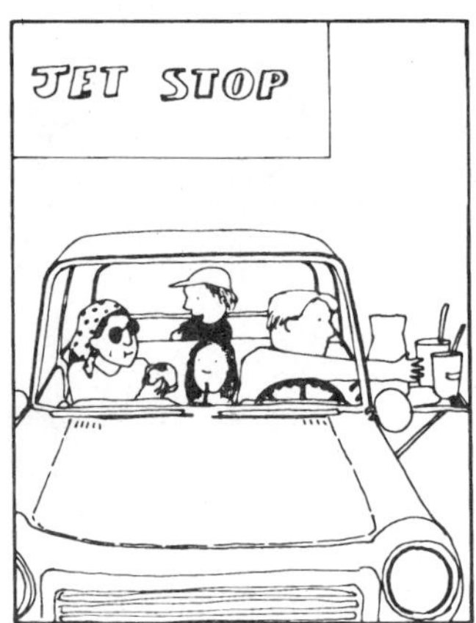

The average U.S. family eats fast food once a week.

Food Feature: Eating Out

So far, this chapter has dealt almost exclusively with foods you buy and cook at home—even if to "cook" means nothing more than to "add water and stir." But if you are like most people you also eat out, perhaps often. What should the nutrition-minded consumer of meals prepared outside the home look out for? Let's begin with the foods typical of fast-paced, modern life: the fast foods.

It won't surprise you to be reminded that the first question to ask about your use of fast foods is, "How often do I use them?" Apparently the average U.S. family visits a fast-food drive-in type of restaurant only a little more often than once a week. This being the case, the food consumed there accounts for only about one meal out of fifteen or twenty and has very little impact on the family's over-all diet. When you do visit a fast-food place, however, you have little choice but to buy a meal more than adequate in protein, several of the B vitamins, and iron. (That's the good news.)

There is more good news. Surprisingly, fast-food meals are not as high in fat as people think. In some, the percentage of calories provided by fat is lower than 35 percent (30 percent is thought to be ideal), and in all but a few it's lower than the 1970s' national average of 42 percent.[18] But if you frequent fast-food places often, here are some hints you may find useful (with a little bad news thrown in):

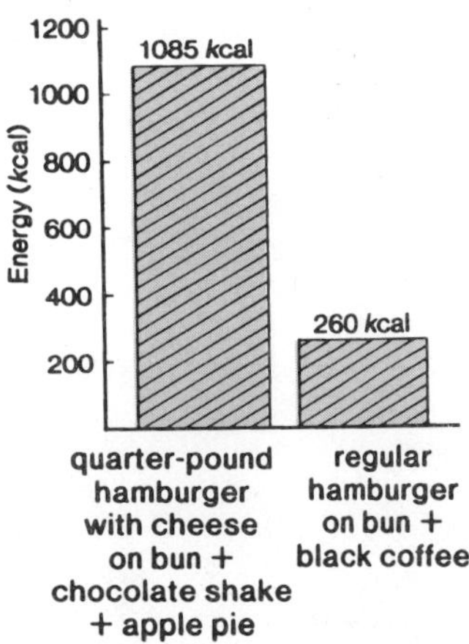

You have to choose carefully to limit calories in a fast-food meal.

The meals are likely to be low in calcium. Choose a milkshake for your beverage or (if you can't afford the calories) make sure to include milk or milk products in your other meals for the day.

They are almost invariably low in vitamin A and folacin. The little leaf of lettuce and slice of tomato provided in a typical fast-food meal don't make a dent on your need for these nutrients. Your next meal should be a large, raw salad or should include a generous serving of dark green vegetables.

They are regrettably high in sodium—so high, in fact, that people on sodium-restricted diets have to stay away from them altogether.

It is possible to vary your calorie intakes widely in a fast-food place (see margin). For women and children, and for men whose energy allowances are low, it's important to learn which are the lower-calorie selections. (You can actually diet and lose weight while using fast foods as part of your diet plan, if you put your mind to it.)

You can find out the calorie values of fast foods from Appendix G. Some fast food meals have been translated into exchanges in Appendix L.

Finally, because they are short on variety, let them be part of a lifestyle in which they complement the other parts. Eat differently, often, elsewhere.

These few suggestions illustrate several points that can be applied to your use of all foods—not just the fast foods. A habit to cultivate is to ask "what's missing?" If you don't think in terms of nutrients (and most people don't, even after taking a nutrition course), think in terms of food groups. Remember the Four Food Group Plan introduced in Chapter 2 and apply its principles here. In a fast-food place, three of the four food groups are well represented. The hamburger is as meaty as any meat can be; the milkshake (if you choose one) is a milk product as surely as is yogurt; and the grain group is represented by the enriched buns used by the franchises—so the only group missing is the fruit-and-vegetable group. You may not realize that vitamin A and folacin are in short supply, but if you think in terms of food groups, you don't need to know this. If you make a point of partaking of generous servings of fruits and vegetables (including dark green or deep orange ones, and some raw ones), at another time in the day, you will get your vitamin A and folacin with or without being conscious of that fact.

Another habit to cultivate is to keep the calories in mind, if calories are a problem for you. This may be an even bigger problem for the eater in a traditional restaurant than it is for the fast-food eater. It may be encouraging to know, however, that the abundance of calories is the only major problem associated with traditional restaurants. Otherwise, their meals—including those of the airlines, school cafeterias, and other such places—are likely to be very nutritious.[19] But restaurants very seldom offer low-calorie choices or small servings. The plate comes with either a large baked potato or a hefty serving of french fries. The vegetables often are swimming in butter. Sometimes no fruits or vegetables are available at all, and the bread-group choices range from pastries rich in sugar to biscuits high in fat. An adult who asks for a "child's plate" is told the restaurant will serve them only to children. Skim milk is seldom available.

Not all restaurants have these faults, and some people choose to avoid those that do. Consumers are learning to assert themselves more forcibly than they did in the past. One can order a plate without the potato, ask the chef to blot the vegetables before serving them, and always request the low-calorie alternatives in the hope that repeated demand will ultimately call forth a supply. Another strategy requires an effort that many consumers find mind-boggling: Leave some food on the plate. (It can be argued that obesity is caused not by restaurants but by obese people themselves.) With practice, you can maximize the benefits of eating out by adopting some of these strategies:

Look for soup and salad restaurants.

Order fruits, juices, vegetables, or salads whenever they are available. Ask for a vegetable plate even if it isn't on the menu as such.

Order from the appetizer or salad sections of the menu; skip the main dishes.

Ask for a "people bag" as soon as you get your food. Cut portions in half, eat half, and take home the other half to enjoy for lunch or supper the next day.

Order fish rather than steak, and ask that it be broiled, not fried.

Request whole-wheat or other whole-grain bread if given a choice, or refuse the bread basket right away when you sit down, before it is brought to the table.

Choose baked potatoes rather than french fries.

Request margarine rather than butter or sour cream for your bread and potatoes or don't use the butter or use only small amounts. (Margarines have 35 calories per pat, just like butter, but most are higher in unsaturated fat.)

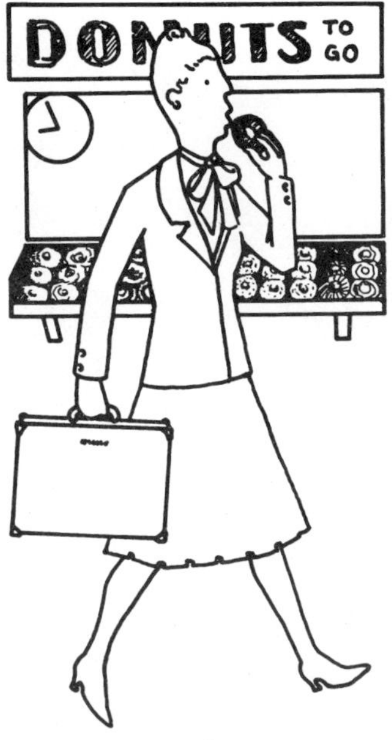

The hurry-up lifestyle may be bad for the health.

Request your salad dressing on the side, or request the salad dry with lemon juice. Ask for dishes without gravy or other sauces.

Leave food on the plate.

There is little question that eating out is a trade-off. One loses in cost and control, but gains in convenience and in pleasure.

That covers the subject of dining out adequately —as far as the foods are concerned. But the spotlight hasn't rested long enough on the most important character in the picture: the diner. While it is possible to find nutritious *foods* in abundance in our fast-food places and restaurants, we do not find well-nourished *people* in such abundance. One survey of 600 people who eat out showed that a fourth of them were lacking in one or more nutrients, that half of them were overweight, and that 20 percent of them were underweight. They had poor breakfast habits and tended to snack on nonnutritious foods, especially sweets and high-calorie foods. They suffered feelings of nausea, dizziness, and headaches before lunchtime and felt fatigued long before the day was over.

These findings suggest that there may be something wrong with eating out, after all. Perhaps persons who eat out depend on others to feed them to the extent that they don't take enough responsibility for seeing to their own needs. Perhaps eating out often is one of many parts of a hurry-up, stressful lifestyle in which attention to health has become a low-priority item. The professor of nutrition who published these findings, Dr. Roslin Alfin-Slater, suggests that the primary problem with these diners-out is that they haven't allowed time in their days to have breakfast.[20] No breakfast means early fatigue, low blood sugar, poor utilization of protein, more snacking later in the day, and overeating at later meals, especially if they are restaurant meals purposely prepared to tempt the appetite. When the spotlight falls on the diner, rather than on the foods served, it becomes clear where the responsibility really lies.

Additives

Controversies are raging over the **additives** in our food supply. On the one hand, articles and books are appearing that tell us we have the safest food supply in the world and shouldn't be concerned about all the furor raised by various consumer groups; on the other hand, scare stories are constantly in the news about the carcinogens or heavy metals that are being allowed to stay in foods because of pressure from Big Business. Many find that the more they read, the less clear the issues become. An apparently objective article on the work of the FDA, published in a reputable journal, turns out to be suspect because the author has been closely associated with the FDA and is now on the staff of a big food company.[21] Moreover, those who want to know what the pure scientists are finding in their laboratories about pollutants, toxicants, carcinogens, or additives are likely to be overwhelmed by the amount of reading involved, because each report deals with only one additive, and there are thousands of additives to consider. Furthermore, there are interactions between additives and nutrients and endless other complications. The best that a textbook in nutrition can do under these circumstances is to define the terminology, to give a brief summary of the laws as they are presently stated, and to clarify some of the issues.

Terminology. Intentional food additives are substances purposely put into foods to give them some desirable characteristic: color, flavor, texture, stability, or resistance to spoilage. Some additives are nutrients added to foods to increase their nutritional value, such as vitamin C added to fruit drinks or potassium iodide added to salt. The most common ones, roughly in order of the quantities used, are listed in the accompanying miniglossary. In addition, there are numerous additives used in still smaller quantities for miscellaneous other purposes.

Incidental food additives are those that get into foods by accident from packaging materials or during processing. Unlike intentional food additives, these are not listed on labels.

Intentional Food Additives

Emulsifiers, stabilizers, thickeners To give texture, smoothness, or other desired consistencies.
Nutrients To improve nutritive value.
Flavoring agents To add or enhance flavor.
Leavening (neutralizing) agents To control acidity or alkalinity.
Preservatives, antioxidants, sequestrants, antimyotic agents To prevent spoilage, rancidity of fats, and microbial growth.
Coloring agents To increase acceptability and attractiveness.
Bleaches To whiten foods such as flour and cheese and to speed up the maturing of cheese.
Humectants, anticaking agents To retain moisture in some foods and to keep others (such as salts and powders) free-flowing.

Regulations governing additives. Consumer demand and government responsibility necessitate that the additives be tested under the conditions and in the amounts in which they are used and that their safety be assessed. The agency charged with this responsibility is the Food and Drug Administration (FDA), and it in turn depends on an alert and informed public. The consumer's responsibility is written into the provisions for adding new substances to the list of additives deemed safe. The 1958 Food Additives Amendment to the Food, Drug, and Cosmetic Act requires that, if food processors wish to add a substance to a food, they must "submit a petition to FDA, accompanied by extensive information on chemistry, use, function, and safety." At public hearings, testimony for and against the substance being added to the food is presented by qualified people. If such a careful review shows that the substance is safe, the FDA will authorize its use under specific conditions.

The responsibilities of the FDA are described in Controversy 11A.

When the Additives Amendment was passed, many substances were exempted from complying with this procedure because there were no known hazards in their use at the time. They were put on what is known as the **GRAS (generally recognized as safe) list**. Any time substantial scientific evidence or public outcry questions the safety of any of the substances on the GRAS list, a special reevaluation is made. Recently the entire GRAS list has been reevaluated and all substances about which any legitimate question was raised have been removed or reclassified.

One of the criteria an additive must meet to be placed on the GRAS list is that it must not have been found to be a **carcinogen** (a cancer-causing agent) in any test on animals or humans. The **Delaney Clause** of the Additives Amendment of 1958 is uncompromising in addressing carcinogens in food and drugs. It states that "no additive shall be deemed safe if it is found to induce cancer when ingested by man or animal."[22]

In recent years, the Delaney Clause has come under fire for not allowing for the different effects on the body of varying dose levels. For example, when the artificial sweetener cyclamate was banned in 1969, it was estimated that a human would have to drink at least 138 12-ounce bottles a day of soft drinks containing cyclamates to ingest an amount of cyclamate comparable to the quantity given animals in the tests that caused the ban.[23] The FDA was criticized for banning the use of cyclamates, but under the law it had no other alternative. It doesn't have the right to make a judgment on dose levels of carcinogens or on the applicability of animal research to humans or even on the reproducibility of an experiment.

The arguments about saccharin are summed up in Controversy 11B, and there's about hyperactivity in Controversy 13.

At present, a similar controversy centers on saccharin. The arguments and counterarguments are many and complex. Meanwhile, additives are also being accused of causing hyperactivity in children. This theory, promoted by Feingold, suggests that the parents of hyperactive children buy only foods that contain no additives. This would necessitate having additive-free foods identified as such on their labels —a measure the FDA says is entirely within the law. However, the question whether additives have any relationship to hyperactivity can probably be answered in the negative in almost all cases.

Incidental food additives, pesticides, and pollutants also fall within the province of the FDA, which must monitor them. It carries out this assignment by conducting a Market Basket Survey: finding the amount and kind of food eaten by a male teenager, buying these foods in the public market, dividing them into categories, and then chemically analyzing the categories for the presence and concentrations of these residues.

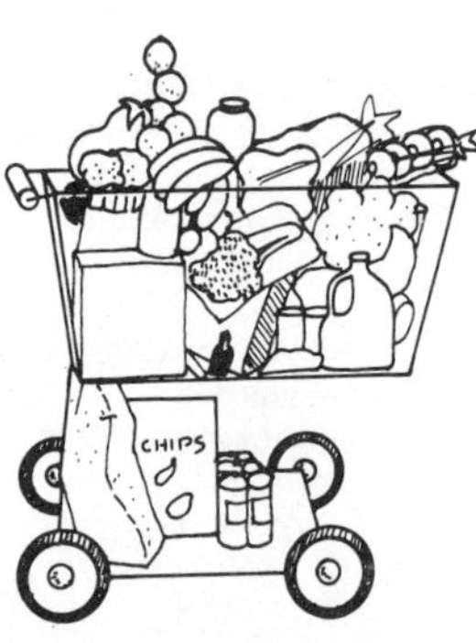

Market basket survey.

The public's fears about additives. Although accidents have happened and scare stories occasionally reflect inadequacies in consumer protection, the dangers associated with the intentional additives in our food supply have been exaggerated. This discussion attempts to present a reasonable and nonalarmist view of these additives in order to counter the scare tactics that have been used against them.

Profits are sometimes made by means of scare tactics. To give but one of hundreds of possible examples, *Nutrition Today* reported in 1975 that a "Sioux City, Iowa, firm is frightening shoppers into buying a product called 'Homaganized Bakon'—exact composition unrevealed except that it contains no nitrites or nitrates," implying that regular bacon would cause cancer.[24] The advertisement for this product appears in the margin. The editorial in that issue of *Nutrition Today*, one of many articles that demolish the panic arguments against additives, is recommended reading for anyone attempting to get a sense of perspective.[25] It concludes, "No one has the right to stand up in our perturbed and restless society and cry, without adequate cause, 'Cancer! Alarm! Cancer!'"

Cancer! Alarm! Cancer!
Here is a special health message!

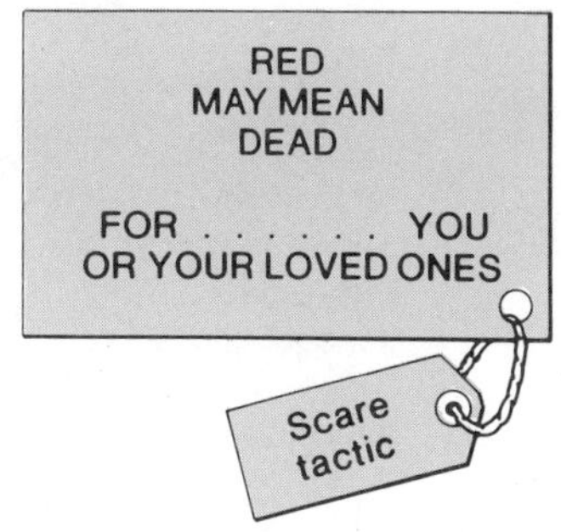

Unfair advertising.

People often ask whether additives are dangerous, and they are reassured to discover that additives are closely regulated by law and probably appear at safe levels in our foods. Later, they object with another doubting question: "But scare stories keep coming up all the time. Some additives really are dangerous. How can I tell which ones to avoid?"

The rest of this chapter presents the many shades of gray in which additives have to be viewed, and it should become apparent that in some cases the answers are still to come. However, there is one situation in which you can clearly discount a scare story: when it is paired with the profit motive. For example, the advertisers crying out, "Cancer! Alarm! Cancer!" were not publishing information for the benefit of the public; they were attempting to sell "Homaganized Bakon." Whenever such a motive clouds the picture, chances are good that the scare story is a fraud based on exaggerated and incomplete evidence.

By contrast, there are people and agencies whose objective in researching possible hazards is to protect the public. They earn their daily wages either way and have nothing (or at least less) to gain from shouting alarms. When a regulatory agency has investigated the possibility that an additive constitutes a hazard and has concluded that it does or does not, there may still be questions left unanswered, but the chances are better that the information made public represents an honest attempt to convey the facts.

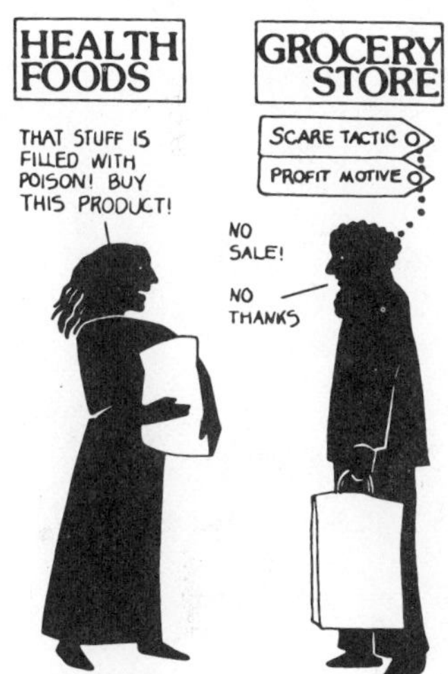
HEALTH FOODS
GROCERY STORE
THAT STUFF IS FILLED WITH POISON! BUY THIS PRODUCT!
SCARE TACTIC
PROFIT MOTIVE
NO SALE!
NO THANKS

The health food promoter capitalizes on the buyer's fears.

One reason for the public's sometimes unreasonable fear of additives is a generalized fear of anything "chemical" or "synthetic." Many deadly poisons are "natural" substances found in foods or produced by living organisms (consider mushrooms). Ironically, contrary to the public's suspicions, it is the processing of food and the introduction of additives that removes toxic substances, prevents the growth of dangerous microorganisms, and makes the food safe for our use. Foods are made of chemicals anyway, as the humorous display of Figure 1 demonstrates.

Another reason why the public has gotten scared about what's in foods is—ironically—that chemists are so much better at their jobs than they used to be, and the analytical techniques they use are so much more powerful than they were in the past. Where once they

Food is a fantastically complex mixture of chemicals, probably numbering in the hundreds of thousands.—F. M. Strong

Toast & Coffee Cake
Gluten
Amino acids
Amylose
Starches
Dextrins
Sucrose
Pentosans
Hexosans
Triglycerides
Monoglycerides and diglycerides
Sodium chloride
Phosphorus
Calcium
Iron
Thiamin (vitamin B_1)
Riboflavin (vitamin B_2)
Niacin
Pantothenic acid
Vitamin D
Methyl ethyl ketone
Acetic acid
Propionic acid
Butyric acid
Valeric acid
Caproic acid
Acetone
Diacetyl
Maltol
Ethyl acetate
Ethyl lactate

Scrambled Eggs
Ovalbumin
Conalbumin
Ovomucoid
Mucin
Globulins
Amino acids
Lipovitellin
Livetin
Cholesterol
Lecithin
Choline
Lipids (fats)
Fatty acids
Lutein
Zeaxanthine
Vitamin A
Biotin
Pantothenic acid
Riboflavin (vitamin B_2)
Thiamin (vitamin B_1)
Niacin
Pyridoxine (vitamin B_6)
Folic acid (folacin)
Cyanocobalamin (vitamin B_{12})
Sodium chloride
Iron
Calcium
Phosphorus

Chilled Cantaloupe
Starches
Cellulose
Pectin
Fructose
Sucrose
Glucose
Malic acid
Citric acid
Succinic acid
Anisyl propionate
Amyl acetate
Ascorbic acid (vitamin C)
B-carotene (vitamin A)
Riboflavin (vitamin B_2)
Thiamin (vitamin B_1)
Niacin
Phosphorus
Potassium

Coffee
Caffeine
Methanol
Ethanol
Butanol
Methylbutanol
Acetaldehyde
Methyl formate
Dimethyl sulfide
Propionaldehyde
Pyridine
Acetic acid
Furfural
Furfuryl alcohol
Acetone
Methyl acetate
Furan
Methylfuran
Diacetyl
Isoprene
Guaiacol
Hydrogen sulfide

Tea
Caffeine
Tannin
Butanol
Isoamyl alcohol
Hexanol
Phenyl ethyl alcohol
Benzyl alcohol
Geraniol
Quercetin
3-galloyl epicatechin
3-galloyl epigallocatechin

Sugar-Cured Ham
Myosin
Actomyosin
Myoglobin
Collagen
Elastin
Amino acids
Creatine
Lipids (fats)
Linoleic acid
Oleic acid
Lecithin
Cholesterol
Sucrose
Glucose
Pyroligneous acid
Phosphorus
Thiamin (vitamin B_1)
Riboflavin (vitamin B_2)
Niacin
Cyanocobalamin (vitamin B_{12})
Pyridoxine (vitamin B_6)
Sodium chloride
Iron
Magnesium
Potassium

Cinnamon Apple Chips
Pectin
Hemicellulose
Starches
Sucrose
Glucose
Fructose
Malic acid
Lactic acid
Citric acid
Succinic acid
Ascorbic acid (vitamin C)
B-carotene (vitamin A)
Cinnamyl alcohol
Cinnamic aldehyde
Potassium
Phosphorus
Acetaldehyde
Amyl formate
Amyl acetate
Amyl caproate
Geraniol

Good Morning

Your "Breakfast Chemicals"

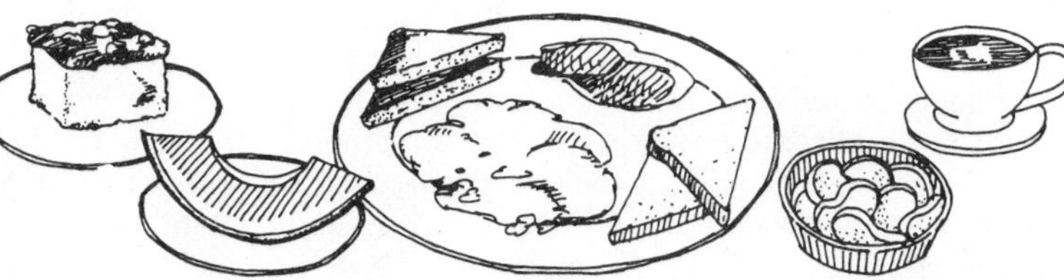

Figure 1. *These chemicals are found naturally in foods. There are no additives present! The chemical listings are not necessarily complete.*

Kindly supplied by the Manufacturing Chemists' Association.

would say there were no detectable levels of a substance in food "down to one part per million," now they have ways of detecting the same substance at one part per *billion.* This makes it seem as if new substances are appearing in our foods while in fact they may have been there all the time but are only now being seen. And the concentrations are so extremely low as to be insignificant. It is ironic, too, that the removal of substances from the GRAS list, which has improved the safety of those permitted, so alarmed the public that the effect seems to have been to make them mistrustful of the entire process. But the main reason for exaggerated alarm about additives is the public's failure to understand the difference between toxicity and hazard.

Toxicity versus hazard. "**Toxicity**—the capacity of a chemical substance to harm living organisms—is a general property of matter; **hazard** is the capacity of a chemical to produce injury under conditions of use. All substances are potentially toxic, but are hazardous only if consumed in sufficiently large quantities."[26] This distinction is readily accepted in other areas—such as air travel: "We fly in airplanes because they are 'safe,' but 'safe' is defined by the low number of deaths per million passenger miles, not the total absence of risk."[27] When chemicals are involved, however, there seems to be an added scare factor.

The consumer should be informed that it is virtually impossible to purchase any food items, including so-called "organic" products, that are totally free of food additives.—L. Peringian, N. Shier, and R. A. Leavitt

In 1975, the Commissioner of Food and Drugs put additives sixth and last among the "broad areas of hazard" with which the FDA was concerned. In order of concern, hazards within the FDA's areas of responsibility were

In the natural foods of our everyday diet there are thousands of toxic substances. This does not imply, however, that a hazard exists in this situation.—J. M. Coon

Food-borne infection, which is increasing because of large-scale operations and multiple transfers involving handling.

Nutrition, which requires close attention as more and more artificially constituted foods appear on the market.

Environmental contaminants, which are increasing yearly in number and concentration and whose consequences are difficult to foresee and forestall.

Naturally occurring toxicants in foods, which occur randomly in arbitrary levels and constitute a hazard whenever people turn to consuming single foods either by choice (fad diets) or by necessity (famine).

Pesticide residues.

Intentional food additives, listed last "because so much is known about them, and all are now, and surely will continue to be, well regulated."[28]

Deaths from food-borne infection can occur whenever batches of contaminated foods escape detection and are distributed. Close monitoring of processing, preparation, and distribution of food is extraordinarily effective, but individual consumers must be vigilant and knowledgeable in order to protect themselves against occasional hazards. Batch numbering makes it possible to recall all food items from a contaminated batch through public announcements on TV and radio.

Risk versus benefit. One of the reasons additives and pesticides are used is, of course, to protect against the spread of infection and food poisoning. Today's highly complex food industry could not have developed without the introduction of additives to ensure stability. Without them, it would be impossible to produce food in one part of the world and have it survive processing, packaging, transportation over great distances, and many months of storage before it is consumed. If these additives were suddenly eliminated, chaos and widespread starvation would result before another system could be evolved. The alternative to eliminating additives, it seems, is to find ways of ensuring that they are safe as used. Some examples will help to illustrate this point: nitrites, DES, and color additives.

Nitrites (for example, sodium nitrite) are added to meats such as bacon, ham, and hot dogs in order to prevent the organisms in them from producing their toxin. **Botulinum toxin** is the most potent biological poison known; an amount as tiny as a single crystal of salt can kill a person within an hour. Once the producing bacteria have released this toxin into a food, cooking won't destroy it, because it is stable at high temperatures. The risk of **botulism** is a hazard (remember the definition of hazard?); that is, it would be likely to occur under the normal conditions of use of these meats—were it not for the additive nitrite. No other additive is presently feasible for use that can effectively and safely prevent botulism.

Average U.S. Consumption of Nitrite per Person per Day

Source	Nitrite (μg)
Vegetables	198
Cured meat	2380
Saliva	8620

Adapted from R. J. Hickey and R. G. Clelland, Hazardous food additives: Nitrite and saliva? (correspondence), New England Journal of Medicine *298 (1978): 1036.*

More about nitrites—Controversy 11B.

On the other hand, there is a theoretical possibility that nitrites can combine with amines in the stomach to form **nitrosamines**, and these can cause cancer. But nitrites occur naturally in nutritious vegetables—and in the body's own saliva—in amounts much higher than those added to meats, so removing them from meats wouldn't effectively remove them from the food supply. Furthermore, the evidence is still not clear on whether they actually do form nitrosamines in the stomach.[29] Viewed in terms of risk versus benefit, their use appears to be justified. At present, we seem to have no better alternative.

On the other hand, when an additive constitutes a risk, no matter how small, that is not outweighed by the benefits, we can afford to do without it. An example is provided by **DES (diethyl stilbestrol)**, a hormone added to cattle feed to promote growth. DES can cause cancer. It was at first not detected in meats from cattle whose feed had contained it, but when tests became sensitive enough to detect it at extraordinarily low levels, its use was banned.[30]

Similarly, when the benefits from an additive are only esthetic, restrictions can be more stringent, as they are with color additives. Attractive colors in food add more appeal than their opponents may give them credit for, but their use is still "only" esthetic. "Today the abundance of our food supply permits the luxury of trying to avoid any and all risk. We can afford to seek the ideal of absolute safety."[31]

Where both benefits and risks are clearly identifiable, the problem is to "quantify risk" and to obtain "a workable definition of the word 'safe.'"[32] At present, the workable definition seems to be based on the concept of a **margin of safety**. Most additives that involve risk are allowed in foods only at levels 100 times below those at which the risk becomes a probability; their margin of safety is 100. Experiments to determine the extent of risk involve feeding test animals the substance at different concentrations throughout their lifetimes. The additive is then permitted in foods at 1/100 the level that can be fed under these conditions without causing any harmful effect whatever. In many foods, naturally occurring substances appear at levels such that the margin of safety is closer to 10. Even nutrients, as you have seen, involve risks at high dosage levels. The margin of safety for vitamins A and D is 25 to 40; it may be less than 10 in infants.[33] For some trace elements, it is about 5. Common table salt is consumed daily by people in amounts only 3 to 5 times less than those that cause serious toxicity.[34]

Salt, perhaps the oldest and most universally used food additive, is the only one known to be toxic under common conditions of use.—T. H. Jukes

Not only are the allowable concentrations of any potentially toxic substances extremely low, but the toxicities also are usually not additive. This is, if you dosed yourself with 100 different compounds, each at 1/100 of what would cause toxicity, you would still have 1/100 the toxic dose. Often there are antagonisms: "The toxicity of one element is offset by the presence of an adequate amount of another."[35] Food itself also protects against toxicity: Carbohydrate in the diet, giving rise to liver glycogen, assists the liver in detoxifying compounds delivered to it.[36] Fiber, amino acids, and trace minerals act to render other compounds harmless.[37] Not in all cases, but in many, combinations of additives are no more harmful than additives used singly, and may even be beneficial. Giving further reassurance, the FAO/WHO Expert Committee on Food Additives has concluded that "an increase in the number of food additives on a permitted list does not imply an over-all increase in the [total amount of] additives used; the different additives are largely used as alternatives . . . there is *less* likelihood of long exposure, or of high or cumulative dose levels being attained if a wide range of substances is available for use" (emphasis ours).[38]

Perspective on additives. From all of this information, it must be apparent that the intentional additives in foods have sometimes been unjustly accused. Understanding the concepts just presented will help to put the additives in perspective. In summary, they are:

All foods are composed of chemicals, even if they have no additives in them.

Additives that might be toxic do not constitute a hazard at the concentrations used.

Additives are allowed in foods only because they confer a benefit in comparison to which the risk, if any, is insignificant.

The presence of several additives in foods is not more hazardous than the presence of any one of them.

If rank-ordered among the problems related to the food supply, the risk from additives falls last below a number of more significant factors.

The value of a varied diet to ensure that the intake of essential nutrients will be adequate for good nutrition has long been accepted. We have now further emphasized the value of a varied diet to ensure that the intake of specific chemical substances in foods will be inadequate to cause injury.
—J. M. Coon

In conclusion, when a normal person eats a normal amount of food and gets sick from it, this is almost invariably because of food poisoning—known to be a hazard and guarded against as vigilantly as possible by our regulatory agencies. However, regulatory agencies can't enforce the washing of home kitchen utensils in hot soapy water with each use or the refrigeration of egg-milk dishes. Otherwise, harm from food almost always results from either abnormally large quantities of a food (as when someone eats tuna three times a day for a year) or from abnormality of the person (allergy, inborn error, or disease).[39]

People who are concerned about the levels of various additives and pollutants in the food supply would be well advised to eat as wide a variety of foods as possible so as to dilute the amount of any one substance. "The wider the variety of food intake, the greater the number of different chemical substances consumed, and the less is the chance that any one chemical will reach a hazardous level in the diet."[40]

It is probably clear from the above discussion that many alarmist views of additives are unjustified. However, there is still an open question that has to do with the long times of exposure to additives that humans experience in their lifetimes. One reviewer puts it this way:

> It is clear that the real challenge that we face is the question of the long-term chronic toxicity, or lifetime effects, of the . . . chemical components of our foods. Such effects that might result from ordinary patterns of consumption are of the greatest potential importance . . . the problem of [cancer] . . . reproductive functions, mutagenesis, cardiovascular-renal diseases, mental disorders and other chronic ills of mankind of which the causes are unknown.[41]

It is also important to point out that this discussion has not dealt with the pollutants and contaminants in foods. It is not yet known to what extent pollutants interact with one another and with nutrients to our possible harm. Some of the fears expressed by consumers about pollutants and toxicants in our food supply are probably unjustified. In some cases, a "new" pollutant arouses alarm; but the pollutant appears new only because modern, more sensitive techniques have enabled investigators to detect extremely small quantities of it. Still, it is on the whole too early to tell whether there are long-term toxic effects caused by food constituents' interacting with one another that will prove significant in the future.

This chapter has addressed three of the areas of greatest concern to today's consumers: the new foods, food labels, and additives. It is to be hoped that what you have read has alerted you to the main things to look for in choosing foods. One question that everyone seems to be asking and that has been a theme throughout this book is "Can a food that is not entirely natural be nutritious?" From what you have read, you might conclude correctly that the answer to this question is "Yes." Another is "Can a food that contains additives be safe?" The answer to this question seems to be yes, too. However, as you have seen, there is an element of judgment, born of learning about nutrition at a level deeper than the superficial, that qualifies both these statements. It seems that, in general, the more nearly a food resembles the original farm-grown animal or plant food from which it is derived, the more likely it is to be nutritious. As for foods with additives, it seems that we are well advised not to rely extremely heavily on any single food to the

exclusion of others—for many reasons, but partly because it is best to avoid accumulations of single additives not familiar to the body.[1]

For Further Information

Recommended references on all nutrition topics are listed in Appendix J. This chapter's notes and the references for the Controversies also contain many references selected for their interest to the general reader. In addition, we suggest the following.

A paperback, delightful to read, that explores these issues further and presents thirty wholesome recipes for "whole foods" (what here are called "farm-grown") is:

- Perl, L. *Junk Foods, Fast Food, Health Food. What America Eats and Why.* New York: Houghton Mifflin/Clarion Books, 1980.

An excellent cookbook of the same general kind was mentioned at the end of Controversy 1.

The best source for the general reader of the latest information on labeling laws, regulations governing additives, and all other areas under the province of the FDA is the *FDA Consumer* magazine, which comes out monthly. Your library probably subscribes, or you can get a subscription of your own (see Appendix J).

For the exact wording of the laws relating to the food supply and of proposals now under consideration, dig into the *Federal Register,* which arrives weekly at your library. Back issues may be found in the U.S. government documents section.

To size up the new foods and to get help in designing a healthful diet, the interested reader will find these useful:

- Fremes, R., and Sabry, Z. *Nutriscore: The Rate-Yourself Plan for Better Nutrition.* New York: Methuen/Two Continents, 1976 (paperback).
- Jacobson, M. F. *Nutrition Scoreboard.* New York: Avon Books, 1974 (paperback).

Consumer Reports frequently publishes evaluations of food products and comments about the additives in them. Although sometimes a trifle alarmist in tone, *CR*'s articles are often valuable because they have impact on the food producers to encourage them to watch over the quality of their products more closely than they might otherwise do.

For help in reading labels, many booklets are available. One we like is:

[1]*Chapter Notes can be found at the end of the Appendixes.*

- Inside information about the outside of the package. This pamphlet is available free from Pillsbury Company, 1177 Pillsbury Bldg., 608 Second Avenue South, Minneapolis, MN 55402.

A leaflet is available free from the American Medical Association to help you learn to prepare foods safely in your kitchen:

- Foodborne illness: The consumer's role in its prevention. Chicago: American Medical Association, 1976. The AMA's address is in Appendix J.

The two opposing views of the safety of additives can be viewed in:

- Hunter, B. T. *The Mirage of Safety*. New York: Scribner's, 1975.
- Whelan, E., and Stare, F. J. *Panic in the Pantry*. New York: Atheneum, 1975.

Short articles on additives that make interesting reading are:

- Hall, R. L. Food additives. *Nutrition Today*, July/August 1973, pp. 20-28.
- Hall, R. L. Safe at the plate. *Nutrition Today*, November/December 1977, pp. 6-9, 28-31. This one pokes fun at all the scare stories.
- Kermode, G. O. Food additives. *Scientific American* 226 (1972), pp. 15-21. This, although older, remains one of the sanest and most balanced views available in short form.

The Nutrition Today Society (address in Appendix J) makes available a teaching aid called *Additives*, by R. L. Hall, which includes a slide set and lecture outline.

Controversy 11A

Freedom of Choice

Is the FDA trying to take it away?

New FDA Commissioner: *I notice the FDA takes a lot of hard knocks in the newspapers. Is there ever any good news about the FDA?*

Outgoing Commissioner: *No, I can't recall any. However, there is sometimes bad news for which we don't get blamed.*

New Commissioner: *For instance?*

Old Commissioner: *Well, there's a report of botulism in borscht on the Trans-Siberian Railroad.*
—*New York Times*, March 12, 1977

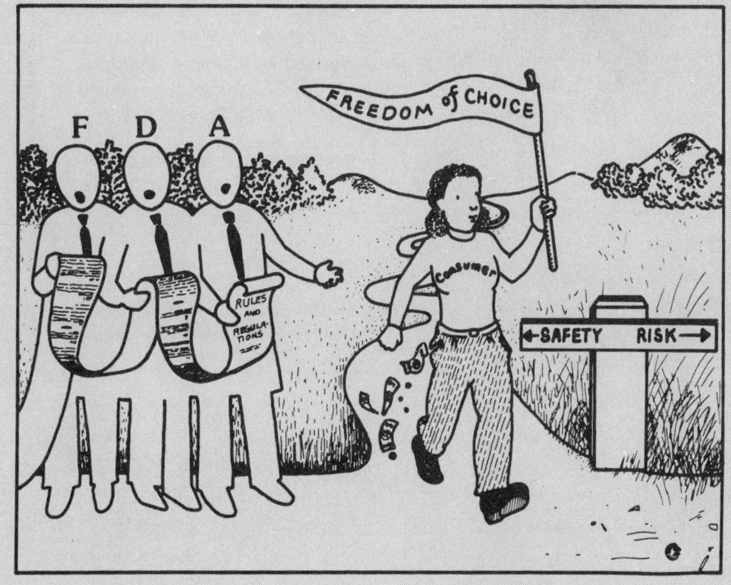

The Food and Drug Administration (FDA) is constantly being shot at from both sides. When it started to consider banning saccharin, consumers got angry because, they said, "You should have done it sooner." At the same time, the diet-food industry said "You shouldn't do it at all. Such an action is capricious, it is not based on scientific findings, it will cause undue alarm." When a new drug is first announced and the FDA is withholding approval pending the results of the final tests, consumers get angry because, they say, "You should do it sooner, the delay is costing lives." Yet those performing the tests insist, "No, wait until later—hurrying is what will cost lives."

So the FDA is in a bind. It has enormous responsibilities. It must ensure that "foods are safe and wholesome, drugs are safe and effective, household products are safe or carry adequate warning labels, and all of the above are honestly and informatively labeled and packaged for the consumer."[1] This involves taking care of the contents, packaging, and labeling of almost all food items except meat, poultry, and eggs (these are the province of USDA, the U.S. Department of Agriculture). In carrying out these responsibilities, the FDA must answer to food consumers—who are increasingly vocal and aggressive about the kind of protection they want. At the same time, it must not handicap industry by imposing so many regulations and such expense that it can't continue to provide safe and nutritious food at a reasonable cost to consumers. Not surprisingly, the FDA can't please everybody.

Miniglossary

adulterated: Contaminated. (Laetrile, for example, is often adulterated with the poison cyanide.)

amygdalin (ah-MIG-duh-lin): The "chemical" name given to laetrile by its promoters.

drug: The FDA has suggested that this term be used to identify foods or vitamin/mineral pills containing vitamins and/or minerals at levels above 150 percent of the U.S. RDA.

laetrile (LAY-uh-trill): A substance purified from apricot pits and advertised (fraudulently) as "vitamin B_{17}"

MDR (minimum daily requirement): A term once used on labels to express vitamin and mineral contents; it proved unsatisfactory because it did not accurately represent people's nutrient needs; now replaced by the more suitable terms, RDA (see Chapter 3) and U.S. RDA (see Chapter 11).

supplement: A term suggested by the FDA to identify foods fortified with vitamins and/or minerals at levels of from 50 percent to 150 percent of the U.S. RDA.

vitamin B_{17}: An alternative name for laetrile, not really a vitamin.

The sale of vitamins. The freedom of choice issue arose when the FDA took upon itself the responsibility of protecting consumers from overdosing on vitamins. Before making a proposal for regulation, the FDA studied the problem for about ten years. Then in the early 1970s it made several decisions. It adopted the U.S. RDA as a standard for labeling (see Chapter 11), believing that consumers would find this a more meaningful term than the MDR (minimum daily requirements) that had been used previously. Then, using the U.S. RDA, it attempted to distinguish among three classes of vitamin- and mineral-containing foods and pills. At this point, the FDA began stepping on several people's toes. Echoes are still resounding from their screams.

To see both sides of the issue, you first have to understand what the FDA was trying to do. It wanted to apply the term *food* to foods containing less than 50 percent of the U.S. RDA of any vitamin or mineral—one of the objectives being to prevent the sellers of "health foods" from claiming that they had any therapeutic (curative) value. It wanted to require the label *supplement* for any food (for example, a breakfast cereal) fortified with vitamins or minerals in amounts between 50 and 150 percent of the U.S. RDA—hoping that consumers would understand from this that in eating a serving of such a food they were, in effect, eating a high-calorie vitamin-mineral pill. And it wanted to attach the term *drug* to any vitamin or mineral being sold in amounts larger than 150 percent of the U.S. RDA per dose.

The health food people may not have liked their items being called mere *foods*, and the breakfast-cereal people may not have liked having to label some of their products *supplements*, but the people who were most upset were those selling and buying large doses of vitamins. Naming these items *drugs* would give the FDA the power to treat them as drugs under the law—and the law is much stricter about drugs than about supplements. If you are a drug you have to prove that you are both "safe" and "effective," and if you can't, then the FDA can take you off the market. The FDA didn't propose to do this with any vitamin or mineral, it only wanted to establish a Standard of Identity for them so that consumers would know what they were getting. But the opponents squawked anyway.

The vitamins the FDA was concerned about primarily were vitamins A and D. Overdosing with these is a real possibility, and as long as pills containing these vitamins in huge doses are available in health food stores and drug stores, many unknowing people are subjected to the risk. The FDA was not planning to take large-dose pills off the market altogether; in fact it was planning to let them be sold over the counter (except for A and D), but it wanted to make them stand up to standards of efficacy and safety, like drugs. A and D would be available too, but by prescription only so that people would have to check with their physicians before they could buy them. The opponents of the FDA's proposal cried out, "They are taking away our vitamins! . . . our freedom of choice!"[2] Actually, the FDA probably didn't have anything against the megadoser; it was merely trying to protect John Doe, the man on the street, who needs a guarantee that the nutrient supplements available are based on a scientifically rational formula. John Doe doesn't much care either way, but he could make a deadly mistake by taking the wrong bottle off the shelf.[3]

It was quite a hullaballoo, and it ended—after a lot of court cases—with a decision by the Senate to ratify the Proxmire bill, a bill that preserves the consumer's freedom of choice. It allows *no* limit to be set on:

The potency, number, combination, amount or variety

Table 1. Safe Doses of Vitamins and Minerals for the Prevention and Treatment of Deficiencies

Minerals	Vitamins
Calcium	**Vitamin C (ascorbic acid)**
For prevention only:	50–100 mg/day prevention
Adults, children 1–10, and 12 and over—400–800 mg/day	300–500 mg/day treatment
Children 10–12 and pregnant and lactating women—600–1,200 mg/day	**Niacin (niacinamide or niacinamide ascorbate)**
Adults over 51—500–1,000 mg/day	10–20 mg/day prevention
Infants 6 months to under 1 year—300–600 mg/day	25–50 mg/day treatment
Infants under 6 months—200–400 mg/day	**Vitamin B_6 (pyridoxine)**
	1.5–2.5 mg/day prevention
	7.5–25 mg/day treatment
Iron	**Vitamin B_2 (riboflavin)**
For prevention only:	1–2 mg/day prevention
Menstruating and lactating women—10–30 mg/day	5–25 mg/day treatment
Pregnant women—30–60 mg/day	**Vitamin B_1 (thiamin)**
Children 6 months to under 5 years—10–15 mg/day	1–2 mg/day prevention
In combination products other than for use in pregnancy: adults and children over 5—10–20 mg/day	5–25 mg/day treatment
	Vitamin A
	1,250–2,500 IU/day prevention
	5,000–10,000 IU/day treatment
Zinc	**Vitamin B_{12}**
For prevention only:	3–10 μg/day prevention
Adults, and children 1 year and over—10–25 mg/day	Not to be used to treat deficiency
Pregnant and lactating women—25 mg/day	**Folic acid (folacin)**
	0.1–1.4 mg/day prevention
	1.0 mg/day for pregnant and lactating women
	Not to be used to treat deficiency
	Vitamin D
	400 IU/day prevention, infants and growing children under 18 years of age
	200 IU/day prevention, adults
	Not to be used to treat deficiency

Adapted from A. Hecht, Vitamins over the counter: Take only when needed, FDA Consumer, *April 1979, pp. 17–19.*

of any synthetic or natural vitamin, mineral, or other nutritional substance or ingredient unless the amount recommended to be consumed is injurious to health.[4]

So now, if you want to know which vitamins are safe, you have to be educated (see Table 1). Meanwhile, you can buy vitamins in any amount you want to—and they are available in amounts up to 33,000 percent of the U.S. RDA.[5] The FDA has no authority to regulate the doses of over-the-counter nutrient supplements except for those designed for use by infants, children, and pregnant women. It is thus up to you to protect yourself from toxic overdoses. The only vitamin that can't be sold over the counter in doses well above the RDA is folacin, because of the risk it poses of delaying the diagnosis of pernicious anemia in vitamin B_{12}-deficient individuals. Even this regulation is resented by those who want to take, or persuade other people to take, massive doses of vitamins:

Nature put folic acid in the B complex but the FDA took it out.[6]

In summary, the freedom-of-choice people have it mostly their way when it comes to the sale of vitamins.

The laetrile furor. One of the angriest arguments over the FDA's authority has involved laetrile, the so-called "vitamin B_{17}" (see Controversy 9). In this situation, as in the fight over vitamins A and D, science and politics got tangled up together and politicians have ended up making decisions scientists wouldn't have made.

Laetrile (amygdalin) is a substance purified from apricot pits and praised by some as a cancer cure. (Its sister, "vitamin B_{15}," was featured in Controversy 9.) The scientific community had pretty well agreed by 1977 that laetrile was not only not a vitamin but was a "hazard," a substance that causes harm under the normal conditions of use. It was dubbed a "toxicant" because it contains the poison cyanide. The FDA had also concluded that laetrile was not effective in cancer treatment, and so it was banned from interstate commerce. But its proponents kept claiming that it was a nutrient, a vitamin. (If you are a vitamin, you don't have to prove that you are either safe or effective, remember.) Its opponents argued that its claim to be a vitamin was a "hoax." Finally, the courts determined that laetrile was an "adulterated food" and that its sale was a "fraud."[7] However, sales continue, and because the FDA has no control over the manufacture and distribution of laetrile, it can only warn the public against it. Batches that contain exceptionally high concentrations of cyanide can't be recalled because lot numbers are seldom used; when an adulterated sample is found there is no way of knowing which other samples came from the same batch.[8]

In this matter, too, the freedom-of-choice people have succeeded in keeping their product available against, under, and around the FDA's efforts to protect the consumer from adulterated foods, mislabeled foods and drugs, and drugs that are unsafe or ineffective. By December 1977, the use of laetrile was legal in twelve states, "despite the failure of those promoting its sale to comply with FDA standards for either safety or effectiveness."[9] Thus legislative action (political) overrode the FDA's (scientific) authority, and a scientific failure became a political success.[10] The FDA had suffered a body blow. An observer noted that the politicians had made it impossible for the FDA to protect the public against frauds and hazards.[11]

Continuing pressure forced the federal government to allocate half a million dollars for large-scale clinical tests of laetrile against the FDA's judgment that the tests would be a waste of public money. However, no alternative would meet the need for definitive, controlled studies of laetrile's effectiveness, and a final answer was urgently needed. In 1977, 50,000 cancer patients were consuming over a million grams of laetrile per month, a major medical and social problem.[12] In 1981 the answer was beginning to come through: Of 156 patients treated with laetrile under controlled conditions, none responded, and 104 died. But the battle was continuing. Laetrile advocates said the tests proved nothing, and twenty-three states were by then allowing the use of laetrile within their borders.[13]

The banning of additives. In 1969, the FDA banned the artificial sweetener cyclamate, because some tests had shown that cyclamate had the potential for causing cancer in human beings. Of the consumers who responded to the ban, the majority (87 percent) were grateful and cooperative. In 1977, when the FDA proposed banning the artificial sweetener saccharin on the same basis, only 16 percent were grateful, and almost half (47 percent) of those who responded felt that their individual rights were being interfered with.[14]

The FDA had no choice in either case; once tests provide evidence that a compound can cause cancer, the law requires that the compound be taken off the market. But taking away the sweetener saccharin would have left the consumer with no widely available, familiar noncaloric sweetener. Consumers wanted to be free to choose artificially sweetened products even if there was a risk of cancer involved. They didn't want to be protected so completely as to have no choice. They felt it was an individual matter.

Again, the FDA was caught in a crossfire and couldn't please everyone. The law required that saccharin be banned; the consumers demanded that it not be. Both were satisfied by means of a technicality: saccharin was banned, but the ban was suspended! The FDA Commissioner remarked in bewilderment:

"Freedom of choice" is used to argue for the legalization both of a substance that causes cancer (saccharin) and of another that does not prevent it (laetrile).[15]

One wag suggested that laetrile should be sold in saccharin-coated pills to make both safe![16]

You have the correct impression if you conclude from all of this that the issue of consumer protection is difficult and complex. The kinds of questions that have to be answered are:

- Should the FDA define the composition of permissible vitamin-mineral formulations and limit the sales of hazardous megadoses to sale "by prescription only"? Or should it leave the formulation up to the producers—no matter who they are—on the basis that some people want to use their own judgment about them (even if misguided)?
- Should the FDA ban a product which may be toxic and which is worthless in treating cancer to protect consumers from hazard and fraud? Or should it leave the product on the market because some cancer victims feel that it will do them some good?
- Should the FDA take off the market an additive which has been proven to have the potential of causing cancer in humans (admittedly at a very low risk level)? Or should it let the product remain available because some consumers protest that, for them, the benefits of using it outweigh the risks and they are entitled to choose for themselves?

The issue these three questions all address is:

- Should the FDA restrict consumers' freedom of choice in order to protect them from the consequences of their own, possibly hazardous, choices?

The FDA—and all of us—have doubtless benefitted from the conflict over this issue. At one time it might have been possible to accuse the FDA of being unduly influenced by industry. "Their sense of public duty is constantly eroded by industry contacts and the considerations of short-term effects on industry instead of long-term effects on consumers."[17] But all the attention and arguments have led to better consumer protection and less willingness to be swayed by industry's lobbying efforts.

In the eyes of other nations, the FDA represents an achievement of high order. Many nations simply copy its decisions on the safety of additives and other compounds in food. The World Health Organization regards the FDA as the best consumer protection agency in the world:

No other nation has citizens who not only desire safety in consumer goods but are also willing to invest a quarter of a billion dollars a year in such regulation.[18]

A case can certainly be made for the view that the FDA serves us well.

Still, in each of the three instances described here, the FDA's efforts to protect consumers have been thwarted and the choice has been made to let people decide for themselves, even though the decisions may be misguided and the consequences may be harmful to health. This puts your protection in your own hands in these matters.

Personal strategy. This Controversy has shown you that in at least three areas—large-dose vitamin-mineral supplements, cancer "cures" such as laetrile, and low-risk carcinogenic additives such as saccharin—there are items available on the market that require the exercise of your good judgment. The strategy to adopt in light of this is obvious: Learn. All consumers of foods, nutrient supplements, household products, drugs, and other items have to stay informed in order to make choices in their own best interest. One way to keep informed is to read the popular and colorful *FDA Consumer* magazine, which lets you know the FDA's position on the issues of the day. Another is to read *Consumer Reports*, put out by private citizens, which often offers a different point of view.

As a consumer, you also have the right to speak up in favor of your own interests. The FDA has periodic consumer exchange meetings so it can listen to your opinion. Watch for the notices of these hearings, and speak up.

Finally, if you enjoy a stressful job, full of challenges, strife, and conflict, go to work for the FDA.

The Controversy Notes and For Further Information follow the Appendixes.

Controversy 11B

Saccharin and Nitrites

Are they going to kill us?

We understand that there is much excitement in the food industry as the rush begins to discover synthetic substitutes for banned additives.—*Changing Times*, July 1977

After the ban on cyclamates, saccharin became the major artificial sweetener used in diet foods and beverages and as a sugar substitute. Then reports were made public that saccharin, too, was a carcinogen. The evidence came from experiments with both rats and human beings. Rats fed large quantities of saccharin in their feed showed a higher incidence of bladder cancer than control animals. Their offspring seemed especially susceptible to this effect. A Canadian follow-up study on humans showed a higher rate of bladder cancer in (male) saccharin users than in sugar users.[1] After much ado,

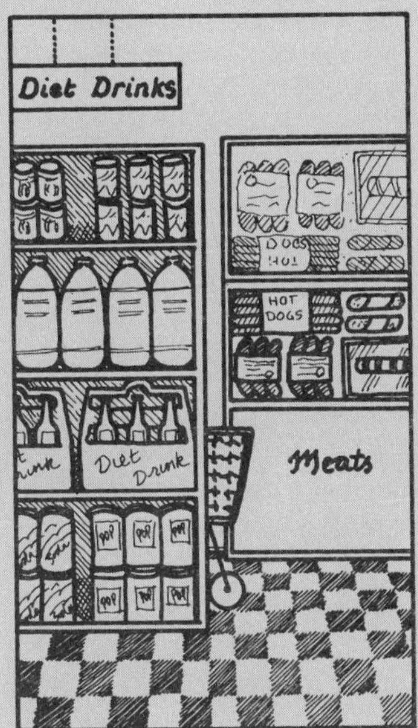

saccharin was banned—and then the ban was suspended so that people who wanted to use it could continue to do so! A warning label was required on all products containing saccharin:

Use of this product may be hazardous to your health. This product contains saccharin, which has been determined to cause cancer in laboratory animals.

The intention was to reduce the use of saccharin by 90 percent and to eliminate the risk to children altogether. This leaves it up to you to decide whether, or how much, to use saccharin. (In Canada, over-the-counter sale of saccharin is now prohibited altogether.)

Meanwhile, alarm arose over nitrite—the antibacterial additive used in cured meats and other products—when a major study involving over 2000 rats concluded that it was also a carcinogen and would have to be banned. As with saccharin, the ban was automatic because the Delaney Clause in the law requires that any additive that causes cancer at any dose level must be removed from foods. But like saccharin, nitrite remained in foods thanks to an escape route (some say a "copout") invoked by the Congress: the ban was suspended.[2]

You may well wonder why—if these substances cause cancer, and if cancer is such a terrible threat that the law of the land demands that all cancer-causing agents be totally eliminated from foods—these two compounds remain in the food supply. Are they killing us? And if not, if there are valid reasons why they should remain in foods, shouldn't the law be changed somehow? A number of considerations bear on these questions, and the person who wishes to make an informed judgment needs to be aware of them.

Miniglossary

aflatoxin (AFF-la-toxin): A potent carcinogen produced by a mold that grows on peanuts.

botulinum toxin: A toxin produced by bacteria that grow in meat, the most potent biological poison known.

carcinogen: A cancer-causing agent.

methemoglobin (meth-EEM-oh-globe-in): A form of the blood protein hemoglobin that cannot carry oxygen. Hemoglobin exposed to excessive nitrite can turn to methemoglobin.

nitrate: Part of a salt containing nitrogen, abundant in vegetables.

nitrite: Part of a salt containing nitrogen which can be produced from nitrate during the processing of vegetables; also such a salt used as an additive to prevent botulism in cured meats.

nitrosamine (nigh-TROH-suh-meen): A compound formed when nitrites and amines combine; a carcinogen.

Perspective on testing methods. An important question is whether, and how far, the results of tests on animals can be extended to apply to human beings. Laboratory animals are much smaller than people, their metabolism is faster, and their life spans are shorter. To test the toxicity of a substance using animals, experiments must be designed so that the total dose received by the animal during the testing period is equivalent to the amount that a person would receive during a whole lifetime. This means giving the animals much larger doses than a person would take but balancing this effect by using a much shorter testing period. This principle involves several assumptions that may or may not be valid.

One of the major assumptions is that the relationship of the dose level to its effects is linear. That is, if 10 units cause 10 episodes of illness, then 100 units will cause 100. This assumption is not valid for a substance such as iodine: Large doses kill, but small amounts are actually required for life. However, with carcinogens, the assumption may be valid.

Another assumption on which animal-cancer experiments are based is that animals and humans will react to carcinogens in the same way. Sometimes the metabolism of a test animal differs importantly from that of a human being. Experiments using rabbits to get information about cholesterol metabolism in humans have had to be discarded, because rabbits' metabolism of cholesterol differs significantly from that of humans. If the animal findings don't apply to people, then all we can conclude from the rat-saccharin experiments is that, as one wit put it:

The Canadians have determined that saccharin is dangerous to your rat's health.—Representative Andrew Jacob (Indiana)

But with cancer, the National Research Council reports, "Virtually every form of human cancer has an experimental counterpart, and every form of multicellular organism is subject to cancer."[3] It seems, from what we know, that it is legitimate to apply rat results to humans in the case of bladder cancers caused by saccharin.

Animal experiments are of great value in predicting the consequences of human intake of certain substances where the direct study of humans would be unethical or would take too long to be of value for the present generation. Each must be scrutinized on its own merits, however. Not treated here have been several questions:

- *The route of administration.*[4] If humans take the substance by mouth, then it should be given by mouth to the animals.

- *The determination of excretion.*[5] Does the substance actually get into the body?
- *The study of metabolism.* If the substance is metabolized in the human to some other substance (for example, nitrites to nitrosamines), then the *metabolite* (nitrosamines) should be tested in animals.
- *The problem of impurities.* It must be demonstrated that it is the compound itself, not something mixed with it in the lab preparations used for animals, that causes the observed effects. (This was a question about the saccharin studies for a while.[6])

To make a long story short, these problems would seem to have been satisfactorily dealt with by the rat-saccharin investigators.

On the basis of present evidence, saccharin does seem able to cause cancer—possibly only in male animals, and certainly only with a very, very low probability. If there is a risk of cancer in females exposed to saccharin it may be a second-generation risk. That is, it is a risk for the offspring of females given saccharin during pregnancy, and only if they have been exposed throughout the entire duration of the pregnancy, from conception on. In comparison with the well-known, potent carcinogen aflatoxin, a sometimes-contaminant of peanut products caused by a mold that can grow in them, saccharin is only about one-millionth as strong. Putting it in more familiar terms, according to a very rough calculation, a diet soft drink is perhaps eighty times less dangerous than a single cigarette.[7] But these are extremely rough approximations. While animal experiments can give us a rough, qualitative (yes-no) answer to a question of carcinogenicity, they can't really tell us anything quantitative (how carcinogenic the substance is):

Depending upon which model for carcinogenic risk is used, the predicted number of cancer cases during the lifetime per million exposed varies from 0.001 to 1,200—a million-fold range! The estimates vary from no significant risk (essentially zero) to a significant, large, real number of 1,200.[8]

As for nitrite, the original experiment which caused the ban has been reviewed and serious doubt has been cast on its validity.[9] Still, it is possible that nitrites can combine in the stomach to form nitrosamines—which are carcinogenic. It is possible that they can, without being converted to anything else by metabolism, cause cancer of the lymphatic system and changes in the immune system of rats. It is also possible that they can reduce the oxygen-carrying protein of the blood, hemoglobin, to an ineffective form, methemoglobin.[10] As with saccharin, there is a continuing debate on the experimental designs that have led to these reports; and like saccharin, nitrite is considered to be at worst a "weak" carcinogen—but still, it seems to be one.

Why are they still on the market? Benefits. Both saccharin and nitrites remain on the market despite their proven carcinogenicity because human beings have made the decision that they should stay. In the case of saccharin, it was largely a matter of freedom of choice, as described in Controversy 11A. The people who would be exposed to the risk were the very same people who would have the benefits, namely, the saccharin users. Wanting to use an artificial sweetener and already barred from using cyclamate, they had no familiar alternative. (Xylitol, which looked like a promising substitute for a while, has now been demonstrated to cause tumors and has been voluntarily removed from chewing gums and foods pending review by the FDA.[11]) Their use of saccharin (except in the case of pregnant women) would affect no one else. "Let us decide," they argued. "We are the ones who will be affected."

The case of nitrite is another matter. Nitrite prevents the formation of botulinum toxin, a deadly poison produced by bacteria that grow in cured meats, poultry, and fish. Nitrite's addition to these foods makes it possible to process, transport, and sell them without fear that a lapse in refrigeration could be catastrophic. If the use of nitrite were forbidden this entire class of foods might be denied to the public because it could not be adequately preserved. And—as if to hammer the point home—there is no other additive available to take its place. Thus there is a clear benefit associated with the use of nitrite; or to put it another way, there is an appreciable risk involved in *not* using it.

Nitrite is different from saccharin in another way, too. It can't be eliminated from the diet. Only about 20 percent of people's daily consumption of nitrite comes from cured food products. The remainder—80 percent—is produced in the body itself by bacteria acting on nitrate, which is a part of the inorganic salts found in plants such as beets, celery, lettuce, carrots, and spinach.[12]

It seems that in the case of both saccharin and nitrite, the decision to keep them was based on a perception that there were benefits involved: freedom of choice, for saccharin, and overwhelming food safety considerations, for nitrite. The law requiring that carcinogens be automatically banished from foods does not take benefits into account.

Should the law be changed? The Delaney Clause, which demands that no additive be permitted in foods "if it is found to induce cancer when ingested by man or animal," is under fire for not being flexible enough to allow for exceptions like those discussed here. For one thing, it doesn't provide for treating additives differently depending on the strength of their effect. For another, it doesn't establish a threshold below which risks can be considered negligible. This was fine when laboratory techniques were crude and any effect that could be detected was worth paying attention to. But when incredibly minute effects can be detected—must alarms be rung?

Still another problem with the Delaney Clause is that it allows for no discretion—no exercise of judgment—on the part of the FDA officials. "If cancer, then ban" is the command, as if there has to be a reflex reaction with no interference from the brain. The FDA, one critic says, bans things "at the drop of a rat."[13]

Finally, still another criticism of the Delaney Clause is that it treats cancer differently from other diseases. If something causes heart disease, shouldn't this be taken equally seriously? Still, Delaney remains in the law, partly because to oppose it is a little like opposing apple pie and motherhood. After all, who wants to appear to be in favor of cancer?[14]

Until the Delaney Clause is modified, additives like saccharin and nitrite will remain in the food supply only by way of some loophole arrangement like the postponed bans described here. But serious discussion is now being devoted to the problem of modifying the law so that it can deal more appropriately with additives. Among the questions being asked are:

- What is an acceptable level of risk?
- Which benefits should be counted, and for how much?
- If the experimental evidence is not sufficient to make a final judgment (and it almost never is), who should make the judgment? How much discretion (for example, by the FDA) should the law allow?
- Should the banning of an additive depend on the availability of others that can do its job?

One conclusion that emerges from all of these considerations is that there cannot be such a thing as "zero risk." When you refuse to tolerate risks at all, you lose too many benefits. (How reasonable would it be, for example, for a bride to say to her husband-to-be, "I will marry you only if you promise me there is no risk involved"?) In the absence of an all-wise witch-doctor to tell us what to do, we need to have confidence in the decision-making *process*, and that process is being thoughtfully worked out.

Perspective on cancer causes. Meanwhile, to put the whole matter in perspective once again, the unavoidable risks of daily living in this society are considerably greater than those being considered here. The risk of skin cancer from exposure to the sun is one that cannot be legislated out of our lives. The risk of crossing the street, of flying in an airplane, of being hit by cosmic rays (which penetrate even lead shielding so that you can't hide from them anywhere)

—these are all real, and much greater, risks. Smoking is at least partly responsible for 38 percent of the deaths from bladder cancer in males, while saccharin can't be conclusively blamed for even one. And in comparison to additives—any additives—there is a dietary factor which looms far larger in relation to cancer: the amount of fat in the diet, as described in Controversy 5B. If you step back and look at the whole picture, saccharin and nitrite will be seen to occupy an almost invisible corner.

Personal strategy. The decision to keep these additives on the market leaves it up to us whether to use them. For most people, moderation is probably the course to adopt. A guideline as to what constitutes moderation in saccharin intake is provided by the Canadian Dietetic Association, which says that an intake of 50 milligrams a day can be considered moderate.[15] This is conservative. A 12-ounce diet drink containing 10 milligrams per ounce provides a total of 120 milligrams of saccharin. Thus we might limit our use to a single dose every other day if we want to be very, very careful.

Weight control, especially by restriction of fat intake, would seem to provide protection against cancer. If saccharin aids you in dieting and satisfies your sweet tooth when you would otherwise eat a high-fat sweet snack such as butter cookies or a chocolate bar, it may be to your advantage to use the saccharin. Undoubtedly, however, you would be better off if you had never developed a taste for fattening foods in the first place. In the interest of the next generation, the best strategy will probably be to develop a taste for nutritious foods that are low in fat and calories in order to avert the obesity problem and avoid altogether the need to make a choice between saccharin and sugar. For the sake of children as well, it is prudent to adopt a diet that is relatively high in complex carbohydrates and low in fat.

As for nitrites, you manufacture nitrites in your own saliva, so you can't avoid them altogether whether you want to or not. And no one suggests that you give up eating vegetables. However, because of the risk of methemoglobin formation in young infants, it is recommended that *home-prepared* carrots, beets, and spinach not be offered to babies under the age of six months, and that ham and cured meats be limited during the first year.[16]

If, as an adult, you wish to exclude cured meats from your diet you can, of course. Or, you could take a more optimistic approach: Eat a variety of fresh meats and only occasionally have cold cuts or ham. As a parent, you may want to limit your children's use of cold cuts for between-meal snacks, and offer cheese and fruits instead. Reserve the cured meats for special occasions, such as times when the whole family wants to enjoy ham. In other words, don't feel compelled to eliminate a class of foods altogether, but enjoy the moderate and appropriate use of all available foods.

The Controversy Notes and For Further Information follow the Appendixes.

PART FOUR

NUTRITION THROUGH LIFE

The preceding three sections have introduced the problem of food choices, provided familiarity with the nutrients and the foods that contain them, and offered guidelines for putting these foods together into healthful, balanced, and adequate diets. This last section views diet from the perspective of the whole person at different stages in the life cycle, where different considerations become important.

Chapter 12 presents the special nutritional problems related to growth, with an emphasis on pregnancy and infancy, and asks what preventive measures can be adopted to promote good health in later life.

Chapter 13 is devoted to the middle years of childhood and the effects of such factors as television on children's eating habits.

Chapter 14 focuses on the years when nutrition becomes the individual's own responsibility and when such factors as alcohol, drugs, and caffeine may complicate the nutrition picture.

Chapter 15 describes the processes of aging and asks what nutritional and food-related measures will enhance the quality of life in the later years.

CHAPTER 12

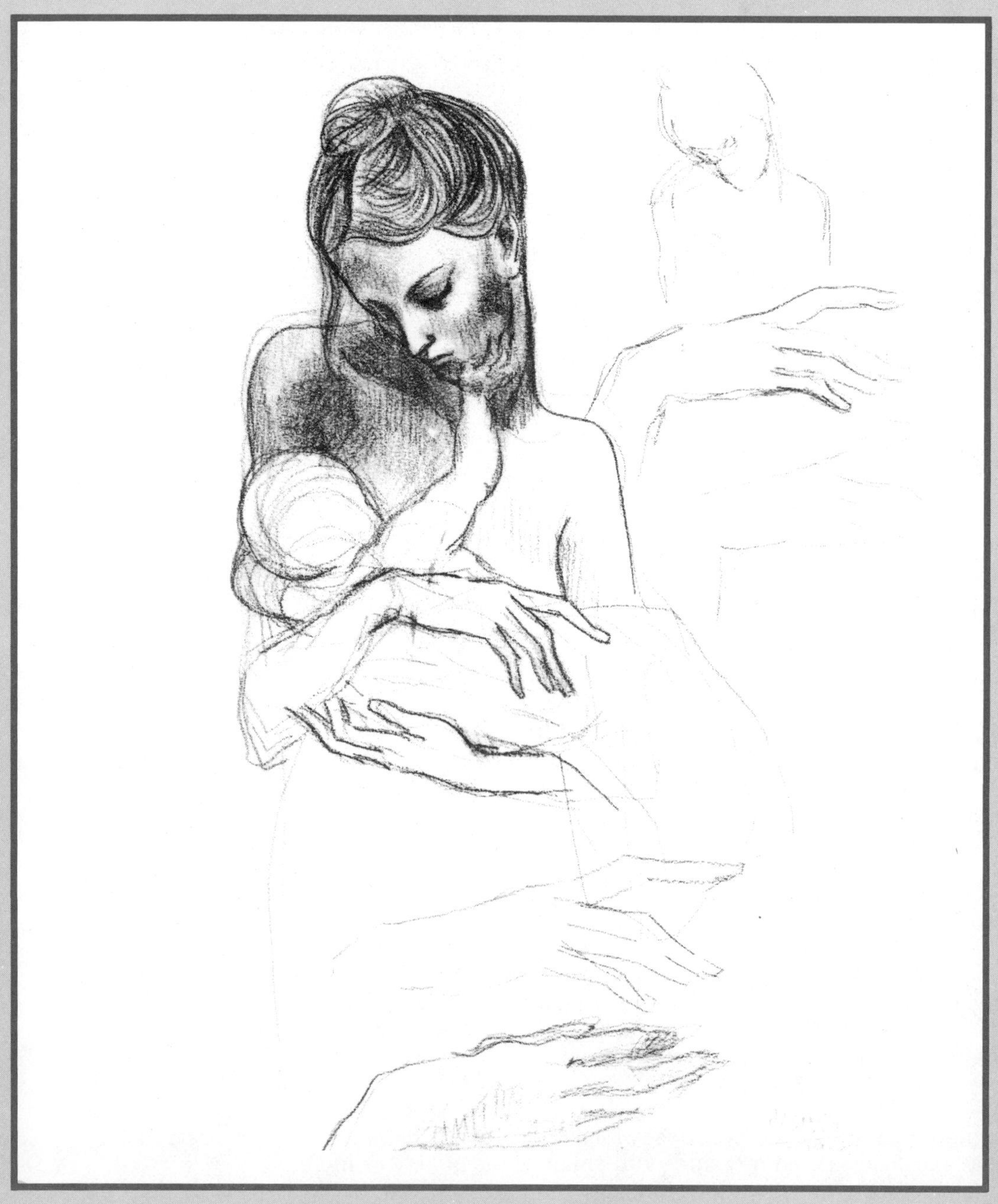

Mother, Infant, and Growth

The preceding chapters have been addressed to the adult. Wherever nutrition information has been relevant to your needs and concerns, examples and illustrations involving adults have been given, with only occasional references to infants, children, and older people. The principles of nutrition apply throughout the life span, but some changes in emphasis are appropriate to these other age groups.

Young people, from infancy through the teen years, are growing—a characteristic not shared by adults. In addition to nutritional needs for maintenance, then, young people have special needs related to the growth process. Furthermore, they are growing psychologically. In considering the nutritional needs and the feeding of infants, children, and teenagers, it is important to keep both kinds of growth in mind.

The Processes of Growth

Growth is not a matter of everything simply getting bigger all at once. From conception to adulthood, different organs differentiate, grow, and mature at different rates and times, each with its own characteristic pattern. A few generalizations hold for all growth processes, however, and an understanding of these generalizations underlies the knowledge of the special nutritional needs imposed by growth. It is helpful to distinguish three growth levels: that of the whole body, that

Opposite: Mother and Child *by Pablo Picasso, Courtesy of the Fogg Art Museum, Harvard University, Bequesta-Meta and Paul J. Sachs.*

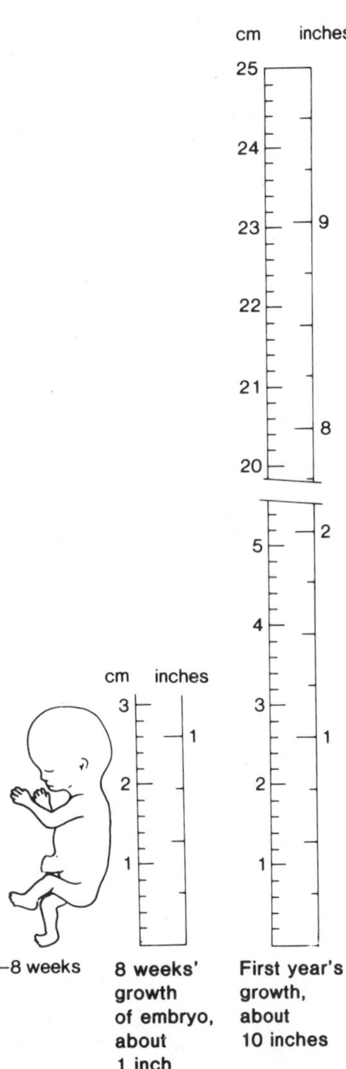

This 8-week-old embryo is shown life-size.

Intensive growth periods:
Prenatal period.
First year.
Adolescence.

of the organs and tissues, and that of the cells of each organ or tissue. At each level, different considerations become important.

Whole body growth. Between conception and birth, a human being's weight increases from a fraction of a gram to 3500 grams. The greatest rate of growth is in the fetal period between eight weeks and term—when the weight increases over five hundred times. After birth, a baby doubles its weight from 7 to 14 pounds in four months, then slows down somewhat and adds another 7 pounds in the next eight months, reaching about 21 pounds at one year. Thereafter, the growth rate slows to 5 pounds a year or less until adolescence, when it increases dramatically again.

A similar pattern holds for height. From a fifth of a millimeter at three weeks of gestation, the embryo reaches 3 centimeters at eight weeks, then 50 centimeters at birth. Thereafter, the increase in height is greatest during the first year (25 centimeters), half that much the second year (12 to 13 centimeters), and then slower still (6 to 7 centimeters) until the adolescent growth spurt. At that time, a sudden increase of some 16 to 20 centimeters is achieved in a two- to two-and-a-half-year period.

What is important to notice about all this is that growth does not proceed at a steady pace, that the maximal rate of growth is in the prenatal period, and that the two postnatal periods during which growth is fastest are the first year and the teen years.

Growth of organs and tissues. The growth of each organ and tissue type has its own characteristic pattern and timing. In the fetus, for example, the heart and brain are well developed at sixteen weeks, even though the lungs are still nonfunctional ten weeks later. During the first year after birth, the brain doubles in weight, but it increases only about 20 percent thereafter. In contrast, the muscles will be more than thirty times heavier at maturity than they are at birth.

Each organ and tissue, then, has its own unique periods of intensive growth. Each organ needs the growth nutrients most during its own intensive growth period. Thus a nutrient deficiency during one stage of development might affect the heart, and at another it might affect the developing limbs.

Cell growth and critical periods. At the level of the cells of a single developing organ, a further point becomes apparent: Each organ has its own specific time for cell division, which may not coincide with its time of growth in size. An interesting case is that of the brain. During development of the fetal brain, there is an early period when the cells are increasing dramatically in *number*. Each time a cell divides, it produces two that are half its size. These two do not grow but divide again, producing four cells that are still smaller. During this time of intense cell division, the size of the brain hardly changes at all. Later, the cells begin to grow and also continue dividing, so that their *size and number* increase simultaneously. It is during these first two periods that the total number of cells to be found in the brain is determined for life. Later still, cell division ceases, and thereafter the total number of cells is fixed, but they continue to increase in *size*. During this last period the brain's growth in size is obvious. The development of almost every organ in the body follows a similar three-stage pattern, but each has different timing.

The third period, during which increase in size is taking place, is the time when the most intensive growth appears to be going on. But actually, the most important events are already over. This fact has important implications for nutrition. The period of cell division is a **critical period**, critical in the sense that the cell division taking place during that time can occur at only that time and at no other. Whatever nutrients and other environmental conditions are needed in this period must be supplied on time if the organ is to reach its full potential. If cell division and the final cell number achieved are limited at this time, later recovery is impossible. Thus malnutrition at an early period can have irreversible effects that may become fully manifest only when the person reaches maturity.

The effect of malnutrition during critical periods is seen in the shorter height of people who were undernourished in their early years; in the delayed sexual development of those undernourished during early adolescence; in the poor dental health of children whose mothers were malnourished during pregnancy;[1] and in the smaller brain size and brain cell number of children who have suffered from episodes of marasmus or kwashiorkor. The irreversibility of these effects is obvious when abundant, nourishing food fed after the critical time fails to remedy the growth deficit. Among the many Korean orphans adopted by U.S. families after the Korean War, for example, several years of catch-up growth have still not made up for the effects of early malnutrition.[2]

An area of active recent research points strongly to the probability that malnutrition in the prenatal and early postnatal periods also affects learning ability and behavior. Much of the severe mental retardation seen in developed countries such as the United States is of unknown cause; certainly many cases may be due to protein deficiency during pregnancy.[3] Clearly, then, it is most critical to provide the best nutrition at early stages of life.

Growth of the person. The concept of critical periods can also be applied, loosely, to personality growth. From the moment of birth (and perhaps even earlier), the human child is learning what to expect from life and how to cope with life's problems. These learning experiences follow one another in a characteristic sequence, and each must reach some degree of completion before the next can proceed. An infant's earliest impressions mold attitudes that in maturity may still affect behavior. A person who nurtures children must understand what is going on psychologically as well as physically. He must supply the nutrients that children need, and equally important, he must encourage learning and behavior that will help them to develop fully as human beings.

There are many ways of understanding and interpreting psychological growth and development. The one we have selected to follow is that of Erik Erikson, whose insightful description of the stages of human growth provides a framework for viewing the whole person.[4] Erikson sees human life as a sequence of eight periods, in each of which the individual has a new learning task. To the extent that individuals master each successfully, they develop a strong foundation from which to proceed to the next. To the extent that they fail, they are handicapped in mastering the task at the next level. The stages in life and their respective learning tasks, as identified by Erikson, are:

Infant. Trust versus distrust.

Toddler. Autonomy versus shame and doubt.

Preschooler. Initiative versus guilt.

School-age child. Industry versus inferiority.

Adolescent. Identity versus role confusion.

Young adult. Intimacy versus isolation.

Adult. Generativity versus stagnation.

Older adult. Ego integrity versus despair.

Whether you agree with Erikson's view or see human development in some other light, we hope you agree with the principle that understanding the whole person is important, even in the providing of food.

Each section that follows is devoted to a special stage in life, its physical growth and development, the related nutrient needs, and a feeding pattern that will supply the needed nutrients. Each section concludes with an attempt to put these nutrient needs in perspective in relation to the needs of the whole person.

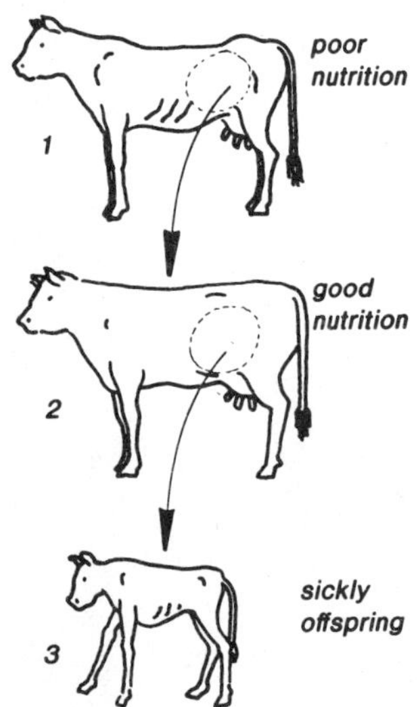

The effects of poor nutrition can extend to the third generation. Here, animal 2 was well nourished after birth, but its prenatal development irreversibly affected its ability to grow a normal placenta. Its offspring, animal 3, was sickly as a result.

Pregnancy: The Impact of Nutrition on the Future

We normally think of the effects of nutrition as being here-and-now: You feel good this afternoon because you ate a good breakfast this morning, and your friend feels sleepy because she had a sweet dessert after lunch. But the effects of nutrition also extend over years. It has been said that the best way to ensure being healthy when you are old is to be thin while you are young. Your eating habits of today, as part of your lifestyle, may help to determine whether you become a victim of cardiovascular disease (perhaps by eating too much salt), of diabetes (if you allow yourself to become obese), even of cancer (if your diet is rich in calories from fat).

At no time is the effect of nutrition on future health more dramatically in evidence than during the early development of an infant in its mother's womb. It is even probable that the nutrition of the infant's *grandmother* during her pregnancy will have permanent effects on the infant when it has become an adult.[5]

Such effects are impossible to demonstrate directly in people, nor would researchers want to experiment on pregnant mothers to see what causes stunting of the body or the brain in their children. But because the questions are important, many of them have been pursued in experiments using animals. We have every reason to believe that most findings from the animal experiments are applicable to human beings. Some have been inadvertently confirmed. Hospital records maintained during the sieges of Holland and Leningrad in World War II gave abundant evidence that the state of the mother's nutrition *prior* to pregnancy was important for the *future* health of her infant.

Growth. Conditions in the uterus at the time of conception determine whether the fertilized egg will successfully implant itself in the uterine wall and begin development as it should. During the two weeks following fertilization, in the **implantation** stage, the egg cell divides into many cells, and these sort themselves into three layers. Very little growth in size takes place at this time; this is a critical period that precedes growth. Adverse influences at this time lead to failure to implant or other disturbances so severe as to cause loss of the fertilized egg, possibly even before the woman knows she is pregnant. Many drugs affect the earliest intrauterine events and later cross the placenta freely. Most health professionals agree that, if possible, a potential mother should be taking no drugs at all, not even aspirin. Nutrition should be, and should have been, continuously optimal.

Implantation: 0-2 weeks.

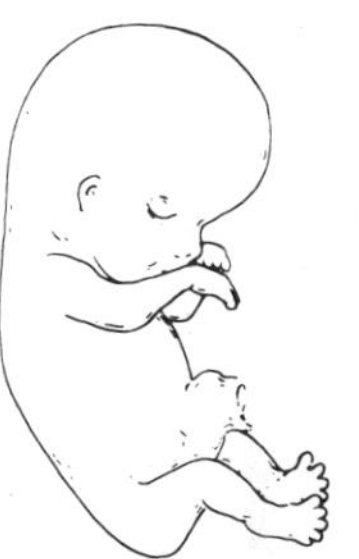

Eight-week-old embryo.

The next five weeks, the period of embryonic development, register astonishing physical changes. From the outermost layer of cells, the nervous system and skin begin to develop; from the middle layer, the muscles and internal organ systems; and from the innermost layer, the glands and linings of the digestive, respiratory, and excretory systems. At eight weeks, the 3-centimeter-long **embryo** has a complete central nervous system, a beating heart, a fully formed digestive system, and the beginnings of facial features. Already the "tail" has formed and almost completely disappeared again, and the fingers and toes are well defined.

Embryo: 2-8 weeks.

The last seven months of pregnancy, the fetal period, bring about a tremendous increase in size. Intensive periods of cell division occur in organ after organ of the **fetus**.

Fetus: 2-9 months.

Meanwhile, the mother's body is undergoing changes. She grows a whole new organ—the **placenta**—a kind of pillow inside her **uterus** (womb). In the placenta, the mother's and infant's blood vessels spread out and intertwine. Nutrients and oxygen leave her bloodstream and cross the vessel walls into the infant's bloodstream. Waste materials (carbon dioxide and urea) leave the infant and are carried away by the mother's blood to be excreted through her lungs and kidneys. The **amniotic sac** fills with fluid to cushion the infant. The mother's uterus and its supporting muscles increase greatly in size, her breasts change and grow in preparation for lactation, and her blood volume almost doubles to accommodate its added load of materials to be carried. The overall gain in weight of mother and child during pregnancy amounts to about 24 pounds (see Table 1).

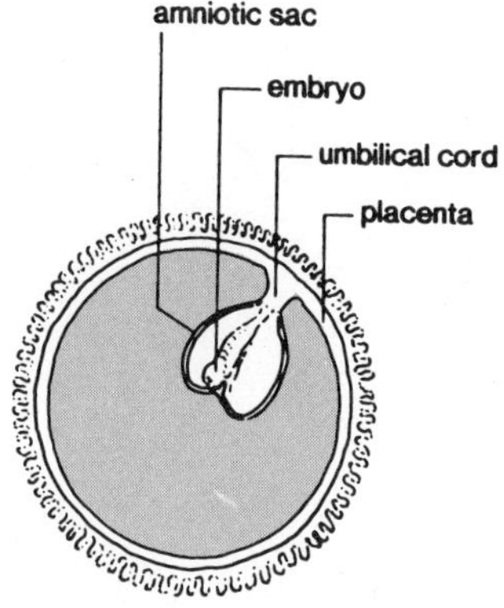

Human embryo in the amniotic sac. Note the attachment to the placenta by a body stalk which will become the umbilical cord.

Nutrient needs. Nutrient needs during periods of intensive growth are greater than at any other time and are greater for certain nutrients than for others, as shown in Figure 1. Whenever intensive growth is going on, the nutrients protein, calcium, phosphorus, and magnesium are of great importance, because of their roles in the structure and functions of rapidly dividing or growing cells and growing bones; but

Table 1. Overall Weight Gain during Pregnancy

Development	Weight Gain (pounds)
Infant at birth	7½
Placenta	1
Increase in mother's blood volume to supply placenta	4
Increase in size of mother's uterus and muscles to support it	2½
Increase in size of mother's breasts	3
Fluid to surround infant in amniotic sac	2
Mother's fat stores	4
Total	24

no nutrient can be overlooked. The extraordinary need for folacin in the pregnant woman is due to the doubling of her blood volume. Folacin-deficiency anemia is more often seen in pregnant women than even iron deficiency, and it is often advisable for the physician to prescribe folacin as a supplement.[6] As you might expect, the vitamin needed in the next highest amount is the other B vitamin associated with the manufacture of red blood cells—B_{12}.

The major route of excretion for iron is menstruation, which ceases during pregnancy. Some of the iron a woman needs to increase her blood stores is saved by having no menstrual losses. As her blood volume increases, so do all its constituents, including the protein that increases absorption of iron from the intestine.[7] An additional adjust-

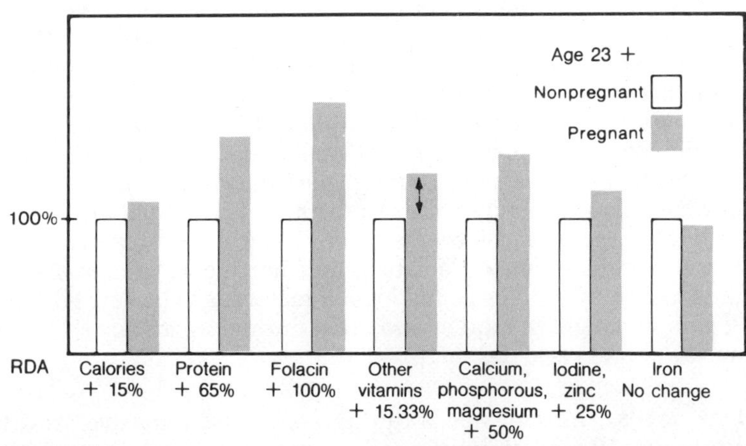

Figure 1. Comparison of the nutrient needs of nonpregnant and pregnant women. ***The nonpregnant woman's needs are set at 100 percent; the pregnant woman's needs are shown as increases over 100 percent. The pregnant woman's iron needs cannot be met by ordinary diets, and she might need to take an iron supplement. (Calculated from the RDA tables, inside front cover.)***

ment is accomplished by the hormones of pregnancy, which act to raise the concentration of iron in the blood, either by increasing absorption still further or by mobilizing iron from its storage places in the bone marrow and internal organs or both. Thus a woman *theoretically* needs no more iron during pregnancy than she has needed all along. However, because many women enter pregnancy with inadequate stores, physicians often prescribe an iron supplement during this time as a kind of insurance.

The 1980 RDAs recommend a 30-60 mg/day iron supplement during pregnancy and for two to three months after delivery to replenish the woman's iron stores.

Eating pattern. If the woman's dietary pattern is already adequate at the start of pregnancy, it can be adjusted to meet changing nutrient needs. The nutrients needing the greatest increase are protein, calcium, phosphorus, magnesium, and folacin, so the foods selected for emphasis should normally be those in the milk, meat, and vegetable categories.

Calorie needs increase less than nutrient needs. To achieve a slight increase in calorie intake with a great increase in nutrient intake, the woman must select foods of high nutrient density. For most women, appropriate choices would be foods like skim milk, cottage cheese, lean meats, eggs, liver, and dark green vegetables. For vitamin C, she should either increase the size of her one serving of a C-rich food, such as citrus fruit or broccoli, or add a second fair C source, such as tomatoes. A suggested food pattern is shown in Table 2.

The pregnant woman must gain weight. Ideally she will have begun her pregnancy at the appropriate weight for her height and will gain about 20 to 24 pounds, most of it in the second half of pregnancy. This sounds like a lot, but if you look again at the components of the pregnant woman's weight gain, you will see that she needs all these pounds—from nutritious calories—to provide for the growth of her placenta, uterus, blood, and breasts, as well as for a strong 7½-pound baby. There is little place in her diet, however, for the empty calories of

Table 2. Daily Food Guide for the Pregnant or Lactating Woman

Food	Number of Servings		
	Nonpregnant Woman	Pregnant Woman	Lactating Woman
Protein foods			
Animal (2 oz serving)	2	2	2
Vegetable (at least one serving of legumes)	2	2	2
Milk and milk products	2	4	5
Enriched or whole-grain breads and cereals	4	4	4
Vitamin C–rich fruits and vegetables	1	1	1
Dark-green vegetables	1	1	1
Other fruits and vegetables	1	1	1

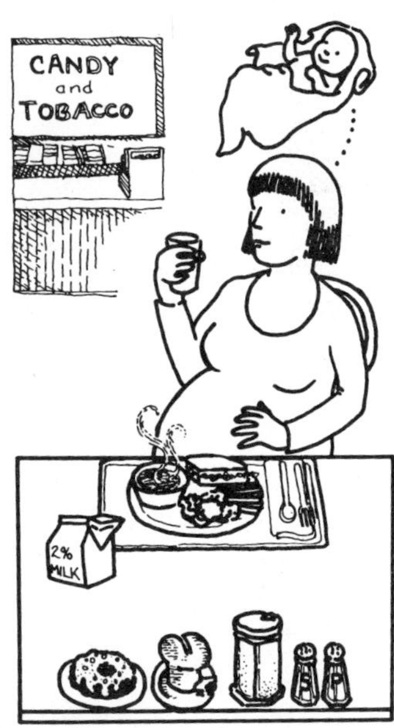

Healthy choices.

sugar, fat, and alcohol, which provide no nutrients to support the growth of these tissues and only contribute to excessive fat accumulation. Much of the weight she gains is lost at delivery; the remainder is generally lost within a few weeks, as her blood volume returns to normal and she loses the fluids she has accumulated.

The underweight woman should try to gain weight before she becomes pregnant, to maximize her chance of having a healthy baby. But all women should be attending to their nutrition before they become pregnant. If nutrient supplementation is needed, the family-planning period is a good time to get it started.

If the pregnant woman is obese at the time of conception, she should not attempt to lose weight during her pregnancy. Even though excess weight is a disadvantage, it is best lost before the beginning of pregnancy. Authorities recommend not only no dieting but also a weight gain in the obese pregnant woman. A report from the Maternal and Child Health Branch of the California Department of Health, based on the available research, clinical data, and combined judgments of various experts, recommends "a smooth and progressive weight gain of at least 24 pounds—just as would be expected in a non-obese woman."[8]

If the mother does not gain the full amount of weight recommended, she may give birth to an underweight baby. To the uninitiated, this may seem like no catastrophe, and in some instances it is not. A small mother may give birth to a small normal baby, and there is nothing wrong in this. However, on the average, the baby's birthweight also reflects the nutritional environment to which it has been exposed, and in general, babies of normal weight can be expected to be more healthy. Nutritionists seeking to find a measure by which they can evaluate the outcome of pregnancy have found no better one than birthweight: It is the most potent single indicator of the infant's future health status. A **low-birthweight** baby, defined as one that weighs less than 5½ pounds (2500 grams), has a statistically greater chance of contracting diseases and of dying early in life. Its birth is more likely to be complicated by problems during delivery than that of a normal baby (defined as one who weighs a minimum of 6½ pounds, or 3000 grams). Low-birthweight infants are sickly, a characteristic often called by health professionals "failure to thrive." Surprisingly, one of the problems some of these infants may later encounter is excessive weight gain and obesity,[9] perhaps because malnutrition interferes with normal development of that part of the brain that controls food intake. About one in every fifteen infants born in the United States is a low-birthweight baby, and about a quarter of these die within the first month of life (see Table 3).[10] Worldwide, it is estimated that one-sixth of all live babies are of low birthweight, more than nine out of ten being born in the underdeveloped countries. Most of them are not premature but are full-term babies; they are small because of malnutrition. The impact of this malnutrition is then seen in the fact that more than half of all the deaths of children under five are caused by low birthweight and nutritional deficiencies.[11]

Low birthweight is often associated with mental retardation, probably by way of deprivation of nutrients and oxygen to the developing brain. It is estimated that about half of all cases of mental retardation

Table 3. Infant Death and Disability in the United States

Category	Number
Total births (1974)	3,159,958
Total low-birthweight infants	233,750
Low-birthweight infants who die in first month of life (1960)	56,865
Low-birthweight infants at risk for lifetime disability	about 60,000

The United States ranks fourteenth among developed nations in infant mortality rate.

could be eliminated by improved programming in maternal and infant care.[12]

Prevention of future health problems. The potential impact of harmful influences during pregnancy cannot be over-estimated. Excessive alcohol consumption can deprive developing nervous tissue of needed glucose and B vitamins and so cause irreversible brain damage and mental and physical retardation in the fetus (**fetal alcohol syndrome**).[13] The damage can occur with as few as two drinks a day, and its most severe impact is likely to be in the first month, before the woman even is sure she is pregnant.[14] Smoking restricts the blood supply to the growing fetus and so limits the delivery of nutrients and removal of wastes. It stunts growth, thus increasing the risk of complications at birth and retarded development.[15] Drugs taken during pregnancy can cause grotesque malformations.

Gathering statistics indicate that [fetal alcohol syndrome] is emerging as the most prevalent combination of birth defects known to modern medicine. Indeed it has been said that the mental retardation due to drinking during pregnancy appears to be becoming the world's most prevalent congenital birth defect.
—Nutrition Today letter, 8 April 1981.

Dieting, even for short periods, is hazardous. Low-carbohydrate diets or fasts that cause ketosis deprive the growing brain of needed glucose and cause congenital deformity. Most serious may be the invisible effects. For example, carbohydrate metabolism may be rendered permanently defective.[16] The consequences of protein deprivation may be still more severe. This has been observed most frequently in the underdeveloped countries, but it is also seen among vegetarians whose children's height and head circumference are markedly and irreversibly diminished.[17] Iron deficiency during pregnancy in animals has been seen to give rise to offspring whose brain cells could never store the needed iron thereafter.[18]

Excessive caffeine consumption (more than 8 cups a day) causes complications in delivery.[19] Saccharin, too, should be avoided, because it has been shown to cause cancer in the offspring of animals exposed to it during pregnancy. Even sugar consumption during pregnancy has been accused of predisposing the infant to obesity.[20]

It is also important not to gain too much weight. Just as brain cell number can be limited by undernutrition, fat cell number may be undesirably increased by overnutrition, predisposing the newborn to obesity. This effect is even more pronounced later on, when the child is about one to three years old.

Diabetes is a condition that can make pregnancy more difficult than usual, and sometimes the symptoms of diabetes first appear when a woman is pregnant. To help women manage their pregnancies with this complication, it is recommended that all pregnant women be screened for diabetes at about the sixth month.[21]

An important consideration for the health of subsequent children is the spacing of offspring to allow the mother's body to regain its nutritional balance. A delay of two to three years between births allows the mother's body to replenish any lost nutrient stores. This is of great benefit to the development of the next child. In the developing countries, where food shortages are common, it is noteworthy that a non-pregnant woman can live three to six months longer than a pregnant woman on the same amount of food.

The profound effects on human life of nutritional and nutrition-related factors during pregnancy are recognized by policy makers all over the world. This recognition has given rise to programs serving pregnant women with education and nutrient supplements where needed. In the United States, the WIC Program (Women's, Infants', and Children's Supplemental Food Program), first funded in 1970, was investing $142 million a year in help to low-income pregnant women by 1977. Among the most active nongovernmental agencies is the March of Dimes, which promotes nutrition education for pregnant women and measures to prevent birth defects. Worldwide, many countries have similar programs.

***There is a distinct relationship between maternal malnutrition and prematurity, which is the leading cause of loss of human life as well as a significant contributor to mental retardation and other disability.*—T. N. Evans**

Not all birth defects are caused by such factors in the newborn's environment as poor maternal nutrition. Some are **inborn errors**: inherited disorders caused by genes received from the parents. Diabetes is a possible member of this group; sickle-cell anemia is another. Another well-known and widespread example is **lactose intolerance**, in which the gene for the intestinal enzyme lactase becomes inactive when the child is about four years old, so that the milk sugar, lactose, cannot be digested. Many inborn errors involve failure to handle specific nutrients, like lactose, and special diets have to be designed to deal with each of them. Any diet therapy book can show you how this is done.

Troubleshooting. Other common problems may be encountered during pregnancy. Edema is not uncommon. In a poorly nourished woman, it is often part of a larger cluster of symptoms known as **toxemia**, a condition involving high blood pressure and kidney problems that requires medical attention. Toxemia causes thousands of infant deaths every year, and babies born of toxemic mothers are likely to have retarded growth, lung problems, and other, more severe birth defects.

Research has shown that toxemia is most common in low-income mothers and pregnant teenagers; it is preventable by good nutrition prior to and in the early stages of pregnancy, because it seems to be most often due to a lack of protein and/or salt. To avert this condition, a pregnant woman should obtain ample protein in her diet, and her salt intake should be above the usual intake.[22] This doesn't mean that she should add any salt; the increased need is normally met by the increased food intake. But she shouldn't have to restrict the salt in her diet, either, unless she has a medical condition that makes it necessary to do so. Even after toxemia has set in, it is likely that the salt intake should not be reduced, and diuretics (to cause sodium excretion) may be harmful.[23] Good nutrition and rest are the cornerstones of treatment.

Another common problem in pregnant women is iron-deficiency anemia. Attention should be paid to getting enough iron during this important time. At birth, a baby is supposed to have enough stored iron to last three to six months; this iron must come from the mother's iron stores, which should be—but seldom are—adequate even before pregnancy.

A problem often encountered by the pregnant woman is nausea, a symptom that can be caused by folacin deficiency. The hormonal changes taking place early in pregnancy may cause transient morning sickness, and a hint some expectant mothers have found helpful is to start the day with a few sips of water and a few nibbles of a soda cracker or other bland carbohydrate food, to get something in the stomach before getting out of bed. Another problem sometimes seen in pregnancy is vitamin B_6 deficiency, which may in some cases cause depression, although depression can of course have other causes.

Later, as the thriving infant crowds the mother's intestinal organs, an expectant mother may complain of constipation; a high-fiber diet and a plentiful water intake will help to alleviate this condition. Calcification of the baby teeth begins in the fifth month after conception; for this and for the bones, fluoride is needed. The woman in a county without fluoridated water may need a prescription from her physician for a supplement that includes fluoride.

What a lot for a woman to remember! And this is only the briefest summary of the nutrient needs in pregnancy. With all of this to worry about, can a woman relax and enjoy expecting her baby?

Psychological needs of the pregnant woman. The developing fetus cannot be said to have many psychological needs (although this can be debated), but pregnancy for many women is a time of adjustment to major changes. The woman who is expecting to bear a baby is a growing person in more ways than one. Not only physically, but also emotionally, her needs are changing. If it is her first baby, she knows her lifestyle will have to change as she takes on the new responsibility of caring for a child. Ideally, she will be encouraged to develop this sense of responsibility by caring for herself during pregnancy. According to Erikson, the psychological events of adolescence culminate in the formation of an identity. Experts from many schools of thought agree that one's self-image begins to form early and ideally is strongly positive: "I'm OK!" The expectant mother needs encouragement in thinking of herself as a thoroughly worthwhile and important person with a new and challenging task that she can and will perform well. She is also, as a young adult, still working out her relationship with her mate, and he and she both know that the coming of a first baby will affect that relationship profoundly. There is a need for sensitive communication and understanding on both parts in this time of transition.

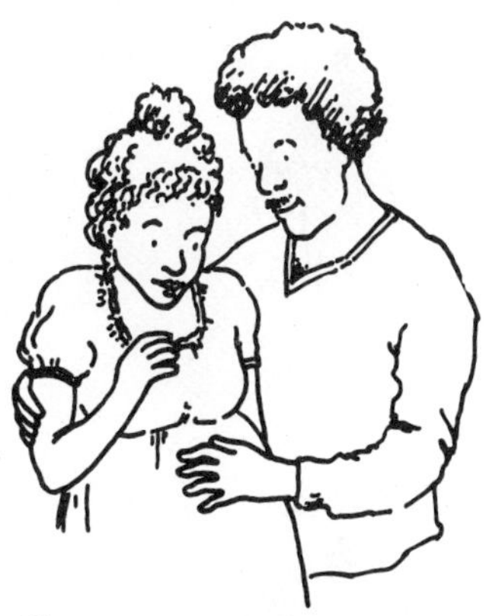

The expectant mother needs emotional, as well as nutritional support.

A question commonly asked is whether the so-called cravings of the pregnant woman reflect physiological needs. They do in only one known instance—in the behavior called **pica**. Pica is the habit of poorly nourished women and children of eating clay, cornstarch, ice, paint, or other substances. This craving has been linked to iron deficiency in some instances and possibly zinc deficiency in others. Other than pica, the only specific messages the body can send to the brain regarding its nutrient needs are for water, possibly salt, and food. In general, the cravings of a pregnant woman seem to be psychological, not physiological. If a woman wakes her husband at 2 in the morning and begs him to go to the nearest all-night grocery to buy her some pickles and chocolate sauce, this is probably not because she lacks a combination of nutrients uniquely supplied by these foods. She is expressing a need, however, as real and as important as her need for nutrients—a need for support, understanding, and love.

Nutrition during Breastfeeding

The secretion of milk by a nursing mother is a beautiful illustration of the ways nature provides for its own. To give but a few examples: The mother's milk supply responds to the infant's needs. If the baby sucks until the breast is empty, a hormone is released that stimulates the mammary glands to produce more milk the next time around; if the baby leaves milk in the breast, the amount secreted is reduced.[24] If a mother is nursing twins, reserving one breast for each, the breasts can even adjust separately to each infant's demands. This same hormone causes the uterus to contract, helping it return to normal size. The infant's crying stimulates a conditioned mother to "let down" her milk (the **let-down reflex**). In anticipation of feeding, the milk moves to the front of the breast and, as the infant begins to suck, flows so freely that the infant may have to gulp fast to keep up with the flow. The milk that flows from the front of the breast at the start of a feeding is dilute, high in water content, so that the infant's thirst will be satisfied. If the baby takes it all and is still hungry, the milk released ten minutes later will be more concentrated and higher in fat to satisfy hunger faster.[25]

Similarly, if a baby is born prematurely, the breast milk will be higher in protein than it is for a full-term baby, and so will meet the premature baby's higher protein need. Its composition changes month by month as lactation continues, always staying appropriate for the developing infant. Like many other designs of living systems, the lactation system is a marvel. But for a mother to succeed in breastfeeding without compromising her own nutritional status, adequate nutrition is important.

Growth and nutrient needs. A comparison between a woman's recommended intakes during pregnancy (second half) and during lactation is shown in Figure 2. The figure reveals that the nursing mother's needs for several nutrients are down, whereas others increase only slightly. A significant increase is needed for calories, both for those that go into her milk and for the energy needed to make the milk. Calcium, phosphorus, magnesium, and protein needs continue to be high. They were going into the baby in the womb; now they are flowing into the baby through the mother's milk. Little iron is secreted in milk, so no

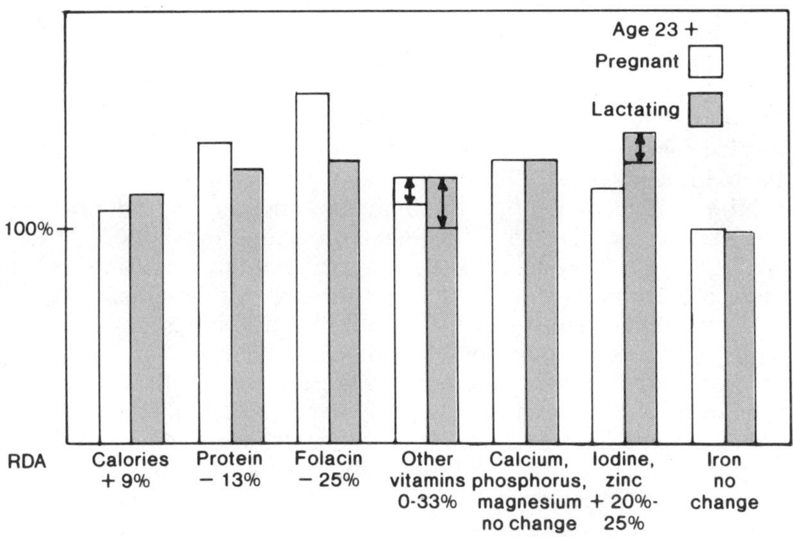

Figure 2. Comparison of the nutrient needs of pregnant and lactating women. ***The nonpregnant woman's needs are set at 100 percent, as in Figure 1. (Calculated from the RDA tables, inside front cover.)***

increase in iron intake is needed, provided, of course, that the mother's iron nutrition has been good all along. The folacin requirement falls as the mother's blood volume declines.

Eating pattern. Logically, because the mother is making milk, she needs to consume something that resembles it in composition. The obvious choice is cow's milk. The nursing mother who can't drink milk needs to find nutritionally similar substitutes like cheese or soy milk and greens. As before, nutritious foods should make up the remainder of the needed calorie increase. Because breast milk is a fluid, the mother's fluid intake should be liberal; a busy new mother often forgets this.

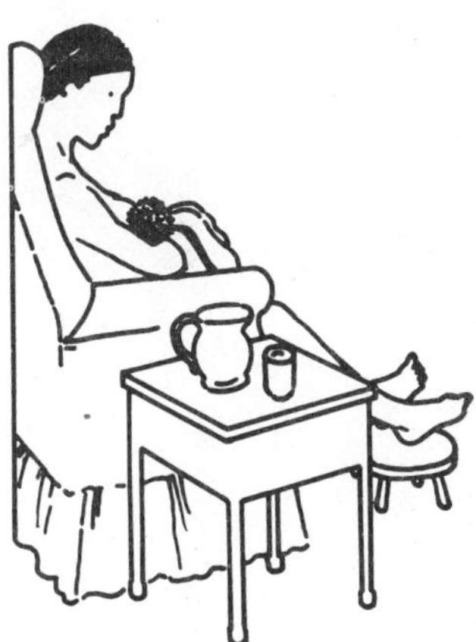

The most important nutrient is water.

The question is often raised whether a mother's milk may lack a nutrient if she is not getting enough in her diet. The answer differs from one nutrient to the next, but in general the effect of nutritional deprivation is to reduce the quantity, not the quality, of the milk. For the energy nutrients and most vitamins and minerals, the milk has a constant composition; if one nutrient is in short supply, correspondingly less milk—but still of the proper composition—will be produced.[26] The mother's diet may make her blood cholesterol higher or lower to some extent, but seems not to affect her breast-milk cholesterol.[27] For some of the water-soluble vitamins and trace minerals, the composition may be more variable, but most evidence seems to indicate that for these ingredients, too, the breast milk concentrations are constant.[28] Even the taking of a vitamin-mineral supplement seems not to raise nutrient concentrations in the breast milk of an otherwise well-nourished mother.[29] A word of warning, however: A too-high intake of vitamin B_6 from pills may have an inhibiting effect on lactation.[30] And to repeat: Water is the major ingredient of milk, and a nursing mother's fluid intake should be ample.

The period of lactation is the natural time for a woman to lose the extra body fat she accumulated during pregnancy. If her choice of foods is judicious, a calorie deficit and a gradual loss of weight can easily be supported without any effect on her milk output. Fat can only be mobilized slowly, however, and too large a calorie deficit will inhibit lactation.[31] On the other hand, if a mother does not breastfeed, she may never lose the fat she gained during pregnancy.[32]

Although there need be no concern about the nutrients in breast milk, a warning is in order for the nursing mother. Chemicals other than nutrients readily enter the milk; in fact, breast milk has been called a "route of excretion" for some compounds. The list of drugs, medical and otherwise, known to be secreted in significant amounts in human milk now numbers over 100 items. Notable among them are nicotine, caffeine, marihuana, morphine, oral contraceptive hormones, and alcohol. A woman who is nursing her baby should abstain from these and all other drugs.

More about breast milk—from the infant's point of view—a few pages further on.

Psychological needs of the nursing mother. To nurse successfully, a woman needs rest and freedom from stress and anxiety. The supportive care of her husband, family, and friends can provide this for her. Many resources are also available to provide her with the information and advice she needs; some are listed in the references at the end of this chapter.

Nutrition of the Infant

The first year is a time of great importance to infants. What they eat during this time, as well as the experience of eating, will influence the rest of their lives.

Growth and Development. A baby grows faster during the first year than ever again, as Figure 3 shows. As mentioned before, the birthweight doubles in four months, from 7 to 14 pounds, and another 7 pounds is added in the next eight months. (If a ten-year-old girl were to do this, her weight would increase from 70 to 210 pounds in a single year.) By the end of the first year, the growth rate has slowed down, and the weight gained between the first and second birthdays amounts to only about 5 pounds. This tremendous growth is a composite of the differing growth patterns of all the internal organs. The generalization that many critical periods occur early still holds.

Changes in body organs during the first year affect the baby's readiness to accept solid foods. At first, all the baby can do is suck (but babies can do that powerfully); then (at six weeks) comes smiling; later (at two months or so) the baby can move the tongue against the palate to swallow semisolid food. Still later the first teeth erupt, but it is not until some time during the second year that a baby can begin to handle chewy food. The stomach and intestines are immature at first; they can digest milk sugar (lactose) but can't manufacture significant quantities of the starch-digesting enzyme, amylase, until somewhat later and so cannot digest starch until perhaps three months.

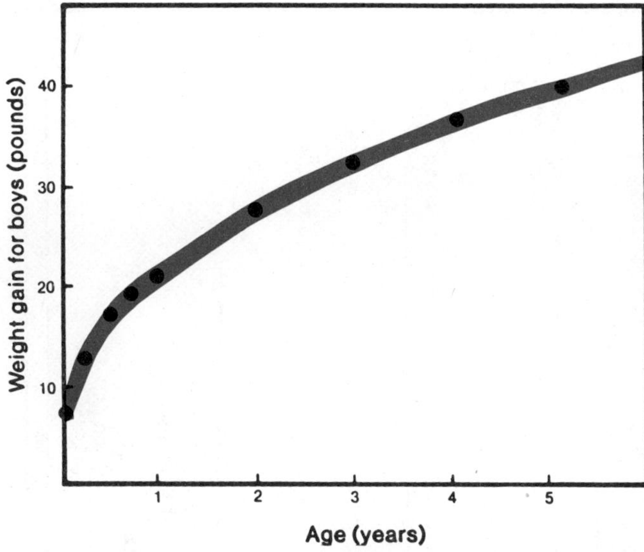

Figure 3. Weight gain of human infants (boys) in the first five years.

The baby's kidneys are unable to concentrate waste efficiently, so a baby must excrete relatively more water than an adult to carry off a comparable amount of waste. This means that dehydration, which can be dangerous, can occur more easily in an infant than in an adult. Because an infant can communicate needs only by crying, it is important to remember that the baby may be thirsty. A baby's metabolism is fast (the infant heart beats 120 to 140 times a minute, and the respiration rate is 20 times a minute, as compared with an adult's 70 to 80 and 12 to 14, respectively), so its energy needs are high.

Nutrient needs. The rapid growth and metabolism of the infant demand ample supplies of the growth and energy nutrients. Babies, because they are small, need smaller total amounts of these nutrients than adults do. But as a percentage of body weight, babies need over twice as much of most nutrients. Figure 4 compares a three-month-old baby's needs with those of an adult man; as you can see, some of the differences are extraordinary. And even though the growth rate slows towards the end of the first year, the baby's calorie needs remain constant throughout that year. The calories not spent growing, as the first birthday nears, are spent in greatly increased activity.

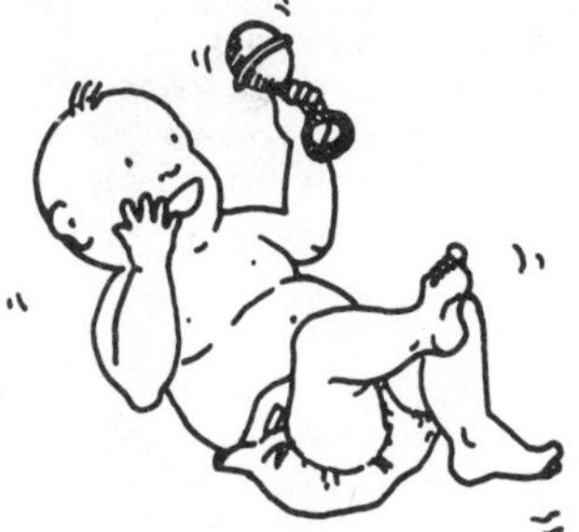

A baby's activity increases as its growth slows, so calorie needs remain high.

Milk for the infant: Breast versus bottle. The obvious food to supply the nutrients most needed by the young infant is milk, and if all other things are equal, breast milk is the milk of choice. Tailor-made to meet the nutritional needs of the human infant during the first year, breast milk offers its carbohydrate as lactose, its fat as a mixture with a generous proportion of polyunsaturated fatty acids, and its protein largely as **lactalbumin**, a protein that the human infant can easily digest. Its vitamin contents are ample. Even vitamin C, for which milk is not normally a good source, is supplied generously by breast milk.

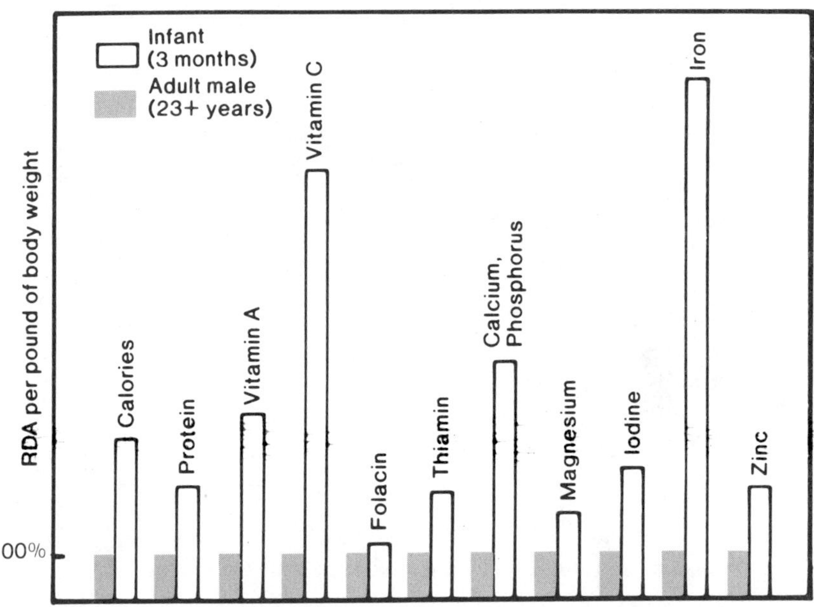

Figure 4. Comparison of the nutrient needs of a three-month-old infant with those of an adult male per unit of body weight.
The adult male's needs are set at 100 percent (see RDA table, inside front cover).

A pair of substantial mammary glands has the advantage over two hemispheres of the most learned professor's brain in the art of compounding a nutritious fluid for infants.—O. W. Holmes, Sr.
(Holmes was right, except in one respect: The breasts do not have to be substantial. Even a woman with small breasts can successfully nurse her baby.)

As for minerals, the calcium-to-phosphorus ratio (two-to-one) is ideal for the absorption of calcium, and both of these minerals and magnesium are present in amounts appropriate for the rate of growth expected in a human infant. Breast milk is also low in sodium. In addition, breast milk contains factors that favor absorption of the iron it contains. On the average, 49 percent of the iron is absorbed from breast milk, as compared with only 4 percent from fortified formula.[33] Zinc, too, is better absorbed from breast milk, which contains a zinc-binding protein necessary for absorption of zinc by the newborn.[34]

Powerful agents against bacterial infection also occur in breast milk. Among them is **lactoferrin**, an iron-grabbing compound, which keeps bacteria from getting the iron they need to grow on and also works directly to kill some bacteria.[35]

Breast milk also contains antibodies against the intestinal diseases most likely to threaten the infant's young life. Entering the infant's body with the milk, these antibodies inactivate bacteria within the digestive tract, where they would otherwise cause harm. Some of the antibodies also "leak" into the bloodstream, because the infant's immature digestive tract cannot completely exclude whole proteins. These antibodies provide additional protection against such diseases as polio.[36] Breast milk also contains a factor (**bifidus factor**) that favors the growth of the "friendly" bacteria, *Lactobacillus bifidus*, in the infant's digestive tract, so that other, harmful bacteria cannot grow there. And recently a new factor has been discovered which stimulates the development of the infant's GI tract.[37]

During the first two or three days of lactation, the breasts produce **colostrum**, a premilk substance whose antibody content is even higher than that of the milk that comes later. Both colostrum and breast milk are sterile as they leave the breast, and the baby cannot contract a bacterial infection from them even if his mother has one. Both contain active white blood cells in the same concentration as in the mother's blood, to devour enemy agents such as bacteria and viruses.[38] Thus, from the start, breast milk protects the infant in many of the same ways that modern medicine (vaccinations) and technology (sanitary water supplies) attempt to do.

Breast milk is nature's original convenience food. The nutrients are mixed with the needs of the consumer in mind. It is always at the right temperature; it is easy to take on trips; and it is kept sterile in handy packages. The directions are easy to follow.—E. M. N. Hamilton

For babies in developed countries, it is said that wealth, education, modern technology, and high-quality formulas have made it a toss-up whether there is any significant advantage to breastfeeding, and this may be true. But there is one baby who, even if born to a wealthy mother in a modern U.S. city, needs the benefits that only breast milk provides: the premature baby. A mother should breastfeed this baby even if she can't. That is, if the baby is being kept sealed away in an incubator in the intensive care unit, the mother should milk herself with her hands or a breast pump and carry the milk to the intensive care unit to be fed to the baby. It may make a life-saving difference.[39]

In the developing countries, breastfeeding is indispensable in protecting all infants' lives against the ravages of disease caused by unsanitary conditions, poverty, and ignorance. When artificial feeding is substituted, as when an infant is brought into a clinic for treatment of diarrhea, it will support the infant's life only as long as competent medical care is given in a sanitary hospital setting. When the baby goes home, the mother will often have nothing but contaminated well water with which to prepare formula and no equipment for sterilizing bottles and nipples. For such a mother to switch to the bottle is to pronounce a death sentence on her baby.[40]

Even in a wealthy nation, breastfeeding is preferable wherever possible, because it is less likely than formula to cause allergy. (For the bottle-fed baby who is allergic to cow's milk, a substitute such as goat's milk or soy milk must be provided.) Breastfeeding also seems to produce fewer fat babies than formula feeding does, perhaps partly because the mother does not force her baby to "finish the breast," since she can't see the milk that's left as she can in a bottle.

The tendency towards early weaning or artificial feeding from birth . . . is now recognized as being nutritionally disastrous for the young of underprivileged communities in all parts of the world.—World Health Organization

Women sometimes hesitate to breastfeed because they have heard that environmental contaminants such as DDT may enter their milk and harm the baby. DDT has been reported in the milk of mothers at higher concentrations than are allowed in cow's milk.[41] The significance of these findings is hard to evaluate, and the decision not to breastfeed on this basis might best be made after consultation with a physician or dietitian familiar with the local circumstances.

The morality of selling formula in the underdeveloped countries is debated in Controversy 12.

It seems to me that one of the dietary goals of infancy should be the universal utilization of breast feeding.—L. A. Barness

Another environmental contaminant that has caused concern is the PCBs, which are found in rivers and waterways polluted by industry. An episode of accidental PCB consumption by pregnant women arose in Japan when the women consumed contaminated cooking oil. Later they gave birth to abnormally small babies whose skin was unusually dark for a while. PCBs are stored in body fat and remain in the body, being excreted only in the fat of breast milk.

According to the Committee on Environmental Hazards of the American Academy of Pediatrics, women in the United States need not fear contamination of their breast milk with PCBs unless they have eaten large amounts of fish caught in PCB-contaminated rivers such as the Saint Lawrence Seaway or have been directly exposed because of their occupations. Should a woman have any question about PCBs in her breast milk, she should ask the advice of the local state health department.[42]

Many mothers choose to breastfeed at first but wean within the first one to six months. This is a nice compromise; the baby gets the advantage of the immunological protection and all the special advantages of breastfeeding during the most critical first few weeks or months, and the mother can choose in good conscience to shift to the bottle after a while. But it is imperative that she wean the baby onto *formula*, not onto plain milk of any kind—white, low-fat, or skim. Only formula contains enough iron (to name but one of many, many factors) to support normal development in the baby's first year.

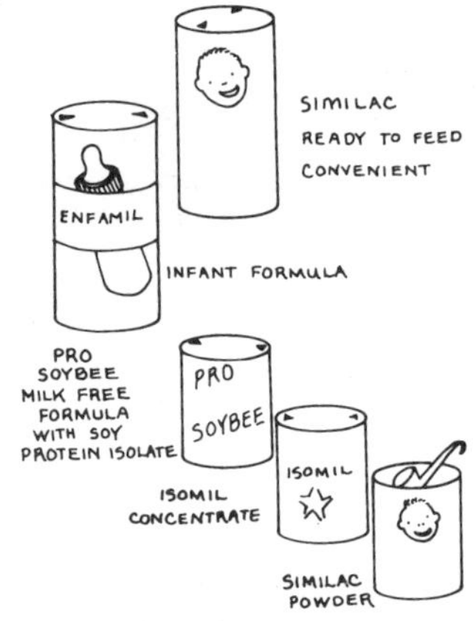

The substitution of formula feeding for breastfeeding involves copying nature as closely as possible. A comparison of the nutrient composition of human and cow's milk shows that they differ. Cow's milk is significantly higher in protein, calcium, and phosphorus, for example, to support the calf's faster growth rate. But a formula can be prepared from cow's milk by first diluting it so that it does not differ significantly from human milk in these respects, then adding lactose and nutrients to make it nutritionally comparable to human milk. The antibodies in cow's milk do not protect the human baby from diseases (they protect the calf from cow diseases), but the high level of preventive medical care (vaccinations) and public health measures achieved in the developed countries, and especially in the United States and Canada, make these considerations less important than they were in the past. Safety and sanitation can be achieved with either mode of feeding by the educated mother whose water supply is reliable.

Infant formula is made as similar to human milk as possible.

Closeness is extremely important in the feeding of a baby. (It has been said that one of the advantages of the breast is that it cannot be "propped.") If bottle feeding is the means chosen, then mother (or father) should be sure to provide the same attention, handling, and play that go naturally with the nursing of a baby. An infant's first impressions of the world relate to emotions felt during feeding; and holding a baby with love and a bottle will do more for its psychological development than holding with resentment at the breast. An advantage of bottle feeding is that it gives the father and other family members a chance to develop a warm, affectionate relationship with the baby, while freeing the mother to work or play more than she could otherwise do.

To assure your baby an adequate diet:

Breastfeed unless there are special problems.

Delay other foods until baby is three to six months old.

Do not add salt or sugar to baby's food.

—USDA Dietary Guidelines

Whichever mode of feeding is chosen, the mother should be supported in her choice. Especially with her first infant, she may be experiencing some problems with adjusting. Heavy pressure against either decision constitutes an avoidable stress.

Supplements for the baby. It is unnecessary to give vitamin-mineral supplements to newborn babies. If they are breastfed, breast milk and their own internal stores will meet their needs until they are well into the second half of the first year, and then the introduction of intelligently chosen juices and foods will keep up with their changing requirements. The only exception to this statement has to do with vitamin D and fluoride. The question is not completely settled, but it seems likely that breast milk doesn't provide enough vitamin D and that its fluoride contents may be somewhat unreliable.[43] The baby's pediatrician is likely to be well informed on this matter and to prescribe appropriate supplementation.

If the baby is formula-fed, the makeup of the formula determines what further supplementation may be necessary. Again, the pediatrician is the expert to consult, and Table 4 gives some suggestions.

First foods. The timing for adding solid foods to a baby's diet depends on several factors. If the baby is breastfed, additions to the diet can probably wait until about six months, but not later. Babies not fed solid foods in the second half of the first year suffer delayed growth.[44] If the baby is formula-fed, a reasonable pattern for adding foods to the diet is shown in Table 4. But all babies are different, and the program of additions should depend on the individual baby, not on any rigid schedule.

The addition of foods to a baby's diet should be governed by three considerations: first, to supply the needed nutrients; second, to supply them in a form the baby is physically ready to handle; and third, to introduce them singly so that allergies can easily be detected.[45] For example, when cereals are introduced, try rice cereal first for several days, because it least often causes allergy. Try wheat cereal last, because it is the most common offender. If a cereal causes an allergic reaction (irritability, misery), discontinue its use before going on to the next food. About nine times out of ten, the allergy won't be evident immediately but will manifest itself in vague symptoms occurring up to five days after the offending food is eaten, so it isn't easy to detect.

About one out of every four people may have an allergy of one kind or another, and about half of these allergies are caused by foods. The foods that most commonly cause allergies are milk, wheat, egg (whites), corn, and pork.[46] If a parent detects allergies in an infant's early life, the whole family can be spared much grief.

More about food allergies in Controversy 13: Hyperactivity.

As for the choice of foods, baby foods commercially prepared in the United States and Canada are generally safe, nutritious, and of high quality. In response to consumer demand, the baby food companies have removed much of the added salt and sugar their products contained in the past,[47] and they also contain few or no additives. They generally have high nutrient density, except for the mixed dinners (which contain little meat) and desserts (which are heavily sweetened). An alternative for the parent who wants the baby to have family foods is to "blenderize" a small portion of the table food at each meal. If this choice is made, the parent should try to be salt-conscious. Parents often salt their table foods, even without meaning to, more than even commercial baby foods are salted. And babies should never be fed canned vegetables; not only is the sodium content too high but also there is a risk of lead contamination.[48] It is also important to take precautions

Table 4. First Foods for the Formula-Fed Baby

Age (months)	Addition
0–1	Supplement (depending on what's in formula)
1–2	Diluted orange juice (for vitamin C)
4–6	Iron-fortified rice cereal followed by other cereals (for iron; baby can swallow and can digest starch now)[a]
5–7	Strained vegetables and/or fruits and their juices, one by one
6–8	Protein foods (cheese, yogurt, cooked beans, meat, fish, chicken, egg yolk)
9	Finely chopped meat (baby can chew now)
Later	Cottage cheese, toast, teething crackers (for emerging teeth)

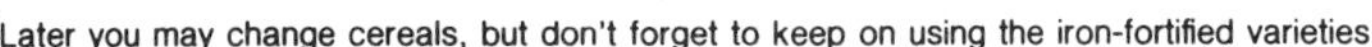

[a]Later you may change cereals, but don't forget to keep on using the iron-fortified varieties.

Adapted from the 1979 Recommendations for Infant Feeding Practices of the California Department of Health Services as presented in Current infant feeding practices, Nutrition and the MD, January 1980.

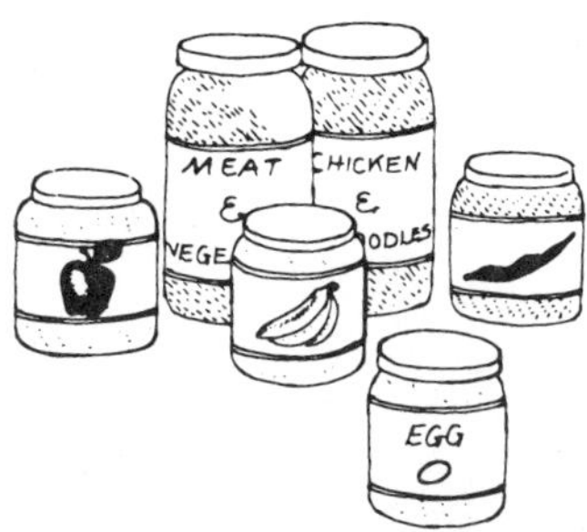

Commercially prepared baby foods are generally safe, nutritious, and of high quality.

Meal plan for a one-year-old

Breakfast
1 cup milk
2-3 tbsp cereal
2-3 tbsp strained fruit
Teething crackers

Lunch
1 cup milk
2-3 tbsp vegetables
Chopped meat
2-3 tbsp pudding

Snack
½ cup milk
Teething crackers

Supper
1 cup milk
1 egg
2 tbsp cereal or potato
2-3 tbsp cooked fruit
Teething crackers

***We are becoming increasingly aware of the unsuspected significance of nutrition during early infancy for the development of certain pathological conditions which only manifest themselves in adulthood.*—L. Rey**

against food poisoning and to avoid the use of vegetables in which nitrites are likely to form (see Controversy 11B). Honey should never be fed to infants because of the risk of botulism.

At one year of age, the obvious food to supply most of the nutrients the baby needs is still milk; 2 to 3½ cups a day are now sufficient. More milk than this would displace foods necessary to provide iron and would cause the iron-deficiency anemia known as **milk anemia**. The other foods—meat, iron-fortified cereal, enriched or whole-grain bread, fruit, and vegetables—should be supplied in variety and in amounts sufficient to round out total calorie needs. A meal plan that meets these requirements for the one-year-old is shown in the margin.

Prevention of future health problems. The first year of a baby's life is the time to lay the foundation for future health. In part, this means taking appropriate measures to avert the likelihood of problems' developing later. From the nutrition standpoint, the relevant problems most common in later years are obesity and dental disease. Prevention of obesity should also inhibit the development of the obesity-related diseases—atherosclerosis, diabetes, and cancer.

Infant obesity should at all costs be avoided. Probably the most important single measure to undertake during the first year is to encourage eating habits that will support continued normal weight as the child grows. Primarily, this means introducing nutritious foods in an inviting way; avoiding concentrated sweets and empty calorie foods; and encouraging plenty of vigorous physical activity. It has been suggested that the early introduction of sweet fruits to a baby's diet might favor the development of a preference for sweets and lessen the liking for vegetables introduced later. To prevent this, the order should perhaps be changed: vegetables first, fruits later. This practice now has a wide following.

The introduction of solid foods should probably wait until the baby has reached the age of about four to six months, when experience with them is first needed to help the normal swallowing reflex develop. Earlier, they might have several undesirable effects: displacing breast milk or formula, which is the most perfectly balanced diet for a young baby; increasing or decreasing overall calorie intake and so upsetting the physiological course toward normal weight in childhood; or establishing the habit of overeating. It is after six months that the transition from breast milk or formula to fluid milk may be made, and at this time, vitamin C and iron need to be supplied from food.

Some parents want to feed solids at an earlier age, on the theory that "stuffing the baby" at bedtime will make him or her more likely to sleep through the night. There is no proof for this theory. Babies start to sleep through the night at the average age of about nine weeks, regardless of when solid foods are introduced.[49]

To discourage development of the behaviors and attitudes that plague the obese, parents should avoid teaching babies to seek food as a reward, to expect food as comfort for unhappiness, or to associate food deprivation with punishment. If they cry for thirst, they should be given water, not milk or juice. A baby has no internal "calorie counter" and stops eating when its stomach is full, so low-calorie foods that provide bulk will be satisfying.[50]

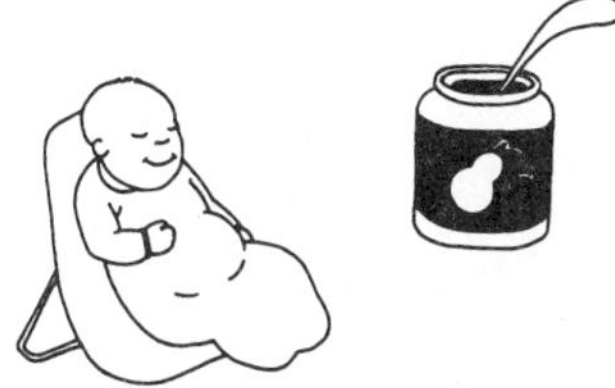

A baby stops eating when its stomach is full.

Beyond these recommendations, there is some thought being given to the idea that infants should be started on a "prudent diet"—designed along the lines recommended for heart patients. This means restricting fat in the diet, increasing the ratio of polyunsaturated to saturated fat, and reducing the cholesterol intake. Such a diet has been tried with infants up to three years of age. It seems to have done them no harm while lowering their serum cholesterol.[51] However, this kind of program is only experimental. Babies need the calories and fat of normal milk, and most experts agree that they should be fed whole or at least low-fat—not skim—milk until after they are a year old. The only exception might be the seriously obese baby, who should perhaps be started on a prudent diet as early as three months of age.[52] Tampering with the amount of protein in a baby's diet could be especially undesirable, because altered amounts of protein affect the baby's body composition with unpredictable consequences.[53]

The ideal diet is one that achieves growth without obesity.
—R. L. Huenemann

Normal dental development is promoted by the same strategies as those outlined above: supplying nutritious foods, avoiding sweets, and discouraging association of food with reward or comfort. In addition, the practice of giving a baby a bottle as a pacifier is strongly discouraged by dentists on the grounds that sucking for long periods of time pushes the normal jawline out of shape and causes the bucktooth profile: protruding upper and receding lower teeth. Once a baby has some teeth, prolonged sucking on a bottle of milk or juice bathes the upper teeth with a continuous flow of carbohydrate-rich fluid that favors the growth of decay-producing bacteria. Babies permitted to do this are sometimes seen with their upper teeth decayed all the way to the gum line.

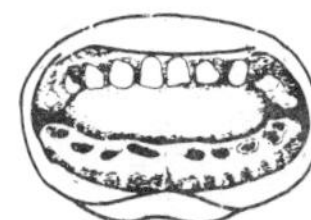

A baby that goes to sleep sucking on a bottle of juice may lose its teeth to decay before two years of age. This is called the nursing bottle syndrome.

Psychological needs. At birth, a baby's needs are simple—warmth, affection, relief from pain, and a consistent feeding schedule to rely on.

A mother may feel, quite rightly, that her major task at the start is to "keep putting it in one end and keep removing it from the other." However, by the time a baby has reached the age of one, his (or her) mother often realizes with consternation that he is no longer the malleable, accepting little creature that he used to be. He is becoming an individual, and the ways he expresses this new development can be exasperating. In recent months he has been "getting into everything"; now that he is learning to walk, his range is broader, and nothing in the house below adult waist level is safe. A toddler explores and experiments endlessly, twisting the knobs on the television set, poking his fingers into the wall sockets, tugging on lamp cords and curtains, pulling all the toilet paper off the roll, stirring the soil in potted plants, and scattering the contents of mother's purse.

He used to be receptive and eager to please; now he is contrary and willful. Whatever mother suggests, he refuses, even if it is something he normally likes to do. When mother tells her little boy to stop hitting the cat with the car keys, he casts an appraising eye at her, hesitates only a moment—and continues hitting the cat.

The wise mother is aware that this is a period in her child's life when these behaviors are normal, natural, and even desirable. The child is developing a sense of *autonomy* that, if allowed to flower, will provide the foundation for later confidence and effectiveness as an individual. A wise mother uses her toddler's short attention span to distract him away from the television set. She absolutely forbids—by force, if necessary—her baby to poke into wall sockets or to eat matches but also avoids punishing too hard. A child's urge to explore and experiment, if consistently denied, can turn to shame and self-doubt.

A one-year-old girl (or boy) behaves the same way at the table as in other settings. She displays her urge to experiment by dipping her bananas into the spaghetti, by fingerpainting with the chocolate pudding, or by pouring her milk over the tabletop and watching, fascinated, as it drips onto the floor. Her sense of autonomy is strengthened when she refuses to eat her cereal and insists on having applesauce instead. The dilemma a mother faces, knowing how important it is for her child to eat a balanced diet, can be resolved if she is prepared for these developments and knows how to handle them to best advantage. Although a mother attempts to feed her baby all the necessary nutrients in good balance and in amounts sufficient to promote optimal growth and health, she at the same time wants to encourage the baby to feel secure, confident, and independent and to avoid the techniques of shaming, blaming, and inhibiting the growing child.

In light of these developmental and nutritional needs, and in the face of the often contrary and willful behavior of the one-year-old, a mother might find a few feeding guidelines helpful. The most typical problem behaviors are listed in the Food Feature, with suggestions for how to handle them.

Food Feature: Setting the Eating Pattern for Life

If a baby spends 2½ hours a day eating, the total will be over 1000 hours a year—as much time as a college student spends in classes in two years of full-time study. Babies are open to new impressions of the world, and the amount of learning that takes place during the feeding hours is astronomical. Not only do they obtain needed nutrients for growth and development, they are also learning about the world—especially about food, about themselves, and about the behaviors that win approval and those that don't. Properly handled, eating times can make a tremendous contribution to a child's future well-being, both physical and psychological. Following are a few problem situations with suggestions for handling them.

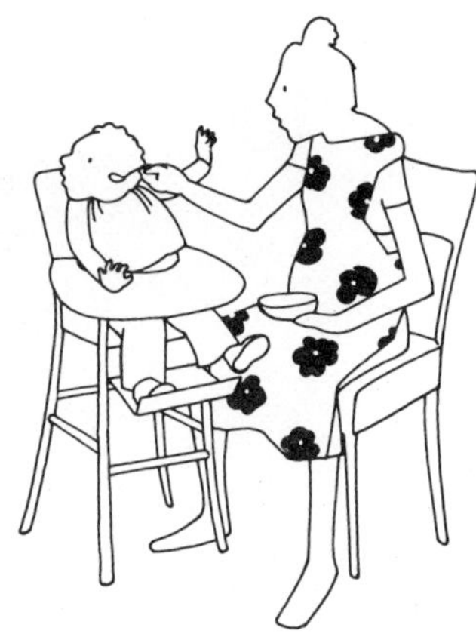

If he refuses food, put him down and let him wait until the next meal.

He stands and plays at the table instead of eating. Don't let him. This is unacceptable behavior and should be firmly discouraged. Put him down and let him wait until the next feeding to eat again. Be consistent and firm, not punitive. If he is really hungry, he will soon learn to sit still while eating. Be aware that a baby's appetite is less keen at a year than at eight months and that his calorie needs are relatively lower. A one-year-old will get enough to eat if he lets his own hunger be his guide.

She wants to poke her fingers into her food. Let her. She has much to learn from feeling the texture of her food. When she knows all about it, she'll naturally graduate to the use of a spoon.

He wants to manage the spoon himself but can't handle it. Let him try. As he masters it, withdraw gradually until he is feeding himself competently. This is the age at which babies can and do learn to feed themselves and are most strongly motivated to do so. They will spill, of course. Mother's best attitude probably is that "one-year-olds don't last forever"; they'll grow out of it soon enough.

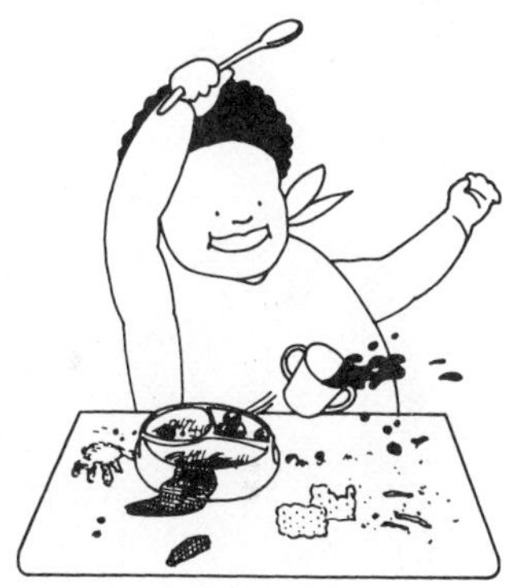

Remember, one-year olds don't last forever.

She refuses food that mother knows is good for her. This way of demonstrating autonomy, one of the few available to the one-year-old, is most satisfying. Don't force. It is in the one- to two-year-old stage that most of the feeding problems develop that can last throughout life. As long as she is getting enough milk and is offered a variety of nutritious foods to choose from, she can and will gradually acquire a taste for different foods—provided that she feels she is making the choice. This is the most important year of a child's life in establishing future food preferences. If a baby refuses milk, an alternative source of the bone- and muscle-building nutrients it supplies must be provided. Milk-based puddings, custards, and cheese are often successful substitutes. For the baby who is allergic to milk, soy milk and other formulas are available.

He prefers sweets—candy and sugary confections—to foods containing more nutrients. Human beings of all races and cultures have a natural inborn preference for sweet-tasting foods. Limit them strictly. There is no room in a baby's daily 1000 calories for the calories from sweets, except occasionally. The meal plan shown before provides more than 500 calories from milk; one or two servings of each of the other types of food provide the other 500. If a candy bar were substituted for any of these foods, the baby would lose out on valuable nutrients; if it were added daily, he would gradually become obese.[1]

For Further Information

Many of the references suggested in Appendix J include good sections or chapters on nutrition of pregnant women and infants. In addition, the following book should be singled out for special mention:

- Worthington, B. S.; Vermeersch, J.; and Williams, S. R. *Nutrition in Pregnancy and Lactation.* St. Louis: Mosby, 1977 (paperback).

A delightful presentation of pregnancy from the fetus's point of view is available from the March of Dimes:

- Inside my mom, a set of about eighty slides with a cassette.

Inquire from your local March of Dimes office or from the National Foundation, March of Dimes, PO Box 2000, White Plains, NY 10602. The March of Dimes has been very active in working to prevent birth defects, and you might inquire what other materials they have available.

The entire issue of *Nutrition and the MD* for November 1980 was devoted to nutrition in pregnancy and contained many valuable pointers.

An excellent ten-minute film on fetal alcohol syndrome, "Born Drunk," is available from ABC, 1330 Avenue of the Americas, New York, NY 10019.

Many good references on breastfeeding are also available. We recommend:

- Jelliffe, D. B., and Jelliffe, E. F. P. "Breast is best": Modern meanings. *New England Journal of Medicine* 297 (1977): 912-915. This article presents the reasons why, in the authors' opinion, breastfeeding is best even in developed countries such as the United States and Canada.
- Smith, G. V.; Calvert, L. J.; and Kanto, W. P., Jr. Breast feeding and infant nutrition. *American Family Physician* 17 (1978): 92-102. This is a fully up-to-date, well-illustrated, scientifically accurate article with useful tips on how to breastfeed.

The USDHEW makes available a short (twenty-two-page) how-to booklet:

[1]*Chapter Notes can be found at the end of the Appendixes.*

- Breast feeding. DHEW publication no. (HSA) 79-5109.

Write to the U.S. Government Printing Office (see Appendix J).

An international organization of women who believe in breastfeeding and who help each other is the LaLeche League, 9616 Minneapolis Avenue, Franklin Park, IL 60131.

FDA Consumer published an update on drugs excreted in breast milk:

- Hecht, A. Advice on breastfeeding and drugs. *FDA Consumer*, November 1979, pp. 21-22.

If you want to learn all there is to know about breastfeeding you can get a giant head start by sending for the National Academy of Sciences' fifty-eight-page booklet prepared by the Committee on Nutrition of the Mother and Preschool Child:

- A selected annotated bibliography on breast feeding, 1970-1977.

Write to the Office of Publications, National Academy of Sciences (address in Appendix J).

In relation to the profound effect that "feeding with love" can have on children, E. M. Widdowson described long ago how this variable "ruined" a nutritional experiment that some investigators tried to carry out. Love and attention had a bigger effect on the children's growth than the food:

- Widdowson, E. M. Mental contentment and physical growth. *Lancet* 1 (1951): 1316-1317.

On nutrition in the first year of life, Fomon's book, *Infant Nutrition*, cited in the chapter notes, is an excellent comprehensive reference.

A tidy four-page statement on the nutritional needs of infants up to a year of age was published in the American Medical Association journal:

- Woodruff, C. W. The science of infant nutrition and the art of infant feeding. *Journal of the American Medical Association* 240 (1978): 657-661.

The whole issue (all six pages) of *Nutrition and the MD*, May 1980, was also devoted to infant nutrition. These resources both rely extensively on the authoritative word of the American Association of Pediatrics, whose Committee on Nutrition published its recommendations in the following article:

- Commentary on breast-feeding and infant formulas, including proposed standards for formulas. *Pediatrics* 57 (1976): 278-285.

According to a recent review, it is "irresponsible to make a dogmatic statement" about the timing or selection of additions of solid food to a baby's diet. This review gives details on what needs to be considered:

- Nutritional adequacy of breast feeding. *Nutrition Reviews* 38 (1980): 145-147.

The USDA has published a manual giving the complete nutritional analysis of many baby foods:

- *Composition of Foods: Baby Foods—Raw, Processed, Prepared.* Agriculture Handbook no. 8-3. Washington, D.C: USDA Science and Education Administration, 1978.

On the rearing of children, Dr. Benjamin Spock's book remains a classic:

- Spock, B. *Baby and Child Care.* New York: Pocket Books, 1977 (paperback). First published as *The Common Sense Book of Baby and Child Care.* New York: Duell, Sloan and Pearce, 1958. The tolerance we recommend for contending with the antics of a young child originated with Spock.

For the parent of a new baby, provided that it's a healthy baby, there's a good paperback available on infant feeding:

- Heslin, J. A., and Natow, A. F. *No-Nonsense Nutrition: For Your Baby's First Year.* Boston: CBI Publishing, 1978.

Controversy 12

Baby Killers

Does infant formula kill Third World babies?

The article was called "The Baby Killer." The first page showed a shriveled baby curled up inside a formula bottle. It was published in 1974 by a charitable organization in London that called itself War on Want, Ltd. It almost did start a war.

The story it told was of thousands of babies dying because their mothers had been persuaded to give up breastfeeding. It charged that the makers of infant formula—Nestle, Bristol Myers, and others—were marketing their cow's-milk-based formula in underdeveloped countries where bottle-feeding wouldn't work. Babies who are bottle fed during the first three months of their lives suffer three times the mortality rates of their brothers and sisters who are exclusively breastfed, it stated. Infection and malnutrition are an almost inevitable result of weaning to formula in the developing countries.

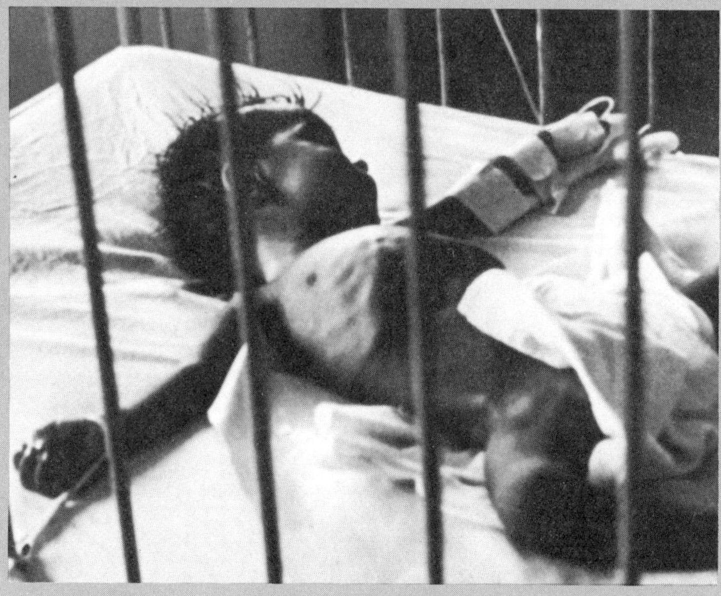

This baby is in the last stages of malnutrition and illness because he was weaned from the breast too soon and inadequately fed thereafter.

The scenario goes like this: A mother in extreme poverty conditions bears a baby and starts breastfeeding it. (She has no other alternative.) The baby thrives, even though the mother becomes somewhat undernourished and exhausted with this drain on her physical resources. Then one day the mother sees a saleslady dressed in white, who looks like a nurse, advertising the virtues of bottles of milk from America or Europe which will make her baby healthy and strong. The nurse has formula samples with pictures of fat, healthy, smiling babies on the packages, and tells the mother that she need only mix the powder with water to feed her baby. The mother accepts a few free samples, and starts looking forward to the time when she can go to work and leave her baby at home to be cared for by its grandmother, the family income will increase, and all will be well.

By the time the free samples are used up, the baby has been weaned and the mother's milk is dried up, so a return to breastfeeding is impossible. Now mother is buying formula, but the baby is beginning to sicken and become weak. The mother hasn't understood how to prepare the formula correctly and has used contaminated water, causing an infection. Or—because the formula is expensive—the mother has diluted it to half strength, not knowing that the baby won't get enough nutrients this way. The baby continues to weaken, becomes malnourished and severely infected, then dies.

A variation of this story is simpler and shorter. The mother comes in to a clinic or hospital to bear her baby. The hospital has been given free samples by an infant formula company, and 90 percent of the newborns are started on bottle feeding at birth. By the time the mother leaves the hospital with a few samples, her milk has dried up and her infant is totally dependent on the bottle. This story ends the same way as the first.

A year after "The Baby Killer," a film made in Kenya—"Bottle Babies"—was shown widely to church audiences and political groups. The final painful scene was of a baby's grave with a headstone shaped like a baby bottle. The stories have spread all over the world: Baby-food makers are killing thousands of babies in the poor countries, preferring to make profits for themselves and their stockholders rather than to support life in these faraway places. Every newspaper has headlined them, TV and radio have picked them up, angered citizens have banded together to inform their neighborhoods and church groups and get organized to stop the killing. The world response climaxed in 1977 with the formation of INFACT—Infant Formula Action Coalition, a community action project which spearheaded a drive to boycott Nestle products. Sixty other groups joined INFACT, including Church Women United, Clergy and Laity Concerned, and many others. Thousands of words have been traded—accusations, denials, arguments, and counterarguments. In 1978 a health and scientific research subcommittee of the U.S. Senate investigated the matter. Later the same year an advisory group to the Nutrition Foundation presented its findings. In 1979 the *Lactation Review* published a study titled "Babies in Poverty, the Real Victims of the Breast/Bottle Controversy." By then, the arguments had all been heard, if not resolved. The two sides of the debate follow.

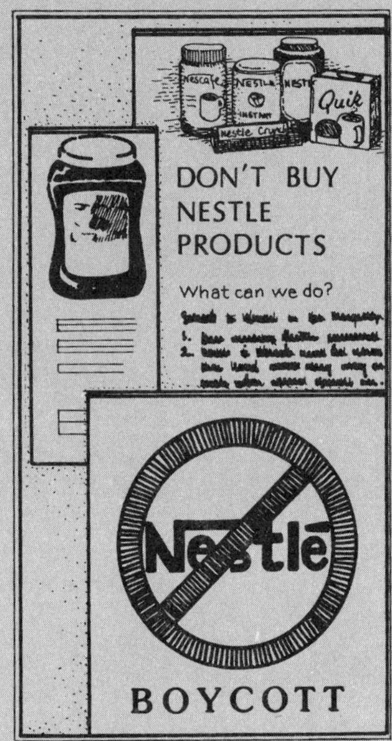
Quik
DON'T BUY
NESTLE
PRODUCTS
What can we do?
Nestlé
BOYCOTT

Opposition to the infant formula companies' actions took the form of a boycott of their other products.

The INFACT argument. Many of those who testified before the Senate subcommittee in 1978 took INFACT's side. According to Dr. Derrick B. Jelliffe, former director of the Caribbean Food and Nutrition Institute in Jamaica, ten million cases of malnutrition and diarrhea in developing countries can be attributed to "inadequate bottle feeding," and most of these could be prevented by a return to breastfeeding. Dr. Allan Jackson of the University of West Indies in Kingston, Jamaica, agreed. He explained that many parents can't afford the price of infant formula so they dilute it to make it last longer. Fatina Petal, a nurse from Lima, Peru, added that mothers often use polluted water to make the formula, "rather than go into the jungle, chop wood, bring it back, and start a fire to boil the water." Dr. Navidad Clavano, a physician from the Philippines, charged that most mothers would breastfeed and wouldn't engage in these unhealthy practices were it not for "overpromotion" by formula manufacturers. The companies offer cocktail parties and free plane flights to medical officers in the developing countries, he said.[1]

In reaction to the hearings, Senator Kennedy, chairman of the Senate subcommittee, seemed persuaded:

Can a product which requires clean water, good sanitation, adequate family income, and a literate parent to follow printed instructions be properly and safely used in areas where water is contaminated, sewage runs in the streets, poverty is severe and illiteracy is high?

Also persuaded were some of the foremost nutrition authorities in the world. One was Dr. S. J. Fomon, professor in the Department of Pediatrics, College of Medicine, University of Iowa and vice president of the Twelfth International Congress on Nutrition. Dr. Fomon said the conditions in developing countries make safe preparation of formula "virtually impossible" and added:

It's hard enough for these babies to survive under the best of circumstances; exploitative marketing and merchandising is tantamount to mass infanticide.

Another was Dr. Michael Latham, director of the Program in International Nutrition at Cornell University. Dr. Latham concluded:

My interpretation of the scientific evidence leaves absolutely no doubt in my mind first that bottle feeding is a major cause of morbidity and mortality in developing countries and secondly that the promotion of formulas by corporations such as Nestle has contributed significantly to this most tragic of problems.[2]

The Senate subcommittee hearing ended with agreement that infant formula companies should not promote their products to the public, that they should not be allowed to sell formula abroad until they had been licensed to do so, that the license should depend on their marketing plans, and that they should be required to provide appropriate instructions with their products in the native language of the buyers—in short, that they should be closely regulated to keep them from unethical and dangerous practices.

By the time the hearings were over, a number of infant formula makers, including Nestle, had reviewed their marketing practices and adopted reforms. But the critics weren't satisfied. Dr. Jelliffe, referring to the fact that infant formula represented $300 million in sales a year to Nestle alone, was quoted:

No company is going to abandon so lucrative a market. It will take major government intervention to do something positive about the misuse of the bottle in the Third World. Meanwhile, as breastfeeding declines, more babies will die.[3]

The battle was not over.

The companies' defense. The makers of infant formula argue that they have done nothing to worsen infant mortality. David O. Cox, president of the Ross Division of Abbott Laboratories, which has about 10 percent of the formula market in the developing countries, said in 1978 that his company promoted its products only to health-care officials and affirmed the superiority of breastfeeding for most infants.[4] Frank Sprole of Bristol-Myers testified at the Senate subcommittee hearing:

Our promotion consists principally of providing infant formula as free goods for hospital use, free samples for distribution at doctors' discretion, the donation of incubators, scales and other equipment for hospital use, and the support of medical symposia . . . any suggestion that professional judgment is compromised by such promotion is unjustified and offensive.[5]

At the same time, the Nestle company circulated thirty-five pages of mimeographed information in defense of its policies to hundreds of U.S. critics. According to Nestle, it had discontinued all direct consumer advertising of infant formula by the end of 1977 except in a few Far Eastern countries where the government health services approved the ads. Nestle promotes breastfeeding in every way it can, it said, and supplies formula only so that mothers who can't breastfeed have a safe alternative. Nestle distributes only limited amounts of free samples and only to the medical profession and to hospitals, clinics, missions, and orphanages that request them. Furthermore, in the countries in which infant formula sales have been rising, infant mortality has been falling. Formula, says Nestle, has helped to lower the infant mortality rate.[6] In April 1979, Doug Grouner of Nestle made the disclaimer on TV:

[Once the manufacturer has sold the product] to a distributor . . . he has no way to assure that the product will be sold where it should be sold and not sold out in the bush somewhere.[7]

Nestle representatives were further quoted as saying "the formula products are usually purchased by people who can afford them" and that "a mother's need or desire to work [is] the principal reason for the breast feeding decline."[8] Clearly there were two opposing views on the matter with very little hard evidence on either side and not much being collected.

The middle ground. Squarely in the middle of all this controversy are bottle-fed babies in developing countries. How well do they fare? Why are they being fed the bottle? If it is harmful to them, who is responsible? And what can be done?

The answer to the first of these questions is clear. The bottle-fed baby is at a real disadvantage. The advantages of breastfeeding for such babies were documented in Chapter 12 and that discussion will not be repeated here, but you may recall that the conclusion was that to take such babies off the breast is to condemn them to probable illness, poor development, and possibly death. The question, then, is: why are these babies being fed formula? And the answer can be approached by asking what it takes to breastfeed successfully.

To breastfeed successfully, a mother needs support. In most traditional societies, she has a network of support from her family and the community. She needs more food when she is lactating, and that means more of the family's resources must be allocated to her. And she needs either to be employed at home where her baby is or to labor in a setting where she can take her baby with her. If she is exposed to outside people such as medical or social personnel, she needs support from them as well, in the form of their recognition that breastfeeding is indeed the best way to feed her baby and their willingness to arrange their interventions to accommodate breastfeeding.[9]

There are many factors in the real world that interfere with this ideal picture. Rural families are moving to cities, where the traditional supporting culture is lacking. Severe poverty interferes with the mother's getting enough food to support lactation, sometimes to the extent of reducing the breast milk supply. Then infant formula, or infant foods introduced as early as three months may be life-saving for the baby. The family may be making an effort to better their situation, moving to the city where they can earn money and where the water flows from pumps or even faucets, but in the process they may experience such disruption of their way of life as to make adequate infant care impossible:

In subsistence economies, there are few obstacles to breast feeding, because the baby remains with his mother all day and she has no money to buy artificial foods. The situation changes with a cash economy, where a mother must often earn money to support the rest of the family, and consequently is separated from the baby for much of the day. This is one explanation for the fact that the incidence of breast feeding has fallen steadily in most countries over the last fifty years, with a concomitant increase in artificial feeding. . . . Arguments about the "economic benefits" of breast feeding are not going to convince a mother who has other hungry mouths to feed, that she should not go out to work.[10]

Then the mother may seek help for her sick baby only to find that there is no medical care available, or that there isn't enough, or that the available medical and social services can't advise her about her infant's nutrition. One of the defenses of the infant formula companies is that they are supplying the next-best food for infants under circumstances where breastfeeding is impossible. One of the retorts made by INFACT is that a mother's need to earn money outside the home accounts for less than 10 percent of the cases of cessation of breastfeeding.[11] Whatever the figure is, at least one thing seems clear: Not all cases of weaning to the bottle can be laid at the door of the formula makers. Other factors make it necessary sometimes, however undesirable; and once weaning has occurred, a good substitute for breast milk is needed.

The question who is responsible for so many of the world's babies' being bottle-fed is not answerable—that is, it isn't a "who" but a whole set of changing circumstances. The *underdeveloped* countries are now *developing*—that is, changing—countries, and the process of change itself is responsible for much of the upheaval in traditional ways of life, including breastfeeding. Benefits may be coming from the changes, but babies are undeniably paying for those changes by suffering inadequate feeding.

What can be done? The World Health Organization met with UNICEF at a major conference in 1979 to ask what could be done to alleviate this problem. It focussed on six issues, two of which are at the core of this Controversy. One was the question how to encourage and support breastfeeding, and another involved the appropriate marketing and distribution of breast milk substitutes.[12] The report of the meeting is included in the selected references at the end of this Controversy and is highly recommended reading. The participants agreed on many issues and made some statements that, for a group of this kind, were remarkably strongly worded:

It is . . . a responsibility of society to promote breastfeeding and to protect pregnant and lactating mothers from any influence that could disrupt it.

All health workers . . . should be committed to the promotion of breastfeeding. . . .

Governments have a duty to ensure the supply and availability of adequate infant food products to those who need them, in ways that will not discourage breastfeeding.

The marketing of breastmilk substitutes . . . should be designed not to discourage breastfeeding.

There should be no sales promotion, including promotional advertising to the public, of products to be used as breastmilk substitutes. This includes the use of mass media and other forms of advertising directed to the mother or general public.[13]

And so on.

These statements by WHO/UNICEF put the focus where it belongs. The infant formula companies may have been advertising their products; they may have been engaging in unethical practices. They may have done so with good motives, sincerely desiring to provide products that would meet the nutritional needs of babies that had to be weaned. Or they may have been pursuing standard marketing practices ("Beat out the competition") with no thought for the consequences to the infants their products would reach. Whatever the companies may have done, the question what to do in the future is more important:

More important [is] the search for ways of getting diverse groups together to save the lives of the world's babies who, while we argue, are being born at the rate of 350,000 a day and many of whom are doomed to die before they learn to speak.[14]

The WHO/UNICEF conference ended with an agreement that companies' marketing practices should be monitored, by both the exporting and the importing countries, under government auspices and with the help of advertising councils, industry, and consumer and professional groups. To this end, a Code of Marketing of Breastmilk Substitutes has since been developed by WHO,[15] and all indications were that it would evolve into a standard for the ethical and humane use of formula where needed and the prevention of its use wherever breastfeeding could be promoted as the rightful first choice.

The conflict was still continuing in 1981, however. In May of that year, ninety-three of the World Health Organization's member nations voted to recommend the breastfeeding code to all the world's governments, with the expectation that they would translate it into national laws and regulations. But the United States voted against it, apparently influenced by the commercial interest of the companies.[16]

Personal strategy. The private citizen, confronted with the realities of the world hunger situation or hearing that ten million babies are suffering malnutrition and sickness each year, is likely to find the problems overwhelming and hopeless. Asking "What can I do?" you may be tempted to conclude, "Nothing. It is too remote and too big a problem for me to handle." Yet in this instance, individuals who cared have achieved a measure of success by banding together. Working with such groups is an experience many conscientious people find rewarding.

On a more impersonal level, it is important for all of us to be well enough informed to help guide our legislators in developing programs intelligently designed to be effective. In the case of "the baby killers," it is suggested that the WHO resolutions are well thought through and should be supported. Infant formula is sometimes a life-saving alternative to starvation, and many of the companies that make it put their best efforts into making the finest possible products. But breastfeeding is life-sustaining in most of the world where formula cannot be properly used. Babies fed breast milk resist disease better, and their mothers, if nutritionally supported, benefit by bearing fewer and healthier children. It is advisable to stop the promotion of infant formula and to restrict its use to those who will make it available with appropriate education and only when there is no alternative.

The Controversy Notes and For Further Information follow the Appendixes.

CHAPTER 13

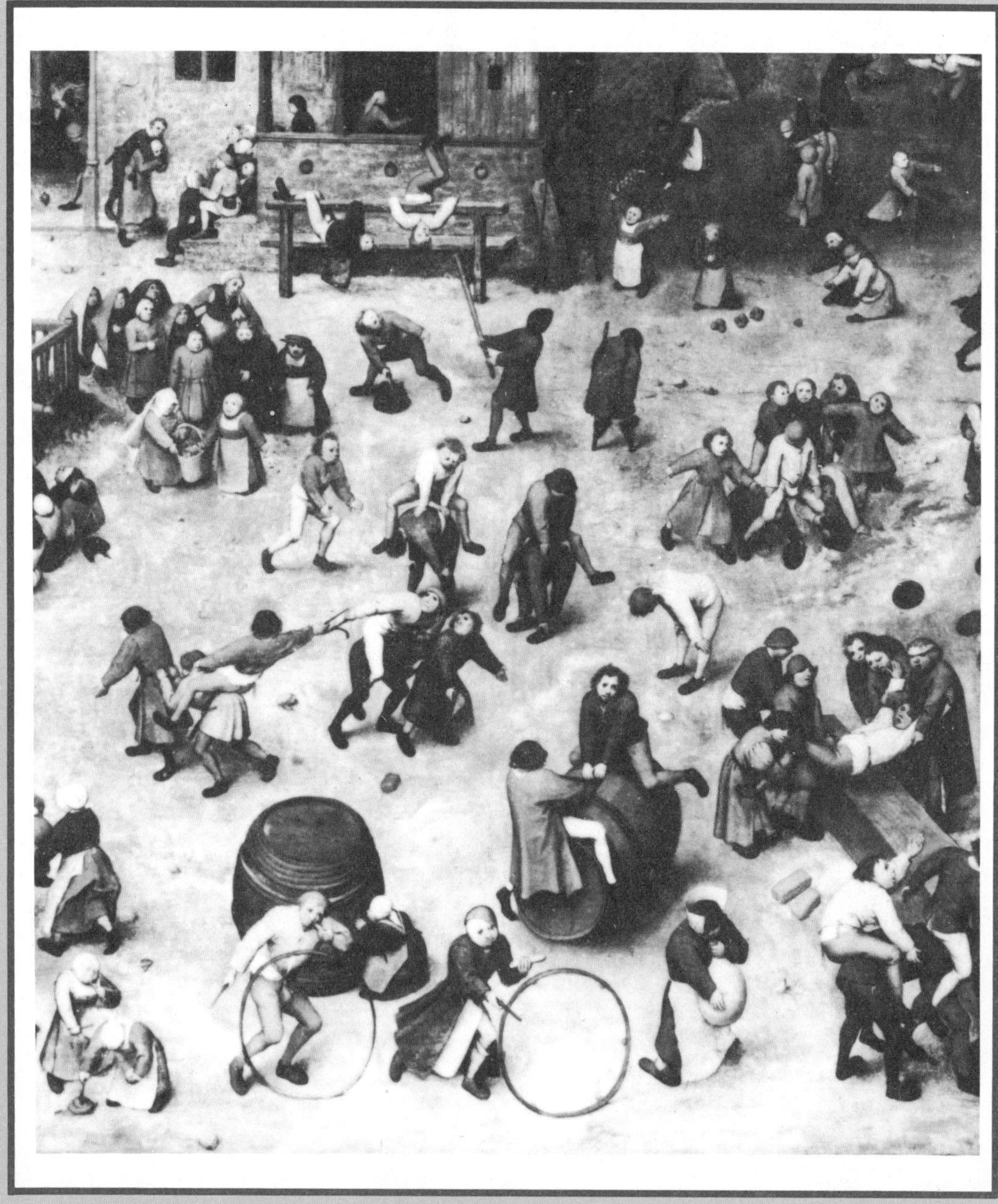

The Early Years

After the age of one, a child's growth rate slows, as shown in the previous chapter. But during the next year, the body changes dramatically. At one, children have just learned to stand erect and toddle, often losing their balance and abruptly sitting down. By two, they can take long strides with solid confidence and are learning to run, jump, and climb. The internal changes that make these new accomplishments possible are the accumulations of a larger mass and greater density of bone and muscle tissue. The changes are obvious in the margin figure: Two-year-olds have lost much of their baby fat; their muscles (especially in the back, buttocks, and legs) have firmed and strengthened, and the leg bones have lengthened and increased in density.

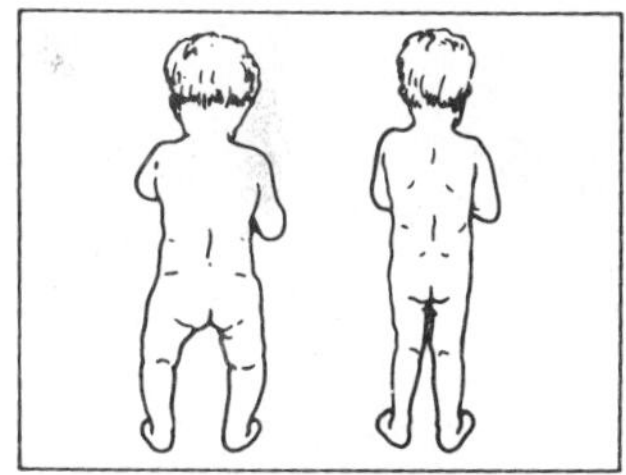

One-year-old and two-year-old reduced to same height.

Thereafter, the same trend—lengthening of the long bones and an increase in musculature—continues, unevenly and still more slowly, until adolescence. Growth comes in spurts; a six-year-old child may wear the same pair of shoes for a year, then need new shoes twice in the next four months.

A factor of importance is that there seems to be a period of rapid cell division in the fat tissue around the age of one or two. As with other critical periods, this is limited in time; later, cell division slows down and the proportion of fat cells becomes fixed. If a baby is overfed during this time, the fat cell number may increase beyond the normal

Opposite: A detail from Children's Games *by P. Breugel. Used with the permission of the Kunsthistorisches Museum, Vienna.*

limit, leaving the child with too many fat cells. If (and this is only theoretical) the number of fat cells is involved in hunger regulation in the adult, this may mean that the fat baby is destined to be abnormally hungry for life and so to have a hard time fighting obesity.

More on the fat-cell theory—Chapter 8.

The validity of this hypothesis is not clearly established for human beings, but it is known that the obesity of childhood differs from adult-onset obesity in several respects. Excess weight in the early years places a demand on the skeletal and muscular tissues so that they, too, grow overly large. Obese children become adults whose bones and muscles are denser than those of their slimmer counterparts. Excess weight is less often successfully and permanently lost by such adults.

Just before adolescence, the growth patterns of girls and boys begin to become distinct. In girls, fat becomes a larger percentage of the total body weight, and in boys the lean body mass—muscle and bone—becomes much greater. Around this time, growth in height may seem to stop altogether for a while, as if the child were settling into a countdown before takeoff. This is the calm before the storm.

Nutritional Needs and Feeding

A one-year-old child needs perhaps 1000 calories a day; a three-year-old needs only 300 to 500 calories more. The appetite decreases markedly around the age of one year, in line with the great reduction in growth rate. Thereafter, the appetite fluctuates; a child will need and demand much more food during periods of rapid growth than during periods of quiescence. The nutrients that need emphasis continue to be protein, calcium, phosphorus, and magnesium, and the food best suited to supply them continues to be milk.

The preadolescent period is the last one in which parental food choices have much influence. As children gather their forces for the adolescent growth spurt, they are accumulating stores of nutrients that will be needed in the coming years. When they take off on that growth spurt, there will be a period during which their nutrient intakes, especially of calcium, cannot meet the demands of rapidly growing bones; then they will be drawing on these stores. The denser their bones are before this occurs, the better prepared they will be.

The gradually increasing needs for all nutrients during the growing years are evident from the RDA table and the Canadian Dietary Standard, which list separate averages for each span of three years. To provide these nutrients, the Four Food Group Plan recommends

3 servings of milk or milk products.

2 servings of meat or meat substitutes.

4 or more servings of fruits and vegetables.

4 or more servings of breads and cereals.

The RDA table appears on the inside front cover. The Canadian Dietary Standard is in Appendix K.

For meat, fruits, and vegetables, a serving is loosely defined as 1 tablespoon per year. Thus, for a four-year old, a serving of any of these foods would be 4 tablespoons (1/4 cup).

Following up on the crucial first year, there is much that a parent can do to foster the development of healthy eating habits. The goal is to teach children to like nutritious foods in all four categories.

The most important task of nutrition education from preschool through the third grade is to introduce many new foods.—B. Rappenthal

Experimentation with children's food patterns shows that candy, cola, and other concentrated sweets must be limited in a child's diet if the needed nutrients are to be supplied. If such foods are permitted in large quantities, there are only two possible outcomes: nutrient deficiencies or obesity. The child can't be trusted to choose nutritious foods on the basis of taste alone; the preference for sweets is innate.[1] The possibility that overfeeding at critical times in children's lives can predispose them to life-long obesity makes this especially important. On the other hand, an active child can enjoy the higher-calorie nutritious foods in each category; ice cream or pudding in the milk group, cake and cookies (whole-grain or enriched only, however) in the bread group. These foods, made from milk and grain, carry valuable nutrients and encourage a child to learn, appropriately, that eating is fun.

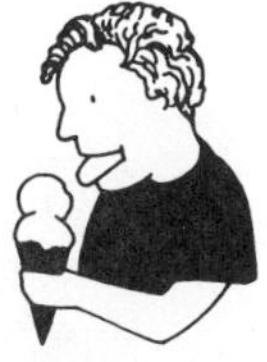

Calcium and riboflavin in a delicious form.

Children sometimes seem to lose their appetites for awhile; this is nothing to worry about. The perfection of appetite regulation in children of normal weight guarantees that their calorie intakes will be right for each stage of growth. A child who wants to eat less is probably taking a normal "time off" from rapid growth. As long as the calories they do consume are from nutritious foods, they are well provided for during this time. (One caution, however: Wandering school-age children may be spending pocket money at the nearby candy store.) An overzealous mother, unaware that her one-year-old is supposed to slow down, may begin a lifelong conflict over food by trying to force more food on the child than the child feels like eating.

Environmental Influences

While parents are doing what they can to establish favorable eating behavior during the transition from infancy to childhood, other factors are entering the picture. At five or so, the child goes to school and encounters foods prepared and served by outsiders.

Nutrition at school. The U.S. government funds several programs to provide nutritious, high-quality meals for children when they are at school. The National School Lunch Act stipulates that every public school must make lunches available to children, and the federal government reimburses the schools for part or all the cost when families can't pay. School lunches are designed to meet certain requirements: They must include specified servings of milk, protein-rich food (meat, cheese, eggs, legumes, or peanut butter), vegetables, fruits, bread or other grain foods, and butter or margarine. The design is intended to provide at least a third of the RDA for each of the nutrients. As of 1978, the school lunch program was available to about 90 percent of all U.S. schoolchildren, and it was expected to continue at that level into 1981. Every day 25 million lunches were served.[2] By 1980, however, funding cuts were being proposed, and concern was being expressed that the families of middle-income children would feel the impact.[3]

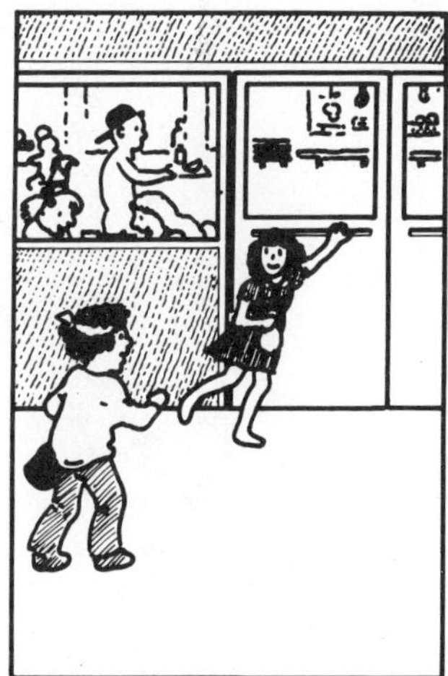

School lunch is available to 90 percent of all U.S. schoolchildren.

Programs similar to the school lunch program operate in day care centers, settlement houses, and recreation programs. School breakfast programs operate in many schools in every state and serve over 2 million youngsters, four-fifths of whom pay little or nothing for the food they receive.

The amount of federal money spent on child nutrition programs has risen explosively since the inception of these programs in the 1940s. To cut costs during the 1970s, experts turned their attention to the problem of "plate waste." Food becomes nutrition only when it passes the lips—and children often refuse to eat the food they are served, thus wasting both food and money and defeating the effort to see that they are well fed. In response to children's differing needs and tastes, the school lunch program and others have been evolving toward better achievement of the objective of feeding the children both what they want and what will nourish them. The trend is:

To increase the variety of offerings and allow children to choose what they are served.

To vary portion sizes, so that little children may take little servings.

To involve students (in secondary schools) in the planning of menus.

To improve the scheduling of lunches so that children can eat when they are hungry and can have enough time to eat well.

A step toward making the lunches more consistent with today's ideals of healthful food has been to drop the requirement for whole milk and to offer low-fat or skim instead. Another alteration has been to eliminate the requirement that butter or margarine be served. Both of these changes have the blessings of the American Dietetic Association, which monitors and offers its judgments about the child nutrition programs.[4]

In many places, the mention of school lunch brings a grimace of dislike to the face of any child. However, some schools have responded to the children's attitudes in creative and imaginative ways that have increased student participation and reduced plate waste. A school in Colorado reports success in feeding its students breakfasts of sandwiches, fish sticks, and tuna salad.[5] A school in Massachusetts offers fast-food cuisine, and students fix their own. As a result, plate waste is greatly reduced, and student participation in the program is up 25 percent. No desserts are offered, but milk is available as milkshakes similar to those at the local fast-food chains.[6] A California school has installed see-through walls so that the students can see the kitchen personnel at work.[7] A school in Georgia offers health foods to meet popular demand.[8] Other schools present ethnic meals and international cuisine on special occasions.

While the schools strive to feed their young clientele nutritious meals, some also seek to educate them in nutritional matters. They are supported by some state programs that provide funds for nutrition education in the classroom. As of 1975, however, nutrition education was mandatory in only seven states, and only two required that the teachers receive instruction in nutrition. The trend was upward, with more states planning to institute nutrition education programs. Still, having read this book, you will probably know more about nutrition than many who teach it in the schools.

Television. For the most part, then, children learn nutrition from parents or teachers who know very little about it. Meanwhile, they hear a great deal about foods from the television set. The very first year of life is probably the most crucial in establishing eating patterns that will persist throughout life, but a great deal is learned and internalized during the years that follow.

Nutrition education is still considered Mommy's business, and chances are that she teaches about nutrition no better than she teaches about sex.—J. Cross

Many authorities are concerned that the influence of television commercials may be less than desirable. It is estimated that the average child sees more than 10,000 commercials a year and that many more than half of them are for sugary foods. Hundreds of millions of dollars are spent in the effort to sell these foods to children.[9] Most of the concern centers on the issue of sugar. You may recall that not all the public disapproval of sugar is based on scientific findings. However, there is widespread agreement on one point: Sticky, sugary foods left in the teeth provide an ideal environment for the growth of mouth bacteria and the formation of cavities.

Who teaches today's preschoolers about nutrition? Television!—J. D. Gussow

More about sugar—Controversy 4A.

A consumer group composed of concerned parents, Action for Children's Television, has urged the Federal Trade Commission to regulate television advertising of these foods. In 1977, this group petitioned the FTC to adopt four measures: (1) to stop the advertising of sticky, sugary foods on children's television programs; (2) to stop "unfair" selling techniques; (3) to require all advertisements to disclose the sugar contents of the products being advertised; and (4) to require the food industries to apply part of their advertising budgets to the support of public service announcements to promote desirable eating habits.[10] A precedent is provided by the Netherlands, where advertisers are required to exhibit an insignia within the last few seconds of every commercial for a sugared product. The insignia shows toothpaste

Table 1. Eating Habits to Favor Good Dental Health

Food Group	Foods to Eat	Foods to Avoid
Milk and milk products	Milk Cheese Plain yogurt	All dairy products with added sugar
Fruit	Fresh fruit Water-packed canned fruit	Dried fruit Sugar-packed canned fruit Jams and Jellies
Juice	Unsweetened	Sweetened
Vegetables	Most vegetables	Candied sweet potatoes Glazed carrots
Grains	Most grain products	Grain products with added sugar

It has been estimated that 70 percent of television messages are not true, and that 70 percent of these are believed by children, creating a hazard to the health of future adults.—C. E. Lewis and M. A. Lewis

being applied to a toothbrush. In the United States, as of 1978, no such regulations were in force,[11] although there is widespread agreement that they would be effective in reducing demand for sugary foods.[12]

It thus remains up to us to determine which food commercials we will believe and which we will not. Dentists, especially, have the obligation to educate their patients individually as long as misleading claims continue to appear on national television. A model eating plan that favors dental health is shown in Table 1.[13] Among the "bad guys" singled out by the dentists are granola bars—a grain food, but so sticky that the dentists consider them no different from candy bars—and fruit yogurt—which the dentists see as the equivalent of ice cream.[14]

Vending Machines. Television is not the only environmental force affecting children's food choices. Another factor that has an impact is vending machines, especially in the schools. The American Dental Association has established a National Task Force for the Prohibition of the Sale of Confections (sticky, sugary foods) in Schools and resolved that the Task Force should seek changes in the School Lunch Act to eliminate the sale of confections as snacks in schools.[15] An experiment in six Canadian schools showed that children would choose more nutritious snacks if they were offered side by side with the sugary foods. When apples were made available in vending machines, there was a 27 percent reduction in the selection of chocolate bars. When milk was made available, soft-drink use dropped by 42 percent.[16] A California school has eliminated all candy and soft drinks from its vending machines and is offering a mixture of orange juice and Hawaiian punch instead; acceptance is reported to be good.[17] And the elimination of vending machines altogether from New Orleans schools increased school lunch participation to 90 percent.[18]

More about caffeine—Chapter 14.

Soft drinks contain not only sugar but also caffeine, which is a matter of some concern to pediatricians.[19] A cup of hot chocolate or a 12-ounce cola beverage may contain as much as 50 milligrams of caffeine; two or more are equivalent in the body of a 60-pound child to the caffeine in eight cups of coffee for a 175-pound man.[20] Chocolate bars also contribute caffeine. Children and young adults who are troubled by irregular heartbeats or difficulty in sleeping may need to control their caffeine consumption.

Prevention of Future Health Problems

Parents look forward to being proud of strong, healthy, competent, and happy sons and daughters who function well in the adult world. To be on the safe side, parents may also think in terms of conditions to avoid. In children, as in infants, eating habits help determine whether development takes place in a positive or in a negative direction.

Obesity. To avoid obesity, the preschool child should be trained to "eat thin." This means that mealtimes should be relaxed and leisurely. Children should learn to eat slowly, pause and enjoy their table companions, and stop eating when they are full. The "clean your plate" dictum should be stamped out for all time. Parents who wish to avoid waste should learn to serve smaller portions or teach their children to serve themselves as much as they truly want to eat. Daily physical activity should be encouraged to promote strong skeletal and muscular development and to establish a habit that will undergird good health throughout life.

With proper education, parents may be led to understand that a "good" eater is not a big eater but a moderate eater.—S. J. Fomon

The child who has already become obese needs careful handling. As in pregnancy, weight loss may easily have a harmful effect on growth. Knittle, who has worked with obese children, recommends that they be fed so as to maintain a constant weight while they grow. The object is to restrict the multiplication of fat cells while promoting normal lean body development. Thus the child can "grow out of his obesity."[21]

Iron-deficiency anemia. Of all nutritional disorders other than obesity found in U.S. children, the most common is iron-deficiency anemia. It is most prevalent in low-birthweight infants, babies from six months to two years of age, and children and adolescents from low-income families.[22]

More on snacking patterns of teenagers—Chapter 14.

Fomon recommends supplementing the diet of infants to ensure an iron intake of 7 milligrams a day and modifying their food intakes as they grow older so that they will receive 5.5 milligrams of iron or more per 1000 calories. To achieve this latter goal, milk must not be overemphasized in the diet, because it is a poor iron source. Too-high milk consumption causes a form of iron-deficiency anemia called milk anemia. If skim or low-fat milk is used instead of whole milk, there will be calories left for investment in such iron-rich foods as lean meats, fish, poultry, eggs, and legumes. Grain products should be whole-grain or enriched only, and children should be steered away from "dairy products (aside from the amount needed to ensure adequate calcium-riboflavin intakes), bakery goods unfortified with iron, candies and soft drinks."[23] Adolescent boys, with their high calorie intakes, can meet their iron needs (6 milligrams of iron per 1000 calories) from their usual dietary intake. Adolescent girls, who need the same amount of iron and who consume fewer calories, probably need iron supplements in most cases.[24]

Most health professionals are aware of the need to promote ample iron intakes in the United States. Pediatricians recommend the use of iron-enriched foods for infants, the school lunch program uses enriched products, and obstetricians frequently prescribe iron supplements for pregnant women.[25] But this is not enough. Teenagers are still left out, perhaps because of their use of "junk foods."[26] Nor does merely being male ensure immunity: 2 to 3 percent of the males in this country are iron deficient.[27] "When simple iron deficiency anemia is observed in adolescent and adult males it is generally accepted that this is a reflection of iron stores never having attained adequate levels."[28] This points up the need to educate women of childbearing age, who are most critically affected by iron deficiency and who are responsible for the storage of iron in the bodies of their infants, both male and female.[29]

More about the dietary need for iron—Chapter 10.

The primary prevention of atherosclerosis is a pediatric problem.—C. L. Williams and E. L. Wynder

If intervention to modify coronary risk factors is put off till adulthood, it may well prove ineffective.—S. Blumenthal and M. J. Jesse

Cardiovascular disease. Many experts seem to agree that early childhood is the time to put into effect practices to prevent cardiovascular disease that until recently were recommended only for adults. Snacking on high-fat, high-sugar, and high-salt food items should be discouraged, because it sets a pattern that favors the development of atherosclerosis and hypertension.[30] Instead, recommendations (like those of the *Dietary Guidelines*) to emphasize foods with a high nutrient density should be followed.

Diabetes and cancer. It seems that the *Guidelines* might also help to prevent or retard the onset of diabetes in children who have the genetic tendency toward it.[31] Those who have been studying the effect of nutrition on cancer have reached the same conclusion: It is suggested that children should follow a "prudent diet," since evidence is increasing that appropriate biological control in terms of fat and cholesterol may be set early in life.[32] The "prudent diet" is a diet originally developed for heart patients, but its outlines are the same as those recommended by nutritionists interested in the prevention of cancer.

Screening. Not everyone agrees that all children should be placed on diets strictly limited in sugar, salt, and fat and high in fruits, vegetables, and whole-grain cereals. However, even those who do not go this far recommend that children be screened early with an eye to determining what conditions each of them might be likely to develop and then paying appropriate attention to diet in each special case. (Figure 1 outlines the screening process.[33]) Thus the child of parents who have high blood pressure should be raised on a diet relatively low in salt; the child whose parents are diabetic should avoid sugar and be encouraged to eat foods high in complex carbohydrate,[34] and the child whose parents have coronary artery disease should eat foods that are

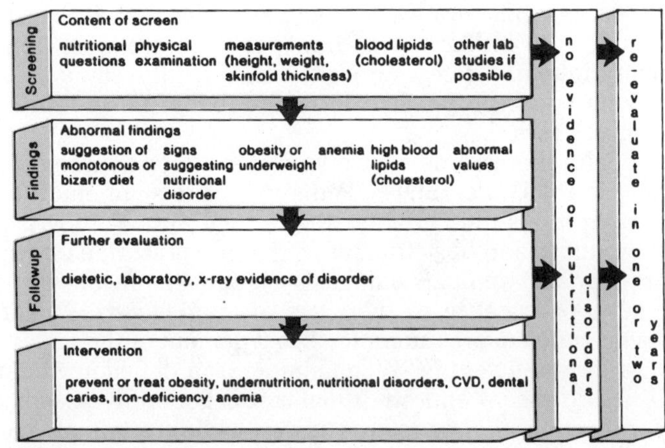

Figure 1. Nutritional screening of children.

From S. J. Fomon, T. A. Anderson, H. Y. W. Stephen, and E. E. Ziegler, Nutritional Disorders of Children: Prevention, Screening, and Followup, DHEW publication no. (HSA) 76-5612 (Washington, D.C.: Government Printing Office), inside front cover.

low in fat, especially saturated fat, and possibly cholesterol. Even acne is better prevented than treated, because success is much more likely if it is caught in the early stages,[35] although in this case the treatment is not primarily nutritional. In all these situations, the greatest success is likely to be achieved if the whole family, and not just the child, follows the recommended dietary guidelines.

Controversy 14A discusses acne in more detail.

Dental health. There is widespread agreement that poor dental health is a preventable condition. The measures recommended for its prevention center around two objectives. First, there is a need to ensure adequate nutrition so that the mouth and teeth develop properly. This means providing an adequate diet, especially in terms of protein, calcium, vitamins A, C, and D, and fluoride. Where local water supplies are not fluoridated, direct application of fluoride to the teeth may be necessary. Second, it is important to restrict the supply of carbohydrate foods to the bacteria that cause tooth decay. This means brushing the teeth or washing the mouth after meals (especially meals high in carbohydrate), avoiding snacks that contain sticky carbohydrate that will linger along the teeth and gumlines, and dislodging persistent particles with dental floss or other devices.

There's more about fluoridation in Controversy 10B.

Other measures. Some parents believe that, like the conditions discussed above, hyperactivity in children can be prevented by nutritional measures such as avoiding sugar and additives. This is questionable.

Hyperactivity is the subject of Controversy 13.

It is desirable for children to learn to like nutritious foods in all of the food groups. With one exception, this liking usually develops naturally. Meats, breads and cereals, fruit, and milk are well accepted by children. The exception is vegetables, which young children frequently dislike and refuse. Even a tiny serving of spinach, cooked carrots, or squash may elicit an expression that registers the utmost in negative feelings (as well as great pride in the ability to make an ugly face). In light of the findings that most people need to learn to eat more vegetables, this chapter's Food Feature is addressed to this problem.

Food Feature: Helping Children Like Vegetables

Do you remember how you felt when first offered a cup of vegetable soup, a serving of runny spinach, or a pile of peas and carrots? If the soup burned your tongue, it brought tears to your eyes. It may have been years before you were willing to try it again. As for the spinach, it was suspiciously murky looking. (Who could tell what might be lurking in that ugly dark-green liquid?) The peas and carrots troubled your sense of order. Before you could eat them, you felt compelled to sort the peas onto one side of the plate and the carrots onto the other. Then you had to separate, into a reject pile, all those that got mashed in the process or contaminated with gravy from the mashed potatoes. Only then might you be willing to eat the intact, clean peas and carrots one by one. You hoped your parents wouldn't notice your picking them up with your fingers. Peas, especially, were so hard to pick up with a fork; they kept rolling off.

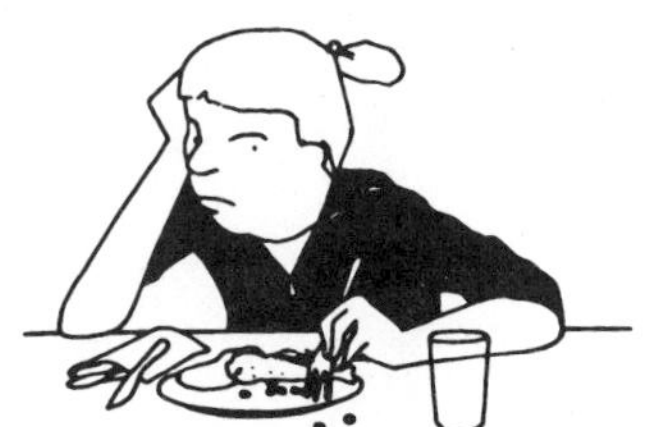

Children can be opinionated about food.

Why children respond in this way to foods that look "off" or "messy" to them is a matter for conjecture. Parents need only be aware that this is how many children feel and then honor those feelings. Children prefer vegetables that are slightly undercooked and crunchy, bright in color, served separately, and easy to eat. They should be warm, not hot, because a child's mouth is much more sensitive than an adult's. The flavor should be mild (a child has more taste buds), and smooth foods such as mashed potatoes or pea soup should have no lumps in them (a child wonders, with some disgust, what the lumps might be). Irrational as the fear of strangeness may seem, the parent must realize that it is practically universal among children and may even have a built-in biological basis.

Little children like to eat at little tables and to be served little portions of food. They also love to eat with other children and have been observed to stay at the table longer and eat much more when in the company of their peers. A bright, unhurried atmosphere free of conflict is also conducive to good appetite. Parents who serve the food in a relaxed and casual manner, without anxiety, provide the emotional climate in which a child's negative emotions will be minimized.

Ideally, each meal is preceded, not followed, by the activity the child looks forward to the most. In a number of schools, it has been discovered that children eat a much better lunch if recess occurs before, rather than after, the meal. With recess after, they are likely to hurry out to play, leaving food on their plates that they were hungry for and would otherwise have eaten. Before sitting down to eat, small children should be helped to clean themselves thoroughly, washing their hands and faces so that they can enjoy the meal with "that clean feeling."[36]

Many little children, both boys and girls, enjoy helping in the kitchen. Their participation provides many opportunities to encourage good food habits. Family tradition often involves letting children help make cookies and lick the mixing bowl, but a child can also help with the preparation of main dishes. A little boy who helps his mother shell peas or cut green beans may eat so many of them raw, before the meal, that his rejection of the cooked equivalent at the dinner table will be a matter of no concern. A little girl who helps break up the lettuce and cut the carrots and celery for a salad may get absorbed in pretending to be a bunny rabbit and nibble a serving or two while she works. Vegetables are pretty, especially when fresh, and provide opportunities to learn about color, about growing things and their seeds, about shapes and textures—all of which are fascinating to young children. Measuring, stirring, decorating, cutting, and arranging vegetables on a plate are skills even a very small child can practice with enjoyment and pride.

When introducing new foods at the table, parents are advised to offer them one at a time—and only a small amount at first. Whenever possible, the new food should be presented at the beginning of the meal, when the child is hungry. If the child is cross, irritable, or feeling sick, don't insist but withdraw the new food and try it again a few days later, just as you would with an adult. Remember, parents have inclinations and dislikes to which they feel entitled; children should be accorded the same privilege. Never make an issue of food acceptance; a power struggle almost invariably results in a confirmed pattern of resistance and a permanently closed mind on the child's part.

Psychological Growth of the Child

The key word (at one year) is *trust*; the parental behavior best suited to promote it is affectionate holding. At two years, the word is *autonomy*; parents should allow children to make their own choices, including giving them the right to say their favorite word (NO!) to offered foods—at the same time providing, of course, other nutritious foods to choose from. (A child may also take great pride in saying no to toilet training by withholding a bowel movement for several days; this is not dangerous.) At four, when the development of *initiative* is their proudest achievement, children can be encouraged to participate in the planning and preparation of meals. At each age, food can be given and enjoyed in the context of growth in its largest, most inclusive sense. If the beginnings are right, children will grow without the kind of conflict and confusion over food that can lead to nutritional problems.

At every age, there is a negative counterpart—distrust, shame, guilt, inferiority—to the desired development. These, too, can be promoted by unaware parents, even if they have the best of intentions. Mealtimes can be nightmarish for the child who is struggling with these issues. If, as she sits down to the table, she is confronted with a barrage of accusations—"Susie, your hands are filthy . . . get your elbows off the table . . . your report card . . . and clean your plate! Your mother cooked that food"—mealtimes may be unbearable. Her stomach may recoil, because her body as well as her mind reacts to stress of this kind.

In the interest of promoting both a positive self-concept and a positive attitude toward good food, it is important for mother and father to help Johnny or Susie remember that they are good kids. Their behavior may need correcting; what they *do* may sometimes be unacceptable; but what they *are*, on the inside, is normal, healthy, growing, fine human beings.[1]

For Further Information

Recommended nutrition references on all topics are listed in Appendix J. In addition, with respect to the information in this chapter, we recommend the following.

[1]*Chapter Notes can be found at the end of the Appendixes.*

On the nutrition of children:

- Fomon, S. J. *Infant Nutrition*, 2d ed. Philadelphia: Saunders, 1974.

- Pipes, P. L. *Nutrition in Infancy and Childhood.* St. Louis: Mosby, 1977 (paperback). This 205-page book is an authoritative, clear, understandable text, one of the best in the field.

On the prevention of later health problems through good nutritional practices in childhood:

- Breslow, L., and Somers, A. R. Lifetime health monitoring: A practical approach to preventive medicine. *New England Journal of Medicine* 296 (1977): 601-608. Breslow and Somers have studied the disorders most likely to appear at every age and have suggested an agenda for screening at intervals throughout life that would detect these disorders.

- Fomon, S. J.; Anderson, T. A.; Stephen, H. Y. W.; and Ziegler, E. E. *Nutritional Disorders of Children: Prevention, Screening, and Followup.* DHEW publication no. (HSA) 76-5612. Washington, D.C.: Government Printing Office, 1976.

- Williams, C. L., and Wynder, E. L. A blind spot in preventive medicine. *Journal of the American Medical Association* 236 (1976): 2196-2197.

On teaching children to resist the allure of television commercials:

- A booklet, "Buy and Buy," to help nine- to thirteen-year-olds learn to see through cereal commercials, is available for 55 cents from MVR Hall, Cornell University, Ithaca, NY 14853.

- A twelve-page foldout, "Children and Television," by Action for Children's Television (ACT), can be obtained for 50 cents from ACT, 46 Austin Street, Newtonville, MA 02160. You might want to inquire what other resources they have.

For people concerned with the nutrition education of children, the national Nutrition Education Clearing House puts out a listing of reference materials. For example:

- *Secondary Teaching Materials and Teacher References.* Rev. ed. Nutrition Education Resource Series 4. Berkeley, Calif.: Society for Nutrition Education, 1977 (address in Appendix J).

For people who feed children:

- Goodwin, M. T., and Pollen, G. *Creative Food Experiences for Children.* Washington, D.C: Center for Science in the Public Interest, 1974 (paperback). Available from Box 3099, Washington, DC 20010. This book encourages children to participate in the preparation of healthful foods.

- Lansky, V. *The Taming of the C.A.N.D.Y. Monster.* Wayzata, Minn.: Meadowbrook Press, 1978 (paperback). This is an unusual cookbook that encourages creativity in the kitchen and helps to solve such problems as what-to-put-in-the-lunchbox.

- McClenahan, P., and Jaqua, I. *Cool Cooking for Kids.* Belmont, Calif.: Fearon-Pitman, 1976. This cookbook for preschoolers and their parents features good ideas for preparing food without using the stove.

- Williams, J., and Smith, M. *Middle Childhood: Behavior and Development.* 2d ed. New York: Macmillan, 1980.

The *School Lunch Journal* and the *School Foodservice Journal* are coming out monthly with creative new ideas. In addition:

- Frederick, L. *Fast Food Gets an "A" in School Lunch.* Boston: Cahner's Books, 1977. This book describes the fast-food style of serving school lunches, which has been proving successful in attracting children away from vending machines and off-campus eating places.

Controversy 13

Hyperactivity

Is it from additives, allergies, sugar, or what?

What makes children hyperactive? If hyperactivity were rare, this would just be an academic question, but it's not rare. It occurs in 5 to 10 percent of young school-age children—that is, one or two in every classroom of twenty children. And it can lead to academic failure and major behavior problems.[1] It is important to identify the cause, wherever possible, and treat it, to avert the untold grief that can otherwise result.

A theory made popular by Dr. B. F. Feingold during the 1970s is that many children are sensitive to the artificial flavors and colors in foods, and especially to those related to aspirin (salicylates). Feingold has stated that, when hyperactive children are fed a diet of natural foods, free of these compounds, 50 percent respond by calming down, two-thirds of them "dramatically."[2] By 1978, Feingold's theory was famous and more than 20,000 children were being fed the Feingold diet.[3]

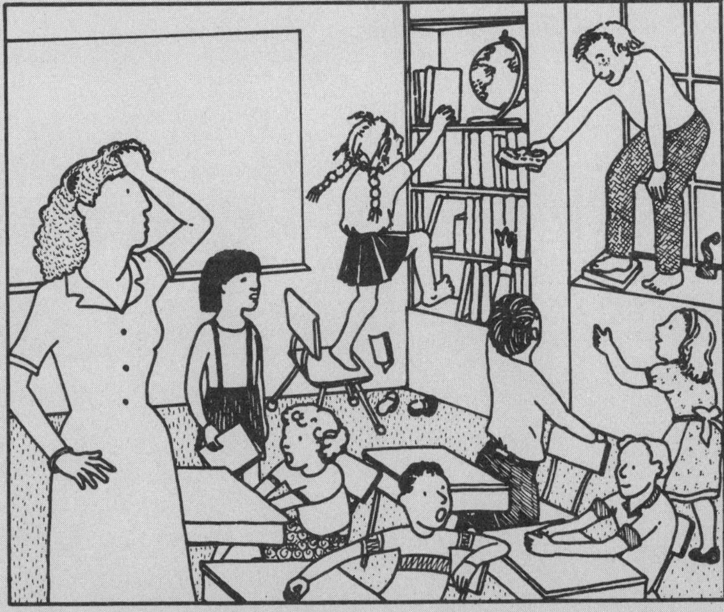

To what extent does the evidence bear out Feingold's hypothesis? If your child or mine appears to be hyperactive, shall we put them on the Feingold diet, or what shall we do about them?

Evidence bearing on Feingold's hypothesis can be sought by asking two questions.

First, do any food additives cause adverse reactions in children? Second, does an additive-free diet relieve symptoms in hyperactive children? The answer to the first question is yes, but the answer to the second appears to be no.

Additives, food allergies, and behavior. Some food additives do cause adverse reactions in some people. One of the best known is MSG (monosodium glutamate), a saltlike powder that, when added to foods, enhances their natural flavor. Known best under the trade name Accent, MSG is widely used in Oriental cookery. People who are sensitive to it may experience a variety of sensations after dining in an Oriental restaurant, from numbness of the back of the neck, arms, and back to weakness, palpitations, and other symptoms. Only a few people are thus affected, and there seem to be no long-term aftereffects.[4] In children, however, MSG has been observed to cause "shudders" that resemble epileptic seizures; in fact, antiepileptic drugs have sometimes been used in the attempt to correct the condition.[5] Increasing familiarity with this phenomenon, the "Chinese restaurant syndrome," has made it appear to be more widespread —perhaps because people are suggestible.

Food allergies also cause adverse reactions that can include hyperactive behavior. Among the symptoms may be "dark circles under the eyes, hyperkinesia (excessive activity), irritability and lack of attention."[6] According to an expert on the subject,

The possibility of a food allergy should be considered in a child with constitutional or generalized signs of easy fatiguability, irritability, insomnia, poor work in school or intermittent headaches and stomach aches. These children oftentimes find it difficult to get along with their siblings or peers.

He goes on to warn: "Dislike of a food may be only a whim or fancy, but it should be regarded as significant until proven otherwise. Aversion to egg or milk in children may be the result of nature's protective effort, often misinterpreted by parents."[7]

Allergies are caused by a tendency of the child's body to produce antibodies against specific proteins found in the foods. It seems that the natural proteins of milk, wheat, and egg white are the worst offenders in this regard,[8] but cane sugar can also cause an allergic reaction.[9] (Perhaps it is an occasional allergy of this kind that has given rise to the rumor that sugar causes hyperactivity.) To diagnose an allergy, you have to remove the suspected food altogether from the diet and watch to see if the symptoms disappear. The clincher is to secretly reintroduce the suspected food and see the symptoms reappear.

A temporary allergy can result from whole proteins leaking from food in the digestive tract into the bloodstream after an upset such as vomiting or diarrhea. This may be a partial explanation for the so-called psychologically caused allergy conditions seen in children. Improper handling of the child can lead to irritability, or overfeeding can cause nausea, and the upset digestive

Miniglossary

Accent: See *monosodium glutamate.*

hyperactivity: Excessive activity, a symptom which can result from any of a multitude of different causes.

hyperkinesia (high-per-kin-EEZ-ee-uh): The medical term for the symptom hyperactivity.

hyperkinesis (high-per-kin-EECE-iss): The syndrome characterized by motor restlessness, short attention span, poor impulse control, learning difficulties, and emotional instability that is responsive to treatment with stimulant drugs. Not the same as minimal brain dysfunction, which is not discussed in this Controversy.

monosodium glutamate (MSG): A flavor-enhancer used widely in Oriental (especially Chinese and Japanese) cookery; it can cause an intolerance reaction (the "Chinese restaurant syndrome") in some individuals. One trade name is Accent.

salicylate (sa-LISS-uh-late): A compound resembling aspirin in chemical structure.

syndrome: A cluster of symptoms.

tartrazine (TAR-truh-zeen): Yellow dye no. 5, a salicylate, which causes occasional allergies.

tract then allows an allergy-causing protein into the bloodstream. In such a case, the psychological problem must be dealt with before the physical system will quiet down and return to normal.[10]

Food allergies are often misdiagnosed, according to a medical authority on the subject, and are less common than some people believe them to be. But they are nonetheless real, being caused by true physical differences in individuals' reactions to the molecules (usually proteins) in foods.[11]

At least one specific food-coloring allergy is known. Yellow No. 5 (tartrazine, a salicylate) causes allergic symptoms, especially in people who are also allergic to aspirin.[12] It was this observation that originally led Feingold to propose an additive-free diet for the treatment of hyperactivity. But this is a distinct, individual reaction, and probably doesn't account for more than about one in a hundred cases of childhood hyperactivity.

In answer to the first question, then (Do any food additives cause adverse reactions in children?), the answer is yes. Moreover, hyperactivity, irritability, and lack of attention are among the symptoms of allergies—the same symptoms that most worry parents and teachers concerned about children's behavior. No wonder Feingold's idea of a natural-food, allergen-free diet as a cure for hyperactivity became so popular so quickly. Does the Feingold diet work?

Experiments on the Feingold diet. The widespread use of Feingold's diet has led to experimentation designed to prove or disprove its usefulness. In 1976, an expert committee of the Institute of Food Technologists undertook to review the evidence. They concluded that no controlled studies had confirmed Feingold's claim. His diet, they said, had not been evaluated for its long-term effects and might not fully meet the nutritional needs of children. They pointed out that, when individual children are singled out for study of the effects of diet on their behavior, diet is not the only thing in their lives that changes. They receive special attention, too, and this may well have beneficial effects on their behavior (the placebo effect). Both the children and their parents and teachers are likely to be influenced by the hope that the experiment will work and by suggestibility—a factor that is difficult to rule out.[13]

The committee designed a double-blind study to avert these problems, and it was conducted over an eight-month period at the University of Wisconsin. The outcome was not conclusive: Some children seemed to have improved while on the additive-free diet, but an equal number had worsened. In general, Feingold's hypothesis was not borne out by these findings, but the possibility remained that some individual children might have benefited from the diet. Further investigation was recommended. Following this study, several others were conducted with similar results, over a million dollars was spent, and as of 1980, no new evidence in favor of Feingold's theory had surfaced.[14] It is disappointing to have to report that, although a few individual cases of salicylate allergy are known, the dietary approach to hyperactivity seems to work mostly by suggestion, if it works at all.

Drug treatment of hyperactivity. The term *hyperactivity* can be used by any person who wants to use it to describe any child's behavior. It can mean noisy, mischievous, energetic, irritable, or whatever the user wants it to mean. It is such a popular term that it is even often shortened to "hyper," and applied to spouses, mothers-in-law, even pet dogs. As such, the term has no useful medical meaning. But there is a term, *hyperkinesis*, that is used medically to describe a special cluster of symptoms, and it is a very useful term for three reasons. First, it describes accurately the behaviors seen in the 5 to 10 percent of school children already mentioned. Second, it can readily be diagnosed by the trained clinician. And third, it responds to treatment by prescription medication.

The symptoms of hyperkinesis are "motor restlessness, short attention span, poor impulse control, learning difficulties, and emotional instability."[15] On encountering a child that fits this description, the clinician makes a tentative diagnosis of hyperkinesis, and prescribes a stimulant drug. If the diagnosis is correct the child will respond by calming down. As with the diagnosis of an allergy, the confirming step is to see the behavior appear and disappear in response to the withdrawal and readministration of the drug, even when the people involved don't know when the drug is in use and when a placebo has been substituted.

Some people oppose violently the use of stimulant drugs with children. If you could listen to a debate between the pros and the cons, it might go like this:

- Pro: The drugs correct the behavior of hyperactive children.
- Con: It is terrible to use drugs with children. It's like brainwashing them, controlling their minds.
- Pro: No, the drugs work specifically on the mechanism that's abnormal in these children. They aren't tranquilizers. They normalize behavior.
- Con: They will lead to later drug abuse.
- Pro: The drugs can't be abused by hyperactive children because they don't get "high" with them, they slow down.
- Con: They have side effects: They cause loss of appetite, they disturb sleep, and they slow growth.
- Pro: That's true, and that's an unfortunate fact about all drugs. That's why they have to be prescribed conservatively after a careful diagnosis. The side effects don't occur in all children, and they can be minimized by discontinuing the medication at night, on weekends, and during summers. In any case, the benefits make them worth using.

A physician experienced in the treatment of hyperkinesis sums up the evidence, "Of the available methods, by far the most effective and the best documented is the use of the stimulant drugs dextroamphetamine and methylphenidate, agents that *in these children* suppress overactivity and impulsivity and lengthen attention span."[16] It seems that *in these children*, prescription medication should indeed be the treatment of choice.

The controversy might be resolved by the conclusion that most hyperactive children can be successfully treated as just described. But the opponents understandably still wish to find a "natural" answer.

Reactions to sugar. A large segment of the public believes that *sugar* is the villain in the case. A television show that "proved" this was aired in 1980 and millions of viewers saw with their own eyes that after eating foods high in sugar, school children were noisy, hyper, and uncontrollable. Seeing is believing, and much of the public is now firmly convinced that sugar causes hyperactivity.

Actually, as of the end of 1980, no significant scientific research had been done on the subject of sugar and hyperactivity. Dr. Lendon Smith, a pediatrician from Oregon, has toured the country suggesting that sugar is responsible for hyperactivity (as well as bedwetting, thumbsucking, criminal behavior, and schizophrenia), but all of his stories are strictly anecdotal. For example, it is noted that "children are more restless than usual . . . on the day after Halloween." To say that this proves anything about sugar is of course absurd. A researcher would instantly identify many "confounding variables" (possible alternative causes that haven't been excluded): fatigue, residual excitement, reluctance to get back to work, and so forth. In reporting on the uproar over sugar, the American Council on Science and Health expresses disappointment that the popular press has given such uncritical coverage to the blaming of sugar and agrees with a sugar newsletter that:

It is essential that members of the media begin to help consumers sort myths from facts in the area of nutrition and health. A terrible disservice is performed in the name of news when . . . [pure speculation] is presented to the public as accurate information.[17]

But there is something to be said for the sugar hypothesis

after all. If you turn it upside-down, it has a kind of validity. The reader of Controversy 4A may remember about sugar that many of the problems it seems to cause are actually caused by the absence of something that is displaced when sugar becomes a major part of the diet. What comes to mind in the case of schoolchildren is food, any food that can be deemed nutritious. And if nutritious food is lacking in a child's diet, problems of all kinds will arise, including behavior problems.

The most common nutrient deficiency in children is iron deficiency. While its effects are hard to sort out from the effects of other factors in children's lives, it is likely that iron deficiency in children manifests itself in a lowering of the "motivation to persist in intellectually challenging tasks," a shortening of the attention span, and a reduction of overall intellectual performance.[18] This description sounds so much like that of hyperkinesis that it seems likely that only a clinical trial using an iron-rich diet or stimulant drugs would distinguish between the two possibilities. If the problem is iron deficiency it will respond to the removal of sugar from the diet and the feeding of nutritious foods in its place. What could be the harm in trying?

Personal strategy. Parents of excitable, rambunctious, and unruly children understandably become impatient and exhausted with them at times, and the question of whether the child is normal may arise and demand attention. "Is my child hyperactive?" "Could her diet be causing some of her problems?" How does one go about determining what is normal child behavior and what is abnormal and requires professional attention?

All children get wild and excitable at times, and the overanxious parent should be aware that there are many normal causes of "hyper" behavior:

- Lack of sleep.
- Overstimulation.
- Too much TV.
- Attention-getting.
- Lack of exercise.

Misbehavior caused by any of these can't be helped by drugs or diet. But if these causes are eliminated and the behavior persists, an obvious thing to check is the child's diet. It costs nothing to ask the question whether the diet is meeting the child's nutrient needs (if you've read this far, you can figure it out for yourself). Any child switched from a high-sugar, high-refined-food, nutrient-dilute diet to one consisting of nourishing, wholesome foods should feel better as a result, and his or her behavior should show improvement.

If the hyperactivity persists, then it's time to go to a competent, trained, experienced, and interested clinician. At least two possibilities should be checked. First, is it drug-responsive hyperkinesis? If the child is indeed hyperkinetic, a treatment regimen based on drugs and possibly behavior modification will be helpful until the child outgrows the problem. It is imperative that an accurate diagnosis be made, however. Self-diagnosis or hasty and incorrect diagnosis by an untrained observer can lead to misuse of drugs and serious consequences. But truly hyperkinetic children can be successfully treated, to their great benefit and that of their families, with prescription medication.

If the diagnosis is not hyperkinesis, the possibility of allergy should be considered. Some of the distinguishing features of allergy were described above. Allergies are difficult to diagnose, because 95 percent of them are of the delayed-reaction type and because people are so suggestible that they often think they have allergies when they don't. According to one expert:

Only through experience with blind food challenges can the amazing power of self-deception be appreciated—only about one-fourth of histories of adverse reactions can be confirmed, the remainder being psychologic or imaginary.[19]

It is important to get help from a doctor who is competent, experienced, and successful with allergy diagnosis. Finally, as for special diets like the Feingold diet, there probably is no need for them—although something may be said in their favor. Parents who care enough to provide nutritious, wholesome foods for their children and who pay attention to them in a loving home atmosphere are providing not only nourishment for the body but also for the mind and soul. To the extent that a diet is a healthy one, providing a balanced and varied selection of nutritious foods, it can only enhance a child's well-being and normal development.

The Controversy Notes and For Further Information follow the Appendixes.

CHAPTER 14

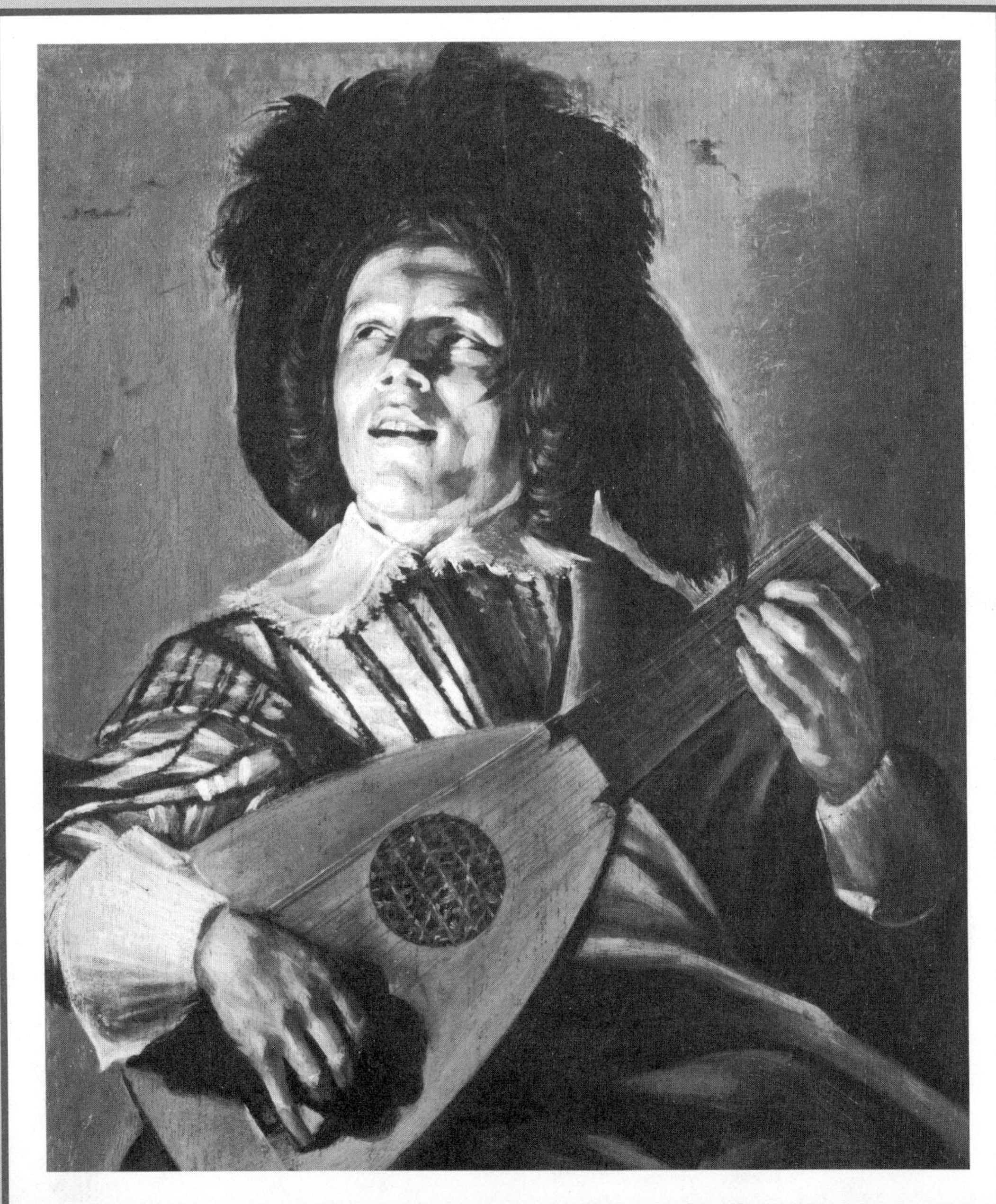

The Young Adult and Adult

Teenagers are not fed; they eat. For the first time in their lives, they assume responsibility for their own food intakes. At the same time, they are intensely involved in day-to-day life with their peers and preparation for their future lives as adults. Social pressures thrust choices at them: to drink or not to drink, to smoke or not to smoke, whether to develop their bodies to meet sometimes extreme ideals of slimness or athletic prowess. Few become interested in foods and nutrition except as part of a cult or fad such as vegetarianism or crash dieting.

After a brief review of the growth and nutrient needs of young adults, this chapter emphasizes the factors that affect their health for good or for ill and the information they need to develop and maintain food habits conducive to good health throughout adulthood.

Growth and Nutrient Needs

At twelve, Russ was a stocky, solid boy; at fifteen he is a tall, long-legged, vigorous young man. The girls who looked down on him three years ago are sizing him up now with a new and mysterious gleam of interest in their eyes, an interest that he reciprocates. His life and theirs are branching and merging in new and unpredictable directions.

Opposite: A detail from Serenade *by Judith Leyster. Used with the permission of the Rijksmuseum, Amsterdam.*

The adolescent growth spurt begins in girls at ten or eleven and reaches its peak at twelve, being completed at about fifteen. In boys it begins at twelve or thirteen and peaks at fourteen, ending at about nineteen. This intensive growth period brings not only a dramatic increase in height but hormonal changes that profoundly affect every organ of the body (including the brain) and that culminate in the emergence of physically mature adults within two or three years. The same nutrition principles apply to this period as to the growth periods previously discussed: The growth nutrients are needed in increased quantities, and there is an added need for iron, caused by the onset of menstruation in girls and by the great increase in lean body mass in boys. These changes, which are taking place in nearly adult-size people, mean that total nutrient needs may increase more during adolescence than during any other time in life. A rapidly growing, active boy of fifteen may need 4000 calories or more a day just to maintain his weight. An inactive girl of the same age, however, whose growth is nearly at a standstill, may need fewer than 2000 calories if she is to avoid becoming obese. Thus, there is a tremendous variation in the nutrient needs of adolescents.

Teenagers as a group do have nutritional problems, however. Nearly every nutrient can be found lacking in one or another group: iron in girls, calories in young men (especially blacks), vitamin A in girls (especially Mexican and Spanish Americans), calcium, riboflavin, vitamin C, even protein. The insidious problem of obesity becomes more apparent, mostly in girls, especially in black girls. Serious nutritional deficiencies often arise in pregnant teenage girls.

Teenagers' Eating Patterns

Teenagers come and go as they choose and eat what they want when they have time. With a multitude of after-school, social, and job activities, they almost inevitably fall into irregular eating habits. The adult becomes a gatekeeper, controlling the availability but not the consumption of food in the teenager's environment. The adult can't nag, scold, or pressure teenagers into eating as they should, because they typically turn a deaf ear to coercion and often to persuasion. To "feed" effectively, the gatekeeper must make every effort to allow these young people independence while providing a physical environment that favors healthy development and an emotional climate that encourages adaptive choices.

In the home, a wise maneuver is to provide access to nutritious and economical energy foods low in sugar and fat and discouraging to tooth decay. Many parents have discovered independently the wisdom of welcoming their teenage sons and daughters and their friends into the kitchen with an invitation to "Help yourselves! There's plenty of food in the refrigerator" (cooked chicken, raw vegetables, milk, fruit juice) "and more on the table" (fruits, nuts, raisins, popcorn). The snacker—and a well-established characteristic of teenagers is that they are snackers—who finds only nutritious foods around the house is well provided for.

Inevitably, teenagers will do a lot of eating away from home—at snack bars, hamburger stands, and corner stores. There, as well as at home, their nutritional welfare can be favored or hindered by the choices they make. A lunch of a hamburger, a chocolate shake, and french fries supplies nutrients in the amounts indicated in Table 1, at a calorie cost of 780. Except for vitamin A, these are substantial percentages of the recommended intakes at a calorie cost many teenagers can afford. Depending on how they adjust their breakfast and dinner choices, teenagers may serve their needs more than adequately with this sort of lunch. They need only supply fruits and vegetables (for vitamin A and associated nutrients like folacin), a good fiber source, and more good iron and vitamin C sources.

For nutritive value of selected fast foods, see Appendix G.

On the average, about a fourth of teenagers' total daily calorie intake comes from snacks. Their irregular schedules may worry adults who think they are feeding themselves poorly, but at least one study shows that the calories they eat are far from empty. They receive substantial amounts of thiamin, protein, riboflavin, and vitamin C. The nutrients found lacking in this study were calcium and iron and, to some extent, vitamin A.[1] This finding indicates that protein need not be stressed in the nutrition education of teenagers but that some should be encouraged to identify and consume more dairy products, for calcium, and more good vitamin A and folacin sources. (Wherever vitamin A is lacking, folacin is too, because both are found in green vegetables.)

The teenager's iron needs are a special problem, caused by several factors. Two already mentioned are the teenager's burgeoning iron need and the lack of iron in traditional snack foods. Other factors are the overemphasis on dairy products by some teenagers, vegetarianism, and the low contribution made by fast foods to iron intakes. A National Academy of Sciences committee, writing on this special problem, finds it doubtful that long-term administration of iron tablets is practical and advises against the measure of fortifying snacks and other foods with iron. Instead, the committee recommends that physicians and clinics screen all teenagers for low levels of iron in the blood. Their report stresses the fact that "the best dietary source of absorbable iron is

The arguments for and against iron superenrichment of foods are summed up in Controversy 10A.

Table 1. Nutrients in a Hamburger, Chocolate Shake, and Fries

Nutrient	Percent of U.S. RDA
Protein	42
Calcium	47
Iron	21
Vitamin A	3
Thiamin	25
Riboflavin	57
Vitamin C	21

meats of all varieties," a point that should in turn be stressed in the nutritional education of teenagers.[2] A later section of this chapter addresses the problem of teaching teens about nutrition.

Anorexia Nervosa

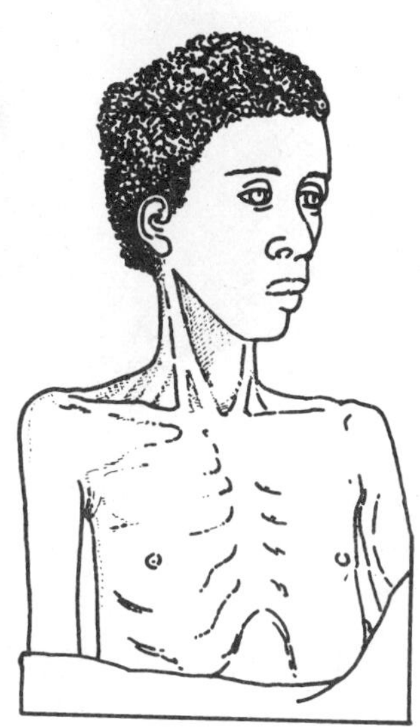

Anorexia nervosa.

Copied from a woodcut accompanying Sir William Gull's article "Anorexia Nervosa" in Lancet 1, 1888.

A concern of teenagers, especially girls, is dieting to maintain a slim and beautiful figure. To accomplish this, many go on fad diets that are neither safe nor effective. The matters of obesity, overweight, and fad diets have been fully discussed elsewhere (see Chapter 8 and Controversy 8) but one special problem should be mentioned here: anorexia nervosa. This is an extreme preoccupation with weight loss and thinness that seriously endangers the health and even the life of the dieter.

Although no two persons with anorexia nervosa are alike, there are certain features considered typical of the condition. The anorexic is almost always female and in her mid-teens. She is usually from an educated, middle-class, success-oriented, weight-conscious family that is proud of her and is surprised to see her develop a problem. She strives to achieve and chooses weight loss as one means of becoming successful herself. Being highly competitive and perfectionistic, she carries the weight-loss effort to an extreme: She will have the slimmest, most perfect body of anyone in her high school class.

So far this description probably fits many young women you know, but this girl develops anorexia nervosa. When she has lost weight to well below the average for her height and is no longer slim but too slim, she still doesn't stop. Weight loss has become an obsession, she is afraid of losing control, and she allows her self-imposed starvation regimen to rule her life. At this point, according to Dr. Hilde Bruch, an authority who has studied and worked with anorexics for a lifetime, starvation has begun to affect her thinking patterns and personality, and physical symptoms are emerging. Although they are the symptoms of starvation, the girl sees them as desirable and prides herself on holding out against her extreme hunger.

Among the physical symptoms are:

Wasting of the whole body, including muscle tissue.

Arresting of sexual development and stopping of menstruation.

Drying and yellowing of the skin, from an accumulation of stored carotene released from body fat.

Loss of health and texture of hair.

Pain on touch.

Lowered blood pressure and metabolic rate.

Anemia.

Severe sleep disturbance.[3]

Simultaneously, some bizarre mental symptoms develop, including an inability to see herself as others see her (she still sees herself as too fat), a preoccupation with death, a frantic pursuit of physical fitness by means of stringent exercise routines, and a manipulative way of dealing with her parents and family such that they make her the center of attention. Diet has become so all-engrossing, now, that she may be quite isolated socially except from friends who stick by her and worry about her without knowing how to help.

Right now I weigh 58 lbs., which isn't too bad for 5′ 2″ though I want to lose a few more pounds—my hips are still fat. Lately I've got it down to no breakfast, a can of mushrooms for lunch, and a can of waxed beans for dinner with lots of iced tea. I reward myself with a big green apple at the end of the day, if I've stuck to The Plan.—A. Ciseaux

By this time, the anorexic has reached an absolute minimum body weight (65 to 70 pounds for a woman of average height) and is on the verge of incurring permanent brain damage and chronic invalidism or death.

Before 1950, the condition was very rare (1 in 2000), and only one out of four such girls could be expected to recover. By 1970, the incidence was increasing and the success rate in treatment was closer to three out of four. During the 1970s anorexia nervosa became still more widespread and familiar to doctors and therapists. Treatment was further improved to the point where success could be expected more often.

Dr. Bruch describes the treatment of the anorexic as a three-stage process. First, she has to have normal nutrition restored, by tube-feeding directly into the stomach if necessary. As she begins to gain weight, some of the family interactions have to be dealt with. With progress in these two areas, she can also begin to be taught some new understanding and clear up some of her misconceptions about nutrition.[4]

Anorexia nervosa is a disease of the developed countries, and becomes more prevalent as wealth increases. The young women who fall victim to it seem to be reacting to the cultural values that emphasize fashion and material success over personal actualization and self-esteem. Whatever its cause, it serves as but one of many possible examples of the ways teenagers feel pressured and of the ways they react to those pressures.

The Pregnant Teenage Girl

A special case of nutritional need is that of the pregnant teenage girl. Even if she were not pregnant, she would be hard put to meet her own nutrient needs at this time of maximal growth. Nourishing the baby doubles her burden. Figure 1 shows that her needs for many nutrients double, although her calorie allowance increases by only a few percent. In the case of a girl who begins pregnancy with inadequate nutrient stores or who lacks the education, resources, and support she needs in order to provide for herself, these problems are compounded.

The complications of pregnancy were briefly discussed in Chapter 12, where it was made obvious that the consequences of poor nutrition are acute and long-lasting. Sickness is common in pregnant teenagers, with toxemia occurring in about one out of every five girls under the age of fifteen. If one pregnancy is followed by another, "the conditions are established for a rapid and irreversible slide from simple toxemia to renal [kidney] damage and hypertensive [heart] disease."[5]

More about toxemia—Chapter 12.

Teenage pregnancy is more common now than it was earlier. About one out of every five babies is born to a mother under nineteen years of age, and more than a tenth of these mothers are fifteen or

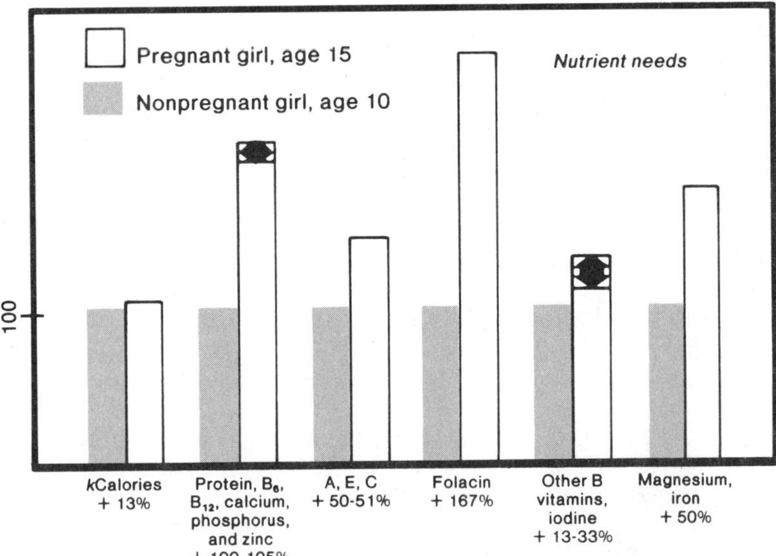

Figure 1. Nutrient needs of a pre-teenager compared with those of a pregnant teenager. *These values were calculated by adding the difference between the RDAs for a ten-year-old and a fourteen-year-old to the difference between the RDAs for a fourteen-year-old and a pregnant woman (see inside front cover).*

younger.[6] The importance of preparing young girls for future pregnancy needs emphasis in public schools and public health programs. Faced with her parents' and classmates' often insensitive reactions, a pregnant girl is likely to wind up alone, with little or no money to buy food and no motivation to seek prenatal care. Programs addressed to all her problems are urgently needed, including medical attention, nutritional guidance, emotional support, and continued schooling.[7] A model program for giving nutritional help to teenage mothers, among others, is the WIC (Women's, Infants' and Children's) program.

More about the WIC program—Chapter 12.

Complicating Factors

The teen years bring exposure to factors not encountered before. Some complicate the nutrition picture: use and abuse of alcohol, prolonged use of prescription medications, drug use (and abuse), caffeine, oral contraceptives, and many more. A section is devoted to each of these, with the object of showing how each contributes to a person's nutritional needs. Because alcohol is by far the most widely used of all drugs in the United States, it receives the heaviest emphasis.

Alcohol. In the mid-teens comes a choice point: whether to drink alcohol or to abstain. A 1975 study showed that more than half of all seventh graders nationwide had tried alcohol at least once within the previous year; nine-tenths of all high school seniors had had experience with alcohol.[8]

The year between the ages of thirteen and fourteen seems to mark the decision point for most white teenagers; and the year between fifteen and sixteen is critical for blacks. Another transitional stage occurs between the ages of seventeen and eighteen, when infrequent drinkers apparently make a decision either to abstain or to drink more heavily. The highest proportion of heavy drinkers by ethnic group is found in Native American youth (16.5 percent), followed by Orientals (13.5) and Spanish (10.9). For whites, the proportion is 10.7 percent; and for blacks, 5.7 percent. Those receiving high grades in school are less likely to become alcohol drinkers; the heavy drinkers characteristically spend more time with peers who also drink.[9]

By the time students get to college, alcohol abuse is frequent and considered part of normal college life. About 90 percent of all college students use alcohol, and heavy drinking is common, with a third or more of all students getting drunk more than once a month.[10] Only a few college students are alcoholics, but 5 to 10 percent will experience serious complications as a result of drinking, and one in twelve will go on to become an adult problem drinker or an alcoholic.[11]

Among adults in the United States, about 100 million drink, and 9 million are estimated to be alcoholics. Because alcohol drinking is more socially acceptable than taking other drugs, alcohol abuse is our most common form of drug abuse.

Much remains to be learned about people's use of alcohol, especially why some people become uncontrolled drinkers (alcoholics) whereas others can drink frequently or even daily for years without ill effects. But much is already known. To clarify the widespread confusion and misconceptions about alcohol, this section presents some important known facts about the body's handling of alcohol, and the Food Feature shows how to apply these facts in handling alcohol responsibly.

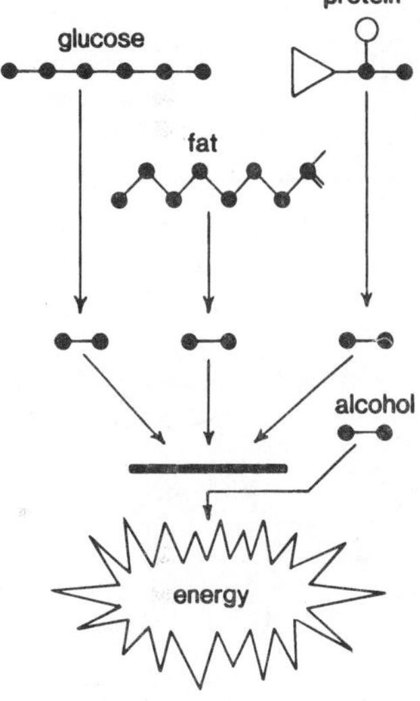

Alcohol gets preferred treatment.

The body's handling of alcohol. Ethyl alcohol, the active ingredient of all alcoholic beverages, is a small organic compound similar in size and composition to the fragments derived from the metabolism of the energy nutrients (carbohydrate, fat, and protein) when they are broken down for energy. Smaller than glucose, alcohol enters the body fluids quickly after a person takes a drink and travels by way of the blood to all organs of the body.

The only organ that can metabolize alcohol is the liver, which converts it to a compound identical to the energy-nutrient fragments mentioned above and then breaks it down the same way these fragments are broken down. The body seems to be in a hurry to accomplish this process. Whenever alcohol is present, it is given top-priority treatment. Glucose, fat, and protein have to wait until after alcohol has been processed.[12]

During the breakdown of alcohol, the energy-containing compound ATP is produced, just as it is from the other energy nutrients. However, the fragments from alcohol cannot be converted to glucose, because there is no machinery in the body that can put these small fragments together in that way. Instead, the fragments derived from alcohol are either used immediately for energy or are converted to fat.

Alcohol is thus, in a sense, an energy nutrient, providing calories the body can use (1 gram of alcohol supplies 7 calories of energy).

glucose
alcohol
fat
energy

The alcohol can go either to energy or to fat, but not to glucose.

1 g alcohol = 7 calories.

Blood Alcohol Level and Effect

2 drinks	0.05 %	Judgment impaired
4 drinks	0.1 %	Control impaired
6 drinks	0.15 %	Muscle coordination and reflexes impaired
8 drinks	0.2 %	Vision impaired
12 drinks	0.3 %	Drunk, totally out of control
14 drinks	0.35 %	Stupor
More	0.5–0.6%	Total amnesia, finally death

However, no cells except those of the liver can use these calories at first, and the liver can turn them only to fat.

Alcohol users who wish to control their weight are resentfully aware that alcohol contains calories. To budget these calories into an adequate diet requires some planning and skill. For a physically large and active young person whose total calorie allowance may be as high as 3000 a day, there may be little problem; but for a smaller, older, or less active person whose calorie needs are less, the problem of compressing the needed nutrients into a reduced allowance may be considerable. The drinker should be reminded that it is nearly impossible to construct an adequate diet within a budget of fewer than 1200 calories of *food* a day. Table 2 shows the calorie values of some alcoholic beverages.

If alcohol overloads the system, with more being supplied than the liver can process right away, the extra alcohol travels around in the bloodstream, waiting its turn. Some of it can be excreted as it is by the kidneys, and some can evaporate when the blood passes through the lungs. These two means of excretion account for about 10 percent of the ingested alcohol. The concentration of alcohol in the breath and in the urine is proportional to the concentration of unmetabolized alcohol circulating in the blood. The "breathalyzer" used by the police department to determine legal drunkenness operates on this principle. Most states consider a person legally drunk at a blood level of alcohol of 0.15 percent, although many have lowered the level to 0.1 percent.

While alcohol is circulating in the bloodstream, waiting to be metabolized, it affects every body organ, including the brain. Contrary to popular belief, it is a depressant, not a stimulant. Like ether, it works as an anesthetic. Sometimes drinkers imagine that they are being stimulated, but that is because the first effect on the brain is to slow down the area that controls judgment and thought. In slowing down this area, alcohol releases the inhibitions which usually guard the drinker's behavior. Being less inhibited and more relaxed may at first make the drinker feel unusually free and easy. But the nervous system is being

Table 2. Calories in Beverages

Beverage	Amount (oz)	Calories
Beer	12	150
Gin, rum, vodka, whiskey (86 proof)	1½	105
Dessert wine	3½	140
Table wine	3½	85
Tonic, ginger ale, other sweetened carbonated water	8	80
Cola, root beer	8	100
Fruit-flavored soda, Tom Collins mix	8	115
Club soda, diet drinks	8	1

depressed, not stimulated, and this depressant action increases as the person continues to drink.

The anesthetic effects of alcohol on the brain take place in a fixed order. This order is determined by the routing of blood through the brain (see the margin). The blood travels first to the forebrain (the frontal lobe), then through the midbrain to the hindbrain, and then leaves the head to be returned to the heart and lungs for more oxygen. When the blood is carrying alcohol, the first cells to feel its effects are those of the frontal lobe, the reasoning part. If additional alcohol continues to enter the bloodstream from the digestive tract before the liver has had time to break down the first, then the speech and vision centers of the brain will be narcotized, and the area that governs reasoning will be more incapacitated. Later the cells controlling the voluntary muscles will be affected. At this point, people "under the influence" will stagger or weave when they try to walk. Finally, the deep brain centers that control respiration and the heartbeat will be anesthetized, but usually the person passes out at about this time, so that breathing and heartbeat continue while the liver gradually does away with the circulating alcohol. Every other organ of the body is also affected, some being stimulated and others being depressed by the drug.

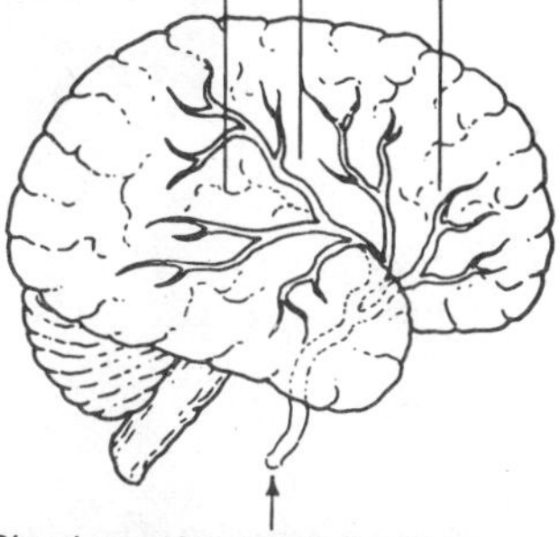

muscular control area
respiration-heart action area
judgment-reasoning area

Blood carrying alcohol enters here. Then blood flow is from front to back of the brain, so that judgment and reasoning are affected first.

Daily consumption of large amounts of alcohol has predictable effects on the body, many of them nutritional. Earlier chapters showed that the breakdown of energy-nutrient fragments requires the participation of the B vitamins thiamin and niacin, among others. These vitamins are also needed to help the liver enzyme that performs the first reaction in alcohol breakdown—the reaction that converts alcohol to a fragment. Thus the breakdown of alcohol uses up these vitamins, leaving fewer to participate in the energy-yielding processes that go on normally, when alcohol is not present. If thiamin and niacin are severely depleted, then even between onslaughts of alcohol, the metabolism of glucose will be impaired; and the supply of its energy, indispensable to the brain and nervous system, will be unreliable. As a result, the heavy drinker often has hypoglycemia.

More about hypoglycemia—Chapter 4.

The liver, after years of handling the calories from alcohol, becomes burdened with an accumulation of fat. Fatty liver partly results from the liver's failure to synthesize the proteins that would wrap the fat for transport in the blood. In addition, the liver cells that are surrounded by fat are shut off from the blood supply. Where the cells die because of this, scar tissue will form.[13] With abstinence and good nutrition, the remaining healthy liver tissue can grow and compensate for the loss. However, with continued drinking and the consequent continued invasion of fat, an irreversible hardening of the liver tissue (cirrhosis) develops, which usually soon leads to death. The sequence of deteriorating events, then, is fatty liver to scarring to liver hardening to death.

Niacin helps break down alcohol by removing hydrogens from it. Once the hydrogens have been attached to niacin, the niacin can't be used until they have been removed again. The niacin passes them on to another body compound, creating an acid, lactic acid. Only after alcohol has left the system can lactic acid be reconverted and disposed of in the normal way. In the meantime, it accumulates in the body. Lactic acid interferes with the excretion of another acid, uric acid, by the kidneys, so that uric acid, too, accumulates. The buildup of these two acids and others necessitates the use of the body's defense system against acidosis: buffering, which depends on the proteins in the blood.

Niacin can't unload its hydrogens if the receiving compound is not available, and the receiving compound is one derived from the breakdown of glucose. Thus, a prior glucose supply is indispensable to the body when it attempts to handle alcohol. Without glucose and its breakdown products, the supply of free niacin runs short. Anyone who has fasted for as little as eight hours before drinking may have a severe enough shortage of free niacin to go into a coma and die because of the lack of glucose for the brain. Sudden death due to massive intakes of alcohol, such as might occur during drinking contests, have been explained by this deficiency, which effectively renders glucose energy unavailable to the brain.[14]

Nutrients especially important for handling of alcohol:
Protein.
Glucose.
B vitamins.

To sum up what has been said so far, the body needs to be well nourished in several ways in order to handle alcohol with a minimum of damage. Protein should be supplied in abundance, so that the buffering action of proteins in the blood will soak up the acids produced by alcohol breakdown and so that the liver enzymes (proteins) will be present and able to work efficiently. The tissues need an ample supply of glucose (normally from carbohydrate) to yield the hydrogen-receiving compound that frees niacin to help process the alcohol. Also, the B vitamins, especially thiamin and niacin, are needed in larger-than-normal quantities when the body is being asked to handle alcohol.

Although good nutrition can help the body handle alcohol and any other drug, it cannot protect against the damage incurred by chronic heavy drinking. Large amounts of alcohol taken daily or frequently damage every body organ, even if a person consumes "the perfect diet" along the way. Good nutrition can prolong good health but can't maintain it against overwhelming odds. Independently of nutrition, alcohol can cause:

High levels of fat in the blood.[15]

Cancer.[16]

Irritation and disease in the esophagus, stomach, and intestine.[17]

Disease of the pancreas and liver.[18]

Muscle disease.[19]

Heart muscle damage and heart disease.[20]

Brain damage, behavior abnormalities, and psychiatric disease.[21]

The most menacing factor in the U.S. nutritional scene today is the health damage caused by alcohol.—G. V. Mann

This is only a partial listing.

Alcohol is entitled to be treated with respect. With an understanding of the way it works, however, most people can use alcohol responsibly and safely and can enjoy its desirable effects while suffering no consequences. The Food Feature provides some pointers for the alcohol user.

Food Feature: Tips for the User of Alcohol

Perhaps the most important message in the discussion of alcohol is to be found in the brain map already displayed. The drinker should be aware that of all the brain centers anesthetized by alcohol, the "judgment center" is the first to go. Thus, for example, a person who goes to a party with every intention of staying sober, of taking only one or two drinks, and of letting their effects wear off before driving home may behave, under the influence of alcohol, in a way that belies all previous sober intentions. After a drink or two, the "judgment," impaired by alcohol, may suggest that the drinker is perfectly well coordinated and can drive normally. Not so. The reaction time and muscular coordination are significantly slowed down. The impairment of judgment by alcohol accounts for the fact that half of all highway fatalities today involve alcohol. Hence the admonition broadcast during the holidays: Don't drive while drinking and don't allow people you care about to drive if they have been drinking.

It takes about 1½ hours for the average 150-pound person's body to rid itself of the alcohol found in one drink. There is no way to sober up quickly. The body processes alcohol at a constant rate. Nothing can hasten this process in a single evening (although years of heavy drinking cause the liver to adapt, so that it can metabolize alcohol at a faster, but still constant, rate). A cold shower or a cup of coffee can have a stimulant effect, so that it will make a drinker feel more awake, but reaction time and judgment are still impaired until the alcohol is gone. The police say, regretfully, "If you give a drunk a cup of coffee, you will make him an awake drunk."

One drink means:
12 oz beer.
5 oz regular wine.
3 oz sherry or port wine.
1½ oz whiskey.
1 highball or cocktail.

Some people believe that walking or exercising will hasten the sobering-up process. This technique is ineffective for two reasons. First, the muscle cells possess no enzymes that can break down alcohol, so exercise can only deplete the available stores of glucose. Second, as already mentioned, the liver breaks down alcohol at a steady rate, so only time can bring about sobriety.

All of this boils down to a single technique: Deliver alcohol to the liver at a rate it can handle. This means sipping each drink so that it will last an hour and a half. It also helps to eat while drinking, because people are less likely to drink too fast if they are not hungry. Moreover, the absorption of alcohol from the stomach will be slowed by the presence of food.

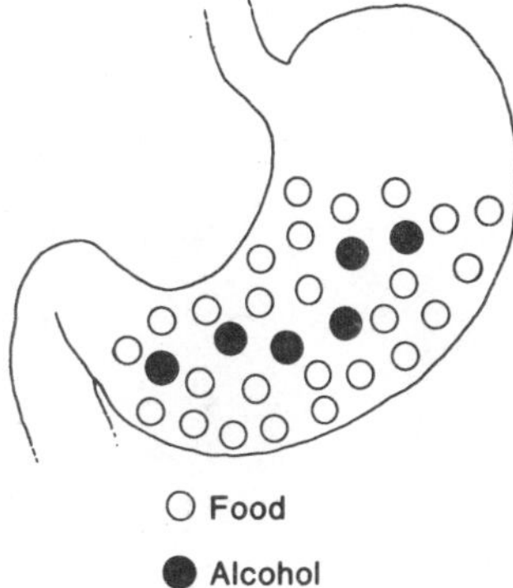

The alcohol in a stomach filled with food has a low probability of touching the walls and diffusing through.

Once the alcohol arrives in the small intestine, the presence of food will no longer slow its absorption. It moves into the bloodstream quickly and completely, taking priority over all other nutrients.[22] Therefore, any method that keeps the alcohol in the stomach longer keeps alcohol from flooding the brain and anesthetizing it. High-fat snacks slow down stomach motility and thus are helpful in regulating the amount of alcohol released into the intestine and bloodstream.

Some people think that if you mix drinks you will get more drunk than if you stick to one kind of drink. The effects of alcohol are strictly additive; and all other factors being equal, only the amount of alcohol consumed affects how drunk you get. (Other factors might be fatigue, stress, mood, and the like.) But because alcoholic beverages are fermented from different plants, they do have different flavors. For some people switching is more likely to cause nausea and vomiting, possibly because of the mixture of these different flavorings.

Alcohol can also make you thirsty, because it depresses the brain's production of a hormone that makes the kidney return water to the bloodstream.[23] Without this hormone, the kidney releases too much water into the urine, causing dehydration and thirst. The drinker, feeling thirsty, takes another drink; if the drink is a highly concentrated cocktail, it may fool the mouth into momentary satisfaction, but it will continue to promote the excretion of water and more thirst. To avoid this cycle, the party goer can drink plenty of water before drinking alcohol, drink tall drinks such as beer or highballs in which the water content is high, or drink short drinks such as martinis or whiskey with a chaser containing water.

One or two drinks daily appear to cause no harm in adults. If you drink, you should do so in moderation.—Dietary Guidelines, USDA

By the use of these techniques, and with practice and experience, about nine out of every ten alcohol users can enjoy the mild, temporary, relaxed state that characterizes social drinking—without risking their permanent well-being. One out of every ten, however, seems destined to become an alcohol addict (alcoholic). This means that, in a college class of fifty people, about four may fall into this category.[24]

Alcohol abuse and alcoholism. There is a great need for the public to know that being an alcohol addict is not a sign of inferiority or something to be ashamed of. It does not reflect failure as a person or moral degeneracy. Like diabetes, alcoholism is now recognized as a disease: a definite process having a characteristic train of symptoms. Although the causes are not yet known, the symptoms have been extensively studied, and the criteria for diagnosis have been completely defined.

Being an alcoholic, like being a diabetic, is probably determined at least to some extent by a person's genes, which can convey a predisposition toward alcohol addiction. People who have every reason to be proud of themselves, their potential, and their achievements may be alcoholic. The typical alcoholic is not a skid row bum.[25] He or she is just as likely to be a doctor, a nurse, a Hollywood star, or a prestigious local businessperson. In fact, there is no such thing as "the typical alcoholic."

The only statement that can be made with certainty about alcoholic persons is they have lost control over alcohol. Intending to drink moderately and responsibly, they repeatedly overconsume alcohol to the point where it damages their family relationships, jobs, social functioning, and self-esteem. Broken promises are a hallmark of the alcoholic. Such a person cannot drink at all: The first drink too often becomes the first of too many.

Many myths and misconceptions surround the public's picture of alcoholism. Four of the most common wrong ideas are the following:

A person who gets drunk is an alcoholic. This is not true. Anyone who loses control over his or her reactions and behavior while drinking alcohol is drunk. This is a temporary state. An alcoholic is an alcohol addict—a person who must have alcohol in order to function or who, in giving it up, suffers severe withdrawal reactions.

An alcoholic person is a drunk. This too is not true. Alcoholic persons may appear to be functioning normally while drinking large quantities of alcohol. Their problem is likely to become apparent when they are not drinking, and thus are feeling the craving that indicates withdrawal, rather than when they are drinking.

A person who never passes out is not an alcoholic. Not true. Passing out is the result when the anesthetic effect of alcohol has reached the part of the brain that controls wakefulness. An alcohol addict may drink to this end point no more often than a nonalcoholic person. What the alcoholic person experiences at a certain stage in the progress toward serious addiction is the blackout. This is temporary loss of memory, not loss of consciousness. No one notices that anything is wrong while the person is drinking—behavior is normal—but the next day the person can't remember what happened beyond a certain point the day before. Blackouts are one of the distinguishing characteristics of alcoholic persons.

A beer drinker can never become an alcoholic. Because beer contains alcohol, it is just as capable of contributing to alcoholism as is wine or "hard" liquor (whiskey, gin, vodka, and the like). It is not the beverage but the constitution of the consumer that determines whether a person will become addicted to alcohol.

Some beer drinkers protest that beer has some redeeming features: It makes people drunk less quickly, and it provides valuable nutrients. True, because the alcohol in beer is diluted, it will reach the bloodstream more slowly than the same amount of alcohol taken straight. But the carbonation in beer stimulates the stomach, hastening the entry of the alcohol into the intestine, where it will immediately be absorbed. As for the nutrient content of beer, an adult male would have to drink at least a six-pack of twelve-ounce cans to meet his recommended niacin intake and nine six-packs to meet his recommended protein intake.

The potential alcohol addict has a hard truth to face: Total avoidance of alcohol is the only sure way to have a chance to lead a normal life. Facing it is made harder by the aura of shame and guilt that surrounds the public's uneducated view of alcoholism. The steps toward recovery are summed up by the experts: Face it, get help, and stop drinking. The selected references at the end of this chapter offer suggestions for further study in this important and much misunderstood area.

Some people choose to abstain from alcohol consumption because they are alcohol addicts; others make the same choice for other reasons. Such people have a hard time in some social settings, because drinking is often not only accepted but even almost demanded of all comers. It is hoped that this discussion will have shown why it is desirable not to pressure other persons to drink. Considerate hosts or social groups will welcome the nondrinker and provide nonalcoholic beverages for his or her enjoyment just as they would provide nonmeat food for a guest who is a vegetarian.

Prescription drugs. The dictionary defines a drug as any chemical compound given to humans to help with the diagnosis or treatment of a disease or the relief from its symptoms. It is thus different in important ways from a nutrient, which only functions to prevent disease caused by a deficiency of that nutrient. Drugs are not natural compounds found in the body when it is functioning normally, and there is no drug that has been shown to be completely without ill effects.

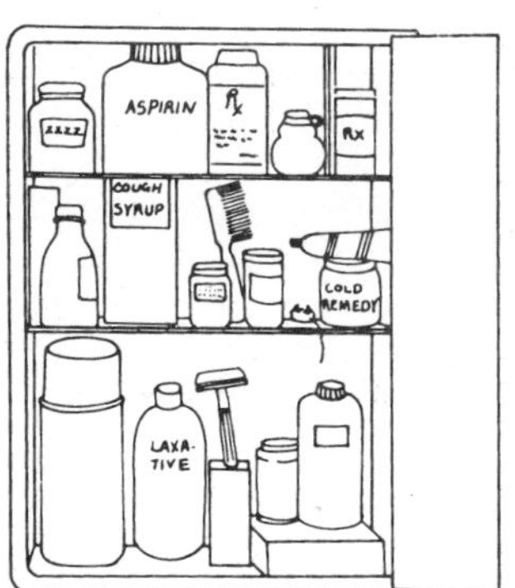

Many drugs affect the body's need for and use of nutrients.

Many drugs affect the body's need for and use of nutrients. Alcohol is a prime example of these effects. Prescription medications can also affect nutritional status by:

Increasing or decreasing appetite.

Causing nausea, vomiting, or an altered sense of taste.

Inhibiting the synthesis of nutrients.

Reducing the absorption or increasing the excretion of nutrients.

Altering the transport, use, or storage of nutrients.

Foods and nutrients can also affect the drugs in the body. For example, some foods interfere with the absorption of medications taken with them, so the medications should be taken between meals. In other cases, the presence of food in the intestine prevents the nausea that might otherwise be caused by the drug; such a drug should be taken with meals. The doctor doesn't always tell you, but your pharmacist will probably be glad to inform you which is which.

Prolonged use of almost any prescription medication can result in gradual nutrient depletion. Aspirin can irritate the intestine and cause bleeding, vitamin C deficiency, and anemia.[26] Antibiotics inhibit iron absorption.[27] Antacids can cause increased excretion of calcium, leading to adult bone loss.[28] Mineral oil depletes fat-soluble vitamins and can cause rickets in children, and other laxatives cause multiple nutrient deficiencies.[29] Many other such effects are known.[30]

The special case of the woman taking oral contraceptives deserves a moment's attention. The Pill alters blood levels of several nutrients, raising some (vitamin A and iron) and lowering others (B vitamins and vitamin C). Women often wonder what vitamin supplements, if any, they should take while on the Pill. The answer seems to be: "None. You are risking a nutritional deficiency only if your diet is grossly inadequate, especially in folacin. And if it is, you need diet counseling more than you need a vitamin pill."[31]

On the other hand, the person who has taken prescription medications for a long time may well have developed nutrient deficiencies. This is most likely in heavy drinkers, in older people who are taking a combination of medications or who abuse laxatives, and in children during the period of active growth.

In addition, many drugs (medications) interact with one another, further complicating the picture. A prime example is the interaction of alcohol with other "downer" drugs such as barbiturates and tranquilizers. The body adapts at first to prolonged alcohol consumption by increasing the rate at which it breaks down alcohol. This adaptation involves increasing the amount of live machinery (enzymes) maintained for alcohol metabolism. Many drugs are processed by that same machinery, so that a dose of these drugs given to an alcohol user may be ineffective; the liver may break it down before it has a chance to reach effective levels in the body. On the other hand, the user who takes alcohol with the drug may swamp the liver metabolizing system, so that it can't handle the drug at all; and the drug may reach unexpectedly high, even toxic, levels in the body. The physician prescribing medications that interact with the body's alcohol system should be fully informed regarding the patient's use of alcohol.

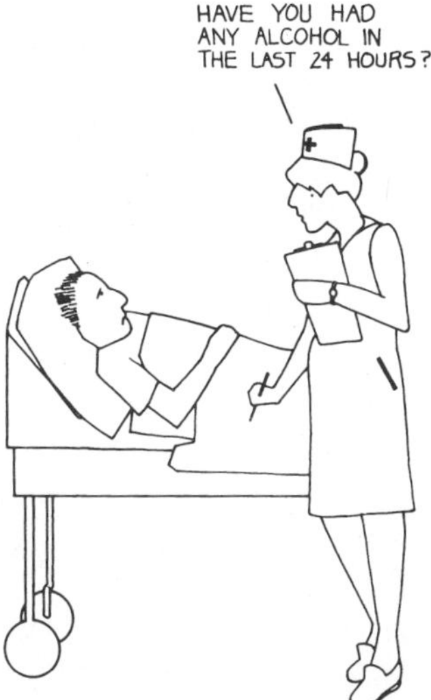

The physician needs complete information on the patient's use of alcohol.

Hundreds of millions of prescriptions are written for mind-altering drugs each year, and billions for other drugs. To protect against the risks of nutrient-drug and drug-drug interactions, one writer on the subject urges:

Avoidance of unnecessary prescriptions.

Limitation of multiple-drug regimens.

Support for control of over-the-counter drug sales.

Education of medical and other health personnel, as well as patients, regarding the nutritional effects of drugs.[32]

"The physician" has been mentioned several times in this chapter, sometimes with the implication that he or she is not always aware of the contributions nutrition makes to health and disease. Whenever we have spoken of medical problems, such as diagnosis and treatment of abnormal conditions, we have urged you to ask your doctor. However, when we have dealt with nutrition-related problems, we have sometimes intentionally suggested that the doctor may not be the most reliable authority. Medical schools often neglect nutrition in their course offerings, and many doctors know as little as, or less than, the average layperson when it comes to the nutrients, the nature of foods, and the adequacy of diets.

We have also tried to convey the notion that, like automobile mechanics, doctors come in all varieties: competent and incompetent, honest and dishonest. In choosing a doctor to consult, you might well want to investigate the reputation, training, and experience of several in relation to the particular problem you have in mind. The questions of how much doctors

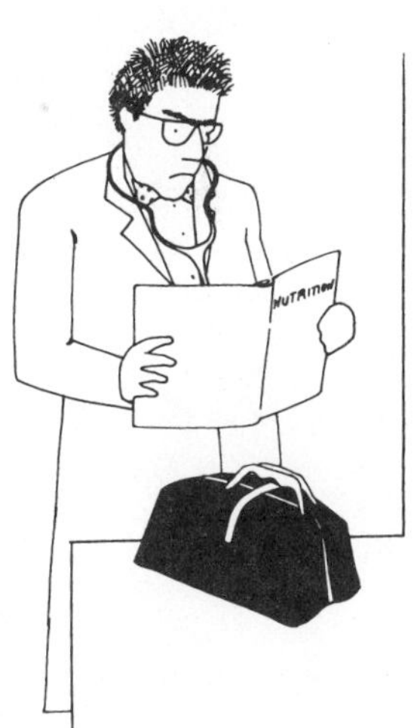

Controversy 14B contains a discussion of doctors and their nutrition knowledge.

know about nutrition and what should perhaps be done to improve their training are important ones in this society, which spends billions of dollars each year on medical care.

Marihuana: alternate spelling, marijuana.

Marihuana. Like alcohol, marihuana has characteristic effects on the body; and like alcohol, it has not been shown to have many pronounced harmful effects even with long-term use, unless the use is very heavy (five to six cigarettes a day for six months). The active ingredients are rapidly and completely (90 percent) absorbed from the lungs.[33] Then, being fat soluble, they are packaged in protein (possibly in lipoproteins[34]) before being transported by the blood to the various body tissues. They are processed by many tissues (not just by the liver), and they persist for several days in body fat, being excreted over a period of a week or more after the smoking of a single cigarette.[35]

Smoking a marihuana cigarette has characteristic effects on hearing, touch, taste, and smell and on perceptions of time, space, and the body; it also produces changes in mental sensations and alterations in the nature of sleep. Among the taste changes apparently induced is a great enjoyment of eating, especially of sweets ("the munchies"), but it is not known how this effect occurs.[36] The drug apparently does not change the blood glucose level.[37] Investigators speculate that the so-called hunger induced by marihuana is actually a social effect caused by the suggestibility of the group in which it is smoked.[38] Prolonged use of the drug does not seem to bring about a weight gain; the members of one small sample of regular users (thirty smokers) have been observed to weigh less than comparable nonsmokers by about seven pounds.[39]

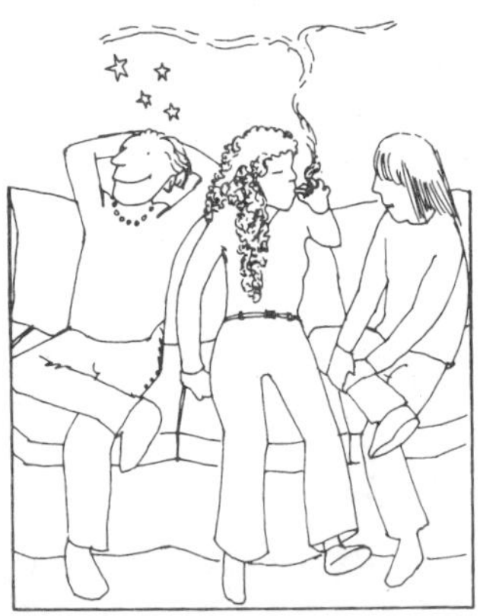

No-one yet knows why marihuana causes "the munchies."

Many young people in the United States are turning to marihuana as an alternative to alcohol. The number of individuals using it at least once a day had grown from half a million in 1971 to over 3 million before 1980.[40] There is much disagreement about the desirability of this trend; and despite much current research, little is known about the possible risks of regular smoking.

It has become clear, however, that even in "socially acceptable" concentrations, the drug brings about a deterioration in some aspects of driving performance such as reaction time and muscular coordination.[41] Another effect widely agreed on is that it causes alterations in heart action, including rapid and sometimes irregular heartbeat.[42] It also reduces the body's immune response and, in young men, reduces the sex hormone level and sperm count after a lag period of about six weeks. Reporting on this effect, the investigator points out that marihuana "is much like other drugs, such as tobacco and liquor, in that the greatest potential hazard exists for those who abuse it. . . . There is still no convincing evidence that casual, infrequent use of marihuana produces any ill effects."[43]

The potency of marihuana preparations reaching this country has been increasing. Before 1970, most marihuana used in the United States was a very weak domestic variety with an average THC content of about 0.2 percent. (THC is tetrahydrocannabinol, the primary active ingredient of marihuana.) During the 1970s, users shifted to a Mexican variety (about 1.5 percent), then to Jamaican and Colombian marihuana (3 to 4 percent). The present trend is toward even higher concentrations. Users looking for a greater "high" then sometimes shift to hashish oil, a much more concentrated form of the active drug (about 40 to 50 percent THC and up to 90 percent), at which point the risks probably increase dramatically.[44]

Most investigators agree that, with moderate use, the hazards of marihuana smoking are few and small. However, it should be remembered that, because possession and use of the drug is not legal, no controls are exerted by any agency, such as the FDA, on the content of preparations sold as marihuana. There is a significant hazard associated with the possibility that they may be contaminated with pesticides or that they may contain "hard" (addictive) drugs such as heroin, concealed in them by the pusher in order to create a demand for a product that can be sold for greater profits. Also, when marihuana use escalates into the use of "hard" drugs, the nutrition and health effects become pronounced, as the next section illustrates.

Drug abuse. The term *drug* has a second meaning, as familiar to most people as the first: a narcotic, especially one that is addictive. Among the drugs in most common use today are heroin, morphine, LSD, PCP, and cocaine. Users of these drugs face multiple problems, not the least of which is nutritional. Their nutrition suffers severely for a multitude of reasons.

They spend their money for drugs rather than for food.

They lose interest in food during "high" periods on drugs.

Some drugs (for example, amphetamines) induce at least a temporary depression of appetite.

Their lifestyle lacks the regularity and routine that would promote good eating habits.

They often have hepatitis (a liver disease caused by the use of contaminated needles), which causes taste changes and loss of appetite.

They often depend on alcohol, especially when withdrawing from drug use.

They often become ill with infectious diseases which increase their need for nutrients.

During their withdrawal from drugs, one of the most important aspects of treatment is to identify and correct these nutritional problems while teaching and supporting adaptive eating habits.[45]

Caffeine. Like alcohol use, the use of caffeine-containing beverages becomes common during the teens. Coffee, tea, and especially cola beverages become permitted drinks.

Caffeine is less likely to be dangerously abused than alcohol, perhaps because its use neither dulls the senses nor impairs judgment.

Caffeine Sources

Source	Caffeine (mg)
Brewed coffee (1 cup)	85
Instant coffee (1 cup)	60
Brewed black tea (1 cup)	50
Brewed green tea (1 cup)	30
Instant tea (1 cup)	30
Decaffeinated coffee	3
Cola beverage (12 oz)	32–65
Aspirin compound (pill containing aspirin, phenacetin, and caffeine)	32
Cope, Midol, etc.	32
Excedrin, Anacin (tablet)	60
Pre-Mens	66
Many cold preparations	30
Many stimulants	100
Cocoa (1 cup)	6–42
No Doz (tablet) or Vivarin	100–200

Adapted from P. E. Stephenson, Physiologic and psychotropic effects of caffeine on man, Journal of the American Dietetic Association 71 (1977): 240-247.

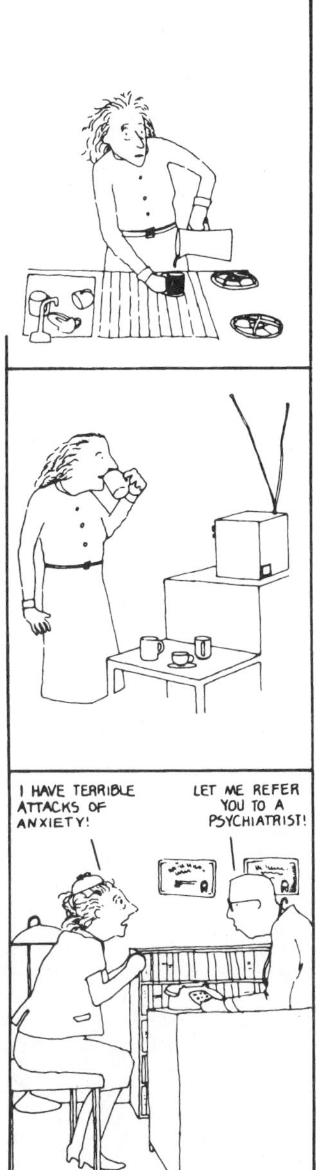
I HAVE TERRIBLE ATTACKS OF ANXIETY!
LET ME REFER YOU TO A PSYCHIATRIST!

Check out your caffeine intake before you go to a psychiatrist for anxiety.

Caffeine is a true stimulant drug, increasing the respiration rate, heart rate, blood pressure, and the secretion of the stress and other hormones.[46] Its "wake-up" effect is maximal within an hour after the dose. In moderate amounts (50 to 200 milligrams a day), caffeine seems to be a relatively harmless drug.

Every human society has made a caffeine-containing food or beverage a staple in its diet: the habitual tea of the English and many other cultures; the coffee of Arabia, Indonesia, Brazil, and others; cola beverages in many South American countries; and many exotic-sounding drinks, chewing gums, and foods elsewhere. The universal human use of caffeine shows that, at least as subjectively perceived, it does something for the user.

Caffeine is not addictive, but it is habit-forming, and the body adapts to its use to some extent. A dose greater than what the body is adapted to causes jitteriness, nervousness, and intestinal discomfort. Sudden abstinence from the drug after long, even if moderate, use causes a characteristic withdrawal reaction; the most frequently observed symptom is a headache. If a person has adapted to a much higher dose level than 50 to 200 milligrams of caffeine per day, then dropping back to this level may cause the same withdrawal reaction.

An overdose of caffeine produces actions in the body that are indistinguishable from those of an anxiety attack.[47] People who drink between eight and fifteen cups of coffee a day, for example, have been known to seek help from doctors for complaints such as "dizziness, agitation, restlessness, recurring headaches, and sleep difficulties." Before prescribing a tranquilizer, the doctor would do well to inquire about the caffeine consumption of such patients.

A large dose of caffeine can also cause extra heartbeats and is believed to have caused heart attacks in people whose hearts were already damaged by degenerative disease.[48] However, neither caffeine nor its vehicle, coffee, can be considered a risk factor for the development of atherosclerosis.[49] Neither the Framingham Study nor a study of 7705 Japanese showed any correlation between coffee drinking and heart attack risk.[50]

Of all people who drink coffee, the pregnant woman is most strongly advised to curtail her consumption. Another person who should perhaps be warned against coffee in particular is the ulcer patient. It has been shown that even decaffeinated coffee stimulates the secretion of stomach acid;[51] thus, there must be compounds in coffee besides caffeine that aggravate ulcers.

Caffeine tolerance decreases with age. As you grow older, you are advised to reduce your caffeine intake gradually. The morning cup of coffee is all right as a "pick-me-up," but the afternoon or evening cup may seriously interfere with your ability to sleep at night.[52] People vary greatly in their responses to caffeine, however; if you think your consumption of caffeine may be causing insomnia, try cutting it down (especially in the afternoon) and see if you sleep better. If you do, better keep it down.

The Self-Determining Young Adult

Adolescence is well known as a time of rebellion. This rebellion extends to foods as well as to all other aspects of lifestyle. The choice of what to eat is up to teenagers themselves. Access points already mentioned include the refrigerator, the school lunch, and vending machines; but other than controlling the contents of these, adults can expect to have little impact on the nutrient intakes of adolescents—especially by such conventional means as education. Still, most young adults in this country are well fed, for reasons perceptively stated by R. M. Leverton: They get hungry; they like to eat; they want energy, vigor, and the means to compete and excel in whatever they do; and they have many good habits, which are just as hard to break as the bad ones.[53]

Nutrition educators who wish to reach the teenager and young adult with nutrition information must find out and pay attention to two factors: why they sometimes are poorly nourished or develop poor food habits and what means of communicating appeals to them.

The young person with a negative attitude toward food and poor food habits is likely to have at least one of the following characteristics:

> He thinks nutrition means eating what you don't like because it's good for you.
>
> She has been criticized for her eating pattern but feels fine and sees no ill effects.
>
> He is uninterested in food, and it plays a negligible role in his very busy life.
>
> The people she is most likely to listen to are not knowledgeable about nutrition.[54]

In the North American food pattern, the father presides over meat and fish, the mother over milk, vegetables, fruit juices and liver, while adolescents tend to demonstrate their independence by refusing to eat what is good for them.—M. Mead

The parent or teacher concerned about a teenager's food habits should be aware of what teenagers feel about themselves (some reflection into your own past may recall painful memories in this connection). They crave acceptance, especially from their peers. They need to fit in. In many cases they are greatly dissatisfied with themselves as they are. One of the most important aspects of their image is the body image. Young men want larger biceps, shoulders, chest, and forearms; young women want smaller hips, thighs, and waists.[55] One study of U.S. teenagers revealed that 59 percent of the young men wanted to gain weight, although only 25 percent actually needed to do so. Similarly, 70 percent of the girls wanted to lose weight, but no more than about 15 percent were obese.[56] Words to the effect that "you look fine as you are" fall on deaf ears. (The same can be said of adults in some cases, up to the age of about ninety-nine.) To be effectively conveyed, nutrition information can be sold as part of a package that will bring about these desired changes. Fortunately, it happens to be true that nutrient-dense, low-calorie foods favor the development of strong biceps in men and a trim figure in women.

No other age group is as concerned about their bodies or as sensitive to or devastated by criticism and comparison as are adolescents. . . . It's not unusual to find these adolescents with distorted body images making inappropriate food choices and thus compromising optimal growth.—B. Lucas

When the young person who is the target of your campaign possesses and cherishes nutrition misinformation, one of the first questions to ask is "whether the practice is beneficial, neutral, or harmful."[57] Opposing a loved ideal is more likely to polarize than to convert the opposition. Practices such as vegetarianism, dieting, or consuming a "muscle-building diet" can be encouraged—with modifications—rather than condemned. Only the most hazardous nutritional practices should be singled out for attention; silence should probably be maintained about the others.

The nutrient needs of the athlete are the subject of Controversy 7.

One of the most effective ways to teach nutrition is by example. When nutrition teachers are moralists who fail to practice what they preach, their words of wisdom fall on deaf ears. The coach and gym teacher, the friendly young French teacher, the admired city recreation director—those who enthusiastically maintain their own health—can have a great impact on teenagers who seek to emulate those they admire. Remember, this is the period of identity formation, the time of seeking and emulating models.

When communicating nutrition information, above all be sure that you have it straight. We make fools of ourselves when we (for example) admonish our students to follow restrictive patterns when their own choices are already as good as ours or better. There may be no harm in using candy bars to meet part of the calorie allowance of an active young adult. It may not be necessary to drink milk if the calcium, vitamin D, and riboflavin needs are being met by cheese or other food sources. Satisfactory diets can be designed on a great variety of different foundations. It is the nutrient content and balance of foods, not the specific foods consumed, that make the difference between "good" and "bad" diets.

Much of the work of "teaching" nutrition can be delegated to the teenagers themselves. Those who are interested and motivated can be guided to reliable sources and allowed to indulge their own desire to benefit their friends and classmates. Among the best materials prepared to teach teenagers the importance of good nutrition are those made by teenagers themselves.

We feel that teenagers may be even more effective teachers of their peers than adults. . . . We must end . . . adult-determined decision making about nutrition education and "teach them what they want to know."—R. Frankle and F. W. Heussenstamm

Finally, hard as it is to accept sometimes, remember that teenagers have the right to make their own decisions—even if they are ones you violently disagree with. You can set up the environment so that the foods available are those you favor, and you can stand by with reliable nutrition information and advice, but you will have to leave the rest to them. Ultimately, they are the ones who make the choices.[1]

For Further Information

Good books for the young adult and adult have been referred to throughout the preceding chapters, in Appendix J, and in this chapter's notes.

The entire February 1981 issue of *Nutrition Reviews* was devoted to adolescent nutrition and included articles on all the topics discussed in this chapter.

Among the most thought-provoking and readable articles available on anorexia nervosa are three that appeared in the *American Journal of Nursing*, August 1980. The first is an account by an anorexic herself:

- Ciseaux, A. Anorexia nervosa: A view from the mirror. Pp. 1469-1470.

[1]*Chapter Notes can be found at the end of the Appendixes.*

- Richardson, T. F. Anorexia nervosa: An overview. Pp. 1470-1471.
- Claggett, M. S. Anorexia nervosa: A behavioral approach. Pp. 1471-1477.

Another excellent short article by the authority H. Bruch is:

- Anorexia nervosa. *Nutrition Today*, September/October 1978, pp. 14-18.

Bruch's book is still the authoritative reference on the subject:

- Bruch, H. *The Golden Cage: The Enigma of Anorexia Nervosa*. Cambridge, Mass.: Harvard University Press, 1978.

Two excellent films on the subject are also available: *Dieting: the Danger Point*, from McGraw-Hill, and *Diet unto Death*, from ABCLearning Corporation.

For the best references on pregnancy, teenage and otherwise, turn to the selected references for Chapter 12.

On alcohol, three references are especially recommended:

- Iber, F. In alcoholism, the liver sets the pace. *Nutrition Today*, January/February 1971, pp. 2-9.
- Lieber, C. S. The metabolism of alcohol. *Scientific American* 234 (1976): 25-33.
- Wolff, P. H. Ethnic differences in alcohol sensitivity. *Science* 175 (1972): 449-450.

The third paper presents one of the possible explanations why some persons do not become alcoholic although others with seemingly similar backgrounds do.

On alcoholism: "Alcoholism," a 1975 pamphlet clarifying some aspects of the problem, is available free from Metropolitan Life (offices in many cities). A highly technical article, intended for use by the diagnosing physician, is:

- Criteria for the diagnosis of alcoholism. *American Journal of Psychiatry* 129 (August 1972): 127-135.

The pamphlet "What are the Signs of Alcoholism?" can be obtained from the National Council on Alcoholism, 733 3rd Avenue, New York, NY 10017. This is a twenty-question quiz that enables alcohol addicts to diagnose themselves. Similar pamphlets are available at local alcohol information centers in most cities and towns. See "alcohol" in your telephone book.

On the interaction between prescription drugs and nutrition, an authoritative but small, easy-to-read book is:

- Roe, D. A. *Drug-Induced Nutritional Deficiencies* (Westport, Conn.: Avi Publishing, 1976).

Controversy 14A

Acne

What's the nutrition connection?

"Acne should never be ignored," says the leaflet on the subject from USDHHS, "especially [in] young persons who are justifiably distressed by their appearance."[1] The young person with acne is sure to agree and is willing to go to considerable trouble and expense to find a remedy. But what's the remedy? To wash constantly? To sunbathe? To have the skin sanded? To take antibiotics? vitamin A? zinc? To spread vitamin A acid on the skin? To stop eating chocolate, drinking cola beverages, eating greasy foods, drinking milk, using iodized salt? Or to try to find relief from "stress"? All of these approaches have been suggested, and each has helped some people in individual cases. But while advances are being made that look hopeful for the treatment of acne in the future, there is as yet no surefire way to get rid of it. The purpose here is to answer the questions you may have about acne and in particular about its relation to foods and nutrients.

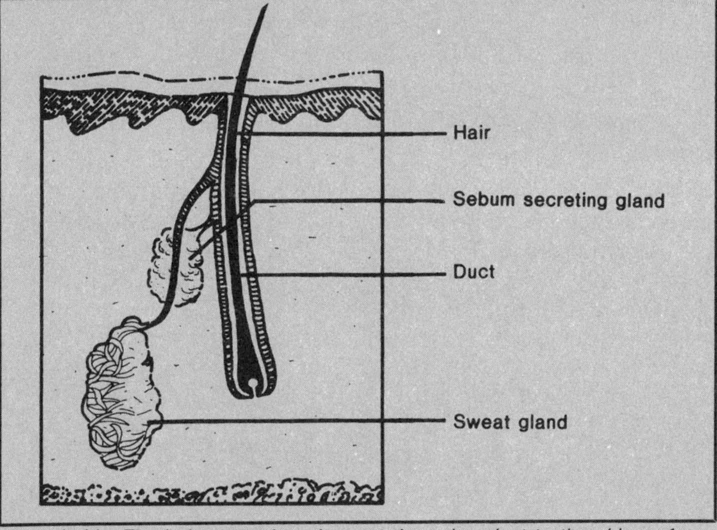

Normal skin. The hair grows from its root through a duct to the skin surface. Beside the duct lies a gland that secretes sebum, a misture of waxes and oils, onto the surface of the skin to help keep it moist. A sweat gland is often associated with the same duct and secretes sweat through the same opening (pore) in the skin.

How acne arises. No one knows why some people get acne while others don't, but there seems to be a hereditary factor involved, because it runs in families. The hormones of adolescence also play a role by increasing the activity of the glands in the skin. The skin's

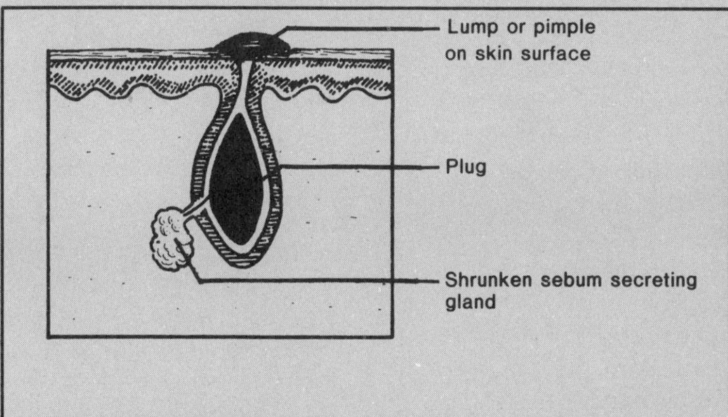

Closed comedo or whitehead. A plug has formed so that the gland contents can't reach the surface of the skin.

natural oil, sebum, is supposed to flow from the deep glands where it is made out through the tiny ducts around the hairs to the skin surface.[2] In acne, the oily secretion is not brought to the surface of the skin.

Inside each of the ducts is a skinlike lining that regularly scales and flakes. The scales or flakes mix with the oil and then are pushed to the surface of the skin. At times, the scale sticks together and forms a plug, which may enlarge and weaken the duct, allowing oil and the skin-surface bacteria to leak into the surrounding skin. The oil is irritating, and the bacteria produce enzymes that make it more irritating, so there is redness, swelling, pus formation—and the beginning of a whitehead or pimple. A cyst may be formed—a sort of enlarged, deep pimple. Or the skin may open above the plug, revealing an accumulation of dark skin pigments just below the surface—a blackhead.

This description should clear up two common mistaken notions about acne. First, it isn't caused by the skin bacteria, although once the process has begun they can make it worse. And secondly, the color of a blackhead is caused by skin pigments, not by dirt. Squeezing or picking at the lesions of acne in an attempt to remove their contents can cause more scars than the acne.

Acne treatment. The careful physician will consider and select from the treatments mentioned at the start. The rationale for washing is to help control the skin-surface bacteria, remove the skin oil, and keep the oil ducts open as much as possible. Surface treatment with antibiotics or peroxides helps control the bacteria. A cream or gel containing retinoic acid (a member of the vitamin A family) can be applied, carefully: Retinoic acid loosens the plugs that form in the ducts and allows the oil to flow again so that the ducts will not burst. But care is necessary because the acid may burn the skin and even cause pimples to form, making the acne look worse rather than better at first. At the end of adolescence, when the acne has subsided, a surgical procedure known as dermabrasion or skin planing can remove the scars—in some cases. (Be sure to request a second opinion before

Miniglossary

acne: A skin condition usually associated with the maturation of young adults, characterized by the eruption of skin lesions (comedones) commonly known as whiteheads, blackheads, pimples, and cysts.

blackhead: An open comedo with an accumulation of the natural, dark pigment of the skin (not dirt) in its opening.

13-cis-retinoic acid: A synthetic derivative of vitamin A; oral doses look promising in preliminary tests with treatment-resistant acne.

comedo (COMM-ee-doh): A blackhead; plural, **comedones** (COMM-ee-DOH-nees).

cyst: An enlarged, deep pimple.

dermabrasion (DERM-uh-bray-zhun): Planing the skin to remove scars, a procedure requiring skill, and one that works on only certain kinds of scars (*dermis* means "skin"; *abrasion* means "sanding, planing").

sebum (SEE-bum): The skin's natural oil, actually a mixture of oils and waxes, that helps keep skin and hair moist.

whitehead: A pimple, caused by the plugging of an oil-gland duct with shed material from the duct lining.

undertaking this and to consult a dermatologist or plastic surgeon known for his or her skill.)

Occasionally a young person, on hearing that "vitamin A acid" helps with acne, has jumped to the conclusion that taking vitamin A internally would help—and has ended up in an emergency room with a toxic overdose of vitamin A.[3] Vitamin A comes in three main forms—retinal, retinol, and retinoic acid—and taking one of them internally is not at all the same as applying another to the skin. As of 1980, some cautious experimentation with oral doses of a synthetic vitamin A derivative, 13-cis-retinoic acid, was under way, and the early results looked promising. A group of patients with severe cystic acne showed clearing of the acne in response to this approach, and the clearing persisted after the drug was discontinued. Much more testing is needed to determine the long-term safety of the drug, however, before it can be submitted to the FDA for approval.[4]

Another nutrient that has been tried with acne in recent years is zinc, and the results with that, too, have been encouraging. The rationale for trying it was that zinc is necessary to maintain normal blood levels of vitamin A, as well as for the working of many enzymes, including some related to the functions of the skin glands. Furthermore, "it is possible that there is an absolute or relative zinc deficiency in puberty." According to the researchers who tried it, zinc brought about a marked improvement in the acne symptoms of their patients in comparison with both placebo and vitamin A (retinol).[5]

Foods and acne. The procedures just described might not be necessary if only we knew how to prevent acne. It has been hoped that certain foods could be blamed and that prevention would then be just a matter of avoiding those foods. Among foods charged with aggravating acne have been chocolate, cola beverages, fatty or greasy foods, milk, nuts, sugar, and foods or salt containing iodine. None of these foods have been shown to worsen acne. Some have been shown not to—notably chocolate and sugar.[6] But the suspicion that foods are related to acne brings forcibly to mind a factor that clearly does relate: stress.

Stress, with its accompanying hormonal secretions, clearly worsens acne.[7] Adolescence is a stressful time anyway, and the pressures of school can make it worse. Vacations help to bring relief. The sun, the beach, and swimming also help, partly because of their relaxing effect and perhaps also because the sun inhibits bacterial activity and water cleanses.[8]

If a physician (or any authority figure) suggests that certain foods will cause acne flareups, the troubled young person forbidden to eat those foods may experience stress when he or she does. It may be the "guilt trip," rather than the foods, that brings on the flareup. The connection between stress and acne is so close that one physician experienced in its treatment has said:

A physician who is not interested in acne nor in the acne patient should not *treat acne. The indifference of an attending physician with such an attitude is felt keenly by the patient and the psychologic reactions to acne can cause the patient's lesions to flare in this situation.*[9]

A sympathetic physician takes a relaxed approach and leaves the decision to the patient: "If you feel these foods increase your tendency toward acne, they can be dropped from your diet without risk." If a food is eliminated, there may be a two-month delay before results are seen.

Personal strategy. Whatever the merits of the various approaches discussed here, one factor always works in favor of the acne sufferer: time. While waiting for it to clear up, as it always does, it is important for the sufferer to try to keep the symptoms under control and, even more, to prevent the scarring that can result from probing or picking at the skin or from leaving the acne untreated. If you have acne you are advised to keep a hopeful eye on the latest developments in the use of 13-cis-retinoic acid and zinc therapy—but under no conditions to try self-medication with these or any other nutrients or drugs. Instead, share with your doctor these references if he or she hasn't seen them and ask his or her advice about pursuing them. As for standard treatments, adopt whatever courses of action promise to give the best results with the fewest undesirable side effects. This, too, is a trial-and-error matter and is best accomplished with the help of an experienced, interested, and sympathetic physician.

The Controversy Notes and For Further Information follow the Appendixes.

Controversy 14B

Doctors

Can you trust your doctor to advise you on nutrition?

"Often doctors are trained in nutrition by doctors who heard it from another doctor who made it up."[1] This statement is typical of many being made today about the nutritional knowledge of doctors. Dr. Philip R. Lee (director of the Health Policy Program, School of Medicine, University of California at San Francisco) has commented:

I would guess 90 percent of the graduates of our medical schools couldn't describe an adequate, nutritious diet.[2]

According to Dr. Myron Winick (professor of pediatrics, professor of nutrition, and director of the Institute of Human Nutrition, Columbia University College of Physicians and Surgeons, New York):

The state of nutrition education in this country as it relates to health is in complete chaos. . . . One cause of that chaos is the medical profession's failure to take responsibility for this area.[3]

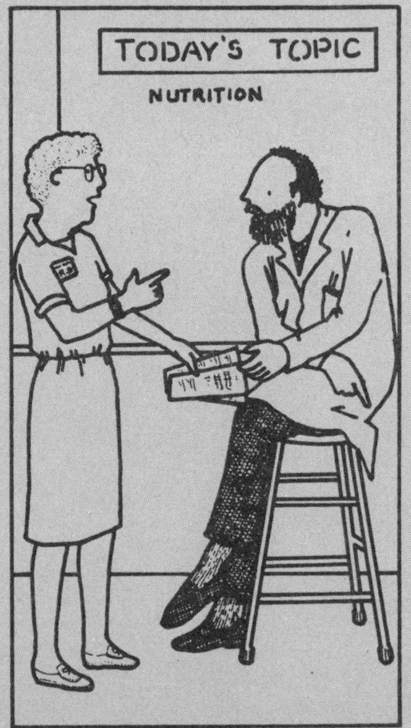

Such statements are upsetting to people who feel that doctors are supposed to know everything and make no mistakes. After all, not only our health but also our life and death are in their hands. Whenever a story is told of a doctor's incompetence, it rapidly travels the grapevine and sometimes even hits the front page of the newspapers. Often the incompetence is medical or surgical, but sometimes it is nutritional. A twenty-three-year-old recently collected $50,000 in damages when his lawyer proved to the court's satisfaction that his doctor caused his mental retardation by putting his mother on a rice-fruit diet during her pregnancy.[4] The public is outraged by stories like this—and rightly so, if the stories are true. Are they? What is the true state of nutritional knowledge among doctors?

Nutrition education in medical schools. Half a century ago, it was routine to teach medical students that starvation of a mother during her pregnancy was a desirable practice, because it produced a tiny baby that was easy to deliver.[5] Medical schools also taught their students that women should drastically restrict their salt intake during pregnancy to avoid developing toxemia. Both of these harmful teachings (see Chapter 12) persisted by tradition and were still being perpetuated by some medical schools in the late 1960s, with little else about nutrition being taught. Only the postgraduate medical training of one class of doctors—pediatricians—emphasized nutrition, and only one medical society—the American Association of Pediatrics—has for decades made efforts to educate the public on nutrition, specifically that of infants.

One of the first popular nutrition writers to make this unfortunate situation known to the public was Adelle Davis, whose *Let's Eat Right to Keep Fit* (first edition, 1946) and other books have sold millions of copies and have contributed greatly to the public's awareness of the importance of nutrition. She also made them aware that an M.D. degree is not evidence of nutritional know-how.[6] In the 1980s it is not uncommon for some doctors to adopt for themselves a nutritionally unsound low-carbohydrate diet or for psychiatrists to treat patients for anxiety and depression with tranquilizers while forgetting to inquire about their daily intakes of food and drink. In one instance, for example, a patient habitually drank twenty-eight cups of coffee a day; her psychiatrist was unaware of this but was medicating her for depression and anxiety.

The public has been growing increasingly aware that it is not traditional to teach nutrition in medical schools, and that awareness has been bringing about change. Still, a survey of forty-two medical schools in 1976, reported in the *Journal of the American Medical Association*, showed that seven of them offered no nutrition instruction of any kind and that thirteen more offered fewer than eleven hours in their four-year curriculum. Only three offered more than twenty hours, and only one had a nutrition department.[7] However, the situation appears to be changing rapidly. A year later, a survey of 102 medical schools reported by the *Journal of Nutrition Education* showed that nutrition training was increasing in the medical schools,[8] a trend reported by another journal to be "a groundswell."[9] As of the beginning of 1977, perhaps one out of every ten medical schools was teaching nutrition adequately.[10]

Nutrition is a relatively new science; medicine is an ancient art. Medicine has been practiced for hundreds of years without knowledge of nutrition. Before that situation would change, there had to be a demand for change, and that demand now exists. The *Journal of the American Medical Association* began publishing articles on nutrition issues in 1973.[11] Efforts are being made to provide nutrition education for doctors who are already practicing, by way of public service announcements and courses on television.[12] About 5000 doctors took such a course in infant nutrition in 1978.[13] *Medical News* reported that, "like sex, nutrition is increasingly discussed among physicians."[14]

New and excellent textbooks for medical students are now available, and reading lists are being offered for them and for doctors already graduated from school. An excellent newsletter for physicians, *Nutrition and the MD*, began coming out monthly in 1974 and was reaching over 900 physicians by the end of 1978 (see the selected references at the end of this Controversy). One medical college reported the successful integration of nutrition education into its curriculum in 1976, and others were expected to follow suit.[15] It seems realistic to expect that, within the next few decades, the public will be able to depend on its doctors for nutrition advice and information as much as it does for the diagnosis and treatment of disease.

But what about now? There must be many doctors now practicing whose nutrition education was inadequate and who have had no opportunity or made no effort to obtain this education on their own. They would be likely to overlook nutritional problems in their patients and might be unable to give specific instructions about changes in diet that would promote good health and prevention of, or recovery from, disease. During the 1970s, as the gaps in medical school curricula were first being widely publicized, a serious situation in the nation's hospitals was also coming to light which suggested that, at present, doctors often do fail in these respects.

Nutrition in the hospital. In 1974, Dr. Charles E. Butterworth published an article in *Nutrition Today* titled "The Skeleton in the Hospital Closet."[16] In it, he reported a high incidence of severe malnutrition in the hospital, which he called "physician-induced." He cited some of the causes: Patients are often deprived of food for days at a time so that they can be given medical tests; they are seldom given vitamin and mineral supplements; and they are often fed inadequate formulas (bottles of glucose and salts without protein, vitamins, or minerals) for long periods. Under these circumstances, they develop protein-calorie malnutrition and iron-deficiency anemia, conditions that severely weaken them—delaying their recovery, prolonging their hospital stays, and increasing the cost of their treatment. Reasons for the neglect of their nutritional care, he reported, include failure to notice low weight and weight loss, frequent staff rotations, diffusion of responsibility, and lack of communication between doctors and dietitians.[17]

Butterworth's report was promptly followed by a report from Boston by two hospital physicians who confirmed his findings. Drs. Blackburn and Bistrian reported that close to half of the patients in their hospitals showed evidence of protein-calorie malnutrition—often caused not by the diseases or conditions that had led to their admission to the hospital but by neglect of their nutritional needs while they were in the hospital.[18]

These findings have since been confirmed and extended by many other investigators. In 1977 the *Journal of the American Medical Association* published a strong statement on the subject, including the directive to physicians: "No patient should be hospitalized without an adequate nutritional profile." It included directions for monitoring patients' nutritional status while they are in treatment.[19]

Like the medical schools, the hospitals have responded to the outcry arising from public knowledge of this situation by conducting surveys and improvement programs of their own.[20] One went to work to improve its height-weight data records.[21] Butterworth and Blackburn published a recommended procedure for detecting and correcting malnutrition in the hospital,[22] and it was instituted with success at a Boston hospital.[23] The great importance of nutrition in recovery from surgery was gaining recognition.[24] A chapter of a medical text published in 1977 was devoted to the management of protein-calorie malnutrition in the hospital.[25]

While change is in the making in this problem area, the situation remains far from ideal. Physicians are being better trained, and dietitians are taking greater initiative and responsibility in the care of hospital patients; but there is much room for improvement. Meanwhile, what is the average person supposed to do if hospitalized and unsure of the doctor's attitude and skill in handling nutritional needs?

Personal strategy. Nearly every Controversy in this book seems to have closed with a statement saying, in effect, "It's up to you." This one is no exception. In seeking competent medical care, you can cross your fingers and hope for the best, but there is much more that you can do. Studying nutrition for yourself and attending to the careful selection of a nutritious diet during times of good health will do much to help reduce your need for medical attention. Still, there are many medical problems that cannot be prevented by nutrition, no matter how devotedly practiced.

When medical help is needed, you are well advised to seek it early and to recognize that, in all matters of diagnosis and treatment, the doctor is far better trained and qualified than any nutritionist or layperson to make decisions and take appropriate action. As for the matter of nutritional support during medical treatment, you might explore the subject with your doctor. Even a brief conversation can give you some idea whether he or she attaches importance to it. If not, you might consult another doctor or turn to a dietitian or nutritionist for supplementary advice.

When you are hospitalized, you are the first to know what food you are receiving and how much you are eating. In almost every disease condition, appropriate nutrition can make a significant difference in the rate and quality of recovery and the duration of hospital stay. The top four causes of death in the United States today are cardiovascular disease, cancer, diabetes, and alcoholism. Both prevention of and recovery from these diseases have strong nutritional components. For cardiovascular disease, control of fat and salt intake often is helpful. For cancer, aggressive nutritional therapy often makes the difference between life and death; patients die more often of the starvation caused by cancer than of the cancer itself. The management of diabetes can often be controlled by diet alone. Alcoholism requires rigid abstinence from alcohol, and recovery is greatly enhanced by the adoption and maintenance of healthful eating habits. Among other major causes of hospitalization are wounds, fractures, and burns; in these instances, too, nutritional therapy greatly speeds the recovery process, whereas poor nutrition delays and prolongs it.

In the hospital, you may need to be your own nutrition advocate. (For the very ill person, it helps greatly to have a friend or relative on hand who can "run interference," reminding the nurse that the tray hasn't arrived, mentioning to the doctor that the patient's weakness might be improved by feeding a meal he or she can eat, and devising other such strategies as needed.) It has often been observed that the ill person who has the will to live and who engages actively and cooperatively in the recovery program stands a better chance of recovering, and recovers faster, than the person who passively leaves the decisions and actions to others who are supposedly responsible. One thing you can do to promote your own health is to eat and to insist on being fed so that you can eat.

The word *cooperatively* needs to be underlined in the above paragraph. It is in your interest as a hospital patient not to antagonize the hospital staff, who have many problems to deal with other than your own. The hostile patient who complains about unimportant small details quickly gains a notoriety that understandably tempts staff to avoid entering the room and to leave it as quickly as possible. A nurse who has just watched a baby die is unlikely to be moved by a patient's demand for cranberry sauce with the turkey slices. While urging that you insist on receiving adequate nutrition, we urge also that you adapt to the absence of frills, be diplomatic, and stay in touch with your feelings of appreciation for the services being offered.

One nonmedical event that almost always takes place under supervision is childbirth, and it deserves a moment's special attention here. Chapter 12 gave heavy emphasis to the importance of healthful nutrition for the mother before she is pregnant and during her pregnancy and to its importance for the infant early in life. Doctors sometimes neglect to provide nutritional advice to expectant and new mothers. A survey of women's nutritional knowledge published in 1977 in the *Journal of Nutrition Education* reported that women who listed their doctors as a source of nutritional information scored lower than others on a nutritional attitudes questionnnaire, showing less knowledge of the need for weight gain and salt during pregnancy and of their infants' nutritional needs.[26] Reasons why breastfeeding may be preferable to bottle feeding, even in the developed countries, were also documented in Chapter 12; yet many doctors are indifferent to breastfeeding and are not taught its relative advantages in medical schools.[27] In this area, too, the consumer has a role to play in keeping herself informed and in seeking medical and nutritional advice from health professionals who are well informed and willing to communicate openly.

In the area of public policy, as in the private practice of

medicine, doctors sometimes overlook the relevance of nutrition to problems in which it may have an important place. For example, in a developing country, doctors may be called on to consult on economic problems. According to knowledgeable critics, they sometimes misadvise because they seldom see the very poor routinely and so are not aware that the diseases recorded in the medical statistics were caused at the outset by malnutrition. According to Drs. Dwyer and Mayer, the worst offenders in this regard are the "influential private physicians or senior academicians" who have long been insulated from exposure to the lower classes whose problems they are called on to solve.[28] Doctors *should* be aware of the role nutrition plays, and other, more knowledgeable experts (public health workers, nutritionists) must participate in policy making.

Although "doctors" have been the subject of this Controversy, other health professionals should be (and in some cases are) contributing to public understanding of nutrition. As of the late 1970s, it seemed apparent that the people most actively involved in consumer health education were the nurses and that they were doing effective work in many instances.[29] Dentists and dental hygienists also were learning and communicating useful nutrition information to their patients, and some pharmacists were taking the opportunity to educate themselves and their customers on nutritional matters.[30] If you are interested and choose to raise the subject of nutrition in conversation with people in these professions, you are likely to be able to collect much interesting and useful information.

The Controversy Notes and For Further Information follow the Appendixes.

CHAPTER 15

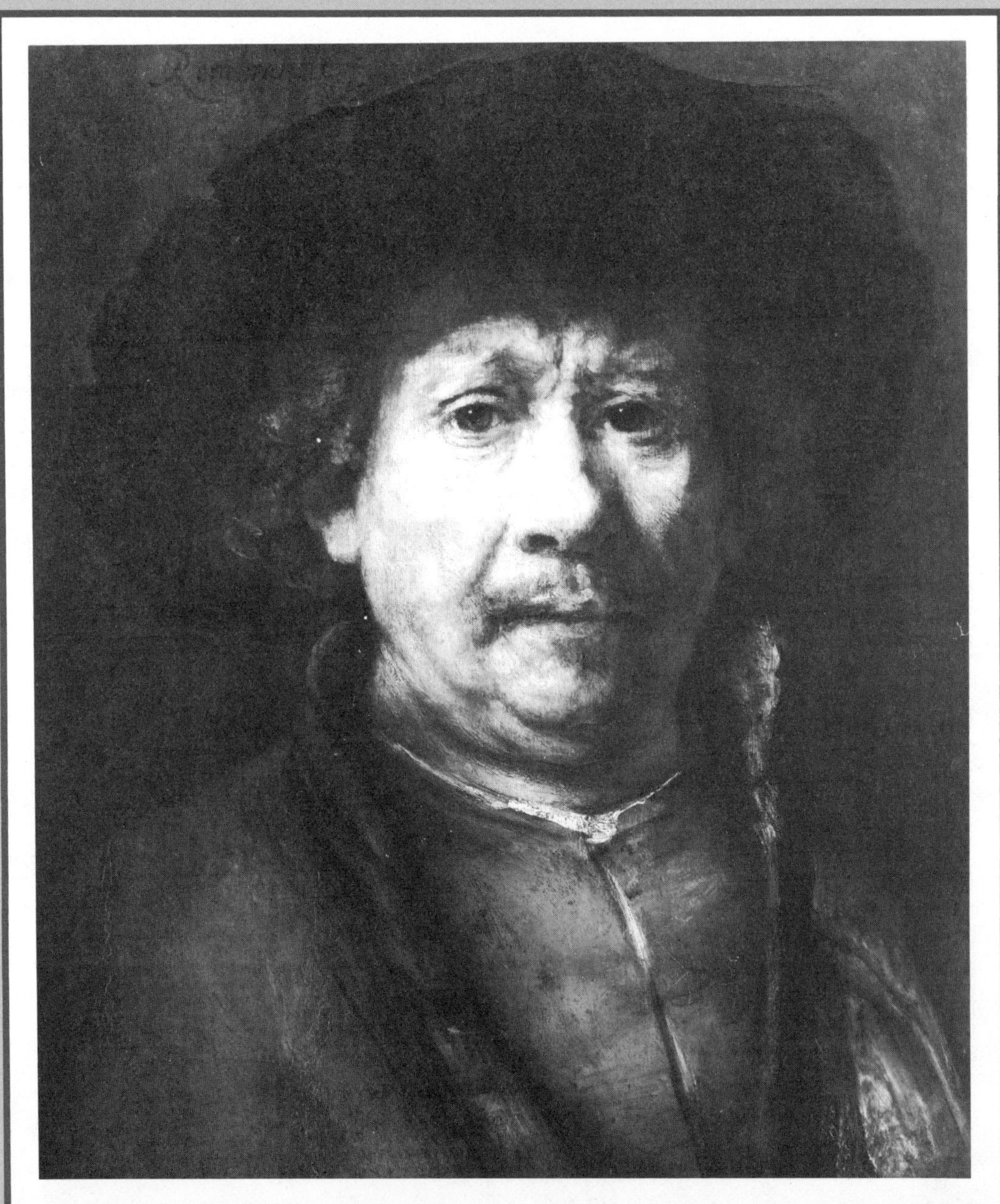

The Later Years

One out of every ten citizens in the United States is above sixty-five years of age, and the percentage is increasing. This fact is evident everywhere. Retirement villages are springing up, especially in the warmer climates. Senior citizen centers are being established for congregate meals and leisure activities. Older adults can be heard on political matters at "silver-haired legislatures." The newspapers tell us the social security fund is nearing bankruptcy because many who were contributors are now retired and receiving from the fund. Civic and church organizations note that there is a preponderance of gray hair in their audiences. The data from recent census reports confirm these observations.

Older people cherish their independence. Of the 6 million who live alone, 1.3 million are men and 4.7 million, women. From 1970 to 1975, the number of older men living alone increased by 9.9 percent and that of women, by 21.1 percent. Contrary to the popular view that older people are mostly in nursing homes, only 5 percent of those over 65 live in institutions. About 80 percent live in the community alone or with nonrelatives, again showing that they have retained a measure of independence.[1] As we will see, this very independence may foster nutritional problems.

Most older citizens are in reasonably good health and have enough money to support themselves, if not in luxury, at least not in

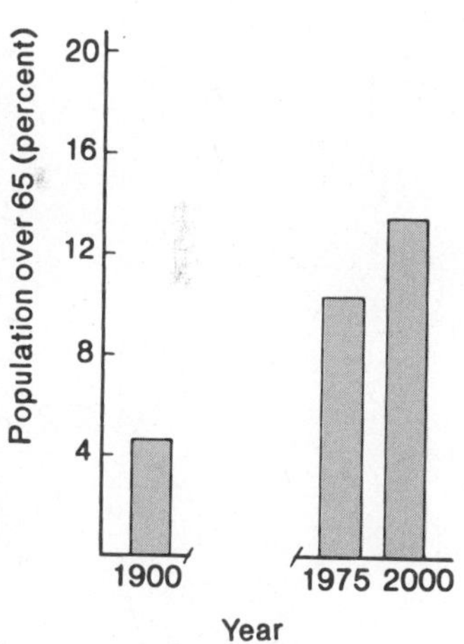

In 1900, 4 percent of the U.S. population were over sixty-five; 10 percent are over sixty-five today; 12.5 percent (30,500,000 people) will be over sixty-five in the year 2000.

Opposite: A detail from Self-Portrait *by Rembrandt. Used with the permission of the Kunsthistorisches Museum, Vienna.*

poverty. When we look around us and see the great needs of some elderly people, we sometimes overlook those who are enjoying their later years. They have leisure to pursue some of their favorite activities and are unencumbered by family responsibilities for the first time in their lives. These facts contradict the popular belief that older people are all poor, lonely, and ill. They are not; they are as individual as members of all other age segments. Grouping them into a stereotype is a disservice to everyone, especially to young adults who might project into their futures a depressing view of old age. Just as only a few teenagers are reckless drivers, only a minority of older-aged persons have the "typical problems" attributed to them. Aunt Charlotte at seventy-seven jets every winter to Europe to enjoy the social life of Paris; Uncle James at eighty-four is out early every morning in his vegetable garden hoeing his cabbages; and it is only Grandma Sadie who at eighty-two is lonely, withdrawn, ill, and forgetful, a problem to her family. Two-thirds of the elderly are relatively free of major problems.

However, the one-third who live at or below the poverty line deserve our attention. The average income of all older single people in the United States is $75 a week. Of aged black women, nearly half have a yearly income of under $1000.[2] Clearly, these people need help in many areas, one of them being nutrition.

In exploring nutrition for the older adult, it will be necessary to remember statistics like these but also to recognize the wide range of individual situations represented in these statistics. It will be helpful to keep three questions in mind:

> What can I do now to prepare myself for the time when I will be an older adult?
>
> What can I do when I am older (or now that I am older) to keep myself healthy and vigorous so I will enjoy these years?
>
> How can I, as a citizen or a relative, help those who are in need?

Theories on Aging

The "increased life span" of people in the twentieth century is not a reality. Most people are not now living much beyond the three-score years and ten that are mentioned in the Bible. In fact, in the last twenty-five years there has been no increase in life expectancy for people who have reached the age of twenty in spite of our miracle drugs and huge medical bills.[3] Since the beginning of the nineteenth century, as mortality from bacterial diseases has been brought under control by modern medicine, deaths from other causes have increased, so that the total life expectancy (for any individual) has remained at about seventy years. It is only the average length of life (for the population) that has increased. This has come about because more infants are surviving to adulthood, and so there are fewer infant deaths to bring the average down. Thus it seems that something built into the human organism (we call it aging) cuts off life at a rather fixed point in time.

Natural selection has not operated in favor of genes that promote longevity.[4] However, the human race, with its superior brain, can collect and store information that helps keep individuals alive after they have reproduced. Longevity can be said to result from evolution only in the sense that the brain has evolved. In today's world, however, older people may contribute accumulated experience and wisdom to the benefit of society long after they have passed their reproductive years and the time when they would contribute genes.

More about natural selection—Appendix A.

We humans have not comprehended what is involved in the aging process, nor have we figured out how to prevent or postpone it. Even our definitions of the process are vague. One writer calls aging a certain kind of change in living systems caused by the passage of time —the increased probability of death with increased chronological age.[5] Another calls it a decrease in viability and an increase in vulnerability.[6] However it is defined, research into aging has been scarce. Much is known about the growth, development, and nutritional needs of the human body from the time of conception until it reaches maturity. But only in recent times has the scientific community become interested in the mechanism by which the human organism ceases to grow once it reaches maturity and then "runs down" and dies. Current interest is increasing, largely because of the rising numbers of older people and the impact they are having on our social and governmental institutions, but answers are still few and far between.

Aging of cells. Cells seem to undergo a built-in (genetic) aging process and also to age in response to outside (environmental) forces. Environmental stresses that promote aging include extremes of heat and cold, disease, lack of nutrients, the wear and tear of hard physical labor, and the lack of stimulation caused by disuse, for example of the muscle cells in the legs of a cripple who can't exercise. But even in the most pleasant and supportive of environments, inevitable changes in the structure and function of the body's cells make them increasingly vulnerable to these environmental stresses.

All theories of aging have one element in common. They agree that at some point the cells become incapable of replenishing their constituents. In a complex organism such as the human body, the cells are interdependent. When some cells die and their function is lost, other cells dependent on the first ones suffer and also eventually die. A consequence of the gradual slowing down of cell function over the years is a reduction in the energy needs of older people.

A second common element seems to be that aging cells are programmed to stop reproducing once a certain stage of development has been reached.[7] Cells have different timetables for reproduction, but each type of cell seems to come to a natural end somehow. For example, red blood cells undergo division only as long as they are in the marrow of the long bones. When they are mature, they move out of the marrow to perform their function in the bloodstream. In the blood, they no longer reproduce; they work for three to six months and then die.

The brain cells are also programmed to stop reproducing, but they all stop within the first two years of life. Many of them maintain themselves without further cell division for about seventy years. Thus, at about fourteen months of age, the human organism already has all the brain cells it will ever have. Thousands die daily, but the daily loss is not noticeable. The accumulated loss over a lifetime is felt only in the slowing of reflexes and in garbled messages going to other organs. It seems strange that the human species should have evolved such a magnificent instrument for receiving, storing, interpreting, and retrieving information and yet not have evolved a method of repairing it. Some scientists view this evolutionary mishap as a "self-destruct" mechanism for the human body.

Some cells seem never to die but only to reproduce. They take in nutrients from their environment and grow; profound changes take place in their internal structure; and the living material within them then divides itself equally between two poles while the cell splits down the middle. Each new daughter cell is an exact replica of the parent cell and contains the same material. Thus the parent cell still lives, in a sense, as two replicas of itself. However, even in optimal conditions, the cells of a multicellular organism seem unable to go on dividing in this manner forever. About fifty to fifty-five replications seem to be the maximum.

A third factor in the aging process seems to be that, with the passage of time, cells become cluttered with debris—partially completed proteins that are never totally dismantled. This intracellular "sludge" interferes with the efficiency of operations within the cells.[8] The material that accumulates in the cells is known as the pigment of old age.[9]

Another factor may be that cells lose their ability to interpret the DNA genetic code words and thus make their proteins incorrectly. As reduced amounts of protein or wrong proteins are produced, cell and organ functions that depend on those proteins also falter. Organs elsewhere in the body may also be adversely affected. A theory that is somewhat allied to this one is that through some environmental stress, such as the continuous bombardment of cosmic rays that penetrate the earth's atmosphere, the DNA code itself may become altered. This, too, would lead to the production of wrong proteins.

If wrong proteins are produced for any reason, another theory states, the body's immune system will react to them as if they were foreign proteins from outside and will produce antibodies to counteract them. Complexes then form between the antibodies and these proteins and accumulate in and among cells as useless debris. This theory—the autoimmune theory—may account in part for the accumulation of deposits in joints, which causes arthritis.[10]

For a picture of the disulfide bridges in a protein, see page 273.

Finally, another theory of aging suggests that cosmic rays bombard molecules in the cells and split them into highly reactive compounds known as free radicals. These free radicals then bind rigidly to other cellular molecules by way of disulfide bridges. This disrupts the informational content of important molecules and so impairs their function. As in other cases, the cells in which this occurs, as well as others that depend on them, then die. (Some investigators have suggested that the formation of free radicals might be retarded by the taking of vitamin E supplements.)

There's more about vitamin E in Controversy 15.

Just as a chain is only as strong as its weakest link, so also is an organism only as long-lived as the least stable of its vital cells. The ability of cells to replenish the substances they need for life or to make fresh copies of themselves after they have reached maturity determines their life spans and ultimately the life span of the entire organism.

An analogy may help to show how all these processes work together to cause aging. A shipbuilding firm must have an office, where the plans and specifications for all the various boats are kept, and a warehouse, where the materials to carry out these orders are stored. There must also be a site where the actual construction takes place. When an order is received for a particular boat to be constructed, the plans on file are duplicated for a working copy, and messengers are sent to bring the materials to the construction site. By following the instructions, workers build the boat.

If, through years of heavy use, the warehouse becomes cluttered and disorganized, then it will become increasingly difficult to fill the orders efficiently. (This parallels the theory that, with age, the cell fluid becomes cluttered with debris.) If some of the messengers take the wrong orders from the files or bring the wrong materials, this too will cause production to slow down or cease. (This parallels the cells' loss of ability to read the genetic code words.) With rain or fire damage to the files themselves, some of the specifications will become unavailable or illegible (like the cellular DNA becoming altered by cosmic ray bombardment). Perhaps a worker instructed to destroy the damaged parts will stack them in corners where they accumulate and get in the way of the work (as in the autoimmune theory). Vandalism (free radicals) might do further damage. With inefficient management of the warehouse, there might be delays in getting supplies. (For the cell, the nutrients might not be present in the blood because they were not taken in, or there might be a breakdown in the ability of the intestinal cells to absorb the nutrients.) Finally, the warehouse might have been set up for a limited order—its destruction, once it had produced a certain number of boats, might have been planned from the beginning. (This represents the idea that cells are programmed to self-destruct after a certain number of generations.)

None of the theories of cellular aging are more than theories, but some interesting work has been done in the attempt to solve the riddle of why cells age. One such experiment was conducted as early as the 1930s. Rats were fed a diet balanced in every respect except that it was severely restricted in calories. A control group was fed the same diet with ample calories. When the control group had reached maturity, the starved rats were still immature. They were then permitted to catch up by being fed ample calories. Surprisingly, the previously starved rats outlived the controls, averaging 1465 days as compared with the controls' 969 days.[11] Similar experiments have since yielded similar results with many different species, and a tentative conclusion is that the key to success is keeping the animals in a juvenile state for longer than the normal period. Obviously, this experiment could not be carried out on human beings, but it suggests some interesting possibilities for explaining longevity.

Aging of organs. The aging of cells is reflected by changes in the organs they are a part of. The most visible changes take place in the skin. As people age, wrinkles increase, partly because of a loss of the fat that underlies the skin and partly because of a loss of elasticity. The scars that have accumulated from many small cuts roughen the texture of the skin. Exposure to sun, wind, and cold hasten the drying process and contribute to wrinkling. The hair disappears also, particularly from the head and face of males.[12]

Another obvious and traumatic change, this one in the digestive system, is painful deterioration of the gums and subsequent loss of teeth. According to the Ten State Survey, gum disease increases with age and exists in 90 percent of the population by age sixty-five to seventy-four.[13] In addition, the senses of taste and smell diminish, which reduces the pleasure of eating.

In other parts of the digestive system, secretion by the stomach of hydrochloric acid and enzymes decreases with age, as does the secretion of digestive juices by the pancreas and small intestine. The large intestine muscles weaken with reduced use, thus allowing the wall to form outpocketings called diverticulosis.

The liver is somewhat different. Liver cells regenerate themselves throughout life; so with normal aging, the loss of liver cells is not a major problem. However, even with good nutrition, fat gradually infiltrates the liver, reducing its work output.[14] The response of the liver to moderate blood glucose levels is not appreciably altered with age, but the response to a large glucose load, as in the glucose tolerance test, is reduced. There may be two reasons for this: First, the blood may not be pushed strongly enough by the heart to reach the pancreas, so that it does not send its insulin message to the liver; second, there may be a reduction in the number of glucose-responsive cells in the pancreas.[15]

The development of atherosclerosis is described in Controversy 5A.

As the heart and blood vessels age, the volume of blood that the heart can pump decreases. The arteries lose their elasticity. The amount of blood going into the networks of capillaries in the various organs decreases. There are deposits of fat in the walls of the arteries, and these deposits may be invaded by calcium salts, which make them hard and inflexible. Because all organs and tissues depend on the circulation of nutrients and oxygen, degenerative changes in this system critically affect all other systems.[16]

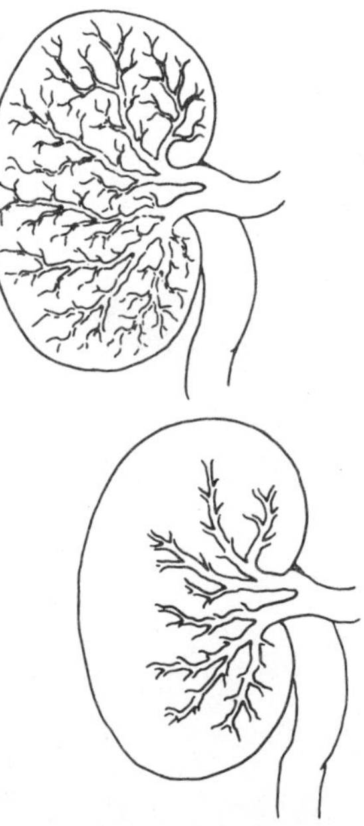

As the heart pumps less blood into an organ, the capillary trees within that organ recede, leaving some of the cells without nourishment.

The decrease in blood flow through the kidneys makes them gradually less efficient at their task of removing nitrogen (amine groups) and other wastes from the blood and maintaining the correct amounts of salts, sugar, and other valuable nutrients in the body fluids. As the heart pumps less blood into the capillary trees of the kidneys, the capillary trees diminish in size, causing some kidney cells to be deprived of their nutrient and oxygen supply. Cells formerly fed by these capillaries then die. Since both the heart rate and the volume of blood pumped into the kidneys depend on the muscular activity of the person, this degenerative process can be retarded by regular exercising.

The ability of the brain to direct the activities of the body decreases during aging. However, the older adult compensates for this with a greater amount of stored information and wisdom. The nerve cells are not replaceable, so any damage by accident permanently diminishes mental ability. This is probably the greatest cause of unhappiness among older people and their relatives, because it decreases the ability to enjoy life. Visual impairment, hearing loss, loss of the senses of smell and taste, and loss of the sense of balance are all evidence of impaired nerve cell function.

Finally, the skeletal system is subject to change. Bone is a structure composed of salts of calcium, phosphorus, and other minerals. Bone is not made of cells but is continuously being laid down by bone-building cells and dissolved or reabsorbed by bone-dismantling cells. With the passage of years, for unknown reasons, the balance shifts in favor of destructive activity, resulting in thinning of the bone and adult bone loss (osteoporosis).

Osteoporosis is more common in women than in men by a ratio of four to one. In our population, it may be severe enough to produce fractures in as many as 30 percent of the people over age sixty-five.[17] A hip fracture caused by osteoporosis may not be a clean break but a shattering of the bone into fragments that can't be reassembled. Surgical repair often requires replacement of the broken bone with an artificial substitute.

The causes of osteoporosis seem to be multiple. Because it occurs more often in women than in men, and because it occurs more predictably after menopause, the cessation of female hormone secretion is thought to be a contributing factor. But it can't be the only factor. If it were, the excretion of calcium would increase after menopause, and it doesn't.[18] Gradual calcium loss may occur because of dietary deficiency, but it would take a large daily deficit (50 milligrams a day) for a long period of time (twenty years) before clinical signs of osteoporosis would appear.[19]

The mass of the skeleton seems to be greatly influenced by the amount of use or the pressure put on the bones. Pressure on the long bones, particularly, causes an increase in the activity of the bone-building cells. Given this stimulation, the skeletal system seems able to repair itself remarkably well into great old age, even though it is subjected to a great deal of wear and tear. However, idleness promotes bone dissolution. Probably the lessened activity of old age, combined with long hospitalizations for age-related problems, contributes to osteoporosis.

More about bones—Chapter 10.

Perhaps the factors that promote or prevent the development of osteoporosis can be traced back to the growing years at the beginning of life. The higher the density of the bones at maturity, the later will be the development of osteoporosis. Heredity also plays some part. Men have denser bones than women, and Mediterranean, Latin American, and African populations have denser bones than Northern European and Asian peoples. Still, the rate at which bone minerals are lost is about the same for all populations.[20] The initial deposit of minerals into bones is responsive to early nutrition, pointing up the importance of prevention of adult bone loss early in life. It may be that, once osteoporosis has developed, it cannot be reversed by the taking of extra calcium.[21] Lifelong adequate intakes of both calcium and fluoride doubtless protect against osteoporosis; the condition is not usually seen in a person who has had a consistently high calcium intake.[22] In fact, patients with osteoporosis give a lifelong history of exceptionally low calcium intakes.[23]

During movement, the bones must rub against each other at the joints. The ends are protected from wear by cartilage and by small sacs of fluid that act as a lubricant. With age, the ends of the bone become pitted or eroded as a result of wear or of diseases such as arthritis. The cause of arthritis, a painful swelling of the joints, is unknown, but it affects millions around the world and is a major problem of the elderly.

The aging of every body system can be accelerated by reducing the flow of nutrients and oxygen to the system. To put this statement more positively, the process of aging can be retarded by maintaining a strong cardiovascular and respiratory system. Exercise, regular and active enough to increase the heartbeat and respiration rate, is one of the keys to good health in the later years. An added benefit of exercise, as you already know, is to prevent the atrophy of all muscles (not only the heart) which would take place with inactivity. A good flow of blood requires a strong heartbeat and strongly flexing muscles to press expelled lymph back into the bloodstream for recirculation. Many older persons believe that they can't participate in strenuous exercise, but studies have shown that they can do more than they think they can. Even modest endurance training can improve the cardiovascular and respiratory function and promote good muscle tone while controlling the accumulation of body fat.[24]

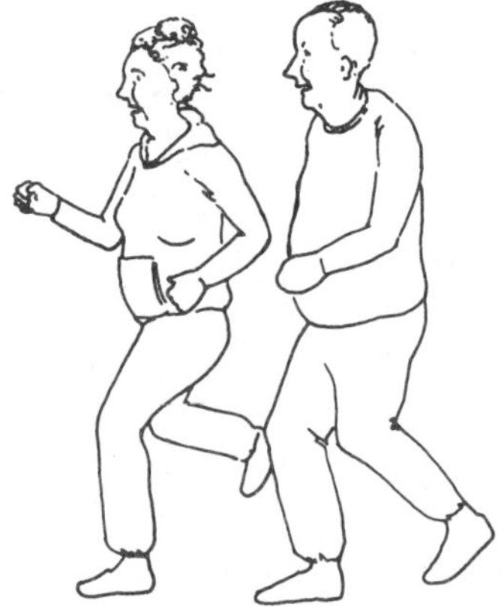
Older people can do more than they think they can.

Eating Pattern Supplying the Recommended Proportions of Protein, Fat, and Carbohydrate for Older People

Food Group	Number of Exchanges: Woman (1500 cal)	Number of Exchanges: Man (2000 cal)
Milk (skim)	3	3
Vegetable	2	4
Fruit	3	9
Bread	10	10
Meat (lean)	4	8
Fat	4	4

Nutritional Implications of Aging

Good health habits, including good nutrition throughout life, are the best guarantee of healthy and enjoyable later years. Many of the nutrient needs of the elderly are the same as for younger persons, but some special considerations deserve emphasis.

Calories. Caloric needs decrease with advancing years—because of the decreased metabolism of all cells and because of decreased muscular activity. About a 5 percent reduction per decade in energy intake is suggested. One study showed that of older persons living alone, 35 percent of the men and 52 percent of the women exceeded their calorie allowances. Caloric needs of each individual vary with metabolic activity, but a rule of thumb for older adults is 1500 calories for women and 2000 calories for men.[25]

Protein-calorie malnutrition is common in older people and often goes unnoticed. The observer, seeing the wasted muscle, weakness, and sometimes swelling of protein deficiency, thinks, "That person looks old," when in fact the person is exhibiting the symptoms of PCM. Older people who have been trying to lose weight or eating monotonous or bizarre diets are most likely to be affected.[26]

Protein foods should contribute about 20 to 25 percent of the calories in the older person's diet, and fats no more than 20 percent, with the remainder coming from complex carbohydrates.[27] On such a limited calorie allowance, all foods must be nutrient dense. There is little leeway for such empty-calorie foods as sugar, sweets, fats, oils, or alcohol.

One side of the energy budget is for calories to be taken in, and the other side is for those calories to be expended. Increase in activity should be emphasized for any person interested in maintaining good health in the later years. Not only would this help control overweight, but also, as already mentioned, it would increase blood flow into all the organs of the body, keeping them more vigorous. DeVries designed an experiment to find out if the trainability of older men depended on their physical prowess in their youth. The answer was no. He decided that their increase in muscle strength during the training was not due to the improvement in their muscles but to the improvement in the nervous system which resulted from the increased blood flow to the brain engendered by the exercise.[28]

Physical activity, such as walking, increases the deposit of calcium in the bones, thus forestalling the development of osteoporosis.[29] People responsible for the care of older adults should encourage more activity of all kinds and shorter recuperation periods in bed following illnesses.

Protein. The need for essential amino acids is the same for older adults as it is for younger adults.[30] However, the older person needs to get these essential nutrients from less food, so care should be taken that the protein is of high quality. The protein should also be spared from being used for energy by the inclusion of complex carbohydrates in the diet.

It has been shown that, for older persons living at home, milk or its equivalent in cheese is one of the foods most often omitted from the diet.[31] Another protein food, meat, is often omitted because it is difficult to chew;[32] in one study, only those with excellent teeth had a high protein intake.[33] Both milk and meat may also be omitted because of difficulties with purchasing and storage. (This chapter's Food Feature presents possible solutions to these problems.) Low hemoglobin levels have been shown to correlate with protein (and iron) content of the diet[34] and may be the cause of the fatigue and apathy so often mentioned as a problem by older persons. It has been recommended that the protein allowance for those over sixty-five be increased to 2 grams per kilogram of ideal weight.[35]

Fat. For many reasons, fat should be limited in the older person's diet. Cutting fat helps cut calories (recall that fat delivers two and a half times as many calories as the other energy nutrients) and may also help retard the development of atherosclerosis. On the limited calorie allowance recommended for older adults, it would be difficult to obtain the many vitamins and minerals that come from protein-rich and complex-carbohydrate foods if too high a percentage of the calories came from fat. Moreover, high fat intake interferes with calcium absorption, promoting osteoporosis.

On the other hand, if fat calories are restricted too greatly, the fat-soluble vitamins and linoleic acid may be deficient. Of the 20 percent of the calories to come from fat, most should be polyunsaturated to contribute linoleic acid, the essential fatty acid, and to displace the saturated fat thought to contribute to high levels of cholesterol in the blood.

Carbohydrate. Another emphasis in the older person's diet should be on securing a wide variety of complex carbohydrate foods to provide the vitamins and minerals contained in these foods. Older people often omit fruits and vegetables from their diets. It is not known whether this is due to earlier consumption patterns or to their finding fruits and vegetables too expensive or too difficult to store and prepare. Any educational campaign conducted to improve the diets of the elderly should emphasize the great amount of essential nutrients, minerals, and fiber contributed by complex carbohydrates. One congregate-meals group furnishes bags so that the participants can take home the fruit that was served for dessert, as a way of encouraging the use of fruit.[36]

Vitamin C Intakes of People Aged Sixty and over (Ten State Survey)

Category	Vitamin C Intake (mg)
White males	30
White females	46
Black males	37
Black females	52
Spanish-American males	28
Spanish-American females	47

Vitamins. Many of the problems seen in the elderly may result from decreased vitamin intakes. Vitamin deficiency is likely unless great care is taken to include foods from each of the food groups. Studies have shown that the one food group omitted most often by the elderly is the vegetable group, which would contribute vitamin A.[37] About 18 percent of older people are reported to eat no vegetables at all. Fruit, a contributor of vitamin C, is lacking in many diets, and 34 percent in one study reported never eating fruit.[38] Some men and women do not eat whole-grain breads and cereals, which would donate the B vitamins; the mental confusion sometimes exhibited by the elderly may be caused not by a loss of brain function but by a B-vitamin deficiency.[39] The destruction of vitamin E by heat processing and oxidation is well known,[40] so the processed and convenience foods so often used by the elderly and nursing homes may contribute to a vitamin E deficiency if their use continues over several years.[41] These statistics have somber implications for the health of older persons.

Not only the omission of food groups that contribute vitamins but also other conditions contribute to vitamin deficiency in the elderly. Many are house- or hospital-bound and thus are deprived of the vitamin D they would get from sunshine on their skin. Many take laxatives regularly (one study says 55 percent[42]), and this causes such a rapid transit time through the intestine that many vitamins do not get absorbed. The use of mineral oil as a laxative especially robs the person of the fat-soluble vitamins. Some drugs regularly taken by older adults interact with vitamins: Some antibiotics kill bacteria in the intestine that produce vitamin K, and the anticonvulsant drugs used in the treatment of epilepsy produce a folacin deficiency.[43]

The recommended intakes for many of the vitamins are thought by some nutritionists to be too low for the over-sixty-five group.[44] They recommend supplements, particularly for the B vitamins and vitamin C, because toxicity from large amounts does not pose a great threat.[45] However, other nutritionists feel that recommending vitamin supplements is a "cop-out" laying the elderly open to exploitation by quacks.[46] Money is better spent, they say, on food of higher quality. The older person would probably be wise to follow the guideline offered in Controversy 2: If your calorie intake is below about the 1500 level, then you should take a vitamin-mineral supplement—not a megavitamin, but just a once-daily type supplement. This means that many older persons, all except those who are very active, should take this precaution, at the same time taking steps to increase their activity.

Minerals. Calcium and iron are the minerals most often low in older adults' diets. Low hemoglobin levels, which correlate with low iron intake, could be the cause of much of the fatigue and apathy experienced by the elderly. Decreased stomach acidity may also contribute, because iron is best absorbed in an acid environment. Serious loss of calcium from the bones, enough to cause osteoporosis, is probably best prevented by a lifelong adequate intake of calcium from infancy. Calcium has other uses besides bone formation, and the need for calcium probably remains constant with advancing age.[47]

Salt, which contains the mineral sodium, should be curtailed, not only by those with hypertension, congestive heart failure, or cirrhosis of the liver, but by all older people. Salt is conducive to the retention of fluid, which results in raised blood pressure. Convenience and processed foods are high in salt content and are widely used by older persons living alone, thus making it difficult for them to restrict their salt intake. Wherever possible, fresh foods should be eaten instead.

For practical suggestions on ways to reduce sodium intake, turn to Chapter 10.

To supply the needed minerals, the same recommendation should be followed as for vitamins: Every food group should be represented in the diet every day. Milk, especially, should be included in some form. If liquid milk causes flatulence (gas), as some older people report, then cheese should be included and dry skim milk should be incorporated into other foods. Suggestions to facilitate this are given in this chapter's Food Feature.

Fiber. The fiber recommendations for the general population should be stressed to older citizens as well: Increase the use of fruits, vegetables, and whole-grain cereals. The fiber content of these food groups is important to the health of the muscles of the intestinal tract. If there is bulk for these muscles to work against, it will be less necessary to resort to the use of laxatives. In addition, some fibers (but not wheat bran) bind cholesterol and carry it out of the body.

Fiber is discussed in more detail in Controversy 4B.

Water. The elderly need to be reminded to drink fluids. They should drink 6 to 8 glasses a day, enough to bring their urine output to about 1500 milliliters (6 cups) per day.[48] A large percentage of foster home operators note that one of the biggest problems with the elderly patients is getting them to use more water and fruit juices.[49]

Those older adults most at risk nutritionally are those who overemphasize one food group to the exclusion of another. Whenever one food group is excluded the vitamins and minerals donated by that group become deficient in the diet. Even small amounts of food from each food group may protect from an overt deficiency. An example of such a skewed diet would be that of a person who, for whatever reason, omitted milk and dairy products. Calcium deficiencies would be expected and osteoporosis would be likely to develop if the omission had been continuing for most of the adult years. In the same manner, someone who excluded meat and cereals might be expected to develop a zinc deficiency, which would impair the sense of taste and slow the healing of wounds.[50] The familiar maxim holds throughout the life cycle: The best dietary guideline is to eat a balanced and varied selection of foods.

All of the above objectives may seem worthwhile, but they may be hard to achieve, especially for the person living alone who has difficulty buying groceries and preparing meals. Packages of meat and vegetables are often prewrapped in quantities suitable for a family of four or more, and even a head of lettuce will perish before one person can use it all. A large package of meat is often a good buy, but dividing and wrapping it in individual portions to be put away in the freezer is time-consuming and hardly seems worth the effort—especially when the packets may get "lost" in the freezer and ruined by freezer burn. For the person who has little or no freezer space, the problem of storage is further compounded. The Food Feature provides suggestions for overcoming some of these problems.

Food Feature: Cooking for One

Following is a collection of ideas gathered from single people who are doing a good job of getting nourishing food:

Buy only three pieces of each kind of fresh fruit: a ripe one, a medium one, and a green one. Eat the first right away and the second soon, and let the last one ripen on your windowsill.

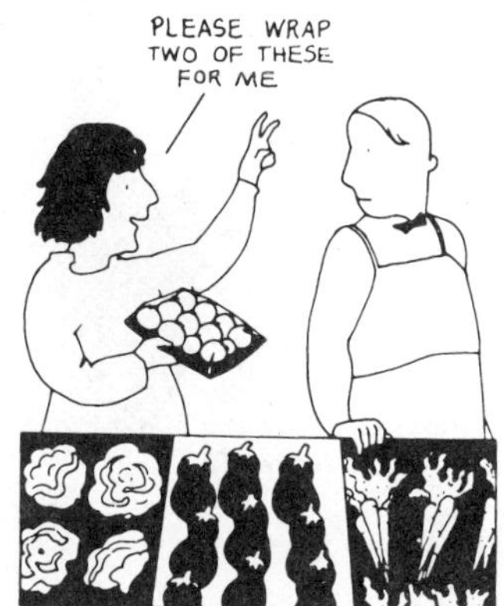
PLEASE WRAP TWO OF THESE FOR ME

Buy only what you will use.

Buy the small cans of vegetables even though they are more expensive. Remember, it is also expensive to buy a regular-sized can and let the unused portion spoil in the refrigerator.

Buy only what you will use. Don't be timid about asking the grocer to break open a package of wrapped meat or fresh vegetables.

Think up a variety of ways to use a vegetable when you must buy it in a quantity larger than you can use. For example, you can divide a head of cauliflower into thirds. Cook one third and eat it as a hot vegetable. Put the other two thirds into a vinegar and oil marinade for use as an appetizer or in a salad. You can keep half-packages of frozen vegetables to be used together in soup or stew.

Make mixtures using what you have on hand. A thick stew prepared from leftover green beans, carrots, cauliflower, broccoli, and any meat, with some added onion, pepper, celery, and potatoes, makes a complete and balanced meal—except for milk. But see the uses of powdered milk that follow: You could add some to your stew.

Buy fresh milk in the size best suited for you. If your grocer doesn't carry pints or half pints, try a nearby service station or convenience store.

You can buy a half-dozen eggs at a time; the carton of a dozen can usually be broken in half. However, eggs keep for long periods in the refrigerator and are such a good source of high-quality protein that you will probably use a dozen before they lose their freshness.

Set aside a place in your kitchen for rows of jars containing shelf staple items that you can't buy in single-serving quantities. These could contain rice, tapioca, lentils or other dry beans, flour, cornmeal, dry skim milk, macaroni, cereal, or coconut, to name only a few possibilities.

This will keep the bugs out of the foods indefinitely. They make an attractive display and will remind you of possibilities for variety in your menus. Cut the directions-for-use label from the package and store it in the jar.

Learn to use dry skim milk. This is the greatest convenience food there is. Dry milk can be stored on the shelf for several months at room temperature. It is fortified with vitamins A and D. It can be mixed with water to make fluid milk in as small a quantity as you like—but once it is mixed, it will sour just like fresh milk. One person says he keeps a jar of dry skim milk next to his stove and "dumps it into everything": hamburgers, gravies, soups, casseroles, sauces, even beverages such as iced coffee. The taste is negligible, but five "dumpings" of a heaping tablespoon each would be the equivalent of a cup of fresh milk. Ask a friend who is a member of Weight Watchers to give you some recipes for delicious milkshakes and ice cream using dry skim milk. Their recipes are for single servings.

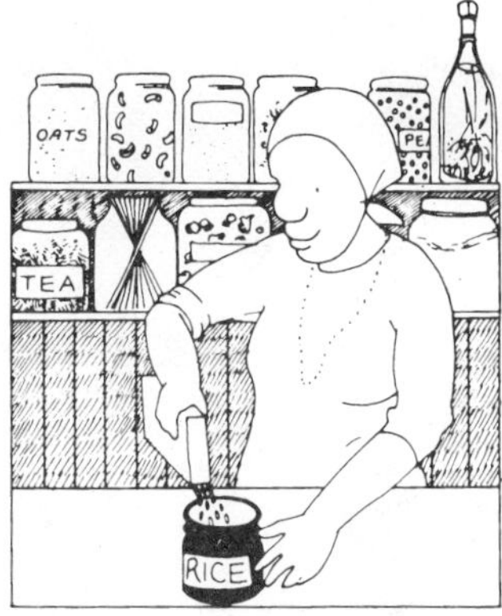

Remember (from the Chapter 9 Food Feature) not to store pastas and grains in glass jars, because light destroys the riboflavin.

Cook for several meals at a time. For example, boil three potatoes with skins. Eat one hot with margarine and chives. When the others have cooled, use one to make a potato-cheese casserole ready to be put into the oven for the next evening's meal. Slice the third one into a covered bowl and pour over it the juice from pickles. The pickled potato will keep several days in the refrigerator and can be used in a salad.

Experiment with stir-fried foods. Use a frying pan if you don't have a wok. Ask your Chinese friends for some recipes. A variety of vegetables and meat can be enjoyed this way; inexpensive vegetables such as cabbage and celery are delicious when crisp-cooked in a little oil with soy or lemon added. Cooked, leftover vegetables can be dropped in at the last minute. There are frozen mixtures of Chinese or Polynesian vegetables available in the larger grocery stores. Bonus: Only one pan to wash.

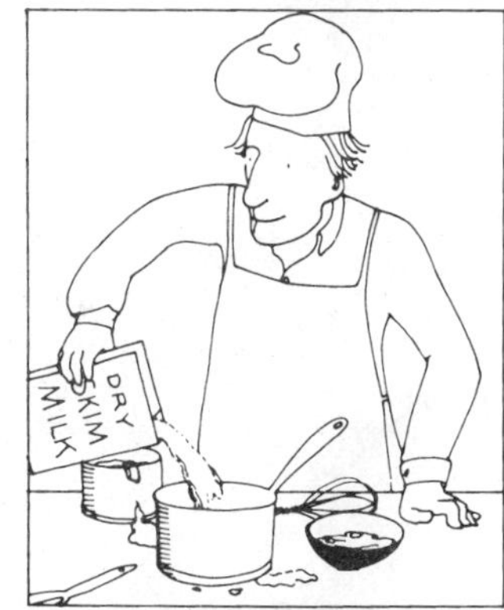

Dump dry skim milk into everything.

Depending on your freezer space, make double or even six times as much as you need of a dish that takes time to prepare: a casserole, vegetable pie, or meatloaf. Save the little aluminum trays from frozen foods and store the extra servings, labeled, in the trays in the freezer. Be sure to date these so you will use the oldest first. Somehow, the work seems worthwhile when you prepare several meals at once.

Learn to connect food with your social life. Cook for yourself with the idea that you are also preparing for guests you might want to invite. Or turn this suggestion around: Invite guests and make enough food so that you will have some left for yourself at a later meal. These suggestions came from a young widow and an eighty-six-year-old widow. The young widow, after her husband's death, purposely cooked generous amounts so she could make her own frozen dinners from the leftovers. With a wide variety of these on hand, she feels free to invite one or another of her single friends on the spur of the moment to "Come over and share my frozen dinners with me tonight." She says she devised this method of managing her food out of the need to manage her "five o'clock loneliness." The eighty-six-year-old widow invites guests for dinner every Sunday, because "it is no fun to cook for one," and she, too, loves having the leftovers.

Buy a loaf of bread and immediately store half, well wrapped, in the freezer. The freezer keeps it fresher than the refrigerator.

If you have space in your freezing compartment, buy frozen vegetables in the very large bags rather than in the small cartons. You can take out the exact amount you need and close the bag tightly with a rubber band. If you return the package quickly to the freezer each time, the vegetables will stay fresh for a long time.

If you have ample freezing space, you can buy large packages of meat such as pork chops, ground meat, or chicken when they are on special sale. Immediately divide the package into individual servings. Wrap in aluminum foil, not freezer paper: The foil can become the liner for the pan in which you bake or broil the meat, thus saving work over the sink. Don't label these individually, but put them all in a brown bag marked "hamburger" or "chicken thighs" or whatever the meat is, along with the date. The bag is easy to locate in the freezer, and you'll know when your supply is running low.

Although these suggestions will help you with the mechanics of food preparation and storage, they are only a part of what you can do for yourself. Loneliness, too, needs to be dealt with if single life in the later years is to be enjoyed. Even for nutrition's sake, it is important to attend to this problem.

The Effect of Loneliness

The concept of old age as being a time of losses is a depressing one, certainly unpleasant to consider. But it is realistic and needs to be faced. As in the poem that follows, many people who arrive at this time of life don't comprehend the universality of the aging experience. They have made no mental preparations for it. Then, when faced with some of the normal experiences of later life—the children wanting to be independent from the parents, for example—they turn inward for the explanation and conclude that there must be something wrong with them. Depression follows such reasoning and compounds the distress of the original problem.

The losses can occur in several areas. Old friends are lost when they die or move away; offspring move away also and are too busy to write; there is loss of income on retirement and loss of status in the community. There is loss of control of the environment, such as finding that the home that was to be a haven in retirement now sits in the middle of a high-crime area so that one can no longer walk the streets or visit with neighbors. The familiar shops and fruit stands where a person knows and is known by the owner may close. The aging person develops a feeling of deep loneliness as the familiar environment constantly shifts. But what place, you may well ask, does such a discussion have in a book on nutrition?

Many authorities believe that malnutrition among the elderly is most often due to loneliness.[51] For the 6 million adults over sixty-five who live alone, the pressing need seems to be for companionship first, then for food. Without companionship, appetite decreases. The association of food with human companionship is built into our genes, and our very first experience with food was combined with human body

OLD AGE IS A TIME OF LOSSES, they say.

Loss of identity

A man before he retired used to say,
"I work for the city."
"I am vice-president of Hometown Nuts and Bolts Co."
"I work for old Mr. Jones."
"This tells you who I am."
But now that he has no job, who is he?

A homemaker used to say,
"My husband is a fisherman."
"My husband is a farmer."
"My husband is a golfer."
But now he is gone. Who is she?

A working woman used to say,
"I am a hair stylist."
"I am a lawyer."
"I am a clerk."
But now she is too old to work. Who is she now?

Loss of control of life

A mother spends twenty-five years learning to be a mother.
"Lynn is a vegetarian. I must be sure she gets some legumes."
"John won't eat pork. I must get him some other meat."
"Must not forget:
To pick up Jake's clothes at the cleaners.
To chauffeur Artie to Cub Scouts.
To be home by 3 o'clock so the plumber can get in."
She gets better and better at her job, then—
She blinks her eyes and they are gone.
They don't need her.
They resent her interference.
They wish she wouldn't phone so often.
They tell her
It's time for her to do what she wants to do.
But what does she want to do?

A father spends twenty-five years earning a living.
"Must do a good job so I'll get that promotion."
"Better work overtime so I can pay the dentist."
"During this year's vacation, I'll repair the roof."
He gets better and better at his job, then—
He blinks his eyes and his job is gone.
The computer takes over.
The company gives him a gold watch.
Friends congratulate him.
They tell him
It's time for him to do what he wants to do.
But what does he want to do?

Loss of people

Young people make friends easily.
Some friends last for many years;
There isn't any need to seek out new ones.
It's comfortable and fun to be around long-time friends.
Then Joe dies and
Margaret and
Good old Butch and
You blink your eyes and the ones that are left are OLD!
And then you lose your spouse.
You are really alone.
Where do you find new long-time friends or make another marriage?

Loss of income

For years you pay the mortgage and
The social security and
The retirement fund and
The insurance premiums and
You dream of Florida's sunny beaches and
Arizona's open spaces but
The reality is
Food prices are up.
Medical costs skyrocket.
Tax assessments rise.
Gas costs more.
Cars cost more.
Electric rates keep rising.
But the retirement check doesn't rise. And you stay at home.
Yes, they're right.
OLD AGE IS A TIME OF LOSSES, BUT
WHEN YOU CONSIDER THE ALTERNATIVE TO OLD AGE,
OLD AGE FEELS PRETTY GOOD.

contact. The social life of the adult is built around food. Most invitations into adults' homes are accompanied by an offer of food or drink. We must admit that feeding is, for human beings, as much a social and psychological event as a biological one.

Having spent a lifetime internalizing the concept of food as part of a social activity, the older adult, alone all day every day, must exert a wrenching effort to place enough importance on the nutrient content of food to prepare it and to eat it alone. The purchase, storage, and preparation of food and kitchen cleanup take a tremendous amount of energy. The lonely, depressed person looking at such a task is likely to forget about the body's needs and say, "What's the use?"

Dr. Jack Weinberg, professor of psychiatry at the University of Illinois, wrote perceptively of this in the *Journal of the American Dietetic Association*:

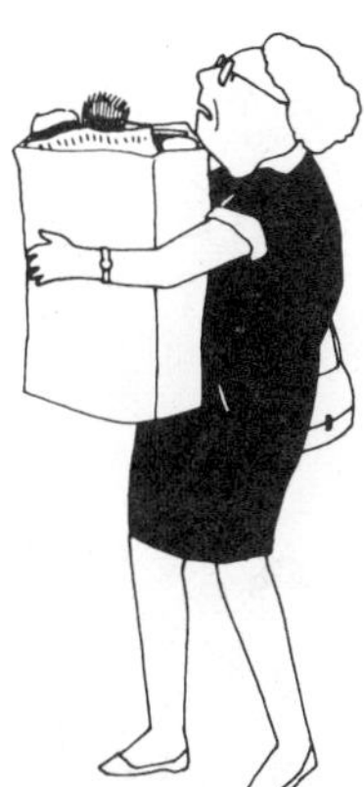

It takes energy to take care of your nutrition.

> In our efforts to provide the aged with a proper diet, we often fail to perceive it is not *what* the older person eats but *with whom* that will be the deciding factor in proper care for him. The oft-repeated complaints of the older patient that he has little incentive to prepare food for only himself is not merely a statement of fact but also a rebuke to the questioner for failing to perceive his isolation and aloneness and to realize that food . . . for one's self lacks the condiment of another's presence which can transform the simplest fare to the ceremonial act with all its shared meaning.[52]

The lack of social interaction is no respector of income. It is equally important in the lives of the financially secure and in the lives of the poverty-stricken. The newspaper occasionally carries a story of a wealthy older person's being discovered in their mansion, alone and without food. The story is newsworthy because people wonder why the victim did not ask for help or make arrangements for someone to take care of her, since she had plenty of money. The answer is simple. Apathy evolves from loneliness; apathy is expressed in inaction. The victim sits for long hours in a chair without the energy even to lift her arms. There is no energy to eat, even when food is just a phone call away. Without adequate food, nutrient deficiencies develop that increase the apathy and depression and eventually result in mental confusion. The downward spiral continues, unless interference of neighbors or friends breaks it at some point.

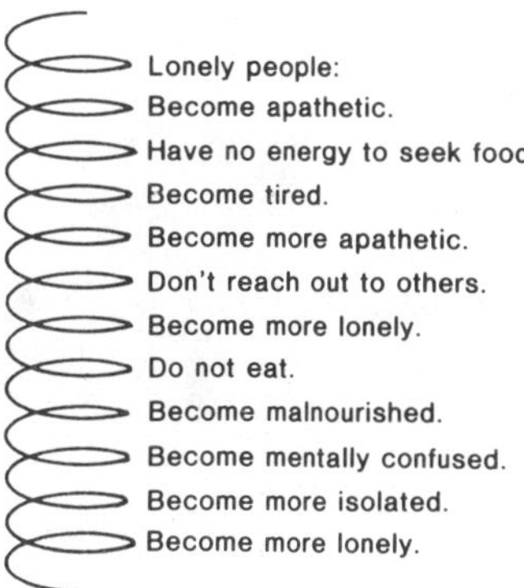

Lonely people:
Become apathetic.
Have no energy to seek food.
Become tired.
Become more apathetic.
Don't reach out to others.
Become more lonely.
Do not eat.
Become malnourished.
Become mentally confused.
Become more isolated.
Become more lonely.

Let's look at what happens when a person receives too little food. In the first place, the body can't tell why it is receiving too few nutrients or calories. The situation is the same for a child dying in a famine in Bangladesh as for a wealthy solitary person who is depressed and refusing food. The B vitamins and vitamin C are quickly depleted because they are needed daily. The first organ to suffer from deprivation is the brain. The B vitamins are necessary for the metabolism of the glucose energy that the brain requires. The brain responds by slowing down all muscular functions. This explains some of the apathy exhibited by the elderly who do not eat. If the carbohydrate calories and the B vitamins are not restored, mental confusion that resembles senility will be manifest and may even progress to hallucinations and insanity.

More about the symptoms of B-vitamin deficiencies—Chapter 9.

If protein foods, protected by complex carbohydrates, are insufficient, then enzymes to digest food and antibodies to protect against infection cannot be synthesized. When iron and vitamin C are absent, the protein hemoglobin cannot be made for the delivery of oxygen, so the feeling of weakness and tiredness grows. With tiredness caused by lack of food added to the apathy from loneliness, there is even less energy with which to make the effort to secure nourishment. If the confusion of vitamin deficiency is diagnosed as senility, the elderly person may be wrongly confined to a nursing home.[53]

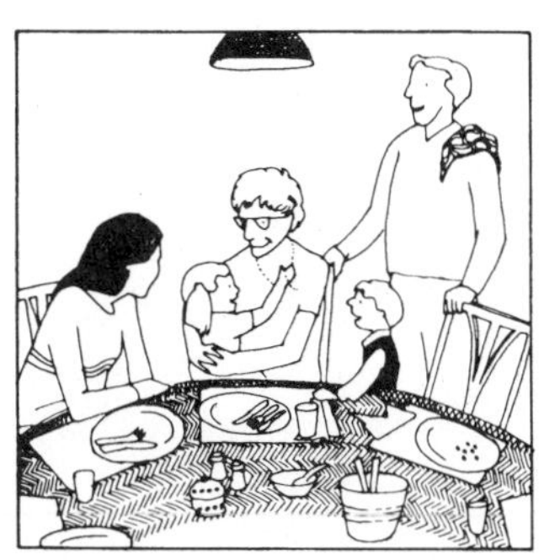

Given a family to love, a "senile" old person may come back to life.

The story is told of a woman who took her mother-in-law to live with her while the older woman waited for a place in a nursing home. The mother-in-law had exhibited the classic signs of senility—mental confusion, inability to make decisions, forgetting to perform important tasks such as turning off a stove burner—so the family had decided she needed institutional care. After several weeks in the daughter-in-law's home—eating good meals and enjoying social stimulation—she became her old self again and returned to her home. This story has been repeated with many variations and serves to remind us to seek a careful medical diagnosis before concluding that a person is senile and needs institutional care. What harm could there be in first trying good, balanced meals served with plenty of tender, loving care?

Money and Other Worries

To add anxiety to their problems, most retired persons have a loss of real income that occurs because the retirement check is fixed while all other expenses are increasing. This has a direct effect on the amount of money spent on food, because food (and clothing) purchases are among the few flexible items in the budget. Costs of shelter, utilities, and medical care must be paid and then the amount left over stretched to cover food and other needs.

Forced to practice economy, the older person usually first eliminates so-called "luxury" items such as fresh fruit, vegetables, and milk. In some cases, transportation to and from the market is both expensive and difficult, so that use is made of a nearby convenience store. The foods offered there are limited in variety and are, for the most part, more expensive than the same items in the larger markets. The amount of food that can be purchased is thus curtailed even further; and eating, one of the few pleasures left to the older person, becomes another reminder of reduced status.

Sometimes older persons fall prey to food fads and fallacies. Led by false claims to believe that health can be improved, aging forestalled, and illness cured by magical food and nutrient preparations, they spend money needlessly on fraudulent health food products, thus depleting their already limited funds.[54]

Two programs are helpful with older people's money problems, although they are not designed specifically for older people but for the poor of all ages. The Food Stamp program enables people who qualify (by way of showing low income or high expenses for dependent children or for medical bills) to stretch their food budgets. A small amount of money buys stamps, which then can be redeemed for more food than the money itself would have paid for. The Supplemental Security Income (SSI) program is aimed at directly improving the financial plight of the very poor by increasing a person's or family's income to the defined poverty level. This sometimes helps older people retain their independence.

WHY WORRY?

There are only two things in the world to worry about—
Whether you are happy or whether you are not happy.
If you are happy, there is nothing in the world to worry
about.
If you are unhappy, there are only two things in the world
to worry about—
Whether you are sick or whether you are well.
If you are well, there is nothing in the world to worry
about.
If you are sick, there are only two things in the world to
worry about—
Whether you will live or whether you will die.
If you are going to live, there is nothing in the world to
worry about.
If you are going to die, there are only two things in the
world for you to worry about—
Whether you are going to heaven or whether you are going to hell.
If you are going to heaven, there is nothing in the world
for you to worry about.
If you are going to hell, you are going to be so busy saying
hello to all your old friends, you are not going to have
time to worry.
So why worry?

Besides loneliness, loss, and limited income, the older person faces an increased likelihood of illness and invalidism. Poor dental health, mental illness, and chronic alcoholism are other problems cited as being prevalent among the elderly.[55] With all of these problems to live with, and with the increasing numbers of people in the older age group, it is not surprising that at least a few individuals and agencies are concerned enough to ask what can be done to help.

Assistance Programs

In recent years, we have come to recognize that the responsibility for support in old age cannot be left entirely to the individual. Two programs arising from this awareness have already been mentioned (the Food Stamp and Supplemental Security Income programs). The first venture into help for older persons grew out of the experiences of the depression years of the 1930s. The Social Security Act was put into effect in 1935. Under this act, employees and employers pay into a fund from which each employee collects benefits at retirement.

A second major political move to benefit the elderly was the Older Americans Act of 1965. Title VII of this act is an amendment, Nutrition Program for the Elderly, which was signed into law by President Nixon in 1972. The major goals of this amendment are:

Low-cost nutritious meals.

Opportunity for social interaction.

Auxiliary nutrition, homemaker education, and shopping assistance.

Counseling and referral to other social and rehabilitative services.

Transportation services.

The nutrition program of Title VII was based on the belief that people living alone are apt to have poor nutrition. If their nutritional status could be improved, they might avoid medical problems, continue living in communities of their own choice, and stay out of institutions. The program was not designed as charity, but during its first years it was found that 80 percent of the participants had incomes less than $200 a month and 34 percent had incomes under $100 a month.[56]

Sites chosen for congregate meals under this program must be accessible to most of the target population. Church or school facilities are often used when they are conveniently located. Providing transportation increases the cost of meals by 20 to 30 percent, but it often is indispensable to the existence of a project. Some projects have been successful in recruiting volunteers to help with the transportation. Volunteers may also deliver meals to those who are homebound either permanently or temporarily: The efforts are known as Meals on Wheels. In 1977 there were about 350 such Meals on Wheels programs in the United States.[57]

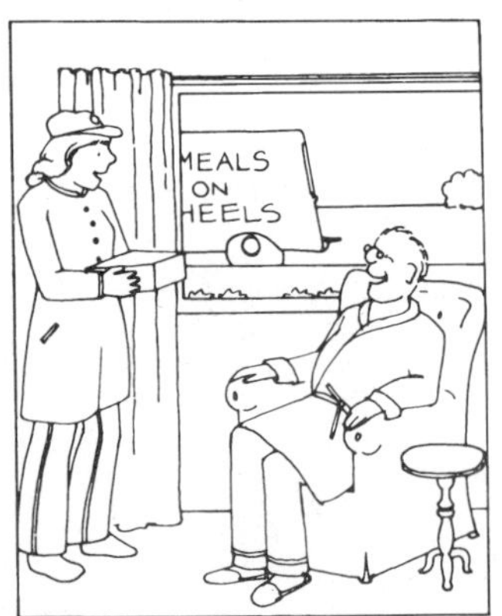

Meals on Wheels reach thousands of home-bound elderly.

Every effort is made to persuade the elderly person to come to the congregate meal sites. The social atmosphere at the sites is as valuable as the nutrition. One participant was heard to remark, "It is better to come to the congregate meal and eat at a table with others, even if no one speaks to me, than it is to sit at home and stare at a wall while I eat."[58]

Independence is rated high by those over sixty-five, and this is usually equated with staying in the home where they have lived many years. But this aloneness may not be a wise choice from a nutritional standpoint. There are alternatives that would enhance the elderly's health without threatening independence. One alternative is covenant living, a lifestyle gaining in popularity. It is patterned after the communes of the young people of the 1960s, although the participants probably would deny this. A number of congenial people, wishing to live in a family group but having no family of their own, agree to live together. Sometimes they buy a house together or rent a house or, in some cases, rent the house of one of the members. The word *covenant* refers to the contractual agreements made among the parties before the arrangement begins. Sometimes it takes several months of talking to hammer out the details of problems that may arise.

The general work of running the house is shared. Either everyone shares equally in the work, taking turns at various jobs, or there is a division based on what each one likes to do or can do well. There are definite economic advantages; but from a nutritional standpoint, the main advantage is in the sharing of meals and the abating of loneliness. One person described covenant living as coming out of "solitary confinement" into a warm family with the sound of laughter and people to touch.

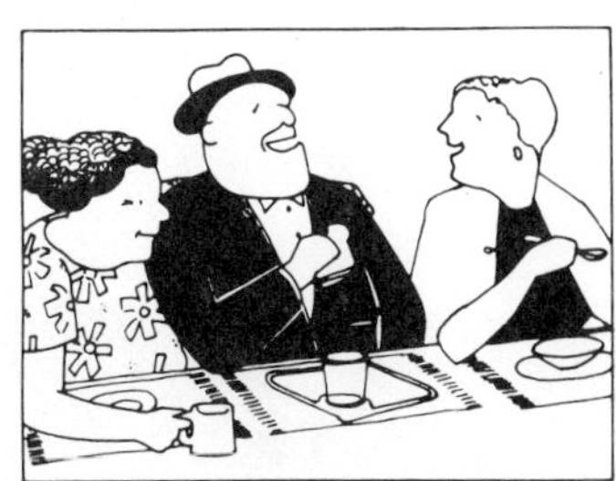

Eating together makes food more enjoyable and so improves nutrition.

Another way of gaining sociability while remaining independent is for several older persons to remain in their own homes but meet together regularly for meals, each one taking a turn at preparing the food. Socializing encourages a better food intake, and the one who prepares the food has leftovers to enjoy the next day. Some of the participants in the congregate meal programs have formed what they call a "diner's club" and go to restaurants in a group on the days when the congregate meal is not served. This kind of arrangement among friends helps improve the dietary intake of many older persons.

Another alternative is to move into a retirement community. Some of these are very expensive, but some have a rule that no one who has an income above a certain moderate amount is eligible. In these, a variety of living arrangements are available, from nursing home space to luxury apartments or separate homes on the grounds. In most, several services are maintained on the premises: an infirmary for slight illnesses, a restaurant, barber shops and beauty salons. A daily check on persons who live alone is one of the valuable services.

Foster home care has proven to be an alternative for people who need some supportive care but do not need medical supervision. Foster homes have the advantage of being located within the community where the older person has lived, so that contact with friends and relatives can be maintained easily. The operators of such homes have no special qualifications and need help from nutritionists for some of their problems. One study of the problems of foster homes, involving 183 operators and 422 residents, showed the biggest problem they faced was the residents' lack of interest in food and other special diet needs. Guidance from nutritionists might help alert them to deterioration that, if allowed to continue, would necessitate more expensive medical care.[59]

Churches and synagogues are ideal organizations to help with the problems of the elderly for a number of reasons: (1) They have neighborhood facilities that lie idle a good portion of the week; (2) they are "caring" organizations; (3) they have a target population, either among their own members or in their neighborhood; and (4) they have a reservoir of volunteers to help cut down on labor costs. Many religious organizations have taken the lead in establishing retirement and nursing homes. However, these facilities are very expensive and usually necessitate the residents' leaving their own communities, which means leaving behind the people who care about them. In addition, a nursing home is a medical solution to what, in many cases, is a social problem.[60]

A group of churches in Kansas City discovered the many needs of older people when they started plans to establish a retirement community.[61] Seven churches met together to build a nursing and retirement home and learned that what was really needed was a community service group capable of helping people remain in their own homes. The Shepherd's Center was the result of their planning. This center is now operated by twenty-two churches in the Kansas City area and has available eight home services, with new ones being made available as the need becomes apparent. The services include congregate meals in neighborhood churches; home delivery of hot meals; a shopping service by which people are taken to shop for groceries or purchases are made for them; a transportation service to take persons to medical appointments; a visitation program in which volunteers keep in personal touch with truly isolated persons; a handyman service to make minor repairs to the home; a crime assistance program; and a team that responds to emergencies at any hour.

In addition to these home services, the Shepherd's Center conducts classes on a wide range of topics taught by skilled or scholarly retired persons. Some 800 are currently enrolled, and there are long waiting lists. The discovery that retired persons are eager to learn new skills and explore new areas of knowledge has been the experience of many other such groups as well. Health care is one topic of prime importance to older persons, and they are especially eager to study nutrition.[62]

For people who need constant medical care, nursing homes provide a less expensive facility than hospitals. Nursing homes are patterned after hospitals in their approach to patients. Sometimes this is detrimental to the patients' attitudes toward themselves and their future. However, for some, especially the crippled, paralyzed, or bedridden, the nursing home offers a valuable service. There has been a great deal of unfavorable publicity of some substandard homes, which makes many older people frightened at the prospect of having to enter one. But investigation by relatives can identify a home that provides the kind of service the individual needs.

The relative inquiring into nursing homes should ask the director or dietitian some questions about the food service. Is a choice given the patient in the selection of food? How often are fresh fruits and vegetables served? Is a plate check conducted regularly, at least once a week, to discover what the patient is consuming? Alternatively, is there good communication between the nursing staff and the dietitian so that what a patient is not eating will be known by the dietitian? Is the patient encouraged and helped to go to the dining room to eat so that some socialization will occur? Are minced meats offered to those who have problems with their dentures? Are religious dietary restrictions honored? How high a proportion of the foods are prepackaged? (No guide can be given for what proportion is desirable, but it should be remembered that processed foods are low in vitamin content and high in salt.) Other questions that the investigator will want to ask have to do with the general atmosphere of the nursing home, in recognition of the effect of social climate on a person's appetite. A nursing home that views residents as persons, not as patients, gets a mark in its favor.

Preparing for the Later Years

The programs just described can do much to help older people adjust to their changing circumstances, but the very best help we could give our elderly citizens would be a change of attitude. As a nation, we value the future more than the present, putting off enjoying today so that tomorrow we will have money or prestige or time to have fun. The elderly feel this loss of future. The present is their time for leisure and enjoyment, but they have no experience in the use of leisure time.

Our culture also values the doers, those concerned with action and achievement. The Mexican mother can enjoy her child's sitting in her lap and laughing in her face; however, the North American mother is more likely preoccupied with how well her child is preparing for tomorrow. The elderly are aware of the status given those who are doing something and of the lack of respect for those who lead a contemplative life in retirement.

It would take a near miracle to change the attitude of a nation, but there is a change in attitude that persons can make toward themselves as they age. Preparation for this period should of course include financial planning, but other lifelong habits should be developed as well. Each adult needs to learn to reach out to others, to forestall the loneliness that will otherwise ensue. Each needs to learn some skills or activities that can continue into the later years—volunteer work with organizations, reading, games, hobbies, or intellectual pursuits—which will give meaning to the activities of the days. One needs to develop the habit of adjusting to change, especially when it comes without consent, so that it will not be seen as a loss of control over life. The goal is to arrive at maturity with as healthy a mind and body as it is possible to have, and this means cultivating good nutritional status and maintaining a program of daily exercise.

Preparation for the later years begins early in life, both psychologically and nutritionally. Everyone knows older people who have gathered around themselves many contacts—through relatives, church, synagogue, or fraternal orders—and have not allowed themselves to drift into isolation. Upon analysis, you will see that their favorable environment came through a lifetime of effort. They spent their entire lives reaching out to others and practicing the art of weaving themselves into other people's lives. Likewise, a lifetime of effort is required for good nutritional status in the later years. A person who has eaten a wide variety of foods, has stayed lean, and has remained physically active will be most able to withstand the assaults of change.[1]

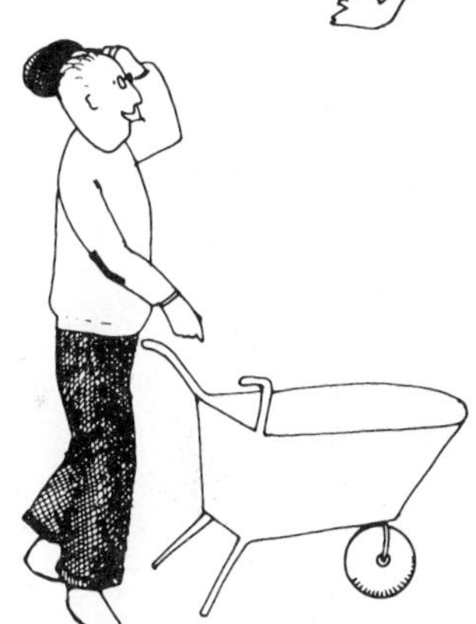

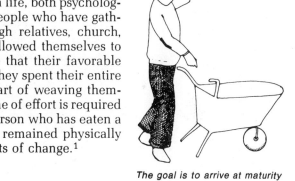

The goal is to arrive at maturity with a healthy body and mind.

For Further Information

Recommended references on all nutrition topics are listed in Appendix J. In addition, we recommend highly the books by Comfort (*A Good Age*) and Puner (*To the Good Long Life*), listed in this chapter's notes.

A book that helps the reader understand the medical and social problems that develop with aging is:

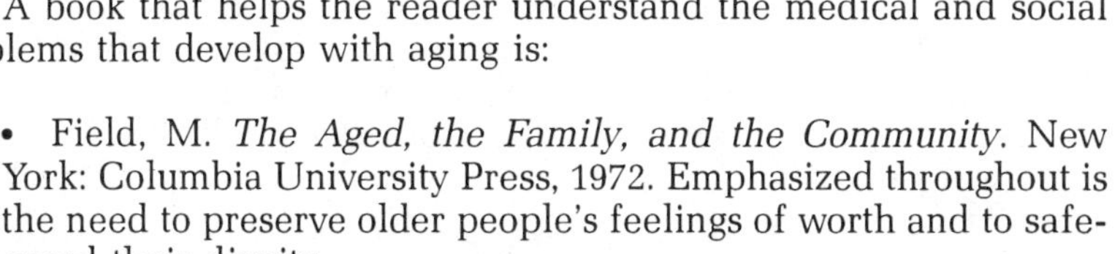

- Field, M. *The Aged, the Family, and the Community.* New York: Columbia University Press, 1972. Emphasized throughout is the need to preserve older people's feelings of worth and to safeguard their dignity.

[1]*Chapter Notes can be found at the end of the Appendixes.*

The *Journal of the American Geriatrics Society* and *The Gerontologist* make good reading for the general reader.

A short article that takes a positive approach toward the nutritional problems of older people and presents up-to-date information on them is:

- Rowe, D. Aging—a jewel in the mosaic of life. *Journal of the American Dietetic Association* 72 (1978): 478-486.

Practical pointers on buying, preparing, and cooking food can be found in:

- Peterkin, B. Your money's worth in foods. This twenty-nine-page pamphlet is available for 60 cents from Home and Garden Bulletin, U.S. Government Printing Office, Washington, DC 20402.
- Nidetch, J. *Weight Watchers Program Cookbook*. Great Neck, N.Y.: Hearthside Press, 1973. Although originally intended for dieters, this book is useful for older people. Many of the recipes are for one or two servings. And they are low in saturated fat and sugar, which enhances their value for someone trying to eat in line with the *Dietary Guidelines*. Nidetch has experimented with standard "down home" recipes to lower saturated fat and sugar content. Her dessert recipes using dry skimmed milk are especially recommended.

The Space Age has brought the development of convenience foods originally intended for use by astronauts but remarkably tasty and handy for the older person living alone. With these freeze-dried foods, which require no refrigeration, hot meals can be prepared for one person in ten minutes. Meals containing a quarter-pound of meat, a vegetable, fruit, dessert, and beverage can be obtained by mail by writing:

- Easy Meal, Oregon Freeze Dry Foods, Inc., PO Box 1048, 770 West 29th Avenue, Albany, OR 97321. The 1978 price was five for $10.

Among films and teaching aids that promote understanding of aging are:

- Pelcovits, J. Nutrition education for older Americans. *Cassette-a-Month*, February 1977. Available from the American Dietetic Association (address in Appendix J).
- *The String Bean*, a fifteen- to twenty-minute-long film, is a hauntingly poetic masterpiece portraying an old lady's devotion to life, love, and beauty. Available from McGraw-Hill Films, in care of Association Films, Inc., 600 Grand Avenue, Ridgefield, NJ 07657.

Controversy 15

Vitamin E

Do large doses of vitamin E retard the aging process?

One of the many, many claims made for vitamin E is the claim that it prevents aging. The theory is that aging is caused by prolonged exposure of cells to such destructive agents as air pollutants, toxins, and peroxides produced when cosmic rays collide with molecules inside the cells. Many of these agents are thought to do their damage by reacting with (oxidizing) cellular constituents, especially polyunsaturated fatty acids in cell membranes. Over the years, the cumulative effect of these agents is believed to cause cell death and reduce efficiency of surviving cells. Doses of up to 2 grams (2000 milligrams) of vitamin E daily, or some 130 times the RDA, are recommended by some to prevent these effects, and thousands of dollars are spent by those who hope to find a miniature fountain of youth in each bottle of vitamin E capsules.

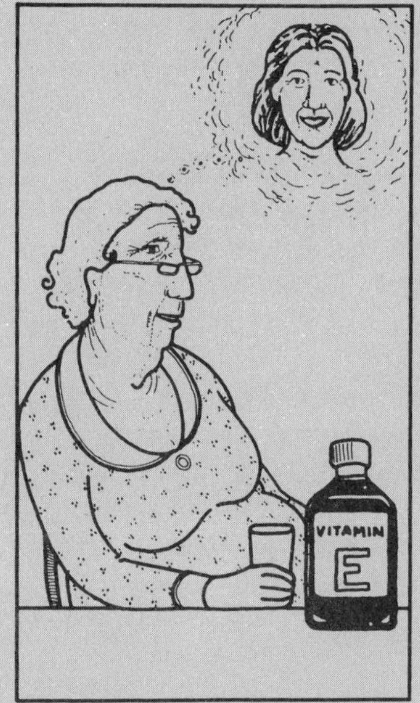

Actually, there is one piece of experimental evidence that is consistent with the notion that vitamin E has something to do with aging. A deficiency of the vitamin causes the accumulation of pigment in the intestinal cell walls, and this same pigment appears in the skin cells of some individuals as they age. Known as "aging spots" or "liver spots," this pigmentation is thought to be retarded or prevented by vitamin E. But if you have read everything in this book so far, you will be astute enough to realize that it is a long, long step from the recognition that the same compound appears in two different places and under two different sets of circumstances in the body to the generalization that aging is a vitamin E-deficiency disease.

Vitamin E does appear in the body in very large quantities, however, and its roles are still somewhat mysterious. It is still too early to say what all of its functions are. An immense amount of recent research reflects the intense interest many investigators have in this vitamin, and some tentative statements can be made about what it does, what it doesn't do, and what happens if you take too much rather than too little.

What vitamin E does. The best-known roles of vitamin E are summed up in Chapter 9. It acts as an antioxidant, protecting red cell (and other) membranes from being destroyed by oxygen. In premature infants, whose immature lungs are especially vulnerable to oxidation, this effect is especially important. It is only at the very end of pregnancy that the mother's blood concentration of vitamin E rises so that the infant will receive protective amounts; the premature baby is born without this extra vitamin E and so has a deficiency. Without supplemental doses, such a baby will develop anemia from breakage of the red blood cells (hemolytic anemia).

The lungs experience a higher oxygen concentration than any other part of the body except the skin. Many of the recently confirmed effects of vitamin E have to do with the antioxidant protection of lung cells and red blood cells (as they pass through the lungs):

- Preventing human red blood cells from the damage done by oxidizing air pollutants (at doses up to 200 IU per day but not higher).[1]
- Promoting survival of infants born with severe respiratory distress.[2]
- Helping to keep the red blood cells from assuming abnormal shapes and losing their usefulness in sickle-cell anemia.[3]
- Improving red cell survival in other rare disorders.[4]

Other cells of the blood may also be dependent on vitamin E for some of their functions. The white cells, which are responsible for fighting off the challenge of infection, function better when they have enough vitamin E—at least, judging from experiments with animals.[5] And the cells of the liver, which are damaged by certain kinds of poisons, can also be protected by vitamin E.[6]

Three other tissues have been seen to respond to vitamin E under very special circumstances. One is the lens of the eye in rats that were made diabetic-like: large vitamin doses given by injection prevented them from getting cataracts, as they would otherwise have done.[7] This may have no application to any human situation but may lead to useful research showing how vitamin E works. The second is the tissue of the human breast. Some women develop lumps which are not cancerous but are composed of fibrous tissue, and this unexplained symptom can be relieved in some cases by large doses (600 IU) of vitamin E.[8] The third is the muscles of the calves, in which cramping can sometimes be relieved by administration of vitamin E.[9]

Finally (while still on the subject of what vitamin E *does*), it is important to remember that any vitamin deficiency causes symptoms that that vitamin can relieve. Vitamin E deficiency in humans is very, very rare, but it does turn up occasionally. It has been seen, as already mentioned, in premature infants, in sickle-cell anemia, and other rare lung and blood disorders. It is also seen in cases where hospital patients (babies and even adults) are fed formulas that don't contain the vitamin, or when people can't absorb fats, or when they have been exposed to poisons that destroy it. Under these conditions, disorders of the brain, the muscles, the eyes, and the heart have occasionally been seen.[10]

What it doesn't do. During the 1960s and 1970s some tremendous claims were made for vitamin E. It was said to improve athletic endurance and skill, to increase potency and enhance sexual performance, to prolong the life of the heart, and to reverse the damage caused by atherosclerosis and even heart attacks. An immense amount of experimentation has discredited these and many similar claims.[11] To give one example: Doses of 1600 IU a day given to forty-eight patients for six months had no effect on chest pain (angina), exercise capacity, heart function, or other factors related to heart disease.[12] Vitamin E also does not help with:

- Lowering high blood lipids, including cholesterol.[13]
- "Hot flashes."[14]
- Bladder cancer.[15]

Nor does it have any effect on other processes of aging, such as the graying of the hair, wrinkling of the skin, and reduced capacity of body organs to perform their functions.

What vitamin E megadoses do. It has been said that, even though the vitamin may not do all that is claimed for it, there can be no harm in taking supplements because it has no harmful effects even in very large doses. In fact, vitamin E does remain one of the few vitamins for which reports of toxicity are rare. There are isolated reports in the medical literature of adverse effects on laboratory animals and of nausea, intestinal distress, and other vague complaints in human beings. However, the impression remains that "for most individuals daily doses below 300 IU are innocuous."[16] But with the recent interest in new research have come new reports of toxicity even for "harmless E."

In one study, 300 IU per day of vitamin E given to men and boys impaired the ability of their white blood cells to respond to a challenge by infection with bacteria.[17] Too high a ratio of vitamin E to vitamin K may interfere with the clotting action of the latter, cause uncontrolled bleeding, and decrease the rate of wound healing.[18] In animals, where more informative experiments can be conducted, vitamin E megadoses have dramatic effects on many body organs including the bones and the heart, effects which the investigators concluded were clearly harmful.[19] Dr. Victor Herbert, whose conscientious research into the nonexistence of "vitamin B_{15}" was described in Controversy 9, has reminded *Nutrition Reviews* readers that, now that so many people are taking megadoses of vitamin E, we are beginning to see cases where damage is real and severe. That damage involves the very same areas people want to improve with their self-dosing: their vision, sex organs, skin, muscles, blood, and nerves.[20]

Personal strategy. It probably remains true that people taking large doses of vitamin E have a better chance of escaping unharmed than they would with many other vitamins and with most of the minerals. For most people, there may be few hazards associated with taking vitamin E supplements other than those to the pocketbook—and if a psychological boost results from the dose, it may be worth the price. Only in one situation is there certain danger: If taking vitamin E lulls a user into postponing a trip to the doctor for correct diagnosis and treatment of a serious condition, then it may cost more than anyone can afford to pay.

But if you actually want to remain young, there are some far more effective strategies than playing games with vitamin pills, and they require taking a broader perspective. Good nutrition is one—but not the only—factor involved in prolonging the body's health and vigor into the later years. It's a matter of lifestyle—all elements relating to health.

A study designed by Belloc and Breslow probed the question of what aspects of lifestyle promote good health and came up with some informative answers. Their study explored the relationship of a number of personal health practices to the state of health in a sample of almost 7000 persons in California. Those who followed all of the "good" practices were in better health at every age than those who followed none or a few.

And what were these health practices? Taking vitamin E capsules was not one of them. They were:

- Getting adequate sleep.
- Eating regular meals.
- Maintaining desirable weight.
- Not smoking.
- Drinking alcohol moderately or not at all.
- Getting regular exercise.[21]

These answers are not surprising. But it is fitting to end this book's presentation by putting nutrition back into perspective as part of a larger picture. The six practices listed here lay the groundwork for the ability to enjoy, in good health, "the best years of life for which the first were made."

A ninety-year-old landscape gardener at his annual checkup asked the doctor, "How am I doing?" Truthfully, the doctor replied, "Well, old man, you're not getting any younger." "But doctor," the old man countered, "I don't ask to get younger. I only ask to get older! I have more trees to plant."

The Controversy Notes and For Further Information follow the Appendixes.

PART FIVE

APPENDIXES

APPENDIX A: The Human Body

The brief anatomy lesson that follows is a lesson in "anatomy for nutrition's sake" to review the body systems and terminology referred to in this book. To make the body's design understandable, the first few paragraphs are devoted to the life needs of the cells and the evolutionary mechanisms that have ensured that they are met.

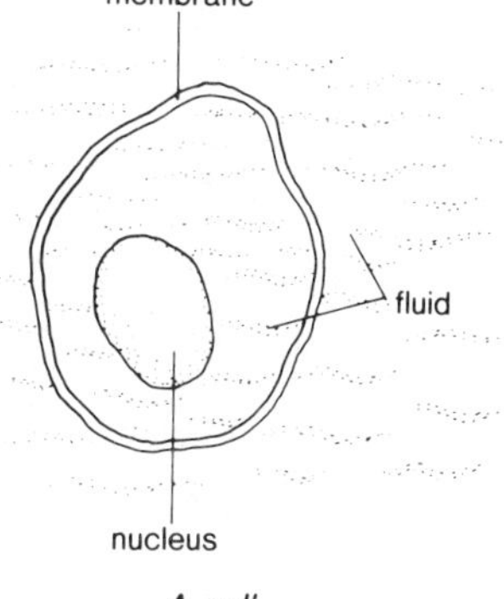

A cell.

The Cells

The body is composed of millions of cells, and not one of them knows anything about food. While you get hungry for meat, milk, or bread, each cell of your body sits in its place waiting until the nutrients it needs pass by. Each cell keeps itself alive just as its single-celled ancestors did, living alone in the ocean 3 billion years ago. The fact that you are alive today means that your cells' ancestors have sustained their lives in an unbroken chain of generations for 3 billion years.

For the cell, death is not the natural end of life. A cell may grow until it has doubled its size and all its parts and then may divide to form two daughter cells. Six generations later, if all goes well, there will be 128 cells, and six generations later still, almost 10,000. The original cell has not died but has produced thousands of replicas of itself. Death comes to any of these only when its needs are not met—when its water supply fails, the temperature becomes extreme, or its integrity is somehow destroyed.

Uncountable daughters of the first living cell are alive and growing and reproducing themselves all over the earth today, in trees, in fish, and in every form of life that we know, including ourselves. Each survives because its predecessors managed to maintain or find the conditions they needed for life or to adapt enough to survive in changing conditions. Often this survival has meant snatching food from others' mouths. The human species endures because we have adapted, so far, to all changing conditions on the earth; other species have died out because they lost the struggle for survival. And where we have competed with another species for the same environment, so far we have proved superior at surviving. This means that every cell has inherited the genes that enable it to work best with all the other cells.

Each **gene** is a blueprint that directs the making of the protein machinery that does the cell's work. Each cell contains a complete set of instructions, but different genes are active in different cells of the body. For example, in the intestinal cells the genes for making digestive enzymes are active; in the red blood cells, the genes for making the protein hemoglobin are active. There are thousands of genes in your cells, and the entire complex is designed for one ultimate purpose—survival to reproductive age. To ensure this survival, each cell cooperates with all the others to maintain the health of the whole. The digestive system breaks foods into nutrients so that all the other cells can use them. The blood system bathes each cell constantly in a nutrient- and oxygen-rich fluid, just as the ancient seas long ago provided the original one-celled ancestor with foods and oxygen. Other systems provide other services to all the cells.

Genes are copied so accurately from one generation to the next that a mistake is made only once every hundred million times. Once made, however, the mistake will be as faithfully copied as the original gene was. Usually, a mistake in a gene (a **mutation**) is a severe disadvantage to the organism, and it dies without reproducing the mistake. But one time in a thousand the mutation turns out to confer some advantage on its possessor. The genes that conferred the greatest advantages on the human species in those ancient days are the ones most likely to appear in your inheritance today.

The process by which undesirable characteristics are weeded out and the most desirable characteristics are handed down to succeeding generations is **evolution**; the force behind it is **natural selection**. Natural selection operates wherever there is both:

Genetic variability—in which genes among the sisters in a species confer different characteristics on them, and

Selection pressure—in which a situation, such as a limited food supply, makes it impossible for all the sisters to survive.

Whenever an organism carrying a particular gene or gene combination turns out to be better adapted to securing or using the food of the area, then that organism will survive in greater numbers. This survivor's offspring will inherit the improved ability to get food. Ultimately, the descendants of that organism take over the area, and the ones that are not so well adapted die out, leaving no progeny. The selected genes are then passed on to all succeeding generations.

Natural selection has been extremely powerful in determining our physical characteristics. But note that:

It has taken eons of time. It is insignificant in mere thousands of years.

It operates to select the better-adapted in the situation of the time—that is, the way we are today is the result of natural selection in the days of the cave dwellers.

It selects organisms most likely to survive to reproductive age. There is no selection pressure in favor of genes that provide advantages for later life.

The significance of these three statements is apparent in many areas in nutrition. If you keep the first two statements in mind, you will see why pure sugar and pure salt are considered so "new" in our world even though you have used them all your life. "New" means "less than several hundred thousand years old," and our bodies may not be equipped to deal easily with such substances

(Controversy 4A and Chapter 10). The third statement shows why the nutritional problems of older people may be different from those of younger people—because the body has not inherited ways of adapting to the process of aging (Chapter 15).

The body's cells have needs similar to those of their single-celled ocean-dwelling ancestors. Their most basic need, always, is for energy fuel and the oxygen with which to burn it. Next, they need water, the environment in which they live. Then they need building blocks to maintain themselves—especially the ones that they can't make for themselves. These building blocks—the **essential nutrients**—must be supplied preformed from food. These are among the limitations of our heredity from which there is no appeal, and they underlie the first principle of diet planning: Whatever foods we choose, they must provide energy, water, and the essential nutrients. In a sense, the body is only a system organized to provide for these needs of its cells. In the body's tissues, organs, and organ systems, the cells have accomplished a division of labor that better guarantees their continued life than when each had to go it alone.

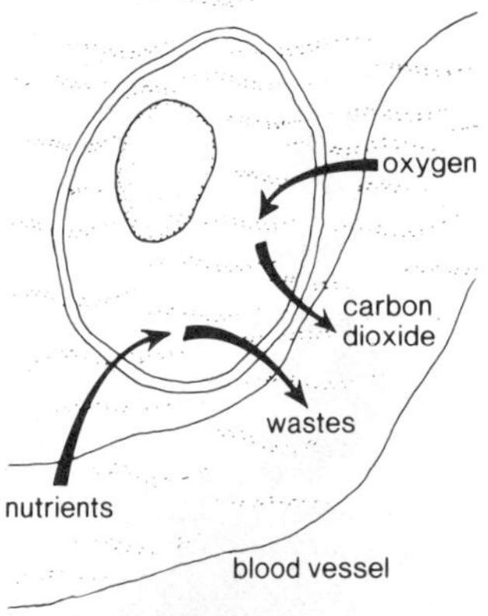

The fluids bathing the cells.

The Body Fluids

Every cell of the body needs a continuous supply of water, oxygen, energy, and building materials. The body fluids supply these, bathing the outside of all the cells much as the ocean water did for their one-celled ancestors. Every cell continuously uses up oxygen (producing carbon dioxide) and nutrients (producing waste products). The body fluids are the brokers for these materials, carrying the oxygen and nutrients to the cells and carbon dioxide and waste away from them. The extracellular fluids must circulate to pick up fresh supplies and deliver the wastes to points of disposal.

The extracellular fluids are the **blood**, contained in the circulatory system, and **lymph**, which is derived from the blood by filtration through the capillary walls. The lymph occurs in the spaces between the cells and in special ducts that comprise the lymphatic system. The blood occurs within the heart, arteries, capillaries, and veins. Both fluids circulate, the lymph squeezing into the spaces between the cells wherever the blood pressure forces it out and making its way back into the blood system through ducts that empty into the veins (see Figure 1).

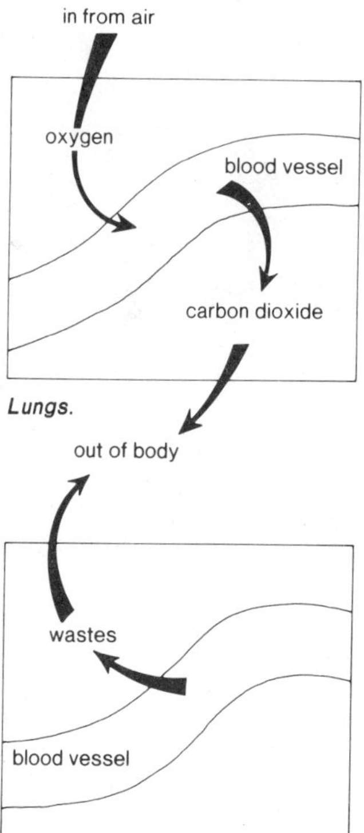

Lungs.

Kidneys.

The Circulatory System

As the blood, pumped by the heart, travels through the circulatory system, it picks up and delivers materials as needed. Its routing ensures that all cells will be served. Oxygen is picked up from the carbon dioxide released in the lungs, and all blood that circulates to the lungs is returned to the heart. From there, it must go to the other body tissues. Thus all tissues receive freshly oxygenated blood.

As it passes the digestive system, the blood delivers oxygen to the cells there and picks up nutrients for distribution elsewhere. All blood leaving the digestive system must go next to the **liver**, which has the special task of altering the composition of the blood to make it better suited for use by other tissues. Then, in passing through the kidneys, the blood is cleansed of its wastes.

As it flows through the skin, the blood is cooled by radiating heat to the surroundings, helping to maintain the temperature of the body's internal organs. Fluid leaving the blood as lymph may ultimately evaporate from the lungs and skin or be used to make body secretions, such as digestive juices, which will be used within the body for various purposes. On returning to the heart, the blood has delivered most of its oxygen and picked up carbon dioxide from the body cells. Its next stop is the lungs once again, to release its carbon dioxide and replenish its oxygen.

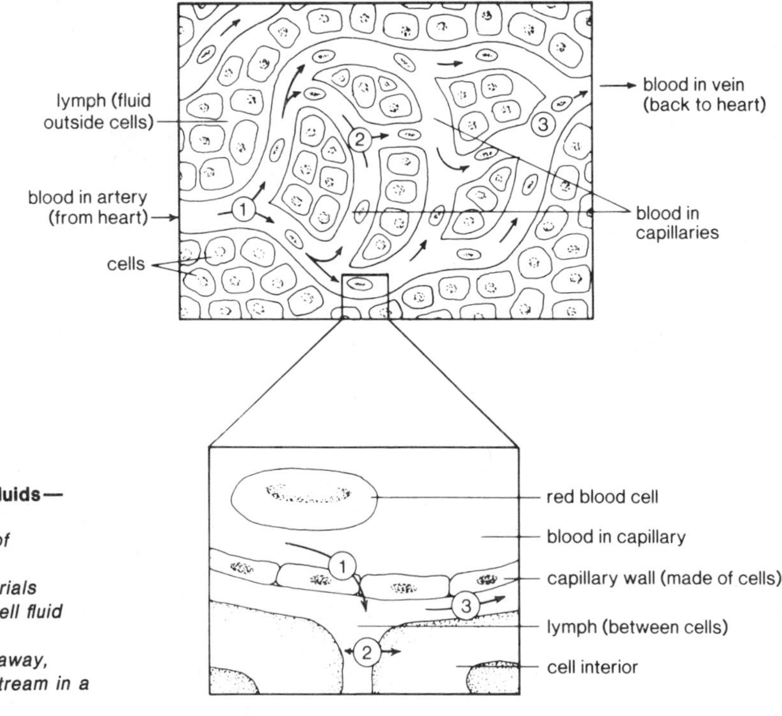

Figure 1a. Portion of body tissue.
1. Blood enters tissues by way of an artery.
2. Blood circulates among cells by way of capillaries.
3. Blood collects into veins for return to heart.

Figure 1b. The body fluids—blood and lymph.
1. Lymph filters out of capillary.
2. Exchange of materials takes place between cell fluid and lymph.
3. Lymph circulates away, later reentering bloodstream in a vein.

In summary, the routing of the blood is heart to body to heart to lungs to heart (repeat). That portion of the blood that flows by the digestive tract travels from heart to digestive tract to liver to heart (see Figure 2).

The Hormonal System

The blood also carries messages, chemical signals from one system of cells to another, that communicate the changing needs of the living system. These chemical messages, or hormones, are secreted by the **endocrine glands**, which release the hormones into the blood. For example, when the pancreas (a gland) experiences a too-high concentration of glucose in the blood, it releases insulin (a **hormone**). Insulin stimulates the liver, muscles, and fat cells to remove glucose from the blood and put it away. When the blood glucose level falls too low, the pancreas secretes another hormone, glucagon. The liver responds by releasing glucose into the blood once again.

More about the blood glucose level—Chapter 4.

Glands and hormones abound in the body, each gland a detector system to monitor a condition in the body that needs regulation and each hormone a messenger to stimulate certain tissues to take appropriate action. Examples of the working of these hormones appear throughout this book.

The Excretory System

To dispose of waste, the **kidneys** straddle the circulatory system and filter each pass of the blood. Waste materials removed with water are collected as urine in tubes that deliver them to the urinary **bladder**, which is periodically emptied. Thus the blood is purified continuously throughout the day, and dissolved minerals are excreted as necessary (including sodium, to keep blood pressure

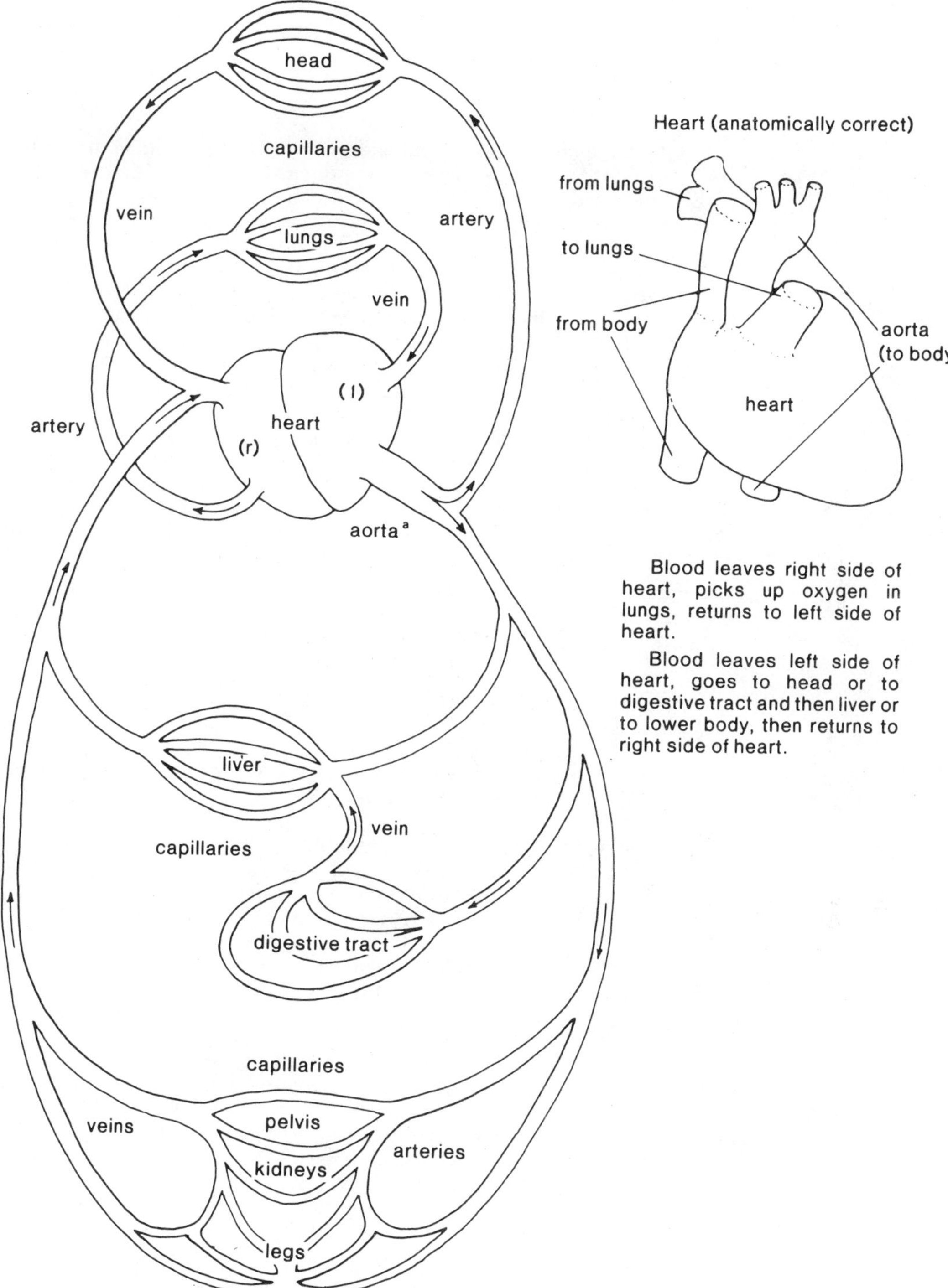

Figure 2. The circulatory system.

[a] The aorta is the main artery that launches blood on its course through the body. The picture is not anatomically correct but is drawn this way for clarity. The aorta actually arises behind the left side of the heart and arcs upwards, then divides. See detail of heart.

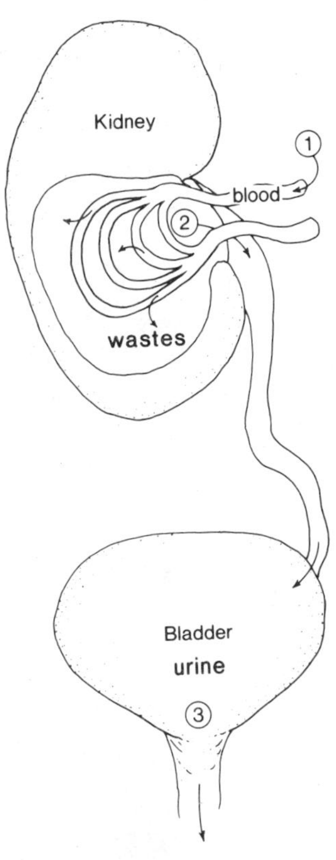

The excretory system.

1. Blood enters kidney by way of arteries.

2. Waste is removed and sent as urine to the bladder.

3. Urine is periodically eliminated.

from rising too high). As you might expect, the kidneys' work is regulated by hormones secreted by glands that are responsive to conditions in the blood.

Temperature Regulation

All the body's cells obtain energy by breaking down the nutrients—carbohydrate, fat, and to some extent protein—and one of the ways this energy is released is as heat. The heat is lost to the air through the skin surface. Temperature regulation involves speeding up or slowing down cellular heat production (**metabolism**) and increasing or decreasing heat loss through the skin. Specialized nerve cells in an area of the brain called the **hypothalamus** serve as a thermostat, measuring the temperature of the blood. These cells signal other cells, near the body surface, to respond appropriately. When the body is too hot, blood vessels immediately under the skin dilate, allowing warm blood to flow near the surface where its heat can radiate away. The sweat glands also are activated to secrete warm fluid onto the skin surface, where its heat can be lost by evaporation. When the body is cold, these mechanisms shut down and shivering is triggered, generating heat.

By means of these systems of transportation, communication, heat regulation, and waste disposal, the cells of the multicellular human animal cooperate to provide one another with a circulating bath of warm, clean, nutritive fluid whose composition is finely regulated to meet their needs.

The Digestive System

You may eat meals only two or three times a day, but your body's cells need their nutrients twenty-four hours a day. Providing the needed nutrients requires the cooperation of millions of specialized cells. When the body's cells are deprived of fuel (glucose), certain nerve cells in the brain (the hypothalamus) detect this condition and generate nerve impulses that signal hunger to the conscious part of the brain, the cortex. They also stimulate the empty stomach to contract with hunger pangs. Becoming conscious of hunger, then, you eat, delivering a complex mixture of chewed and swallowed food to the intestinal tract.

Many of the cells lining the intestinal tract are organized into **exocrine glands**, which secrete powerful juices and enzymes to disintegrate carbohydrate, fat, and protein into their component parts—sugars, glycerol and fatty acids, and amino acids. The presence of these digestive juices and enzymes requires that still other cells specialize in protecting the digestive system. They secrete a thick, viscous substance known as **mucus**, which coats the intestinal tract lining and ensures that it will not itself be digested.

Perhaps most amazing of all the cells of the digestive system are those of the intestinal lining. They can recognize the nutrients needed by the body and absorb enough of them to nourish all the body's cells. Every nutrient that enters the body fluids must traverse one of these cells.

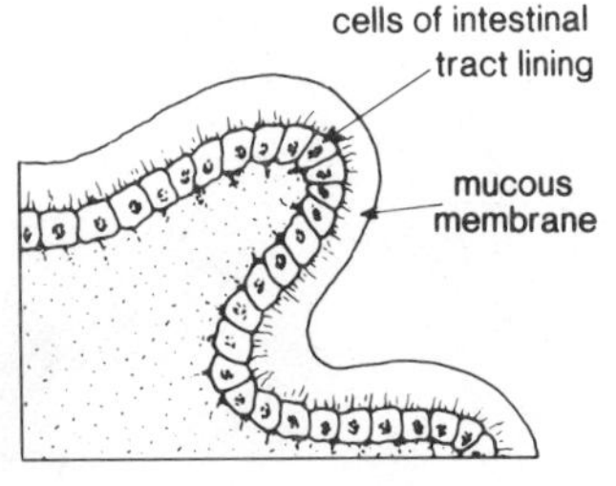

To work efficiently, each cell has a velvety covering of tiny hairs (**microvilli**), which can trap the nutrient particles. The intestinal tract lining is composed of a single sheet of these cells, and the sheet pokes out into millions of finger-shaped projections (**villi**). Each villus is lined with muscle so it can actively wave about, stirring and making contact with the intestinal contents. And each villus has its own capillary network and a lymph vessel so that nutrients transferred across its selective cells immediately mingle into the body fluids.

The process of rendering foods into nutrients and absorbing these into the body fluids is remarkably efficient. In a healthy body, more than 90 percent of the carbohydrate, fat, and protein that pass through the intestinal tract are digested to sugar, glycerol and fatty acids, and amino acids in time to be absorbed. The total surface area of the small intestine with its villi has been estimated at a quarter of an acre. Its cells, weighing perhaps 4 to 5 pounds, absorb enough nutrients in a few hours a day to nourish the other 100 to 200 pounds of cells in the body.

The complete digestive system is shown in Figure 3. The first part, the mouth, is designed for physically breaking down foods. The teeth cut off a bite-size portion and then, aided by the tongue, grind it finely enough to be mixed with saliva and swallowed. The **esophagus** carries the mixture to the stomach. The stomach is supplied with several sets of muscles to mix and grind it further and secretes numerous chemicals that will begin to break it apart chemically.

During the preparatory stage, as the complex carbohydrate known as starch is released from a food (such as bread), an enzyme present in the saliva starts to break it down chemically to smaller units. But this action is stopped when the carbohydrate units reach the stomach, because glands in the stomach wall exude hydrochloric acid. The salivary enzyme that breaks up starch is not active in an acid medium. Further dismantling of carbohydrate occurs after it leaves the stomach.

Fats and oils, taken as part of such complex foods as meats or nuts or in relatively pure form as butter or oil, are thoroughly mixed with the stomach fluids but are not much affected otherwise until after leaving the stomach.

Proteins are eaten as part of such foods as meat, milk, or soybeans. Although no chemical action on them takes place in the mouth, chewing and mixing protein with saliva is an important part of preparing it for the chemical action that begins in the stomach. There, enzymes and hydrochloric acid break

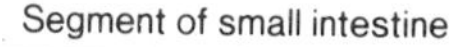

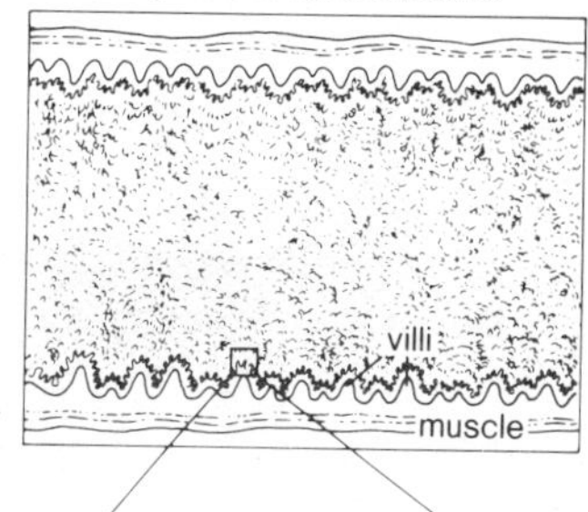

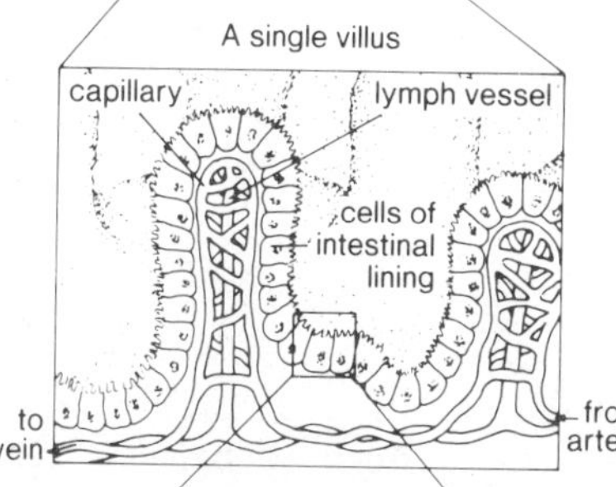

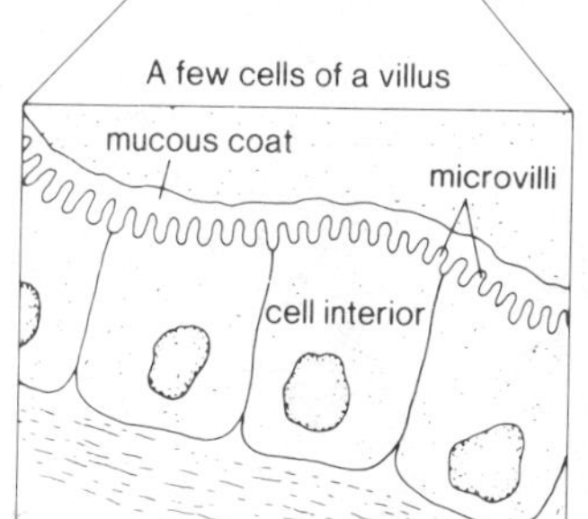

The digestive tract lining.

Digestive tract glands and their secretions:
Salivary glands:
Saliva.
Salivary amylase (enzyme, breaks down starch).
Stomach (gastric) glands:
Gastric juice.
Hydrochloric acid (uncoils protein).
Gastric protease (enzyme, breaks down protein).
Intestinal glands:
Intestinal juice.
Enzymes (break down carbohydrate, fat, and protein).

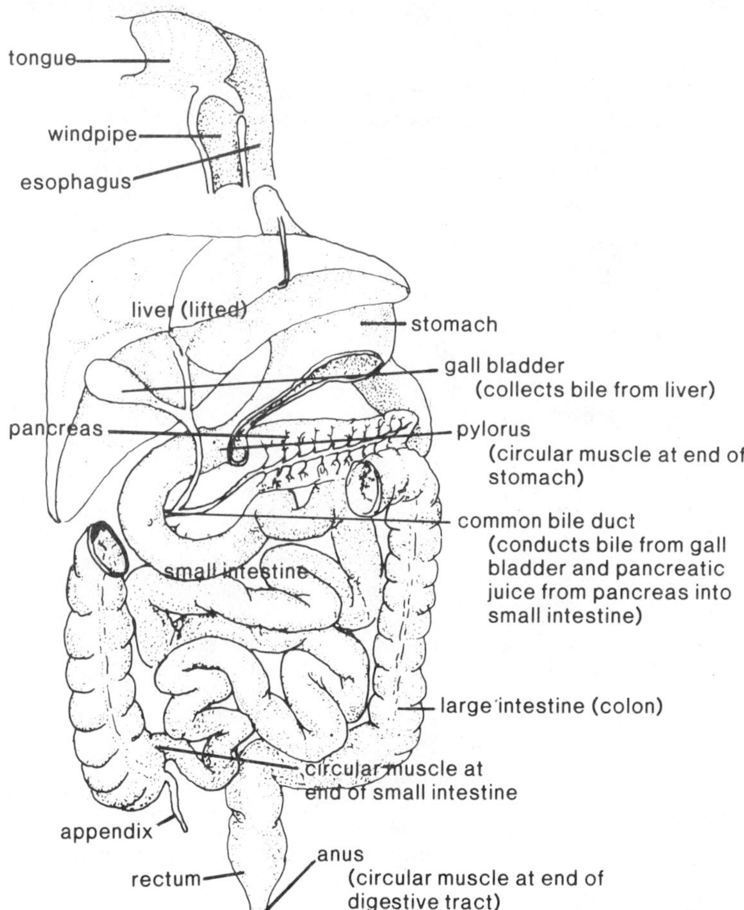

Figure 3. The digestive system.

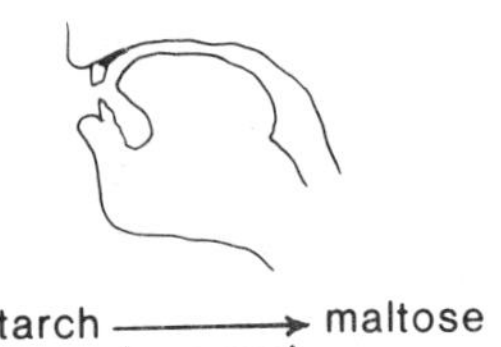

starch —(enzyme)→ maltose

Digestion in the mouth.

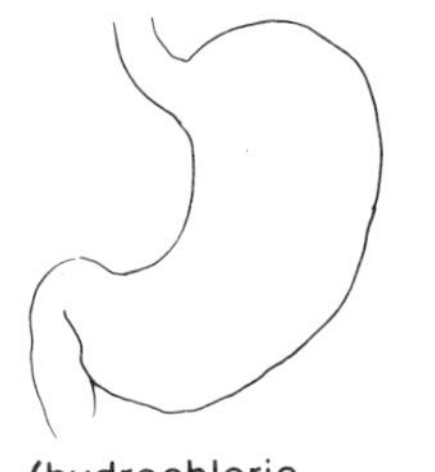

protein —(hydrochloric acid) (enzymes)→ peptides amino acids

Digestion in the stomach.

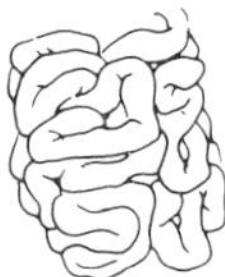

carbohydrate —(enzymes)→ monosaccharides

fat —(bile) (enzymes)→ glycerol monoglycerides fatty acids

protein —(enzymes)→ amino acids

Digestion in the small intestine.

apart the large, very complex protein molecules into smaller proteins known as peptides and finally into dipeptides, tripeptides, and amino acids.

Some of the early stages of digestion, such as chewing and swallowing, are under conscious control. Action in the esophagus and in the stomach requires no thought, although it does make us aware that something is happening there. After swallowing, the digestive apparatus works in a manner too complicated for the conscious brain (**cortex**) to be bothered with; at this juncture, we must relinquish all awareness and put our trust in the ability of each cell to perform its own specialized job.

The complicated chemical dismantling that takes place beyond the stomach requires that very small amounts be processed at one time. To accomplish this, the **pylorus**, a circular muscle surrounding the lower end of the stomach, controls the exit of the contents, allowing only a little at a time to be squirted forcefully into the small intestine. Gradually the stomach empties itself by means of these powerful squirts; once empty, it will rest until hunger pangs signify that it's time to eat again.

The **small intestine** is "the" organ of digestion and absorption; it finishes the job the mouth and stomach have started. It is actually about twenty feet long, but it is called small because its diameter is small compared with that of the large intestine. Its contents must touch its walls in order to make contact with the secretions and in order to be absorbed at the proper places. At the end of the small intestine, a circular muscle (similar in function to the pylorus at the end of the stomach) controls the flow of the contents going into the large intestine (**colon**).

The small intestine works with the precision of a laboratory chemist. As the thoroughly liquefied and partially digested nutrient mixture arrives there, hormonal messages tell the **gall bladder** to send its **emulsifier**, **bile**, in amounts matched to the amount of fat present. Other hormones notify the **pancreas**to release **bicarbonate** in amounts precisely adjusted to neutralize the stomach acid as well as enzymes of the appropriate kinds and quantities to continue dismantling whatever large molecules remain. Such messages also keep the strong muscles imbedded in the walls of the intestine contracting, in a squeezing activity called **peristalsis**, so that the contents will be pressed along to the next region. Peristalsis is stimulated by the presence of roughage or fiber and is quieted by the presence of fat, which requires a longer time for digestion.

Meanwhile, as the pancreatic and intestinal enzymes act on the bonds that hold the large nutrients together, smaller and smaller units make their appearance in the intestinal fluids. Finally, units that the cells can use—glucose, glycerol, fatty acids, and amino acids, among others—are released. These are contacted and absorbed through the intestinal villi. Nutrients released early, such as simple sugars, and those requiring no special handling, such as the water-soluble vitamins, are absorbed high in the small intestine; nutrients that are released more slowly are absorbed further down. The lymphatic and circulatory systems then take over the job of transporting them to the cell consumers. The lymph at first carries most of the products of fat digestion and the fat-soluble vitamins, later delivering them to the blood. The blood carries the products of carbohydrate and protein digestion, the water-soluble vitamins, and the minerals. By the time the remaining mixture reaches the end of the small intestine, little is left but water, indigestible residue (mostly fiber), and dissolved minerals. The cells lining the colon are specialized for absorbing these minerals and retrieving the water for recycling. The final waste product, the **feces**, a smooth paste of a consistency suitable for excretion, is stored in the colon until **defecation**. Such a system can adjust to whatever mixture of foods is presented.

Although a meal may be eaten in half an hour, the nutrients it provides reach the body fluids over a span of about four hours. However, as already mentioned, the cells of the body need their nutrients around the clock. Providing a constant supply requires that there be systems of storage and release to meet the cells' needs between meals.

Storage Systems

All nutrients leaving the digestive system by way of the blood are collected in thousands of capillaries in the membrane that supports the intestine. These converge into veins and then into a single large vein. This vein conveys its contents to the liver and there breaks up once again into a vast network of capillaries that weave among the liver cells, allowing them access to the newly arriving nutrients. The liver cells process the digestive products of all three classes of energy nutrients: carbohydrate, fat, and protein. The sugars from carbohydrate they convert mostly into the body's sugar, glucose, and if there is a surplus, they store some as glycogen and convert the remainder to fat. The fatty acids and glycerol from fat they reassemble into larger fats and package in protein coats for transport to other parts of the body. As for the amino acids from protein, the liver cells alter these as needed, making glucose from some if necessary and fat from others if there is an excess or converting one amino acid into another to use in making proteins.

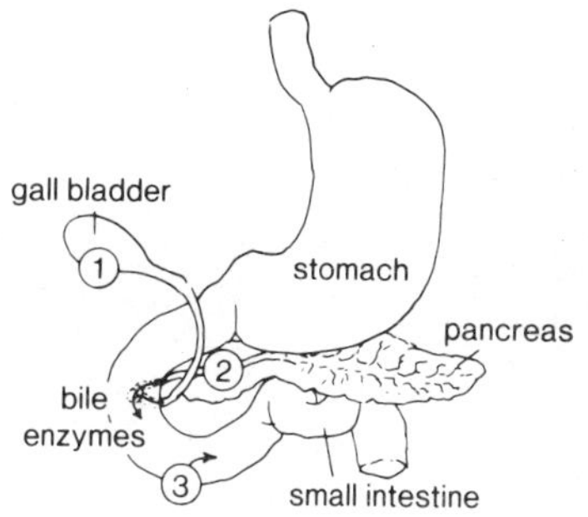

Small intestine—details.
1. The gall bladder sends bile into the small intestine by way of a duct.
2. The pancreas sends enzymes (and bicarbonate).
3. The small intestine also secretes enzymes.

The new products of liver metabolism—glucose, fat packaged in protein coats (lipoproteins), and amino acids—are released into the bloodstream again and circulated to all other cells of the body. Surplus fat is then removed by cells specialized for its storage; these fat cells are located in deposits all over the body.

More about liver glycogen—Chapter 4.

More about lipoproteins—Chapter 5.

The liver glycogen provides a reserve supply of the body's sugar, glucose. The liver can store about three to six hours' worth of glycogen and thus sustain cell activities if the intervals between meals become so long that glucose absorbed from ingested food is used up. Similarly, the fat cells store reserves of fat, the body's other principal energy nutrient. Unlike the liver, however, the fat cells have virtually infinite storage capacity and can sustain the body for days, weeks, or even months when no food is eaten.

More about fasting—Chapter 7.

These storage systems for glucose and fat ensure that the cells will not go without energy nutrients even if the body is hungry for food, except under extreme conditions. Body stores also exist for many other nutrients, each with a characteristic capacity. For example, the third energy nutrient, protein, is held in an available pool (the amino acids in the liver and blood) that is rather rapidly depleted during protein deficiency. The liver and fat cells store many vitamins, and the bones provide reserves of calcium, sodium, and other minerals that can be drawn on to keep the blood levels constant and to meet cellular demands.

More about protein deficiency—Chapter 6.

Other Systems

In addition to the systems described above, the body has many others: the bones, the muscles, the nerves, the lungs, the reproductive organs, and others. All of these cooperate so that each cell can carry on its own life. Each assures, through hormonal or nerve-mediated messages, that its needs will be met by the others, and each contributes to the welfare of the whole by doing the work it is specifically designed for.

Of the millions of cells in the body, only a small percentage comprise the cortex of the brain, in which the conscious mind resides. These receive messages from other cells of the body when they require you to "become conscious" of a need for decision and action. In modern life the need may be as complex as, for example, to notice that you feel anxious and to decide to consult an adviser, or it may be such a "simple" need as "I'm tired, I think I'll go to bed," or "I'm hungry, I guess I'd better eat."

Most of the body's work is done automatically and is finely regulated to achieve a state of well-being. But when your cortex does become involved, you would do well to "listen" to your body and to cultivate an understanding and appreciation of its needs. Then when you make decisions you will act to promote your body's health.

For Further Information

For further reading on the fascinating and beautiful balances maintained by the human body, we recommend:

- Cannon, W. B. *The Wisdom of the Body.* New York: Norton, 1932 (paperback). This is the early classic in physiology, in which Cannon reveals and marvels at the ways the body maintains its balances.
- Clegg, P. C., and Clegg, A. C. *Hormones, Cells and Organisms: The Role of Hormones in Mammals.* Palo Alto, Calif.: Stanford University Press, 1969. This is a brief and accurate introduction to the study of hormones.
- Curtis, H. *Invitation to Biology.* New York: Worth, 1972 (paperback). This is an unusually clear and beautiful presentation of the study of life. Curtis's recommended references provide additional excellent reading material.
- Loewy, A. G., and Siekevitz, P. *Cell Structure and Function.* 2d ed. New York: Holt, Rinehart and Winston, 1969 (paperback). This is a short, clear explanation of cell biology, recommended for the student who is unfamiliar with the subject.
- Oparin, A. I. *Origin of Life.* New York: Dover, 1973 (paperback). A classic in the literature of the history of life on earth, revealing facets of the intimate relationship between environmental water and the life of cells.
- Schmidt-Neilson, K. *Animal Physiology.* 2d ed. Englewood Cliffs, N.J.: Prentice-Hall, 1964 (paperback). This is a brief exposition of physiology for the beginner. The three pages on the digestive system are unusually clear and concise.
- Smith, H. W. *From Fish to Philosopher.* Garden City, N.J.: Doubleday, 1959 (paperback). This little book presents an admiring description of the anatomy, physiology, and evolution of the kidney by a man who devoted his life to its study.
- Wald, G. The origin of life. *Scientific American* 190 (1956): 44-53 (available from *Scientific American* as offprint no. 47). Like the Oparin book, this is a classic. Wald makes the assembly of the first living molecules particularly clear and understandable.

APPENDIX B: Glossary

These are the key terms used in this book and include all those printed in boldface type in the text. Some words are included that do not appear in the book because people often want to know what they mean. The pronunciations and roots are simplified versions of those you might find in a dictionary.

Accent: See *monosodium glutamate.*

acid-base balance: Equilibrium between acid and base concentrations in the body fluids.

acidosis (a-ci-DOSE-iss): Blood pH below the normal range of 7.35-7.45 (*osis* means "too much in the blood").

acid: A water solution in which there are more hydrogen ions (H^+) than hydroxyl (OH^-), or base, ions. See Chapter 10

acne: A skin condition usually associated with the maturation of young adults, characterized by the eruption of skin lesions (comedones) commonly known as whiteheads, blackheads, pimples, and cysts.

additive: A chemical substance added to food, either intentionally, in processing, or incidentally (as an accident such as contamination from the environment or packaging material). See *intentional food additive; incidental food additive.*

adequate diet: A diet that provides all of the essential nutrients and calories in quantities adequate to maintain good health and ideal body weight.

adult-onset obesity: Obesity arising after adolescence; sometimes called "reactive obesity" if it appears to arise in response to a specific traumatic or stressful life event.

adulterated: Contaminated. (Laetrile, for example, is often adulterated with the poison cyanide.)

aerobic: Refers to processes requiring oxygen. Aerobic exercise is exercise performed at an intensity that causes oxygen intake and transport (breathing and heartbeat) to be speeded up (*aero* means "air, oxygen").

aflatoxin (AFF-la-toxin): A potent carcinogen produced by a mold that grows on peanuts.

alkalosis (al-ka-LOCE-iss): Blood pH above the normal range of 7.35-7.45 (*alka* means "base"; *osis*means "too much in the blood").

amenorrhea (ay-men-or-REE-uh): Failure to menstruate, reflecting a halted ovulatory cycle (*a* means "without"). *Athletic amenorrhea* refers to this problem in women athletes.

amine group (a-MEEN): The nitrogen-containing portion of an amino acid.

amino acid (a-MEEN-o): A building block of protein: a compound containing an amine group and an acid group attached to a central carbon, which also carries a distinctive side chain. About twenty amino acids are found in the protein of living tissues.

amniotic sac (am-nee-OTT-ic): The "bag of waters" in the uterus, in which the fetus floats.

amygdalin (ah-MIG-duh-lin): The "chemical" name given to laetrile by its promoters.

anabolic steroids: Hormones, produced normally in males during puberty, that bring about maturation; dangerous when used by athletes to try to promote muscular development (*anabole* means "building up"). Also known as **androgens** (*andro* means "man"; *gen* means "building").

anaerobic: Refers to processes that do not require oxygen, like the first steps in the breakdown of glucose for energy (*an* means "without").

anemia (a-NEE-me-a): Any disease in which the size or shape of red blood cells is altered and their number is reduced (*an* means "without"; *haima* means "blood").

aneurysm (AN-yoo-rism): The ballooning out of an artery wall where the wall is weakened by deterioration and the pressure is high (*ana* means "throughout"; *eurus* means "wide").

angina (an-JYE-nuh; some people say ANN-juh-nuh): Pain in the heart region caused by lack of oxygen.

anorexia (an-oh-REX-ee-uh): Lack of appetite (*an* means "without"; *orex* means "mouth").

anorexia nervosa (nerv-OH-sa): A dangerous condition of intentional underweightness requiring skilled professional treatment (*nervosa* means "of the nerves; neurotic").

anthropometric measures: Measurements of the body including height and weight and often others such as arm circumference and fatfold thickness; used in the evaluation of nutritional status.

antibody (ANT-ee-BOD-ee): Large protein of the blood, produced in response to invasion of the body by foreign protein; inactivates foreign protein.

antioxidant (anti-OX-ih-dant): A compound that protects other compounds from oxygen by itself reacting with oxygen (*anti* means "against"; *oxy* means "oxygen").

aorta: The major artery carrying blood from the heart to the arteries and capillaries. See Figure 2 in Appendix A.

appendicitis: Inflammation and/or infection of the appendix, a sac protruding from the large intestine.

appetite: The desire to eat that normally accompanies hunger.

arteries: The vessels that carry blood from the heart towards the capillaries. See Figure 2 in Appendix A.

ascorbic acid (ass-KOR-bic): Vitamin C (*a* means "without"; *scorb* means "scurvy").

atherosclerosis (ATH-er-oh-scler-OH-sis): The most common kind of hardening of the arteries, characterized by plaque formation in their inner walls (*athero* means "porridge"; *scleros* means "deterioration"). (The general term for hardening of the arteries from all causes is **arteriosclerosis** (ar-TEER-ee-oh-scler-OH-sis.)

balance study: A laboratory study in which a person is fed a controlled diet and the intake and excretion of a nutrient are measured. Balance studies are valid only for nutrients like calcium that don't change while they are in the body.

balanced diet: A diet in which each nutrient is supplied in appropriate quantities relative to the others; also a diet in which the members of each food group are represented in appropriate quantities relative to the others.

basal metabolism: The ongoing metabolic work of the body's cells.

basal metabolic rate (BMR) (BAY-zal meh-ta-BOLL-ic): The rate of energy output of a body at rest after a 12-hour fast.

base: A water solution with more hydroxyl (OH^-) ions than hydrogen (H^+), or acid, ions.

behavior modification: The systematic substitution of one set of behaviors for another by the selective rewarding of the desired behaviors.

beriberi (berry-berry): The thiamin-deficiency disease.

bicarbonate: A commonly occurring chemical that neutralizes acid; a secretion of the pancreas.

bifidus factor (BIFF-id-us, by-FEED-us): A factor in breast milk that favors the growth, in the infant's intestinal tract, of the "friendly" bacteria *Lactobacillus* (lack-toh-ba-SILL-us) *bifidus*, so that other less desirable intestinal inhabitants will not flourish.

bile: A mixture of salts made from cholesterol by the liver, stored in the gall bladder, and secreted into the small intestine. It emulsifies lipids to ready them for enzymatic digestion and helps transport them into the intestinal wall cells.

biological value (BV): A measure of protein quality, assessed by determining the extent to which a given protein supports nitrogen retention.

biotin (BYE-oh-tin): One of the B vitamins.

blackhead: An open comedo with an accumulation of the natural, dark pigment of the skin (not dirt) in its opening.

bladder: The sac in which urine is collected and held for excretion after filtration from the blood by the kidneys.

blood: The fluid of the circulatory system—water, red and white blood cells and other formed particles, proteins, nutrients, oxygen, and other constituents.

body type: A largely outmoded system of classification by height and build into three types: ectomorph (tall and thin); mesomorph (medium); endomorph (short and stout).

botulinum toxin: A toxin produced by bacteria that grow in meat, the most potent biological poison known.

botulism (BOTT-you-lizm): Food poisoning by the toxin produced by a certain species of bacteria (*Clostridium botulinum*).

bran: The fiber of wheat, notable for its effectiveness against constipation and also notable for *not* being effective in lowering blood cholesterol. Its principal constituent is cellulose.

brown fat: A kind of fat found in hibernating mammals, and to some extent in humans, in which futile cycles take place so that energy nutrients are oxidized and generate heat without their energy being stored or used to do work.

brown sugar: Sugar crystals contained in molasses syrup with natural flavor and color, 91 to 96 percent pure sucrose. (Some refiners add syrup to refined white sugar to make brown sugar.) See Controversy 4A.

buffer: A compound that can stabilize pH by picking up or releasing hydrogen ions as needed.

CAD (coronary artery disease): Another term for CHD.

calorie: A measure of the amount of energy in food. The nutritionist's calorie is actually a kilocalorie (*k*calorie or *k*cal), 1000 times as large as the physicist's calorie, but the two terms are often used interchangeably with reference to foods. Accurately speaking, a *k*calorie is the amount of heat energy necessary to raise the temperature of 1000 grams of water 1° Centigrade (*calor* means "heat"; *kilo* means "1000").

capillaries: The smallest of the blood vessels; constituents of blood and body fluids filter across their walls to and from the tissues. See Figure 2 in Appendix A.

carbohydrate: A compound composed of carbon, hydrogen, and oxygen arranged as monosaccharides or multiples of monosaccharides (*carbo* means "carbon"; *hydrate* means "water," H_2O).

carcinogen (car-SIN-oh-jen): A cancer-causing substance (*carcin* means "cancer"; *gen* means "gives rise to").

carotene (CARRA-teen): The vitamin A precursor, a yellow pigment found in plants. Technically, this compound is known as beta (BAY-tah) carotene.

cellulose: The indigestible polysaccharide composed of glucose (see Chapter 4); it is the principal constituent of bran (the fiber of wheat) and is also found in fruits and vegetables.

cell salts: A mineral preparation sold in health food stores supposed to have been prepared from living, healthy cells. It is not necessary to take such preparations and it may be dangerous.

CF: See crude fiber.

chamomile (CAM-oh-meel): One of a number of plants whose leaves, flowers, or other parts are popularly used for the making of herbal teas. Hazards arise from the overuse of this, ginseng, sassafras, and others.

CHD (coronary heart disease): Atherosclerosis in the arteries feeding the heart muscle.

chlorophyll: The green pigment of plants, which absorbs energy from sunlight and transfers this energy to other molecules, initiating photosynthesis.

cholesterol (koh-LESS-ter-all): One of the sterols, manufactured in the body for a variety of purposes and also found in animal foods.

chylomicron (KIGH-low-MY-cron): A type of lipoprotein (very low in density) made by the cells of the intestinal wall; serves as a means of transporting lipids from the intestine through lymph and blood. Chylomicrons are cleared from the blood by liver cells.

***cis*-fatty acid:** See *trans-fatty acid.*

13-*cis*-retinoic acid: A synthetic derivative of vitamin A; oral doses look promising in preliminary tests with treatment-resistant acne.

clinical test: Also called a laboratory test or biochemical test; a test of a body tissue (most often blood or urine) used to detect abnormalities that may reflect abnormal nutritional status.

cobalamin (co-BAL-uh-min): Vitamin B_{12} (*cobal* means "cobalt-containing"; *amin* means "vitamin").

cocarcinogen: A carcinogen helper; see *promoter.*

coenzyme (co-EN-zime): A small molecule that works with an enzyme to promote the enzyme's activity (*co* means "with"). Many coenzymes have B vitamins as part of their structure.

collagen (COLL-uh-gen): A water-insoluble protein; the main constituent of supportive tissues such as tendons and blood vessel walls (*kolla* means "glue"; *gen* means "to produce").

colostrum (co-LAHS-trum): A milklike secretion from the breast, rich in protective factors, that precedes milk during the first day or so after delivery.

colon: The large intestine; see Figure 3 in Appendix A.

comedo (COMM-ee-doh): A blackhead; plural, **comedones** (COMM-ee-DOH-nees).

complementary proteins: Two or more proteins whose amino acid assortments complement each other in such a way that the essential amino acids missing from each are supplied by the other.

complete protein: A protein containing all the essential amino acids.

complex carbohydrate: The polysaccharides—starch, glycogen, and cellulose.

constipation: Hardness and dryness of bowel movements, associated with discomfort in passing them.

convenience food: A food preprepared or packaged in such a way that it is easy to cook and serve at home.

corn sweeteners: A term that refers to corn syrup and sugars derived from corn. See Controversy 4A.

corn syrup: A syrup produced by the action of enzymes on cornstarch. High-fructose corn syrup may contain as little as 42 percent or as much as 90 percent fructose; dextrose makes up the balance. See Controversy 4A.

cornea (CORN-ee-uh): The transparent membrane covering the outside of the front of the eye.

cortex: Outer covering; the part of the brain in which conscious thought takes place.

cretinism (CREE-tin-ism): Severe mental retardation of an infant caused by iodine deficiency during pregnancy.

critical period: A finite period during development. Certain events may occur during such a period but not later, and these will impact irreversibly on later developmental stages. A critical period is usually a period of cell division in a body organ.

crude fiber: The indigestible material found in food when it is subjected to a laboratory procedure; more technically, "the residue of plant food left after extraction by dilute acid followed by dilute alkali." Sometimes abbreviated *CF.*

CVA (cerebrovascular accident): A stroke or aneurysm in the brain.

CVD (cardiovascular disease): A general term for all diseases of the heart and blood vessels. Atherosclerosis is the main form of CVD.

cyst: An enlarged, deep pimple.

deep-vein thrombosis (throm-BOH-sis): Clot formation inside an interior vein in a body organ.

defecation (deff-uh-CAY-shun): Excretion of the feces.

dehydration (de-high-DRAY-shun): Loss of water from the body; a dangerous condition.

Delaney Clause: A clause in the Food Additive Amendment to the Food, Drug, and Cosmetic Act that states that no substance shall be added to foods that is known to cause cancer in animals or humans at any dose level, no matter how small.

denaturation: The change in shape of a protein brought about by heat, acid, base, alcohol, or heavy metals.

dermabrasion (DERM-uh-bray-zhun): Planing the skin to remove scars, a procedure requiring skill, and one that works on only certain kinds of scars (*dermis* means "skin"; *abrasion* means "sanding, planing").

DES (diethyl stilbestrol): A hormone added to cattle feed to promote growth; a carcinogen, now no longer in use.

dessicated liver: Dehydrated liver, a powder sold in health food stores and supposed to contain in concentrated form all the nutrients found in liver. Possibly not dangerous, this supplement has no particular nutritional merit, and grocery-store liver is considerably less expensive.

dextrose: The technical name for glucose.

DF: See *dietary fiber.*

diabetes (dye-uh-BEET-eez): An hereditary metabolic disease characterized by an inadequate supply of effective insulin, which renders a person unable to regulate the blood glucose level normally. See also note 6 of Chapter 4.

dietary fiber: The indigestible material actually remaining when food passes through the intestinal tract; more technically, the residue of plant food resistant to hydrolysis [splitting] by human digestive enzymes. Sometimes abbreviated *DF.*

diet history: An interview used to determine the adequacy of a person's dietary intake of nutrients, used as one means of evaluating nutritional status.

dipeptide (dye-PEP-tide): A protein fragment two amino acids long.

disaccharide (dye-SACK-uh-ride): A pair of monosaccharides bonded together; sucrose, maltose, or lactose (*di* means "two"; *saccharide* means "sugar").

diuretic (dye-you-RET-ic): A medication causing increased water excretion (*dia* means "through"; *ouron* means "urine").

diverticulitis (dye-ver-tic-you-LYE-tiss): Inflammation or infection of diverticular pockets in the intestine; a disease condition which can lead to rupture.

diverticulosis (dye-ver-tic-you-LOCE-iss): Outpocketings of weakened areas of the intestinal wall; can lead to diverticulitis.

drug: The FDA has suggested that this term be used to identify foods or vitamin/mineral pills containing vitamins and/or minerals at levels above 150 percent of the U.S. RDA.

ectomorph (EK-toh-morf): See *body type.*

edema (uh-DEEM-uh): The swelling of body tissue caused by leakage of fluid from the blood vessels, seen in (among other conditions) protein deficiency.

electrolyte balance (ee-LEC-tro-lite): Distribution of electrolytes (salts) among the body fluids.

embolus (EM-boh-lus): A clot (thrombus) that has broken loose from one location and traveled until it has lodged in a small artery cutting off the blood flow. Once the embolus has lodged (embolism) it has the same effect as a thrombosis.

embryo (EM-bree-oh): The developing infant during its second to eighth week after conception. Before the second week it is called an ovum (OH-vum) or zygote (ZYE-goat).

empty calorie food: A popular term used to denote foods that contain no nutrients, only calories. Actually, all foods contain some nutrients. Therefore most nutritionists prefer to say "food of low nutrient density." See *nutrient density.*

emulsifier (ee-MULL-si-fire): A compound with both water-soluble and fat-soluble portions that can attract lipids into water solution.

endocrine: A term to describe a gland or hormone: secreting or being secreted into the blood (*endo* means "into").

endomorph (EN-doh-morf): See *body type.*

energy: The capacity to do work.

energy nutrient: A nutrient that provides energy the body can use—carbohydrate, fat, or protein. (Alcohol provides energy but is not a nutrient.)

engineered food: A food subjected to a complex technical process, such as extraction of certain components.

enriched: Refers to a process by which the nutrients thiamin, riboflavin, niacin, and iron are added to refined grains and grain products at levels specified by law. After enrichment, a grain product has approximately the same amount of thiamin, niacin, and iron, and about twice as much riboflavin, as the original whole-grain product would have had.

enzyme (EN-zime): A protein catalyst. A **catalyst** is a compound that facilitates (speeds up the rate of) a chemical reaction without itself being altered in the process.

epithelial tissue (ep-i-THEE-lee-al): The cells of most body surfaces, including the eyes and skin and the linings of the lungs, urinogenital tract, and intestinal tract.

ergogenic: A term used to refer to foods that are supposed to have unusual energy-producing power (*ergo* means "work"; *genic* means "gives rise to"). Actually, no foods are ergogenic.

esophagus (es-SOFF-uh-gus): The muscular tube that conveys swallowed food from the mouth to the stomach. See Figure 3 in Appendix A.

essential amino acid: An amino acid that cannot be synthesized at all or that cannot be synthesized in amounts sufficient to meet the physiological need of the body.

essential fatty acid: A fatty acid that cannot be synthesized in the body.

essential nutrient: A compound that can't be synthesized by the body in amounts sufficient to meet physiological needs. Many nutrients are needed by the body, but the word *essential* in this term refers only to those that must be supplied by eating food.

evolution: The process by which undesirable or maladaptive inherited characteristics (mutations) are weeded out and desirable or adaptive characteristics are handed down to succeeding generations.

exchange: A food serving equivalent in energy nutrient composition and calorie content to those on one of the exchange lists. For example, one small potato is a bread exchange: It is equivalent to one slice of bread in protein-fat-carbohydrate content and calories.

exocrine: A term used to describe a gland or hormone: secreting or being secreted out of the blood into the small intestine or onto the skin (*exo* means "out").

external cue theory: The theory that some persons eat in response to such external factors as the presence of food or the time of day rather than to such internal factors as hunger.

extrinsic factor (ex-TRIN-sic): A factor found outside a system; the name given to vitamin B_{12} at the time when it was known only as an unidentified substance in liver that would cure pernicious anemia. See also *intrinsic factor.*

fabricated food: A food put together from highly processed ingredients, such as substitute-meat-burgers made from textured vegetable protein.

fast food: Food prepared quickly in a fast-food restaurant such as a hamburger stand or fried-chicken place.

fat: A lipid that is solid at room temperature (70° F or 25° C).

fatfold test: A clinical test of body fatness in which the thickness of a fold of skin on the back of the arm (triceps), below the shoulder blade (subscapular), or in other places is measured with an instrument called a caliper.

fatty acid: An organic acid composed of a carbon chain with hydrogens attached and an acid group at one end.

feces (FEECE-eeze): The bowel movement, the excretion product of the GI tract.

fetal alcohol syndrome: The cluster of symptoms seen in an infant or child whose mother consumed excess alcohol during her pregnancy; includes mental and physical retardation with facial and other body deformities.

fetus (FEET-us): The developing infant from the eighth week after conception until its birth.

fiber: The indigestible residue of plant food, composed of the carbohydrates cellulose, pectin, and hemicellulose and the noncarbohydrate lignin. More precisely, crude fiber (CF) is the residue of plant food left after extraction by dilute acid followed by dilute alkali. Dietary fiber (DF), a new term, is the residue of plant food resistant to hydrolysis (splitting) by human digestive enzymes.

fibrin (FYE-brin): A water-insoluble protein, the principal protein material in a blood clot.

fight-or-flight reaction: The body's response to danger or threat, mediated by the stress hormones, the effect of which is to make every body system maximally ready for physical exertion.

fluid balance: Appropriate distribution of fluid among body compartments.

folacin (FOLL-uh-sin): One of the B vitamins; also known as folic acid.

folic acid (FOLL-ick): See *folacin.*

food: Nutritive material taken into the body to keep it alive and enable it to grow (*nutritive* means "containing nutrients").

fortified: Refers to the addition of nutrients to foods—for example, vitamins A and D to milk, iodine to salt, iron to breakfast cereals. See also *enriched.*

frame size: The size of a person's bones and musculature. This is a vague term; frame-size standards have not been established.

fructose (FROOK-toce): A monosaccharide sometimes known as fruit sugar (*fruct* means "fruit"; *ose* means "sugar").

futile cycle: A metabolic activity of the body's cells in which chemical reactions take place with a loss, and no storage, of energy. Futile cycles are believed to account for some people's "fast metabolism" and their ability to consume calories without the expected weight gain.

galactose (ga-LACK-toce): A monosaccharide; part of the disaccharide lactose.

gall bladder: The storage organ for bile; see Figure 3 in Appendix A.

gene: A unit of a cell's inheritance, made of a chemical, DNA, that is copied faithfully so that every time the cell divides both its daughters get identical copies. Genes direct the cells' machinery to make the proteins that form the cell's structures and do its work.

ginseng (JINN-seng): See *chamomile.*

glucose (GLOO-coce): A monosaccharide sometimes known as blood sugar, sometimes as grape sugar; also called dextrose.

glucose tolerance factor (GTF): An organic compound containing chromium; found in foods.

glycerol (GLISS-er-all): An organic alcohol composed of a three-carbon chain, each with an alcohol group (-OH) attached; forms the backbone of triglycerides.

glycogen (GLIGH-co-gen): An animal polysaccharide composed of glucose, manufactured in the body and stored in liver and muscle.

goiter (GOY-ter): Enlargement of the thyroid gland due to iodine deficiency (simple goiter).

granola: A cereal made from mixed oats and other grains.

GRAS (generally recognized as safe) list: A list of food additives, established by the Food and Drug Administration (FDA), that had long been in use and were believed safe. The list is subject to revision as new facts become known.

hard water: Water with a high calcium and magnesium concentration.

hazard: State of danger; used to refer to any circumstance in which toxicity is possible under normal conditions of use. See also *toxicity.*

HDL (high-density lipoproteins): Lipoproteins that return cholesterol from the storage places to the liver for dismantling and disposal.

health food: A misleading term used on labels, usually of organic or natural foods, to imply unusual power to promote health. This term had no legal definition as of 1981.

hemicellulose: A carbohydrate fiber that occurs in the same foods as cellulose.

hemoglobin (HEEM-o-globe-in): The oxygen-carrying protein of the blood; found in the red blood cells (*hemo* means "blood"; *globin* means "spherical protein").

hemorrhoids (HEM-or-oids): Varicose veins in the rectum, sometimes caused by the pressure resulting from constipation.

hiatal hernia (hye-AY-tal): An outpocketing at the top of the stomach at the point of entry of the esophagus. Such a hernia can slide up and down through the diaphragm (see Figure 3 in Appendix A), becoming irritated, and can be most uncomfortable when the stomach is full and when a person is lying down so that the stomach contents put pressure on it.

homeopathy (home-ee-OPP-path-ee): A branch of medicine (supposedly) that focuses on prevention of disease, promotion of health, and restoration of disturbed body balances by feeding needed nutrients. Homeopathic "physicians" may or may not have M.D. degrees.

honey: Invert sugar formed by an enzyme from nectar gathered by bees. Composition and flavor vary, but honey usually contains fructose, glucose, maltose, and sucrose.

hormone: A chemical messenger, secreted by one organ (an endocrine gland) in response to a condition in the body, that acts on another organ or organs and elicits a specific response that will change the condition.

hunger: The physiological need for food.

hydrogenation (high-droh-gen-AY-shun): The process of adding hydrogen to unsaturated fat to make it more solid and more resistant to chemical change.

hyperactivity: Excessive activity, a symptom which can result from any of a multitude of different causes. See also *hyperkinesis.*

hyperglycemia (HIGH-per-gligh-SEEM-ee-uh): An abnormally high blood glucose concentration (above about 170 mg per 100 ml) (*hyper* means "too much"; *glyce* means "glucose"; *emia* means "in the blood").

hyperkeratinization: See *keratinization.*

hyperkinesia (high-per-kin-EEZ-ee-uh): The medical term for the symptom hyperactivity.

hyperkinesis (high-per-kin-EECE-iss): The syndrome characterized by motor restlessness, short attention span, poor impulse control, learning difficulties, and emotional instability that is responsive to treatment with stimulant drugs. Not the same as minimal brain dysfunction.

hypertension: High blood pressure (*hyper* means "too much"; *tension* means "pressure").

hypoglycemia (HIGH-po-gligh-SEEM-ee-uh): An abnormally low blood glucose concentration (below about 60 to 70 mg per 100 ml) (*hypo* means "too little"; *glyce* means "sugar"; *emia* means "in the blood"). **Reactive hypoglycemia** is a temporary hypoglycemia that may be experienced by any normal person in response to an overload of sugar. **Spontaneous hypoglycemia** is a rare chronic hypoglycemia seen in people with abnormal carbohydrate metabolism which requires diagnosis, medical treatment, and a special diet.

hypothalamus (high-poh-THALL-uh-mus): A part of the brain that senses a variety of conditions in the blood, such as temperature, salt content, glucose content, and others, and signals other parts of the brain or body to change those conditions when necessary.

ideal weight: The average weight given in tables for insured persons of a given sex and height—not necessarily ideal for a given individual.

imitation food: A food nutritionally inferior to the food it imitates. This term must by law appear on the label of a food if it contains 10 percent less of the U.S. RDA of an essential nutrient than the food it imitates.

immunity: The specific disease resistance conferred by the ability of the body to manufacture antibodies promptly against a given disease agent when there has been prior exposure to that agent.

implantation: The stage of development in which the fertilized egg embeds itself in the wall of the uterus and begins to develop, during the first two weeks after conception.

inborn error (of metabolism): An inherited disorder caused by a defective gene, usually the gene for a specific enzyme.

incidental food additive: An additive unintentionally added to a food by an accident of contamination such as by packaging materials or chemicals used during processing.

incomplete protein: A protein lacking one or more of the essential amino acids.

INQ (index of nutritional quality): A measure of the nutritional quality of a food, derived by comparison of selected nutrient contents (relative to the RDA) with calorie value (relative to the RDA).

insulin: A hormone secreted by the pancreas in response to increased blood glucose concentration.

intentional food additive: An additive intentionally added to food, such as nutrients or colors.

international unit: See *IU.*

intrinsic factor: A factor found inside a system; the name given to the factor, synthesized in the stomach, that attaches to vitamin B_{12} to facilitate its absorption. See also *extrinsic factor.*

invert sugar: A mixture of glucose and fructose formed by the splitting of sucrose in a chemical process. Sold only in liquid form, sweeter than sucrose, invert sugar is used as an additive to help preserve food freshness and prevent shrinkage.

ion (EYE-on): An electrically charged particle, such as sodium (positively charged) or chloride (negatively charged).

iron-deficiency anemia: Reduction of the size of red blood cells and loss of their color because of iron deficiency.

iron overload: The state of having more iron in the body than it needs or can handle. Iron can become toxic in this situation.

ischemia (iss-SHE-me-uh): The deterioration and death of tissue (for example, of heart muscle), often caused by atherosclerosis. Ischemic heart disease (IHD) is another term for atherosclerosis and its relatives.

IU (international units): A measure of fat-soluble vitamin activity, now being phased out but still appearing in tables of food contents of vitamin A.

junk food: A popular term used to denote foods that are "bad" for one—for example, foods high in salt, sugar, or fat content.

juvenile-onset obesity: Obesity arising in childhood; also called "developmental obesity."

kcalorie: See *calorie.*

kelp: : A kind of seaweed used by the Japanese as a foodstuff. Kelp tablets are made from dehydrated kelp.

keratin (KER-uh-tin): A water-insoluble protein; the principal material of hair and nails (*kerat* means "horn").

keratinization: The process by which the epithelial cells, deprived of vitamin A, fill with keratin instead of producing mucus; also called hyperkeratinization.

ketones (ketone bodies): Molecules produced by condensing together the incompletely oxidized fragments of fat formed when carbohydrate is not available to assist fat to be oxidized in the normal way.

ketosis (kee-TOH-sis): An undesirably high concentration of ketones, such as acetone, in the blood and urine (*osis* means "too much in the blood").

kidneys: The organs that filter the blood to remove waste material to be delivered to the bladder for excretion.

kwashiorkor (kwash-ee-OR-core, kwash-ee-or-CORE): The deficiency disease suffered by newly weaned children whose calorie supply is adequate but whose protein supply is not.

lactalbumin (lact-AL-byoo-min): The chief protein in human breast milk, as opposed to casein (CAY-seen), the chief protein of cow's milk.

lactic acid: An acid produced when oxygen is not available to oxidize pyruvic acid all the way to carbon dioxide and water. Lactic acid accumulates in hard-working muscles and makes them sore.

lactoferrin (lak-toe-FERR-in): A factor in breast milk that binds iron and keeps it from supporting the growth of the infant's intestinal bacteria.

lacto-ovo-vegetarian: A vegetarian who excludes animal flesh but eats such animal products as milk and eggs (*lacto* means "milk"; *ovo* means "eggs").

lactose: A disaccharide composed of glucose and galactose; commonly known as milk sugar (*lact* means "milk"; *ose* means "sugar").

lactose intolerance: An inborn error of metabolism that becomes apparent at about the age of four and involves failure of the intestinal enzyme lactase to digest milk sugar. Symptoms include abdominal pain, nausea, and/or diarrhea after drinking milk.

laetrile (LAY-uh-trill): A substance isolated from apricot pits, advertised as a cancer cure and sold under the trade-name "vitamin B_{17}" but actually not a vitamin and never shown to be either safe or effective as a cancer cure. See Controversy 11A for the details.

LDL (low-density lipoproteins): Lipoproteins that transport lipids from liver to other (muscle, mammary gland, fat) tissues.

lecithin (LESS-ih-thin): A phospholipid, a major constituent of cell membranes, manufactured by the liver and also found in many foods.

legume (leg-GYOOM, LEG-yoom): A plant of the bean and pea family having roots with nodules that contain bacteria that can fix atmospheric nitrogen. The seeds are rich in protein that is of high quality as compared with that of most other plant foods.

let-down reflex: The reflex that forces milk to the front of the breast when the infant begins to nurse.

levulose: The technical name for fructose.

lignin: A noncarbohydrate fiber that occurs in grains, especially wheat and rye, cabbage and other vegetables, apples and strawberries and other fruits, and nuts.

linoleic acid (lin-o-LAY-ic): A fatty acid essential for humans.

lipids (LIP-ids): A family of compounds soluble in organic solvents, which includes the triglycerides (fats and oils), phospholipids, and sterols; commonly called **fat**.

lipoprotein (LIP-o-PRO-teen): A cluster of lipids wrapped in protein that otherwise would not be soluble in blood or lymph. The four main types of lipoproteins are chylomicrons, VLDL, LDL, and HDL; IDL (intermediate density lipoproteins) are sometimes identified as a fifth type.

liver: The large, many-lobed organ that lies under the ribs on both sides of the body and filters the blood, removing, processing, and readying for redistribution many of its materials.

low birthweight: A birthweight of 5½ pounds (2500 grams) or less, used as a predictor of poor health in the newborn and as an indicator of probably poor nutritional status of the mother during and/or before pregnancy. Normal birthweight is 6 ½ pounds (3500 grams) or more.

lymph: The fluid outside the circulatory system that bathes the cells, derived from the blood by being pressed through the capillary walls; similar to the blood in composition but without red blood cells.

macronutrient element: See *major mineral.*

major mineral: (macronutrient element): An essential mineral nutrient found in the human body, constituting more than 0.005 percent of the body weight (*macro* means "large").

maltitol: See *sorbitol.*

maltose: A disaccharide composed of two glucose units; sometimes known as malt sugar.

mannitol: See *sorbitol.*

marasmus (ma-RAZ-mus): The calorie-deficiency disease; starvation.

margin of safety: As used when speaking of food additives, a zone between the concentration normally used and that at which a hazard exists. For common table salt, for example, the margin of safety is fivefold (five times the concentration normally used would be hazardous).

MDR (minimum daily requirement): A term once used on labels to express vitamin and mineral contents; it proved unsatisfactory because it did not accurately represent people's nutrient needs; now replaced by the more suitable terms, RDA (see Chapter 3) and U.S. RDA (see Chapter 11).

megaloblastic anemia (MEG-ah-low-BLAS-tic a-NEE-mee-uh): A kind of anemia (blood disease) in which the red blood cells are large and immature (*megalo* means "great"; *blast* means "cell"); can be caused by a deficiency of vitamin B_{12} or folic acid. When caused by a B_{12} deficiency, it is pernicious anemia.

menadione (men-uh-DYE-own): A synthetic compound similar to vitamin K.

mesomorph (MEZZ-oh-morf): See *body type.*

metabolism: The sum total of all the chemical reactions that go on in living cells.

methemoglobin (meth-EEM-oh-globe-in): A form of the blood protein hemoglobin that cannot carry oxygen. Hemoglobin exposed to excessive nitrite can turn to methemoglobin.

MI: See *myocardial infarct.*

micronutrient element: See *trace mineral.*

microvilli (MY-croh-vill-eye): Tiny hairlike projections on each cell of the intestinal tract lining that can trap nutrient particles and translocate them into the cells (singular: **microvillus**).

milk anemia: Iron-deficiency anemia caused by drinking so much milk that iron-rich foods are displaced in the diet.

mineral: A naturally occurring, inorganic, homogeneous substance; an element.

monoglyceride (monn-oh-GLISS-er-ide): One of the products of digestion of lipids; a glycerol molecule with one fatty acid attached to it (*mono* means "one" (fatty acid); *glyceride* means "a compound of glycerol").

monosaccharide (mon-oh-SACK-uh-ride): A single sugar—glucose, fructose, or galactose (*mono* means "one").

monosodium glutamate (MSG): A flavor-enhancer used widely in Oriental (especially Chinese and Japanese) cookery; it can cause an intolerance reaction (the "Chinese restaurant syndrome") in some individuals. One trade name is Accent.

mucus (MYOO-cus): The thick, slippery inner coating of the intestines (and other organs) which protects the cells (for example, from exposure to digestive juices). The adjective form is *mucous.*

mutation: An event that alters a gene so that it codes for a slightly different protein; a very rare event but one that makes possible variation among organisms (*muta* means "change").

mutual supplementation: The strategy, used by vegetarians, of combining two protein foods in a meal so that each food provides the essential amino acid(s) lacking in the other. See also *complementary proteins.*

myocardial infarct (MI) (my-oh-CARD-ee-ul in-FARKT): The sudden shutting off of the blood flow to the heart muscle by a thrombus or embolism; the same as a heart attack (*myo* means "muscle"; *cardium* means "heart"; *infarct* means "blocking off").

myoglobin (MYE-o-globe-in): The oxygen-holding protein of the muscles (*myo* means "muscle").

natural food: A food that has been altered as little as possible from the original farm-grown state. As used on labels, this term may misleadingly imply unusual power to promote health. Not legally defined as of 1981.

natural selection: The means by which evolution takes place: Among the varied offspring in a generation, those that are best adapted survive to reproduce and pass on the genes that gave them the adaptive advantage so that the next generation has a different gene pool.

natural sweeteners: A term that refers to any of many sugars. See the Miniglossary in Controversy 4A.

NCBR (nutrient-calorie benefit ratio): A measure of the nutritional quality of a food; similar to INQ.

neuritis (nyoo-RYE-tis): Inflammation or infection of the nerves (*neur* means "nerve"; *itis* means "inflammation"); a symptom of deficiency of thiamin (among other things). Beriberi is sometimes known as polyneuritis—neuritis of many nerves (*poly* means "many").

niacin (NIGH-uh-sin): One of the B vitamins (formerly vitamin G or B_3). Active forms include nicotinic acid, nicotinamide, or niacinamide.

niacin equivalents: The unit of measure of the niacin activity in food, computed by adding the amount of niacin preformed in the food to that theoretically obtainable from the tryptophan present.

niacinamide, nicotinamide, nicotinic acid: Active forms of niacin.

nicotine (NICK-oh-teen): A toxic substance found in tobacco; not related to nicotinic acid.

night blindness: A symptom of vitamin A deficiency. After being bleached by bright light at night, the visual purple pigment regenerates slowly, with a lag time during which the person is unable to see.

nitrate: Part of a salt containing nitrogen, abundant in vegetables.

nitrite: Part of a salt containing nitrogen which can be produced from nitrate during the processing of vegetables; also such a salt used as an additive to prevent botulism in cured meats.

nitrogen balance: The amount of nitrogen consumed (nitrogen-in) as compared with the amount excreted (nitrogen-out) in a given period of time. In nitrogen equilibrium, nitrogen-in equals nitrogen-out. In positive balance, nitrogen-in exceeds nitrogen-out; in negative nitrogen balance, nitrogen-in is less than nitrogen-out.

nitrosamine (nigh-TROH-suh-meen): A compound formed when nitrites and amines combine; a carcinogen.

nutrient: A substance obtained from food and used in the body to promote growth, maintenance, or repair.

nutrient density: A characteristic of a food such that it provides a high quantity (relative to need) of one or more essential nutrients, with a small quantity (relative to need) of calories.

nutritious food: A food with high nutrient density.

obesity: Body weight more than 15 to 25 percent above desirable weight; excessive body fatness.

occlusion (ock-CLOO-zhun): Shutting off the blood flow in an artery.

oil: A lipid that is liquid at room temperature (70° F or 25° C).

oleic acid (oh-LAY-ic): A mono-unsaturated fatty acid found in animal and vegetable oils.

organic (chemist's definition): Containing carbon atoms or, more precisely, containing carbon-carbon or carbon-hydrogen bonds.

organic (popular definition): Referring to foods and nutrients, produced without the use of chemical fertilizers, pesticides, or additives. As used on labels, this term may misleadingly imply unusual power to promote health. Not legally defined as of 1981. See Controversy 1.

osteomalacia (oss-tee-oh-ma-LAY-shuh): The vitamin D- and calcium-deficiency disease in adults; "adult rickets" (*osteo* means "bone"; *malacia* means "softening").

osteoporosis (oss-tee-oh-pore-OH-sis): A disease of older persons in which the bone becomes porous (*poros* means "porous"); also known as adult bone loss.

overweight: Body weight more than 10 percent above desirable weight.

P:S ratio: The ratio of polyunsaturated to saturated fat in the diet, a factor that influences blood cholesterol level.

pancreas: A gland that secretes the endocrine hormone insulin and also produces the exocrine secretions that aid digestion in the small intestine. See Figure 3 in Appendix A.

pangamic acid/pangamate: A name used for a substance supposed to be isolated from apricot pits. Actually, pangamate has no particular chemical identity. See also vitamin B_{15}.

pantothenic acid (pan-toe-THEN-ic): One of the B vitamins.

PCM: See *protein-calorie malnutrition*.

pectin: The fiber of apple, citrus fruits, and other fruits, notable for its effectiveness in lowering blood cholesterol.

pellagra (pell-AY-gra): The niacin-deficiency disease.

peristalsis (perri-STALL-sis): The wave-like squeezing motions of the stomach and intestines that push their contents along.

pernicious anemia (per-NISH-uss a-NEE-mee-uh): The vitamin B_{12}-deficiency disease.

pH: A measure of the acid-base balance. A low pH means strong acid, as in the stomach (about pH 2). Neutral pH is 7; pH above 7 is basic. The pH of the blood and other body fluids is slightly above neutral (for example, blood pH is 7.35 to 7.45).

phospholipid (FOSS-foe-LIP-id): One of the three main classes of lipids; a lipid similar to a triglyceride but having a phosphorus-containing acid in place of one of the fatty acids.

photosynthesis: The synthesis of carbohydrates by green plants from carbon dioxide and water using the sun's energy (*photo* means "light"; *synthesis* means "making").

physical examination: A technique used in the evaluation of nutritional status, which includes examination of accessible body parts such as the skin, eyes, teeth, tongue, and hair, and also includes anthropometric measures.

pica (PYE-ka): The eating of clay, ice, cornstarch, paint, or other nonnutritious substances; often a symptom of iron deficiency.

placebo (pla-SEE-bo): An inert, harmless medication given to provide comfort and hope.

placebo effect: The healing effect that faith in medicine, even inert medicine, often has.

plaque (PLACK): A mound of lipid material, smooth muscle cells, and calcium that accumulates in the inner artery wall, causing atherosclerosis.

plasma (PLAZ-muh): Unclotted blood with only the cells removed. The terms *blood, plasma,* and *serum* mean about the same thing when referring to concentrations of substances in the blood like glucose or cholesterol, but they refer to different laboratory procedures used to measure those concentrations.

point of unsaturation: A site in a molecule where the bonding is such that additional hydrogen atoms can easily be added.

polyneuritis (polly-nyoo-RYE-tis): A symptom of beriberi. See *neuritis.*

polysaccharide (polly-SACK-uh-ride): Many (ten or more) monosaccharides chemically linked together (*poly* means "many").

polyunsaturated fat: A triglyceride in which one or more of the fatty acids is polyunsaturated.

polyunsaturated fatty acid (PUFA): A fatty acid in which two or more points of unsaturation occur.

polyunsaturated:saturated fat ratio: See *P:S ratio*

precursor (PRE-curse-er): The forerunner of a compound in a chemical pathway; an inactive compound which can be converted into an active compound. For example, a provitamin is the precursor of (can be converted into) a vitamin.

primary deficiency: A nutrient deficiency caused by inadequate dietary intake of the nutrient.

processed food: Any food subjected to a process such as enrichment, refining, fortification, alteration of texture, mixing, or cooking.

promoter: A substance that does not initiate cancer but that favors its development once the initiating event has taken place.

prostate gland: A gland associated with the male reproductive organs.

protein: A compound—composed of carbon, hydrogen, oxygen, and nitrogen —arranged as amino acids linked in a chain, usually about 300 units long. Some amino acids also contain sulfur.

protein efficiency ratio (PER): A measure of protein quality assessed by determining the extent to which a given protein supports weight gain in a growing child.

protein-calorie malnutrition (PCM): The world's most widespread malnutrition problem, including both kwashiorkor and marasmus and states in which they overlap.

protein-sparing action: The action of carbohydrate and fat, which by providing energy allows protein to be used for other purposes.

protein synthesis (SIN-thuh-sis): The process by which amino acids are assembled into proteins by the cells (*synthesis* means "making, putting together").

prothrombin (pro-THROM-bin): One of the proteins involved in blood clotting.

provitamin: A compound that the body can convert into an active vitamin.

P:S ratio: The ratio of polyunsaturated to saturated fat in the diet, a factor that influences blood cholesterol level.

pure vegetarian: See *vegan*.

pylorus (pye-LORE-us): The circular muscle that regulates the opening at the bottom of the stomach. See Figure 3 in Appendix A.

pyridoxal, pyridoxamine, pyridoxine: (peer-uh-DOX-al, peer-uh-DOX-uh-meen, peer-uh-DOX-in): Different chemical forms of vitamin B_6.

pyruvic acid (pye-ROO-vic): A breakdown product of glucose. Glucose can be oxidized to pyruvic acid without the help of oxygen, but pyruvic acid can be further oxidized only when oxygen is available and is shunted to lactic acid whenever oxygen is in short supply.

raw sugar: The residue of evaporated sugar cane juice, tan or brown in color. Raw sugar can only be sold in the U.S. if the impurities (dirt, insect fragments, and the like) have been removed. See Controversy 4A.

RDA (Recommended Dietary Allowances): Nutrient intakes suggested by the Food and Nutrition Board of the National Academy of Sciences/National Research Council for the maintenance of health in people in the United States.

RE (retinol equivalents): The newer units in which vitamin A is measured, now replacing IU. See Chapter 9.

refereed journal: A journal that refuses to publish research or review articles submitted to it until they have been approved by two or more referees, experts in the specific subject area of the articles and in the research methods used.

reference man: A theoretical "average" figure used by the Food and Nutrition Board for calculating nutrient and calorie needs. He is 5 feet 9 inches tall, 154 pounds (70 kilograms), age 23 to 50.

reference protein: Egg protein, designated by the FAO as the highest-quality protein (BV = 94 percent), the standard against which other proteins are measured.

reference woman: A theoretical "average" figure used by the Food and Nutrition Board for calculating nutrient and calorie needs. She is 5 feet 5 inches tall, 128 pounds (58 kilograms), age 23 to 50.

refined: Refers to the process by which the coarse parts of the food products are removed. For example, the refining of wheat into flour involves removing three of the four parts of the kernel—the chaff, the bran, and the germ—leaving only the endosperm (starch).

requirement: That amount of a nutrient that will just prevent the development of specific deficiency signs; distinguished from the RDA, which is a recommended and generous allowance.

residue: A term not used here, residue is sometimes confused with fiber but actually refers to whatever material still remains solid when the intestinal contents reach the colon. Milk, for example, contains no fiber, but its curds form a residue in the intestines.

retina (RET-in-uh): The layer of light-sensitive cells lining the back of the inside of the eye.

retinoic acid: A form of vitamin A. See Controversy 14A.

retinol (RET-in-all): The chemical name for an active form of vitamin A.

retinol equivalents: See *RE.*

riboflavin (RYE-bo-flay-vin): Vitamin B_2.

rickets: The vitamin D- and calcium-deficiency disease in children.

roughage (RUFF-idge): The coarse material in food that remains undigested in the intestine and aids in maintaining the tone of the intestinal muscles by stimulating them, a term that has now been largely replaced by the term *fiber.*

salicylate (sa-LISS-uh-late): A compound resembling aspirin in chemical structure.

salt: A compound composed of a positive and a negative ion. For example, sodium chloride (Na^+Cl^-) is table salt.

salt balance: See *electrolyte balance.*

sassafras: See *chamomile.*

satiety (sat-EYE-uh-tee): The feeling of fullness or satisfaction after a meal. Fat provides more satiety than carbohydrate or protein, because it slows the stomach's motility.

saturated fatty acid: A fatty acid carrying the maximum possible number of hydrogen atoms (having no points of unsaturation).

scurvy: The vitamin C-deficiency disease.

SDE (specific dynamic effect): The energy needed for assimilating nutrients from food (including the energy for digestion, immediate absorption of nutrients into the body, and immediate transfer of those nutrients into the cells). Also known as **specific dynamic activity**.

sebum (SEE-bum): The skin's natural oil, actually a mixture of oils and waxes, that helps keep skin and hair moist.

secondary deficiency: A nutrient deficiency caused by something other than diet, like a disease condition that reduces absorption, increases excretion, or causes destruction of the nutrient.

serum (SEER-um): The watery portion of the blood that remains after the cells and clot-forming material have been removed. See *plasma.*

set point: A term used to describe the point around which regulation takes place, as on a thermostat—the setting below which conservation measures are initiated and above which wasting measures take over. In body weight, the set point is considered to be the body's preferred weight, that to which it tends to return naturally after any disturbance.

shock: An emergency reaction of the body in which the blood pressure drops suddenly; a dangerous condition.

simple carbohydrate: The monosaccharides (glucose, fructose, and galactose) and the disaccharides (maltose, lactose, and sucrose).

skinfold test: See *fatfold test.*

small intestine: The organ in which most of the major digestive events take place. See Figure 3 in Appendix A.

soft water: Water with a low calcium and magnesium concentration.

sorbitol, mannitol, maltitol, xylitol: Sugar alcohols, that can be derived from fruits or produced from dextrose.

spastic colon: A condition in which the colon is irritable and tends to tighten, causing constipation. Stimulation by fiber makes this kind of constipation worse, not better.

specific dynamic activity/effect: See *SDE.*

spermatogenesis (sperm-at-oh-JEN-uh-sis): The process of manufacturing sperm, a function that can be disturbed by the use of anabolic steroids.

Standard of Identity: A legal statement of the ingredients required in such standard products as mayonnaise. These products must conform to the listings if they use the standard name on the label.

staple: With respect to food, one which is used frequently or daily in the diet; for example, potatoes (in Ireland) or rice (in the Far East).

starch: A plant polysaccharide composed of glucose, digestible by humans.

sterol (STEER-all): One of the three main classes of lipids; a lipid with a structure similar to that of cholesterol.

subclinical deficiency: : A nutrient deficiency that has no visible or otherwise detectable (clinical) symptoms. It is possible for such a deficiency to develop (see the discussion of loss of iron from body stores in Chapter 3), but the term is often used as a scare tactic to persuade consumers to buy nutrient supplements they don't need.

sucrose: Table sugar or powdered (confectioner's) sugar, 99.9 percent pure; a disaccharide composed of glucose and fructose, also known as beet sugar or cane sugar (*sucr* means "sugar").

sugar: A monosaccharide or disaccharide; a simple carbohydrate.

supplement: : A preparation (such as a pill, powder, or liquid) containing nutrients that can be used to supplement the diet. Breakfast cereals that contain "100 percent of the U.S. RDA" for certain nutrients are also considered dietary supplements.

syndrome: A cluster of symptoms.

tartrazine (TAR-truh-zeen): Yellow dye no. 5, a salicylate, which causes occasional allergies.

testicular degeneration: Wasting of the testicles, can be a side effect of the use of anabolic steroids.

thiamin (THIGH-uh-min) Vitamin B_1.

thrombosis (throm-BOH-sis): The closing off of an artery by a growing clot. A cerebral thrombosis is such an event in the brain—a stroke (*cerebrum* means "brain"). A coronary thrombosis is such an event in the arteries that feed the heart muscle—a heart attack (*coronary* means "crowning" the heart).

thrombus (THROM-bus): A clot that forms in an artery. See also *embolus.*

thyroxin (thigh-ROX-in): A hormone secreted by the thyroid gland; regulates the rate of the body's metabolic activity (that is, the rate at which the body uses energy from food); also known as thyroid hormone.

tocopherol (toe-COFF-er-all): The chemical name for a class of compounds with vitamin E activity. Alpha tocopherol is the most active of these.

toxicity: The ability of a substance to be toxic (cause harmful effects). All substance are toxic if high enough concentrations are used. See also *hazard.*

trace mineral (micronutrient element): An essential mineral nutrient found in the human body, constituting less than 0.005 percent of the body weight (*micro* means "small").

***trans*-fatty acid:** An unsaturated fatty acid that has assumed an unusual shape, often as a result of heat processing (*trans* means "opposite sides" and refers to the arrangement of the parts of the molecule around one of the double bonds.) The natural form is *cis* ("same sides").

triglycerides (try-GLISS-er-ides): The major class of dietary lipids. A triglyceride is a compound in which three fatty acids are attached to a molecule of glycerol.

tripeptide (try-PEP-tide): A protein fragment three amino acids long.

tryptophan (TRIP-toe-fane): An amino acid essential for human beings; convertible to niacin in the body.

U.S. RDA: The RDA figures used on labels; in most instances, the highest RDA suggested in the U.S. RDA tables for any age-sex group for each nutrient.

underweight: Body weight more than 10 percent below desirable weight.

unsaturated fat: A lipid (triglyceride or phospholipid) in which one or more of the fatty acids is unsaturated.

unsaturated fatty acid: A fatty acid in which one or more points of unsaturation occur.

urea (yoo-REE-uh): The principal nitrogen-excretion product of metabolism, generated mostly by removal of amine groups from unneeded amino acids or from those being sacrificed to a need for energy.

varicose veins (VAIR-ih-kose): Veins that have become hard and knotted because of high pressure in them.

vegan (VAY-gun, VEJ-an): A strict vegetarian; one who excludes all animal flesh and animal products, eating only plant foods.

veins: The vessels that carry blood from the capillaries back to the heart. See Figure 2 in Appendix A.

villi (VILL-eye): Poked-out parts of the sheet of cells that line the GI tract; the villi make the surface area much greater than it would otherwise be (singular: **villus**).

visual purple: The visual pigment of the retina used in dim light; also called rhodopsin.

vitamin (VITE-a-min): A potent, indispensable, noncaloric organic compound needed in very small amounts in the diet, which performs specific and individual functions to promote growth or reproduction or to maintain health and life.

vitamin B_3: See *niacin.*

vitamin B_6: One of the B vitamins. Active forms include pyridoxal, pyridoxine, and pyridoxamine.

vitamin B_{12}: One of the B vitamins, also known as cobalamin.

vitamin B_{15}: Trade-name for pangamic acid. The term *vitamin* in this name does not signify that B_{15} is an essential nutrient.

vitamin B_{17}: See *laetrile.*

vitamin G: See *niacin.*

VLDL (very-low-density lipoproteins): Lipoproteins made in intestine and liver that transport lipids to other body organs.

whitehead: A pimple, caused by the plugging of an oil-gland duct with shed material from the duct lining.

whole grain: Refers to a grain that retains its edible outside layers (has not been refined).

xerophthalmia (zee-roff-THAL-me-uh): A condition of extreme thickening of the cornea of the eye due to vitamin A deficiency; causes blindness.

xylitol: See *sorbitol.*

APPENDIX C: Fiber

If you are attempting to evaluate your fiber intake, it is important to be aware of the distinction made in Chapter 4: The fiber in the colon is not the same as the fiber found in foods when they are analyzed in the laboratory. In the colon, the fiber that remains is whatever has resisted the action of human GI tract enzymes. This is dietary fiber (DF). But when foods are analyzed in a laboratory, they are exposed to stronger agents—dilute acid and dilute alkali. What remains after these treatments is crude fiber (CF). For every gram of crude fiber, there may be 2 to 3 grams of dietary fiber.

Diets in the United States and Canada probably provide an average of about 4 grams of crude fiber a day, as compared with about 6 grams back in 1900. Some fiber enthusiasts recommend intakes higher than these, but there may be hazards in overdosing with fiber, as with any other food constituent. Even conservative authorities, however, seem to agree that there would be no harm in aiming at a crude fiber intake from foods of about 6 grams a day.

Table 1 shows estimates of the crude fiber contents of foods.[1] Table 2 shows approximations of the dietary fiber contents of foods.[2] We recommend that you read the article it came from for an understanding of the limitations on the accuracy of the numbers in the table and for a breakdown of the fiber types into cellulose, lignin, and other sources.

Table 1. Approximate Crude Fiber Content per Serving of Food

Food	Serving Size	Crude Fiber (g)
Cereals	½–⅔ c	
All bran		3.0
Wheat bran		0.8
40 percent bran		0.9
Most other cooked or ready-to-eat		trace–0.3
Breads	1 slice	
Whole wheat, pumpernickel		0.4
Raisin, rye, French, Italian, enriched white		0.05–0.2
Fruits	medium or ½ c	
Watermelon		1.5
Apple (with skin)		2.0
Prunes, dried peaches		1.5
Honeydew melon, banana		1.0
Berries		1.0
Peaches, apricots, citrus fruits, fruit cocktail		0.5
Fruit juice		0.2
Vegetables	½–⅔ c	
Parsnips, peas, brussels sprouts		2.0
Pork and beans		2.0
Lima beans		1.5
Kidney beans		1.0
Broccoli, carrots		1.0
Green beans, corn, celery, turnip, tomato, greens		0.5–1.0
Potato (with skin)		0.8
Potato chips, spinach		<0.5
Nuts	½ c	1.0–2.0
Sunflower Seeds	1 c	2.0

Table 2. Dietary Fiber in Selected Foods

Food	Total dietary fiber (g/100 g)
Flour	
White, bread-making	3.15
Brown	7.87
Whole-meal	9.51
Bran	44.0
Breads	
White	2.72
Brown	5.11
Hovis	4.54
Whole-meal	8.50
Cereals	
All-Bran	26.7
Cornflakes	11.0
Grapenuts	7.00
Readibrek	7.60
Rice Krispies	4.47
Puffed Wheat	15.41
Sugar Puffs	6.08
Shredded Wheat	12.26
Swiss breakfast (mixed brands)	7.41
Weetabix	12.72
Biscuits	
Chocolate digestive (half-coated)	3.50
Chocolate (fully coated)	3.09
Crispbread, rye	11.73
Crispbread, wheat	4.83
Ginger biscuits	1.99
Matzo	3.85
Oatcakes	4.00
Semisweet	2.31
Short-sweet	1.60
Wafers (filled)	1.62
Leafy vegetables	
Broccoli tops (boiled)	4.10
Brussels sprouts (boiled)	2.86
Cabbage (boiled)	2.83
Cauliflower (boiled)	1.80
Lettuce (raw)	1.53
Onions (raw)	2.10
Legumes	
Beans, baked (canned)	7.27
Beans, runner (boiled)	3.35
Peas, frozen (raw)	7.75
garden (canned)	6.28
processed (canned)	7.85
Root vegetables	
Carrots, young (boiled)	3.70
Parsnips (raw)	4.90
Swedes (raw)	2.40
Turnips (raw)	2.20
Potatoes	
Main crop (raw)	3.51
Chips (fried)	3.20
Crisps	11.9
Canned, drained	2.51
Peppers (cooked)	0.93
Other vegetables	
Peppers (cooked)	0.93
Tomatoes, fresh	1.40
canned, drained	0.85
Sweet corn, cooked	4.74
canned, drained	5.69
Fruits	
Apples, flesh only,	1.42
peel only	3.71
Bananas	1.75
Cherries (flesh and skin)	1.24
Grapefruit (canned)	0.44
Guavas (canned)	3.64
Mandarin oranges (canned)	0.29
Mangoes (canned)	1.00
Peaches (flesh and skin)	2.28
Pears, flesh only	2.44
peel only	8.59
Plums (flesh and skin)	1.52
Rhubarb (raw)	1.78
Strawberries, raw,	2.12
canned	1.00
Sultanas	4.40
Nuts	
Brazils	7.73
Peanuts	9.30
Preserves	
Jam, plum,	0.96
strawberry	1.12

Table 2. Dietary Fiber in Selected Foods *(continued)*

Food	Total dietary fiber (g/100 g)	Food	Total dietary fiber (g/100 g)
Lemon curd	0.20	**Beverages (concentrated)**	
Marmalade	0.71	Cocoa	43.27
Mincemeat	3.19	Drinking chocolate	8.20
Peanut butter	7.55	Coffee and chicory essence	0.79
Pickle	1.53	Instant coffee	16.41
Dried soups (as purchased)		**Extracts**	
Minestrone	6.61	Bovril	0.91
Oxtail	3.84	Marmite	2.69
Tomato	3.32		

Notes

1. Table 1 adapted from K. W. McNutt, Perspective: Fiber, *Journal of Nutrition Education* 8 (1976): 150-152, from unpublished data of Harland and Oberless and *USDA Handbook No. 8.* Used here with the permission of the authors and publisher.

2. Table 2 adapted from D. A. T. Southgate, B. Bailey, E. Collinson, and A. F. Walker, A guide to calculating intakes of dietary fibre, *Journal of Human Nutrition* 30 (1976): 303-313, with the permission of the authors and publisher.

Suggested References

For further information on the nonnutritive ingredients of foods, check the twelfth edition of the following:

Church, C. F., and Church, H. N. *Bowes and Church's Food Values of Portions Commonly Used.* 12th ed. Philadelphia: Lippincott, 1975.

APPENDIX D: Fats: Cholesterol and P:S Ratios

To adopt a "prudent diet," you are advised to control calories and salt intake; to avoid empty-calorie foods, especially those high in concentrated sugars; and to make sure that fat intake is kept in line. To manage fat consumption, three measures are recommended: (1) cut total fat; (2) reduce cholesterol intake; and (3) adjust the ratio of polyunsaturated to saturated fat so that it balances in favor of the polyunsaturates (and mono-unsaturates).

For the first objective, total fat intake can be calculated from Appendix H, as explained in the Chapter 5 Self-Study.

For the second, cholesterol intake can be estimated from Table 1.[1] A cholesterol intake of 300 milligrams a day or less is often recommended, although there is much disagreement about the recommendation (see Controversy 5A).

As for the third objective, nutritionists tend to think in terms of the P:S ratio (the ratio of polyunsaturated to saturated fat). In general, according to present thinking, the higher the P:S ratio (and the more polyunsaturated fat there is in comparison to the amount of saturated fat), the better. The P:S ratio of a day's food intake or menu can be precisely calculated using the ratio of linoleic acid grams to saturated fat grams (from Appendix H), but you can get a general idea of the fat quality of common fat-containing foods from Table 2.

Table 1. Cholesterol Content of Foods

Food	Serving size	Cholesterol (mg)
Meat, fish, poultry		
Beef, cooked, lean, trimmed of separable fat	3 oz	77
Lamb, lean, cooked	3 oz	83
Pork, cooked, lean, trimmed	3 oz	77
Veal, cooked, lean	3 oz	86
Chicken, dark meat	3 oz	76
Chicken, light meat	3 oz	54
Turkey, dark meat	3 oz	86
Turkey, light meat	3 oz	65
Rabbit, domestic	3 oz	52
Variety meats		
liver (beef, calf, lamb), cooked	3 oz	372
chicken liver	3 oz	480
heart	3 oz	274
sweetbreads	3 oz	396
brain	3 oz	1,810
kidney	3 oz	690
Fish		
caviar (fish roe)	1 tbsp	48
cod	3 oz	72
haddock	3 oz	51
halibut	3 oz	51
flounder	3 oz	43
herring	3 oz	83
salmon, cooked	3 oz	40
trout	3 oz	47
tuna, packed in oil	3 oz	56
sardines	1 can (3 3/4 oz)	109
Shellfish		
abalone	3 oz	120
crab	3 oz	85
clams	3 oz	55
lobster	1/2 c	57
oysters	3 oz	40
scallops	1/2 c (scant)	45
shrimp	3 oz	96

Food	Serving size	Cholesterol (mg)
Eggs		
Yolk	1 medium	240
White		0
Dairy products		
Milk, whole	1 c (8 oz)	34
Milk, low-fat (2%)	1 c	22
Milk, nonfat (skim)	1 c	5
Buttermilk	1 c	14
Yogurt, low-fat plain	1 c	17
Yogurt, low-fat flavored	1 c	14
Sour cream	1 tbsp	8
Whipped cream	1 tbsp	20
Half and half	1 tbsp	6
Ice milk	1 c	26
Ice cream	1 c	56
Butter	1 tsp	12
Cheese		
American	1 oz	26
Blue or roquefort	1 oz	25
Camembert	1 oz	28
Cheddar, mild or sharp	1 oz	28
Cottage		
creamed (4% fat)	1 c	48
uncreamed	1 c	13
Cream cheese	1 tbsp	16
Mozzarella, low moisture, part skim	1 oz	18
Muenster	1 oz	25
Parmesan	1 oz	27
Ricotta, part skim	1 oz	14
Swiss	1 oz	28
Nondairy fats		
Lard or other animal fat	1 tsp	5
Margarine, all vegetable		0
Margarine, 2/3 animal fat, 1/3 vegetable fat	1 tsp	3

Table 2. P:S Ratios of Foods

High (more than 2½ times as much polyunsaturated as saturated fat)	Almonds Corn oil Cottonseed oil Linseed oil Margarine, soft Mayonnaise (made with any of the oils in this group)	Safflower oil Sesame oil Soybean oil Sunflower oil Walnuts
Medium-high (about twice as much polyunsaturated as saturated fat)	Chicken breast, skin, thigh Freshwater fish	Peanut oil Semisolid margarines
Medium (about equal amounts of polyunsaturated and saturated fat)	Beef, heart and liver Chicken heart Hydrogenated or hardened vegetable oils	Peanut butter Pecans Saltwater fish Solid margarines
Low (about a tenth to a half as much polyunsaturated as saturated fat)	Chicken liver Lard Olive oil	Palm oil Pork
Very Low (less than a tenth as much polyunsaturated as saturated fat)	Beef, both lean and fat Butter Coconut oil	Egg yolk Milk and milk products Mutton, both lean and fat

Notes

1. Table 1 from E. N. Whitney and E. M. N. Hamilton, *Understanding Nutrition*, 2d ed. (St. Paul, Minn.: West, 1977), pp. A39-A40. These figures are probably high and can be used only to obtain a "ballpark estimate" of cholesterol intake.

APPENDIX E: Sodium and Potassium

Tables 1 and 2 are shown so that you can compare your sodium intake with the U.S. Dietary Goals.[1] The goals recommend restricting salt intake to about 5 grams a day, which effectively means reducing sodium intake to about 2 grams (2000 milligrams). No recommendation is made for the daily consumption of potassium, but people who take diuretics are instructed by their physicians to eat foods high in potassium to replace losses and may be interested to see from Table 3[2] what foods contain large amounts of this mineral.

Table 1. Average Sodium and Potassium Content of Common Foods

Food	Weight (g)	Sodium (mg)	Potassium (mg)
Meat, fish, or poultry, cooked without added salt			
Average	30	33	125
Clams, soft	100	36	239
Clams, hard	100	205	311
Crab, canned	100	1000	110
Crab, steamed	100	456	271
Flounder	100	237	587
Frankfurters (2)	100	1100	220
Frozen fish (cod)	100	400	400
Haddock	100	177	348

Table 1. Average Sodium and Potassium Content of Common Foods *(continued)*

Food	Weight (g)	Sodium (mg)	Potassium (mg)
Kidneys, beef	100	253	324
Lobster, canned	100	210	180
Lobster, fresh	100	325	258
Oysters, raw	100	73	121
Salmon, canned	100	522	349
Salmon, salt-free, canned	100	48	391
Scallops, fresh	100	265	476
Shrimp, raw	100	140	220
Shrimp, frozen or canned	100	140	200–312
Sweetbreads	100	116	433
Tuna, canned	100	800	240
Tuna, salt-free, canned	100	46	382
Cheese			
American cheese	30	341	25
Cream cheese	30	75	22
Cottage cheese	30	76	28
Cottage cheese, unsalted	30	6	—
Low-sodium cheese (cheddar)	30	3	120
Egg			
Whole, fresh and frozen (1)	50	61	65
Whites, fresh and frozen	50	73	70
Yolks, fresh	50	26	49
Milk			
Buttermilk, cultured	120	135	192
Condensed sweetened milk	120	135	377
Evaporated milk, undiluted	120	142	364
Powdered milk, skim	30	160	544
Low-sodium milk, canned	120	6	288
Whole	240	120	346
Yogurt (skim milk)	100	51	143
Potato			
White, baked in skin	100	4	323
White, boiled	100	2	285
Instant, prepared with water, milk, fat	100	256	290
Sweet (canned solid pack)	100	48	200
Breads			
Bakery white	25	127	26
Bakery, whole wheat	25	132	68
Bakery, rye	25	139	36

Table 1. Average Sodium and Potassium Content of Common Foods *(continued)*

Food	Weight (g)	Sodium (mg)	Potassium (mg)
Low-sodium (local)	25	4	25
Plain muffin	40	132	38
English muffin	57	215	57
A-proten rusk (1)	11	4	5
Graham crackers (2)	14	93	53
Low-sodium crackers (2)	9	10	11
Vanilla wafers (5)	14	35	10
Yeast doughnut	30	70	24
Cake doughnut	35	160	32
Cereal, dry			
Kellogg's Corn Flakes	30	282	15
Puffed Rice	15	trace	7
Rice Krispies	30	267	15
Special K	30	244	17
Puffed Wheat	15	trace	21
Shredded Wheat	20	1	52
Kellogg's Sugar Frosted Flakes	30	200	19
Sugar Pops	30	67	22
Bran Flakes	30	118	151
Cereal, cooked without added salt			
Corn grits, enriched, regular	100	1	11
Farina, enriched, regular	100	2	9
Farina, instant cooking	100	7	13
Farina, quick cooking	100	190	10
Oatmeal or rolled oats	100	2	61
Pettijohn's Wheat	100	trace	84
Rice	100	5	28
Rice, instant	100	trace	trace
Wheat, rolled	100	trace	84
Wheatena	100	trace	84
Fat			
Bacon (1 strip)	7	73	17
Butter	5	49	3
Margarine	5	49	1
Mayonnaise	15	90	5
Mayonnaise, low-sodium	15	17	1
Low-sodium butter	15	1	3
Unsalted margarine (Fleishman's)	5	1	1
Vegetable oil	15	0	0

Table 1. Average Sodium and Potassium Content of Common Foods *(continued)*

Food	Weight (g)	Sodium (mg)	Potassium (mg)
Cream			
Coffee Mate	1[a]	4	27
Half-and-half	30	14	39
Heavy whipping cream (30 percent)	30	10	27
Poly-perx	30	—	—
Sour cream (Sealtest)	30	13	43
Table cream (18 percent)	30	13	37
Whipped topping	30	4	6
Gravy			
Low sodium	30	10	25
Regular	30	210	28
Peanut butter			
Cellu, salt free	15	1	100
Regular, made with small amounts of added fat and salt	15	91	100
Desserts			
Baked custard (Delmark)	120	128	174
D'zerta	120	35	0
Gelatin	120	51	1
Ice cream (4-oz cup)	60	23	49
Sherbet	60	6	14
Water ice	60	trace	2
Cakes			
All varieties except gingerbread and fruit cakes (both mixes and recipes)	50[b]	123	50
With low-sodium shortening and baking powder	50[b]	10–20	75–150
Pies			
All varieties except raisin, mince (⅛ of 9-inch pie)	320[b]	375	180
Candy			
Hard candy (1 equals 5 g)	100	32	4
Gum drops (8 small equals 10 g)	100	35	5
Jelly beans	100	12	1
Salt			
(1 g NaCl—1 packet salt)	—	400	—
(5 g NaCl—1 tsp)	—	2,000	—

[a]In teaspoons.
[b]Average serving.

Table 1. Average Sodium and Potassium Content of Common Foods *(continued)*

Food	Weight (g)	Sodium (mg)	Potassium (mg)
Salt substitutes			
Diamond Crystal	500[c]	1	220
Co-salt	500[c]	0	185
Adolph's	500[c]	0	241
McCormick's	500[c]	0	234
Morton	500[c]	0	250
Sugar substitutes			
Saccharine (¼-gr tablet)	1	1	0
Sucaryl	500[c]	0	0
Sweet-10	500[c]	0	0
Adolph's	500[c]	0	0
Morton	500[c]	0	0
Diamond Crystal	500[c]	0	0
Beverages			
Beer	100	7	25
Chocolate syrup (2 tsp)	10	5	29
Coca-Cola	100	4	1
Coffee, instant (beverage)	—	1	50
Cranberry juice	100	1	10
Diet Seven-Up	100	10	0
Egg nog, reconstituted	240	250	630
Fresca	100	18	0
Frozen lemonade, reconstituted	100	trace	16
Ginger ale	100	6	2
Hot chocolate (Carnation 1 pack—6 oz water)	100	104	190
Kool-Aid, reconstituted	240	trace	0
Meritene, reconstituted	240	250	740
Pepsi Cola	100	2	4
Royal Crown Cola	100	3	trace
Seven-Up	100	9	0
Sprite	100	16	0
Tab	100	5	0
Tea, instant (beverage)	—	trace	25

Fresh fruits and fruit juices are naturally very low in sodium and thus are not listed individually in this table.
[c]In milligrams

Table 2. Sodium Content of Vegetables (100-gram Portions)[a]

Food	Sodium (mg)
Group I vegetables (0–20 mg/100 g, average 7.4 mg)	
Asparagus	7
Broccoli	12
Brussel sprouts	14
Cabbage, common	14
Cauliflower	9
Chicory	7
Collards	16
Corn	2
Cow peas	1
Cucumbers	6
Eggplant	1
Endive	14
Escarole	14
Green peppers	13
Kohlrabi	6
Leeks	5
Lentils	3
Lettuce	9
Lima beans, not frozen	1
Mushrooms, raw	15
Mustard green	10
Navy beans	7
Okra	2
Onions	7
Parsnips	8
Peas, dried, split, cooked	13
Peas, green	1
Potatoes, baked in skin	4
Potatoes, boiled, pared before cooking	3
Radishes	18
Rutabagas	4
Squash, summer or winter	1
String beans	2
Sweet potato	10
Tomatoes	4
Turnip greens	17
Wax beans	2
Yams	4

Note: This table assumes the use of fresh vegetables without salt added in cooking. The amount of salt added to canned and frozen vegetables can vary. *Agricultural Handbook No. 8* from the USDA estimates that canned vegetables average 235 milligrams sodium per 100 grams edible portion. Frozen vegetables range from almost no sodium to as high as 125 milligrams sodium per 100 grams edible portion.

[a]A 100-gram portion for most vegetables is about a half-cup to a one-cup serving.

Table 2. Sodium Content of Vegetables (100-gram Portions) *(continued)*

Food	Sodium (mg)
Group II vegetables (23-60 mg / 100 g, average 40 mg)	
Artichoke	30
Beets	43
Black-eyed peas, frozen only	39
Carrots	33
Chinese cabbage	23
Dandelion greens	44
Kale	43
Parsley	45
Red cabbage	26
Spinach	50
Turnips	34
Watercress	52
Group III vegetables (75-126 mg / 100 g, average 81 mg)	
Beet greens	76
Celery	88
Chard, Swiss	86

Table 3. Sodium and Potassium Content of Selected Fruits and Vegetables (100-gram Portions)

		Potassium (mg)	Sodium (mg)
Fruits and Fruit Juices 100-gram servings			
Apple			
Raw	with peel	95	0.5
Juice	canned	85	2.2
Sauce	canned, drained	70	16
Apricots	canned, drained	170	22
Banana	ripe	405	2.9
Blueberries	water-pack, drained	45	0.9
Cantaloupe		295	33
Cherries, Royal Anne	canned, drained	155	1.2
Grapes			
Fresh	with peel	230	<0.5
Juice	canned	125	2.2
Grapefruit			
Juice	canned	125	2.2
Sections			

Table 3. Sodium and Potassium Content of Selected Fruits and Vegetables *(continued)*

		Potassium mg	Sodium mg
Fresh	skinless	170	<0.5
Canned	drained	100	3.6
Orange			
Juice	frozen, reconstituted	185	1.8
Sections	skinless	135	<0.4
Pineapple			
Crushed	canned, drained	95	3.6
Juice	canned	145	0.9
Peach, cling	canned, drained	100	1.6
Pear	canned, drained	73	9.0
Prunes			
Cooked		340	3.6
Juice	canned	170	1.3
Watermelon		95	1.6
Vegetables			
Asparagus spears	frozen, uncooked	300	3.3
Beans			
Baked with pork		240	427
Green	frozen, uncooked	148	0.9
Lima, baby	frozen, uncooked	560	136
Wax	canned, salt-free, drained	90	7
Beets	canned, salt-free, drained	148	69
Broccoli	frozen, uncooked	220	25
Brussels sprouts	frozen, uncooked	475	14
Cabbage	uncooked	199	6.9
Carrots	uncooked	315	109
Cauliflower	frozen, uncooked	310	12
Celery	fresh	245	87
Corn, whole kernel	canned, salt-free, drained	117	<0.5
Cucumber		148	0.7
Lettuce		139	7.6
Mushrooms, stems and pieces	canned	98	355
Onions	fresh, mature	141	2.2
Peas	canned, salt-free, drained	118	5.4
Potatoes			
Fresh	uncooked	280	1.45

Table 3. Sodium and Potassium Content of Selected Fruits and Vegetables ***(continued)***

		Potassium mg	Sodium mg
Instant	uncooked	625	124
Pumpkin	canned	176	0.7
Spinach	frozen, uncooked	575	140
Squash	frozen, cooked	172	0.9
Sweet potato	canned	164	16
Tomato			
Fresh		178	1.45
Juice	canned, salt-free	250	2.2

Notes

1. Tables 1 and 2 from Select Committee on Nutrition and Human Needs, *Dietary Goals for the United States*, 2d ed. (Washington, D.C.: Government Printing Office, 1977), pp. 80-83. The Senate's tables are taken from information in U.S. Department of Agriculture, Agricultural Research Service, Composition of foods: Raw, processed, prepared, *Agricultural Handbook No. 8* (Washington, D.C.: Government Printing Office, 1963).

2. Table 3 adapted from A. Gormican, Inorganic elements in foods used in hospital menus, *Journal of the American Dietetic Association* 56 (1970): 397-403.

APPENDIX F: Sugar

Table 1 presents the refined-sugar contents, in teaspoon measures, of common foods. No one will be surprised to see that cola beverages contain a large quantity of refined sugar, but it may be a surprise that sugar is added to dried fruits, hamburger buns, and other items. This table is adapted from a listing developed at the University of Iowa.[1]

Table 2 expands the section on cereals by showing which brand names have the most, and which the least, refined sugar. Adapted from a publication in which the sugar contents of cereals were not presented in teaspoons per serving but as a percentage of dry weight, this table gives only a rank order. The dentists who published this information suggested, tentatively, that to avoid promoting the development of dental decay the consumer should choose cereals containing less than 20 percent refined sugar.[2]

Table 1. Refined Sugar in Common Foods

Food	Portion Size	Approximate Sugar Content (tsp)
Beverages		
Cola drinks	12 oz	9
Ginger ale	12 oz	7
Orangeade	8 oz	5
Root beer	10 oz	4½

Measured in teaspoon equivalents of granulated sugar.

Table 1. Refined Sugar in Common Foods *(continued)*

Food	Portion Size	Approximate Sugar Content (tsp)
Seven-Up	12 oz	9
Soda pop	8 oz	5
Sweet cider	1 cup (8 oz)	4½
Desserts		
Apple cobbler	½ cup	3
Custard	½ cup	2
French pastry	1 (4 oz)	5
Jello	½ cup	4½
Apple pie	1 slice (average)	7
Junket	⅛ qt (½ cup)	3
Berry pie	1 slice	10
Cherry pie	1 slice	10
Cream pie	1 slice	4
Custard pie	1 slice	10
Coconut pie	1 slice	10
Lemon pie	1 slice	7
Peach pie	1 slice	7
Pumpkin pie	1 slice	5
Rhubarb pie	1 slice	4
Raisin pie	1 slice	13
Banana pudding	½ cup	2
Bread pudding	½ cup	1½
Chocolate pudding	½ cup	4
Plum pudding	½ cup	4
Rice pudding	½ cup	5
Tapioca pudding	½ cup	3
Brown betty	½ cup	3
Plain pastry	1 (4 oz)	3
Sugars and syrups		
Brown sugar	1 tbsp	3[a]
Granulated sugar	1 tbsp	3[a]
Corn syrup	1 tbsp	3[a]
Karo syrup	1 tbsp	3[a]
Honey	1 tbsp	3[a]
Molasses	1 tbsp	3½[a]
Chocolate sauce	1 tbsp	3½[a]
Jams and jellies		
Apple butter	1 tbsp	1

[a] Actual sugar content.

Table 1. Refined Sugar in Common Foods *(continued)*

Food	Portion Size	Approximate Sugar Content (tsp)
Jelly	1 tbsp	4–6
Orange marmalade	1 tbsp	4–6
Peach butter	1 tbsp	1
Strawberry jam	1 tbsp	4
Candies		
Milk chocolate bar (Hershey bar)	1½ oz	2½
Chewing gum	1 stick	½
Chocolate cream	1 piece	2
Chocolate mints	1 piece	2
Fudge	1 oz square	4½
Gum drop	1	2
Hard candy	4 oz	20
Lifesavers	1	⅓
Peanut brittle	1 oz	3½
Marshmallow	1	1½
Fruits and canned juices		
Raisins	½ cup	4
Currants, dried	1 tbsp	4
Prunes, dried	3–4 medium	4
Apricots, dried	4–6 halves	4
Dates, dried	3–4 stoned	4½
Figs, dried	1½-2 small	4
Fruit cocktail	½ cup	5
Rhubarb, stewed, sweetened	½ cup	8
Canned apricots	4 halves and 1 tbsp syrup	3½
Applesauce, unsweetened	½ cup	2
Prunes, stewed, sweetened	4–5 medium and 2 tbsp juice	8
Canned peaches	2 halves and 1 tbsp syrup	3½
Fruit salad	½ cup	3½
Fruit syrup	2 tbsp	2½
Orange juice	½ cup	2
Pineapple juice, unsweetened	½ cup	2⅗
Grape juice, commercial	½ cup	3⅖
Canned fruit juices, sweetened	½ cup	2
Breads and cereals		
White bread	1 slice	½

Table 1. Refined Sugar in Common Foods *(continued)*

Food	Portion Size	Approximate Sugar Content (tsp)
Cornflakes, Wheaties, Krispies, etc.	1 bowl and 1 tbsp sugar	4–8
Hamburger bun	1	3
Hot dog bun	1	3
Cakes and cookies		
Angel food cake	4 oz	7
Applesauce cake	4 oz	5½
Banana cake	2 oz	2
Cheesecake	4 oz	2
Chocolate cake, plain	4 oz	6
Chocolate cake, iced	4 oz	10
Coffeecake	4 oz	4½
Cupcake, iced	1	6
Fruitcake	4 oz	5
Jelly-roll	2 oz	2½
Orange cake	4 oz	4
Pound cake	4 oz	5
Sponge cake	1 oz	2
Strawberry shortcake	1 serving	4
Brownies, unfrosted	1 (¾ oz)	3
Molasses cookies	1	2
Chocolate cookies	1	1½
Fig Newtons	1	5
Ginger snaps	1	3
Macaroons	1	6
Nut cookies	1	1½
Oatmeal cookies	1	2
Sugar cookies	1	1½
Chocolate eclair	1	7
Cream puff	1	2
Donut, plain	1	3
Donut, glazed	1	6
Snail	1 (4 oz)	4½
Dairy products		
Ice cream	⅓ pint (3½ oz)	3½
Ice cream bar	1 (depending on size)	1–7
Ice cream cone	1	3½
Eggnog, all milk	1 (8 oz)	4½
Ice cream soda	1	5

Table 1. Refined Sugar in Common Foods *(continued)*

Food	Portion Size	Approximate Sugar Content (tsp)
Cocoa, all milk	1 cup (5 oz milk)	4
Ice cream sundae	1	7
Chocolate, all milk	1 cup (5 oz milk)	6
Malted milk shake	1 (10 oz)	5
Sherbet	½ cup	9

Table 2. Refined Sugar (Sucrose) in Breakfast Cereals

Cereal	Sucrose (percent)
Less than 10 percent sucrose	
Shredded wheat, large biscuit	1.0
Shredded wheat, spoon-size biscuit	1.3
Cheerios	2.2
Puffed rice	2.4
Uncle Sam Cereal	2.4
Wheat Chex	2.6
Grape nut flakes	3.3
Puffed wheat	3.5
Alpen	3.8
Post Toasties	4.1
Product 19	4.1
Corn Total	4.4
Special K	4.4
Wheaties	4.7
Corn flakes, Kroger	5.1
Peanut Butter	5.2
Grape Nuts	6.6
Corn Flakes, Food Club	7.0
Crispy Rice	7.3
Corn Chex	7.5

Note: The glucose content of these cereals is less than 5 percent, except for Special K and Kellogg Corn Flakes (6.4 percent). Kellogg Raisin Bran (14.1 percent), and Heartland with raisins (5.6 percent). Other sugars, such as fructose, were not analyzed.

Table 2. Refined Sugar (Sucrose) in Breakfast Cereals *(continued)*

Cereal	Sucrose (percent)
Corn Flakes, Kellogg	7.8
Total	8.1
Rice Chex	8.5
Crisp Rice	8.8
Raisin bran, Skinner	9.6
Concentrate	9.9
10 to 19 percent sucrose	
Rice Krispies, Kellogg	10.0
Raisin bran, Kellogg	10.6
Heartland, with raisins	13.5
Buck Wheat	13.6
Life	14.5
Granola, with dates	14.5
Granola, with raisins	14.5
Sugar-frosted corn flakes	15.6
40% bran flakes, Post	15.8
Team	15.9
Brown Sugar–Cinnamon Frosted Mini Wheats	16.0
40% bran flakes, Kellogg	16.2
Granola	16.6
100% bran	18.4
20 to 29 percent sucrose	
All Bran	20.0
Granola, with almonds and filberts	21.4
Fortified Oat Flakes	22.2
Heartland	23.1
Super Sugar Chex	24.5
Sugar Frosted Flakes	29.0
30 to 39 percent sucrose	
Bran Buds	30.2
Sugar Sparkled Corn Flakes	32.2
Frosted Mini Wheats	33.6
Sugar Pops	37.8
40 to 49.5 percent sucrose	
Alpha Bits	40.3
Sir Grapefellow	40.7
Super Sugar Crisp	40.7
Cocoa Puffs	43.0
Cap'n Crunch	43.3
Crunch Berries	43.4
Kaboom	43.8

Table 2. Refined Sugar (Sucrose) in Breakfast Cereals *(continued)*

Cereal	Sucrose (percent)
Frankenberry	44.0
Frosted Flakes	44.0
Count Chocula	44.2
Orange Quangaroos	44.7
Quisp	44.9
Boo Berry	45.7
Vanilly Crunch	45.8
Baron Von Redberry	45.8
Cocoa Krispies	45.9
Trix	46.6
Froot Loops	47.4
Honeycomb	48.8
Pink Panther	49.2
50 to 59 percent sucrose	
Cinnamon Crunch	50.3
Lucky Charms	50.4
Cocoa Pebbles	53.5
Apple Jacks	55.0
Fruity Pebbles	55.1
King Vitamin	58.5
More than 60 percent sucrose	
Sugar Smacks	61.3
Super Orange Crisp	68.0

Notes

1. Table 1 from Hidden sugars in foods, a three-page typescript (Iowa City: Department of Pedodontics, College of Dentistry, University of Iowa, March 1974). Developed by Arthur J. Nowak, D.M.D., Professor, College of Dentistry, Department of Pedodontics, University of Iowa, and reprinted with his permission.

2. Table 2 from I. L. Shannon, Sucrose and glucose in dry breakfast cereals, *Journal of Dentistry for Children*, September/October 1974, pp. 17-20. Shannon's data are used here with his permission and that of the publisher. The reader who wants to pursue the subject further might find another article interesting: I. L. Shannon and W. B. Wescott, Sucrose and glucose concentrations of frequently ingested foods, *Journal of the Academy of General Dentistry*, May/June 1975, pp. 37-43. This article presents sucrose and glucose contents for diet soft drinks (less than 0.1 percent); commercially available cheeses (less than 2.0 percent); fresh fruits and vegetables (from 0 to about 5 percent); commercially available luncheon meats (less than 1 percent for those analyzed); commercially available crackers and wafers (from about 1 to 10 percent, except for graham crackers, Cinnamon Treats, Cinnamon Crisp, and glazed Sesame Crisp, which contained from 10 to 30 percent); commercially available breads (less than 1 percent for those analyzed, except for old-fashioned cinnamon loaf); and commercially available snack foods (from 0 to 3 percent except for Morton's Kandi-roos, which contained almost 50 percent sucrose).

APPENDIX G: Fast Foods

The following table is reprinted from a publication by Ross Laboratories.[1] We appreciate their permission, and that of the authors, to use this information.

Notes

1. Table 1 from E. A. Young, E. H. Brennan, and G. L. Irving, Update: Nutritional analysis of fast foods, *Dietetic Currents, Ross Timesaver* 8 (March-April 1981).

Table 1. Nutritional Analyses of Fast Foods (Dashes indicate no data available. X = less than 2% RDA; tr = trace)

	Weight (g)	Energy (cal)	Protein (g)	Carbo-hydrate (g)	Fat (g)	Cholesterol (mg)	Vitamin A (IU)	Thiamin (mg)	Riboflavin (mg)	Niacin (mg)	Vitamin C (mg)	Calcium (mg)	Iron (mg)	Sodium (mg)
ARBY'S®														
Roast beef	140	350	22	32	15	45	X	0.30	0.34	5	X	80	3.6	880
Beef and cheese	168	450	27	36	22	55	X	0.38	0.43	6	X	200	4.5	1220
Super roast beef	263	620	30	61	28	85	X	0.53	0.43	7	X	100	5.4	1420
Junior roast beef	74	220	12	21	9	35	X	0.15	0.17	3	X	40	1.8	530
Ham and cheese	154	380	23	33	17	60	X	0.75	0.34	5	X	200	2.7	1350
Turkey deluxe	236	510	28	46	24	70	X	0.45	0.34	8	X	80	2.7	1220
Club sandwich	252	560	30	43	30	100	X	0.68	0.43	7	X	200	3.6	1610

Source: Consumer Affairs, Arby's, Inc., Atlanta, Georgia. Nutritional analysis by Technological Resources, Camden, New Jersey.

	Weight (g)	Energy (cal)	Protein (g)	Carbo-hydrate (g)	Fat (g)	Cholesterol (mg)	Vitamin A (IU)	Thiamin (mg)	Riboflavin (mg)	Niacin (mg)	Vitamin C (mg)	Calcium (mg)	Iron (mg)	Sodium (mg)
BURGER CHEF®														
Hamburger	91	244	11	29	9	27	114	0.17	0.16	2.7	1.2	45	2.0	—
Cheeseburger	104	290	14	29	13	39	267	0.18	0.21	2.8	1.2	132	2.2	—
Double cheeseburger	145	420	24	30	22	77	431	0.20	0.32	4.4	1.2	223	3.2	—
Fish filet	179	547	21	46	31	43	400	0.23	0.22	2.7	1.0	145	2.2	—
Super Shef® sandwich	252	563	29	44	30	105	754	0.31	0.40	6.0	9.3	205	4.5	—
Big Shef® sandwich	186	569	23	38	36	81	279	0.26	0.31	4.7	1.0	152	3.6	—
TOP Shef® sandwich	138	661	41	36	38	134	273	0.35	0.47	8.1	0	194	5.4	—
Funmeal® feast	—	545	15	55	30	27	123	0.25	0.21	4.6	12.8	61	2.8	—
Rancher® platter[a]	316	640	32	33	42	106	1750[a]	0.29	0.38	8.6	23.5	66	5.3	—
Mariner® platter[a]	373	734	29	78	34	35	2069[a]	0.34	0.23	5.2	23.5	63	3.3	—
French fries, small	68	250	2	20	19	0	0	0.07	0.04	1.7	11.5	9	0.7	—
French fries, large	85	351	3	28	26	0	0	0.10	0.06	2.4	16.2	13	0.9	—
Vanilla shake (12 oz)	336	380	13	60	10	40	387	0.10	0.66	0.5	0	497	0.3	—
Chocolate shake (12 oz)	336	403	10	72	9	36	292	0.16	0.76	0.4	0	449	1.1	—
Hot chocolate	—	198	8	23	8	30	288	0.93	0.39	0.3	2.1	271	0.7	—

[a] Includes salad. Source: Burger Chef Systems, Inc., Indianapolis, Indiana. Nutritional analysis from *Handbook No. 8*. Washington: US Dept of Agriculture.

	Weight (g)	Energy (cal)	Protein (g)	Carbo-hydrate (g)	Fat (g)	Cholesterol (mg)	Vitamin A (IU)	Thiamin (mg)	Riboflavin (mg)	Niacin (mg)	Vitamin C (mg)	Calcium (mg)	Iron (mg)	Sodium (mg)
CHURCH'S FRIED CHICKEN®														
White chicken portion	100	327	21	10	23	—	160	0.10	0.18	7.2	0.7	94	1.0	498
Dark chicken portion	100	305	22	7	21	—	140	0.10	0.27	5.3	1.0	15	1.3	475

Source: Church's Fried Chicken, San Antonio, Texas. Nutritional analysis by Medallion Laboratories, Minneapolis, Minnesota.

	Weight (g)	Energy (cal)	Protein (g)	Carbo-hydrate (g)	Fat (g)	Cholesterol (mg)	Vitamin A (IU)	Thiamin (mg)	Riboflavin (mg)	Niacin (mg)	Vitamin C (mg)	Calcium (mg)	Iron (mg)	Sodium (mg)
DAIRY QUEEN®														
Frozen dessert	113	180	5	27	6	20	100	0.09	0.17	X	X	150	X	—
DQ cone, small	71	110	3	18	3	10	100	0.03	0.14	X	X	100	X	—
DQ cone, regular	142	230	6	35	7	20	300	0.09	0.26	X	X	200	X	—
DQ cone, large	213	340	10	52	10	30	400	0.15	0.43	X	X	300	X	—
DQ dip cone, small	78	150	3	20	7	10	100	0.03	0.17	X	X	100	X	—
DQ dip cone, regular	156	300	7	40	13	20	300	0.09	0.34	X	X	200	0.4	—
DQ dip cone, large	234	450	10	58	20	30	400	0.12	0.51	X	X	300	0.4	—
DQ sundae, small	106	170	4	30	4	15	100	0.03	0.17	X	X	100	0.7	—
DQ sundae, regular	177	290	6	51	7	20	300	0.06	0.26	X	X	200	1.1	—
DQ sundae, large	248	400	9	71	9	30	400	0.09	0.43	0.4	X	300	1.8	—
DQ malt, small	241	340	10	51	11	30	400	0.06	0.34	0.4	2.4	300	1.8	—
DQ malt, regular	418	600	15	89	20	50	750	0.12	0.60	0.8	3.6	500	3.6	—
DQ malt, large	588	840	22	125	28	70	750	0.15	0.85	1.2	6	600	5.4	—
DQ float	397	330	6	59	8	20	100	0.12	0.17	X	X	200	X	—
DQ banana split	383	540	10	91	15	30	750	0.60	0.60	0.8	18	350	1.8	—
DQ parfait	284	460	10	81	11	30	400	0.12	0.43	0.4	X	300	1.8	—
DQ freeze	397	520	11	89	13	35	200	0.15	0.34	X	X	300	X	—
Mr. Misty® freeze	411	500	10	87	12	35	200	0.15	0.34	X	X	300	X	—
Mr. Misty® float	404	440	6	85	8	20	100	0.12	0.17	X	X	200	X	—
"Dilly"® bar	85	240	4	22	15	10	100	0.06	0.17	X	X	100	0.4	—
DQ sandwich	60	140	3	24	4	10	100	0.03	0.14	0.4	X	60	0.4	—
Mr Misty Kiss®	89	70	0	17	0	0	X	X	X	X	X	X	X	—
Brazier® cheese dog	113	330	15	24	19	—	—	—	0.18	3.3	—	168	1.6	—
Brazier® chili dog	128	330	13	25	20	—	—	0.15	0.23	3.9	11.0	86	2.0	939
Brazier® dog	99	273	11	23	15	—	—	0.12	0.15	2.6	11.0	75	1.5	868

Table 1. Nutritional Analyses of Fast Foods *(continued)*

	Weight (g)	Energy (cal)	Protein (g)	Carbo-hydrate (g)	Fat (g)	Cholesterol (mg)	Vitamin A (IU)	Thiamin (mg)	Riboflavin (mg)	Niacin (mg)	Vitamin C (mg)	Calcium (mg)	Iron (mg)	Sodium (mg)
DAIRY QUEEN® *(continued)*														
Fish sandwich	170	400	20	41	17	—	tr	0.15	0.26	3.0	tr	60	1.1	—
Fish sandwich with cheese	177	440	24	39	21	—	100	0.15	0.26	3.0	tr	150	0.4	—
Super Brazier® dog	182	518	20	41	30	—	tr	0.42	0.44	7.0	14.0	158	4.3	1552
Super Brazier® dog with cheese	203	593	26	43	36	—	—	0.43	0.48	8.1	14.0	297	4.4	1986
Super Brazier® chili dog	210	555	23	42	33	—	—	0.42	0.48	8.8	18.0	158	4.0	1640
Brazier® fries, small	71	200	2	25	10	—	tr	0.06	tr	0.8	3.6	tr	0.4	—
Brazier® fries, large	113	320	3	40	16	—	tr	0.09	0.03	1.2	4.8	tr	0.4	—
Brazier® onion rings	85	300	6	33	17	—	tr	0.09	tr	0.4	2.4	20	0.4	—

Source: International Dairy Queen, Inc., Minneapolis, Minnesota. Nutritional analysis by Raltech Scientific Services, Inc. (formerly WARF), Madison, Wisconsin. (Nutritional analysis not applicable in the state of Texas.)

	Weight (g)	Energy (cal)	Protein (g)	Carbo-hydrate (g)	Fat (g)	Cholesterol (mg)	Vitamin A (IU)	Thiamin (mg)	Riboflavin (mg)	Niacin (mg)	Vitamin C (mg)	Calcium (mg)	Iron (mg)	Sodium (mg)
JACK IN THE BOX®														
Hamburger	97	263	13	29	11	26	49	0.27	0.18	5.6	1.1	82	2.3	566
Cheeseburger	109	310	16	28	15	32	338	0.27	0.21	5.4	<1.1	172	2.6	877
Jumbo Jack® hamburger	246	551	28	45	29	80	246	0.47	0.34	11.6	3.7	134	4.5	1134
Jumbo Jack® hamburger with cheese	272	628	32	45	35	110	734	0.52	0.38	11.3	4.9	273	4.6	1666
Regular taco	83	189	8	15	11	22	356	0.07	0.08	1.8	<0.9	116	1.2	460
Super taco	146	285	12	20	17	37	599	0.10	0.12	2.8	1.6	196	1.9	968
Moby Jack® sandwich	141	455	17	38	26	56	240	0.30	0.21	4.5	1.4	167	1.7	837
Breakfast Jack® sandwich	121	301	18	28	13	182	442	0.41	0.47	5.1	3.4	177	2.5	1037
French fries	80	270	3	31	15	13	—	0.12	0.02	1.9	3.7	19	0.7	128
Onion rings	85	351	5	32	23	24	—	0.24	0.12	3.1	<1.2	26	1.4	318
Apple turnover	119	411	4	45	24	17	—	0.23	0.12	2.5	<1.2	11	1.4	352
Vanilla shake[a]	317	317	10	57	6	26	—	0.16	0.38	0.5	<3.2	349	0.2	229

	Weight (g)	Energy (cal)	Protein (g)	Carbo-hydrate (g)	Fat (g)	Cholesterol (mg)	Vitamin A (IU)	Thiamin (mg)	Riboflavin (mg)	Niacin (mg)	Vitamin C (mg)	Calcium (mg)	Iron (mg)	Sodium (mg)
JACK IN THE BOX® *(continued)*														
Strawberry shake[a]	328	323	11	55	7	26	—	0.16	0.46	0.6	<3.3	371	0.6	241
Chocolate shake[a]	322	325	11	55	7	26	—	0.16	0.64	0.6	<3.2	348	0.7	270
Vanilla shake	314	342	10	54	9	36	440	0.16	0.47	0.5	3.5	349	0.4	263
Strawberry shake	328	380	11	63	10	33	426	0.16	0.62	0.5	<3.3	351	0.3	268
Chocolate shake	317	365	11	59	10	35	380	0.16	0.60	0.6	<3.2	350	1.2	294
Ham and cheese omelette	174	425	21	32	23	355	766	0.45	0.70	3.0	<1.7	260	4.0	975
Double cheese omelette	166	423	19	30	25	370	797	0.33	0.68	2.5	1.7	276	3.6	899
Ranchero style omelette	196	414	20	33	23	343	853	0.33	0.74	2.6	<2.0	278	3.8	1098
French toast	180	537	15	54	29	115	522	0.56	0.30	4.4	9.2	119	3.0	1130
Pancakes	232	626	16	79	27	87	488	0.63	0.44	4.6	<26.2	105	2.8	1670
Scrambled eggs	267	719	26	55	44	259	694	0.69	0.56	5.2	<12.8	257	5.0	1110

[a] Special formula for shakes sold in California, Arizona, Texas, and Washington. Source: Jack-in-the-Box, Foodmaker, Inc., San Diego, California. Nutritional analysis by Raltech Scientific Services, Inc. (formerly WARF), Madison, Wisconsin.

	Weight (g)	Energy (cal)	Protein (g)	Carbo-hydrate (g)	Fat (g)	Cholesterol (mg)	Vitamin A (IU)	Thiamin (mg)	Riboflavin (mg)	Niacin (mg)	Vitamin C (mg)	Calcium (mg)	Iron (mg)	Sodium (mg)
KENTUCKY FRIED CHICKEN®														
Original Recipe® dinner[a]														
Wing and rib	322	603	30	48	32	133	25.5	0.22	0.19	10.0	36.6	—	—	—
Wing and thigh	341	661	33	48	38	172	25.5	0.24	0.27	8.4	36.6	—	—	—
Drum and thigh	346	643	35	46	35	180	25.5	0.25	0.32	8.5	36.6	—	—	—
Extra crispy dinner[a]														
Wing and rib	349	755	33	60	43	132	25.5	0.31	0.29	10.4	36.6	—	—	—
Wing and thigh	371	812	36	58	48	176	25.5	0.31	0.35	10.3	36.6	—	—	—
Drum and thigh	376	765	38	55	44	183	25.5	0.32	0.38	10.4	36.6	—	—	—
Mashed potatoes	85	64	2	12	1	0	<18	<0.01	0.02	0.8	4.9	—	—	—
Gravy	14	23	0	1	2	0	<3	0.00	0.01	0.1	<0.2	—	—	—
Cole slaw	91	122	1	13	8	7	—	—	—	—	—	—	—	—
Rolls	21	61	2	11	1	1	<5	0.10	0.04	1.0	0.3	—	—	—
Corn (5.5-inch ear)	135	169	5	31	3	X	162	0.12	0.07	1.2	2.6	—	—	—

[a] Includes two pieces of chicken, mashed potato and gravy, coleslaw, and roll. Source, Kentucky Fried Chicken, Inc., Louisville, Kentucky. Nutritional analysis by Raltech Scientific Services, Inc. (formerly WARF), Madison, Wisconsin.

Table 1. Nutritional Analyses of Fast Foods *(continued)*

	Weight (g)	Energy (cal)	Protein (g)	Carbo-hydrate (g)	Fat (g)	Cholesterol (mg)	Vitamin A (IU)	Thiamin (mg)	Riboflavin (mg)	Niacin (mg)	Vitamin C (mg)	Calcium (mg)	Iron (mg)	Sodium (mg)
LONG JOHN SILVER'S®														
Fish with batter (2 pc)	136	366	22	21	22	—	—	—	—	—	—	—	—	—
Fish with batter (3 pc)	207	549	32	32	32	—	—	—	—	—	—	—	—	—
Treasure Chest®	143	506	30	32	33	—	—	—	—	—	—	—	—	—
Chicken Planks® (4 pc)	166	457	27	35	23	—	—	—	—	—	—	—	—	—
Peg Legs® with batter (5 pc)	125	350	22	26	28	—	—	—	—	—	—	—	—	—
Ocean Scallop (6 pc)	120	283	11	30	13	—	—	—	—	—	—	—	—	—
Shrimp with batter (6 pc)	88	268	8	30	13	—	—	—	—	—	—	—	—	—
Breaded oysters (6 pc)	156	441	13	53	19	—	—	—	—	—	—	—	—	—
Breaded clams	142	617	18	61	34	—	—	—	—	—	—	—	—	—
Fish sandwich	193	337	22	49	31	—	—	—	—	—	—	—	—	—
French Fryes	85	288	4	33	16	—	—	—	—	—	—	—	—	—
Cole slaw	113	138	1	16	8	—	—	—	—	—	—	—	—	—
Corn on the cob (1 ear)	150	176	5	29	4	—	—	—	—	—	—	—	—	—
Hushpuppies (3)	45	153	3	20	7	—	—	—	—	—	—	—	—	—
Clam chowder (8 oz)	170	107	5	15	3	—	—	—	—	—	—	—	—	—

Source: Long John Silver's Food Shoppes, Lexington, Kentucky. Nutritional analysis by L. V. Packett, PhD, Department of Nutrition and Food Science, University of Kentucky.

	Weight (g)	Energy (cal)	Protein (g)	Carbo-hydrate (g)	Fat (g)	Cholesterol (mg)	Vitamin A (IU)	Thiamin (mg)	Riboflavin (mg)	Niacin (mg)	Vitamin C (mg)	Calcium (mg)	Iron (mg)	Sodium (mg)
McDONALD'S®														
Egg McMuffin®	138	327	19	31	15	229	97	0.47	0.44	3.8	<1.4	226	2.9	885
English muffin, buttered	63	186	5	30	5	13	164	0.28	0.49	2.6	0.8	117	1.5	318
Hotcakes with butter and syrup	214	500	8	94	10	47	257	0.26	0.36	2.3	4.7	103	2.2	1070
Sausage (pork)	53	206	9	tr	19	43	<32	0.27	0.11	2.1	0.5	16	0.8	615
Scrambled eggs	98	180	13	3	13	349	652	0.08	0.47	0.2	1.2	61	2.5	205
Hashbrown potatoes	55	125	2	14	7	7	<14	0.06	<0.01	0.8	4.1	5	0.4	325
Big Mac®	204	563	26	41	33	86	530	0.39	0.37	6.5	2.2	157	4.0	1010
Cheeseburger	115	307	15	30	14	37	345	0.25	0.23	3.8	1.6	132	2.4	767
Hamburger	102	255	12	30	10	25	82	0.25	0.18	4.0	1.7	51	2.3	520

	Weight (g)	Energy (cal)	Protein (g)	Carbo-hydrate (g)	Fat (g)	Cholesterol (mg)	Vitamin A (IU)	Thiamin (mg)	Riboflavin (mg)	Niacin (mg)	Vitamin C (mg)	Calcium (mg)	Iron (mg)	Sodium (mg)
McDONALDS® *(continued)*														
Quarter Pounder®	166	424	24	33	22	67	133	0.32	0.28	6.5	<1.7	63	4.1	735
Quarter Pounder® with cheese	194	524	30	32	31	96	660	0.31	0.37	7.4	2.7	219	4.3	1236
Filet-O-Fish®	139	432	14	37	25	47	42	0.26	0.20	2.6	<1.4	93	1.7	781
Regular fries	68	220	3	26	12	9	<17	0.12	0.02	2.3	12.5	9	0.6	109
Apple pie	85	253	2	29	14	12	<34	0.02	0.02	0.2	<0.8	14	0.6	398
Cherry pie	88	260	2	32	14	13	114	0.03	0.02	0.4	<0.8	12	0.6	427
McDonaldland® cookies	67	308	4	49	11	10	<27	0.23	0.23	2.9	0.9	12	1.5	358
Chocolate shake	291	383	10	66	9	30	349	0.12	0.44	0.5	<2.9	320	0.8	300
Strawberry shake	290	362	9	62	9	32	377	0.12	0.44	0.4	4.1	322	0.2	207
Vanilla shake	291	352	9	60	8	31	349	0.12	0.70	0.3	3.2	329	0.2	201
Hot fudge sundae	164	310	7	46	11	18	230	0.07	0.31	1.1	2.5	215	0.6	175
Caramel sundae	165	328	7	53	10	26	279	0.07	0.31	1.0	3.6	200	0.2	195
Strawberry sundae	164	289	7	46	9	20	230	0.07	0.30	1.0	2.8	174	0.4	96

Source: McDonald's Corporation, Oak Brook, Illinois. Nutritional analysis by Raltech Scientific Services, Inc. (formerly WARF), Madison, Wisconsin.

	Weight (g)	Energy (cal)	Protein (g)	Carbo-hydrate (g)	Fat (g)	Cholesterol (mg)	Vitamin A (IU)	Thiamin (mg)	Riboflavin (mg)	Niacin (mg)	Vitamin C (mg)	Calcium (mg)	Iron (mg)	Sodium (mg)
TACO BELL®														
Bean burrito	166	343	11	48	12	—	1657	0.37	0.22	2.2	15.2	98	2.8	272
Beef burrito	184	466	30	37	21	—	1675	0.30	0.39	7.0	15.2	83	4.6	327
Beefy tostada	184	291	19	21	15	—	3450	0.16	0.27	3.3	12.7	208	3.4	138
Bellbeefer®	123	221	15	23	7	—	2961	0.15	0.20	3.7	10.0	40	2.6	231
Bellbeefer® with cheese	137	278	19	23	12	—	3146	0.16	0.27	3.7	10.0	147	2.7	330
Burrito Supreme®	225	457	21	43	22	—	3462	0.33	0.35	4.7	16.0	121	3.8	367
Combination burrito	175	404	21	43	16	—	1666	0.34	0.31	4.6	15.2	91	3.7	300
Enchirito®	207	454	25	42	21	—	1178	0.31	0.37	4.7	9.5	259	3.8	1175
Pintos 'n cheese	158	168	11	21	5	—	3123	0.26	0.16	0.9	9.3	150	2.3	102
Taco	83	186	15	14	8	—	120	0.09	0.16	2.9	0.2	120	2.5	79
Tostada	138	179	9	25	6	—	3152	0.18	0.15	0.8	9.7	191	2.3	101

Sources: (1) *Menu Item Portions* (San Antonio, Texas: Taco Bell Co., July 1976); (2) Adams, C. F., Nutritive value of American foods in common units, in *Handbook No. 456* (Washington, D.C.: USDA Agricultural Research Service, November 1975); (3) Church, E. F., Church, H. N., eds. *Food Values of Portions Commonly Used,* 12th ed. (Philadelphia: J. B. Lippincott Co., 1975); (4) Valley Baptist Medical Center, Food Service Department, *Descriptions of Mexican-American Foods* (Fort Atkinson, Wisconsin: NASCO).

Table 1. Nutritional Analyses of Fast Foods *(continued)*

	Weight (g)	Energy (cal)	Protein (g)	Carbo-hydrate (g)	Fat (g)	Cholesterol (mg)	Vitamin A (IU)	Thiamin (mg)	Riboflavin (mg)	Niacin (mg)	Vitamin C (mg)	Calcium (mg)	Iron (mg)	Sodium (mg)
WENDY'S®														
Single hamburger	200	470	26	34	26	70	94	0.24	0.36	5.8	0.6	84	5.3	774
Doubie hamburger	285	670	44	34	40	125	128	0.43	0.54	10.6	1.5	138	8.2	980
Triple hamburger	360	850	65	33	51	205	220	0.47	0.68	14.7	2.0	104	10.7	1217
Single with cheese	240	580	33	34	34	90	221	0.38	0.43	6.3	0.7	228	5.4	1085
Double with cheese	325	800	50	41	48	155	439	0.49	0.75	11.4	2.3	177	10.2	1414
Triple with cheese	400	1040	72	35	68	225	472	0.80	0.84	15.1	3.4	371	10.9	1848
Chili	250	230	19	21	8	25	1188	0.22	0.25	3.4	2.9	83	4.4	1065
French fries	120	330	5	41	16	5	40	0.14	0.07	3.0	6.4	16	1.2	112
Frosty	250	390	9	54	16	45	355	0.20	0.60	X	0.7	270	0.9	247

Source: Wendy's International, Inc., Dublin, Ohio. Nutritional analysis by Medallion Laboratories, Minneapolis, Minnesota.

	Weight (g)	Energy (cal)	Protein (g)	Carbo-hydrate (g)	Fat (g)	Cholesterol (mg)	Vitamin A (IU)	Thiamin (mg)	Riboflavin (mg)	Niacin (mg)	Vitamin C (mg)	Calcium (mg)	Iron (mg)	Sodium (mg)
PIZZA HUT®[a] serving size: 2 slices of medium (13") pizza/ 4 servings per pizza														
THIN 'N CRISPY®														
Standard cheese	—	340	19	42	11	22	600	0.45	0.51	4	X	500	3.6	900
Superstyle cheese	—	410	26	45	14	30	750	0.53	0.60	4	X	800	3.6	1100
Standard pepperoni	—	370	19	42	15	27	700	0.45	0.43	4	X	400	3.2	1000
Superstyle pepperoni	—	430	23	43	19	34	800	0.60	0.43	5	X	550	3.6	1200
Standard pork with mushrooms	—	380	21	44	14	35	750	0.53	0.51	6	X	120	4.5	1200
Superstyle pork with mushrooms	—	450	26	46	19	40	750	0.60	0.60	6	1.2	150	6.3	1400
Supreme	—	400	21	44	17	13	750	0.68	0.51	6	2.4	400	4.5	1200
Super supreme	—	520	30	46	26	44	1100	1.05	0.68	8	3.6	550	5.4	1500
THICK 'N CHEWY®														
Standard cheese	—	390	24	53	10	18	800	0.75	1.19	8	X	600	4.5	800
Superstyle cheese	—	450	31	54	14	21	1000	0.83	0.68	8	1.2	950	4.5	1000
Standard pepperoni	—	450	25	52	16	21	1500	0.83	0.68	5	X	500	4.5	900
Superstyle pepperoni	—	490	27	52	20	24	1000	0.83	0.68	6	1.2	500	3.6	1200
Standard pork with mushrooms	—	430	27	53	14	21	1000	0.90	0.60	11	2.4	400	5.4	1000

	Weight (g)	Energy (cal)	Protein (g)	Carbo-hydrate (g)	Fat (g)	Cholesterol (mg)	Vitamin A (IU)	Thiamin (mg)	Riboflavin (mg)	Niacin (mg)	Vitamin C (mg)	Calcium (mg)	Iron (mg)	Sodium (mg)
PIZZA HUT® *(continued)*														
Superstyle pork with mushrooms	—	500	30	54	18	21	1000	0.90	0.68	12	2.4	550	6.3	1200
Supreme	—	480	29	52	18	24	1000	0.90	0.77	10	3.6	550	5.4	1000
Super supreme	—	590	34	55	26	38	1000	1.20	0.94	12	3.6	550	6.3	1400

[a] "PIZZA HUT, THIN 'N CRISPY, and THICK 'N CHEWY are all registered trademarks of Pizza Hut, Inc., and are being used with permission." Source: Pizza Hut, Inc., Wichita, Kansas. Nutritional analysis determined in 1979 by Raltech Scientific Services, Inc. (formerly WARF), Madison, Wisconsin.

	Weight (g)	Energy (cal)	Protein (g)	Carbo-hydrate (g)	Fat (g)	Cholesterol (mg)	Vitamin A (IU)	Thiamin (mg)	Riboflavin (mg)	Niacin (mg)	Vitamin C (mg)	Calcium (mg)	Iron (mg)	Sodium (mg)
BEVERAGES														
Coffee[a]	180	2	tr	tr	tr	—	0	0	tr	0.5	0	4	0.2	2
Tea[a]	180	2	tr	—	tr	—	0	0	0.04	0.1	1	5	0.2	—
Orange juice	183	82	1	20	tr	—	366	0.17	0.02	0.6	82.4	17	0.2	2
Chocolate milk	250	213	9	28	9	—	330	0.08	0.40	0.3	3.0	278	0.5	118
Skim milk	245	88	9	13	tr	—	10	0.09	0.44	0.2	2.0	296	0.1	127
Whole milk	244	159	9	12	9	27	342	0.07	0.41	0.2	2.4	188	tr	122
Coca-Cola®	246	96	0	24	0	—	—	—	—	—	—	—	—	20[b]
Fanta® ginger ale	244	84	0	21	0	—	—	—	—	—	—	—	—	30[b]
Fanta® grape	247	114	0	29	0	—	—	—	—	—	—	—	—	21[b]
Fanta® orange	248	117	0	30	0	—	—	—	—	—	—	—	—	21[b]
Fanta® root beer	246	103	0	27	0	—	—	—	—	—	—	—	—	23[b]
Mr. Pibb®	245	95	0	25	0	—	—	—	—	—	—	—	—	23[b]
Mr. Pibb® without sugar	236	1	0	tr	0	—	—	—	—	—	—	—	—	37[b]
Sprite®	245	95	0	24	0	—	—	—	—	—	—	—	—	42[b]
Sprite® without sugar	236	3	0	0	0	—	—	—	—	—	—	—	—	42[b]
Tab®	236	tr	0	tr	0	—	—	—	—	—	—	—	—	30[b]
Fresca®	236	2	0	0	0	—	—	—	—	—	—	—	—	38

[a] 6-oz serving; all other data are for 8-oz serving.

[b] Value when bottling water with average sodium content (12 mg/8 oz) is used.

Sources: (1) Adams, C. F., Nutritive value of American foods in common units, in *Handbook No. 456* (Washington, D. C.: USDA Agricultural Research Service, November 1975); (2) The Coca-Cola Company, Atlanta, Georgia, January 1977; (3) *American Hospital Formulary Service* (Washington, D. C.: American Society of Hospital Pharmacists, March 1978) Section 28:20.

APPENDIX H: Table of Food Composition

The table presented here is the standard table found in all nutrition textbooks and references. It presents the calorie content, energy-nutrient composition, and vitamin and mineral contents of 615 common foods by household measure.[1] It can be purchased from the U.S. Government Printing Office (address in Appendix J) as a separate softcover booklet.

Of the minerals, only calcium and iron are included in this table. You might also be curious about zinc, but we have chosen not to present information here on the zinc contents of foods. A few references that do are available.[2]

Of the vitamins, vitamin A, thiamin, riboflavin, niacin, and ascorbic acid (vitamin C) are included. An expanded version of this table, presently being published in installments by the U.S. Department of Agriculture, Agricultural Research Service, includes folacin and other vitamin information, as well as the amino acid analyses of foods.

The nutrient content of brand-name products—cookies, snack foods, cookie mixes, canned fruit, TV dinners, condiments, and so on—not found in this table can be obtained from *Consumer Guide*.[3] The composition of foods used by various ethnic groups, also not found in this table, can be requested from the U.S. Department of Agriculture.[4]

Notes

1. U.S. Department of Agriculture, Nutritive values of the edible parts of foods, *Nutritive Value of Foods*, Home and Garden Bulletin no. 72 (Washington, D.C.: Government Printing Office, 1971), Table 1.

2. K. A. Haeflein and A. I. Rasmussen, Zinc content of selected foods, *Journal of the American Dietetic Association* 70 (1977): 610-616; E. W. Murphy, B. W. Willis, and B. K. Watt, Provisional tables on the zinc content of foods, *Journal of the American Dietetic*

Association 66 (1975): 345-355; and J. H. Freeland and R. J. Cousins, Zinc content of selected foods, *Journal of the American Dietetic Association* 68 (1976): 526-529.

3. Food: *The Brand Name Game* (Skokie, Ill.: Consumer Guide, 1974).

4. *Composition of Foods Used by Ethnic Groups—Selected References to Sources of Data* can be requested from Dr. Louise Page, Food and Diet Appraisal Group, Consumer and Food Economics Institute, U.S. Department of Agriculture, Agricultural Research Service, Hyattsville MD 20782. For Japanese-American food equivalents, a reprint is available from the American Dietetic Association (address in Appendix J).

Appendix H Table of Food Composition

[Dashes in the columns for nutrients show that no suitable value could be found although there is reason to believe that a measurable amount of the nutrient may be present]

	Food, approximate measure, and weight (in grams)			Water	Food energy	Protein	Fat	Fatty acids: Saturated (total)	Fatty acids: Unsaturated: Oleic	Fatty acids: Unsaturated: Linoleic	Carbohydrate	Calcium	Iron	Vitamin A value	Thiamin	Riboflavin	Niacin	Ascorbic acid
			Grams	Percent	kCalories	Grams	Grams	Grams	Grams	Grams	Grams	Milligrams	Milligrams	International units	Milligrams	Milligrams	Milligrams	Milligrams
	MILK, CHEESE, CREAM, IMITATION CREAM; RELATED PRODUCTS																	
	Milk:																	
	Fluid:																	
1	Whole, 3.5% fat	1 cup	244	87	160	9	9	5	3	Trace	12	288	0.1	350	0.07	0.41	0.2	2
2	Nonfat (skim)	1 cup	245	90	90	9	Trace	---	---	---	12	296	.1	10	.09	.44	.2	2
3	Partly skimmed, 2% nonfat milk solids added.	1 cup	246	87	145	10	5	3	2	Trace	15	352	.1	200	.10	.52	.2	2
	Canned, concentrated, undiluted:																	
4	Evaporated, unsweetened.	1 cup	252	74	345	18	20	11	7	1	24	635	.3	810	.10	.86	.5	3
5	Condensed, sweetened.	1 cup	306	27	980	25	27	15	9	1	166	802	.3	1,100	.24	1.16	.6	3
	Dry, nonfat instant:																	
6	Low-density (1 1/3 cups needed for reconstitution to 1 qt.).	1 cup	68	4	245	24	Trace	---	---	---	35	879	.4	[1]20	.24	1.21	.6	5
7	High-density (7/8 cup needed for reconstitution to 1 qt.).	1 cup	104	4	375	37	1	---	---	---	54	1,345	.6	[1]30	.36	1.85	.9	7
	Buttermilk:																	
8	Fluid, cultured, made from skim milk.	1 cup	245	90	90	9	Trace	---	---	---	12	296	.1	10	.10	.44	.2	2
9	Dried, packaged	1 cup	120	3	465	41	6	3	2	Trace	60	1,498	.7	260	.31	2.06	1.1	---
	Cheese:																	
	Natural:																	
	Blue or Roquefort type:																	
10	Ounce	1 oz.	28	40	105	6	9	5	3	Trace	1	89	.1	350	.01	.17	.3	0
11	Cubic inch	1 cu. in.	17	40	65	4	5	3	2	Trace	Trace	54	.1	210	.01	.11	.2	0

[1] Value applies to unfortified product; value for fortified low-density product would be 1500 I.U. and the fortified high-density product would be 2290 I.U.

Table of Food Composition (continued)

[Dashes in the columns for nutrients show that no suitable value could be found although there is reason to believe that a measurable amount of the nutrient may be present]

	Food, approximate measure, and weight (in grams)			Water	Food energy	Protein	Fat	Fatty acids: Saturated (total)	Fatty acids: Unsaturated: Oleic	Fatty acids: Unsaturated: Linoleic	Carbohydrate	Calcium	Iron	Vitamin A value	Thiamin	Riboflavin	Niacin	Ascorbic acid
	MILK, CHEESE, CREAM, IMITATION CREAM; RELATED PRODUCTS—Con.																	
	Cheese—Continued																	
	Natural—Continued		Grams	Percent	kCalories	Grams	Grams	Grams	Grams	Grams	Grams	Milligrams	Milligrams	International units	Milligrams	Milligrams	Milligrams	Milligrams
12	Camembert, packaged in 4-oz. pkg. with 3 wedges per pkg.	1 wedge	38	52	115	7	9	5	3	Trace	1	40	0.2	380	0.02	0.29	0.3	0
	Cheddar:																	
13	Ounce	1 oz.	28	37	115	7	9	5	3	Trace	1	213	.3	370	.01	.13	Trace	0
14	Cubic inch	1 cu. in.	17	37	70	4	6	3	2	Trace	Trace	129	.2	230	.01	.08	Trace	0
	Cottage, large or small curd:																	
	Creamed:																	
15	Package of 12-oz., net wt.	1 pkg.	340	78	360	46	14	8	5	Trace	10	320	1.0	580	.10	.85	.3	0
16	Cup, curd pressed down.	1 cup	245	78	260	33	10	6	3	Trace	7	230	.7	420	.07	.61	.2	0
	Uncreamed:																	
17	Package of 12-oz., net wt.	1 pkg.	340	79	290	58	1	1	Trace	Trace	9	306	1.4	30	.10	.95	.3	0
18	Cup, curd pressed down.	1 cup	200	79	170	34	1	Trace	Trace	Trace	5	180	.8	20	.06	.56	.2	0
	Cream:																	
19	Package of 8-oz., net wt.	1 pkg.	227	51	850	18	86	48	28	3	5	141	.5	3,500	.05	.54	.2	0
20	Package of 3-oz., net wt.	1 pkg.	85	51	320	7	32	18	11	1	2	53	.2	1,310	.02	.20	.1	0
21	Cubic inch	1 cu. in.	16	51	60	1	6	3	2	Trace	Trace	10	Trace	250	Trace	.04	Trace	0
	Parmesan, grated:																	
22	Cup, pressed down	1 cup	140	17	655	60	43	24	14	1	5	1,893	.7	1,760	.03	1.22	.3	0
23	Tablespoon	1 tbsp.	5	17	25	2	2	1	Trace	Trace	Trace	68	Trace	60	Trace	.04	Trace	0
24	Ounce	1 oz.	28	17	130	12	9	5	3	Trace	1	383	.1	360	.01	.25	.1	0
	Swiss:																	
25	Ounce	1 oz.	28	39	105	8	8	4	3	Trace	1	262	.3	320	Trace	.11	Trace	0
26	Cubic inch	1 cu. in.	15	39	55	4	4	2	1	Trace	Trace	139	.1	170	Trace	.06	Trace	0

	Pasteurized processed cheese:																	
	American:																	
27	Ounce	1 oz.	28	40	105	7	9	5	3	Trace	1	198	.3	350	.01	.12	Trace	0
28	Cubic inch	1 cu. in.	18	40	65	4	5	3	2	Trace	Trace	122	.2	210	Trace	.07	Trace	0
	Swiss:																	
29	Ounce	1 oz.	28	40	100	8	8	4	3	Trace	1	251	.3	310	Trace	.11	Trace	0
30	Cubic inch	1 cu. in.	18	40	65	5	5	3	2	Trace	Trace	159	.2	200	Trace	.07	Trace	0
	Pasteurized process cheese food, American:																	
31	Tablespoon	1 tbsp.	14	43	45	3	3	2	1	Trace	1	80	.1	140	Trace	.08	Trace	0
32	Cubic inch	1 cu. in.	18	43	60	4	4	2	1	Trace	1	100	.1	170	Trace	.10	Trace	0
33	Pasteurized process cheese spread, American.	1 oz.	28	49	80	5	6	3	2	Trace	2	160	.2	250	Trace	.15	Trace	0
	Cream:																	
34	Half-and-half (cream and milk).	1 cup	242	80	325	8	28	15	9	1	11	261	.1	1,160	.07	.39	.1	2
35		1 tbsp.	15	80	20	1	2	1	1	Trace	1	16	Trace	70	Trace	.02	Trace	Trace
36	Light, coffee or table	1 cup	240	72	505	7	49	27	16	1	10	245	.1	2,020	.07	.36	.1	2
37		1 tbsp.	15	72	30	1	3	2	1	Trace	1	15	Trace	130	Trace	.02	Trace	Trace
38	Sour	1 cup	230	72	485	7	47	26	16	1	10	235	.1	1,930	.07	.35	.1	2
39		1 tbsp.	12	72	25	Trace	2	1	1	Trace	1	12	Trace	100	Trace	.02	Trace	Trace
40	Whipped topping (pressurized).	1 cup	60	62	155	2	14	8	5	Trace	6	67	-----	570	-----	.04	-----	-----
41		1 tbsp.	3	62	10	Trace	1	Trace	Trace	Trace	Trace	3	-----	30	-----	Trace	-----	-----
	Whipping, unwhipped (volume about double when whipped):																	
42	Light	1 cup	239	62	715	6	75	41	25	2	9	203	.1	3,060	.05	.29	.1	2
43		1 tbsp.	15	62	45	Trace	5	3	2	Trace	1	13	Trace	190	Trace	.02	Trace	Trace
44	Heavy	1 cup	238	57	840	5	90	50	30	3	7	179	.1	3,670	.05	.26	.1	2
45		1 tbsp.	15	57	55	Trace	6	3	2	Trace	1	11	Trace	230	Trace	.02	Trace	Trace
	Imitation cream products (made with vegetable fat):																	
	Creamers:																	
46	Powdered	1 cup	94	2	505	4	33	31	1	0	52	21	.6	[2] 200	-----	-----	Trace	-----
47		1 tsp.	2	2	10	Trace	1	Trace	Trace	0	1	1	Trace	[2] Trace	-----	-----	-----	-----
48	Liquid (frozen)	1 cup	245	77	345	3	27	25	1	0	25	29	-----	[2] 100	0	0	-----	-----
49		1 tbsp.	15	77	20	Trace	2	1	Trace	0	2	2	-----	[2] 10	0	0	-----	-----
50	Sour dressing (imitation sour cream) made with nonfat dry milk.	1 cup	235	72	440	9	38	35	1	Trace	17	277	.1	10	.07	.38	.2	1
51		1 tbsp.	12	72	20	Trace	2	2	Trace	Trace	1	14	Trace	Trace	Trace	Trace	Trace	Trace
	Whipped topping:																	
52	Pressurized	1 cup	70	61	190	1	17	15	1	0	9	5	-----	[2] 340	-----	0	-----	-----
53		1 tbsp.	4	61	10	Trace	1	1	Trace	0	Trace	Trace	-----	[2] 20	-----	0	-----	-----

[2] Contributed largely from beta-carotene used for coloring.

Table of Food Composition (continued)

[Dashes in the columns for nutrients show that no suitable value could be found although there is reason to believe that a measurable amount of the nutrient may be present]

	Food, approximate measure, and weight (in grams)			Water	Food energy	Protein	Fat	Fatty acids: Saturated (total)	Fatty acids: Unsaturated: Oleic	Fatty acids: Unsaturated: Linoleic	Carbohydrate	Calcium	Iron	Vitamin A value	Thiamin	Riboflavin	Niacin	Ascorbic acid
	MILK, CHEESE, CREAM, IMITATION CREAM; RELATED PRODUCTS—Con.		Grams	Per-cent	kCalories	Grams	Grams	Grams	Grams	Grams	Grams	Milli-grams	Milli-grams	Inter-national units	Milli-grams	Milli-grams	Milli-grams	Milli-grams
	Whipped topping—Continued																	
54	Frozen	1 cup	75	52	230	1	20	18	Trace	0	15	5	---	² 560	---	0	---	---
55		1 tbsp.	4	52	10	Trace	1	1	Trace	0	1	Trace	---	² 30	---	0	---	---
56	Powdered, made with whole milk.	1 cup	75	58	175	3	12	10	1	Trace	15	62	Trace	² 330	.02	.08	.1	Trace
57		1 tbsp.	4	58	10	Trace	1	1	Trace	Trace	1	3	Trace	² 20	Trace	Trace	Trace	Trace
	Milk beverages:																	
58	Cocoa, homemade	1 cup	250	79	245	10	12	7	4	Trace	27	295	1.0	400	.10	.45	.5	3
59	Chocolate-flavored drink made with skim milk and 2% added butterfat.	1 cup	250	83	190	8	6	3	2	Trace	27	270	.5	210	.10	.40	.3	3
60	Dry powder, approx. 3 heaping tea-spoons per ounce.	1 oz.	28	3	115	4	2	---	---	---	20	82	.6	290	.09	.15	.1	0
61	Beverage	1 cup	235	78	245	11	10	---	---	---	28	317	.7	590	.14	.49	.2	2
	Milk desserts:																	
62	Custard, baked	1 cup	265	77	305	14	15	7	5	1	29	297	1.1	930	.11	.50	.3	1
	Ice cream:																	
63	Regular (approx. 10% fat).	½ gal.	1,064	63	,055	48	113	62	37	3	221	1,553	.5	4,680	.43	2.23	1.1	11
64		1 cup	133	63	255	6	14	8	5	Trace	28	194	.1	590	.05	.28	.1	1
65		3 fl. oz. cup	50	63	95	2	5	3	2	Trace	10	73	Trace	220	.02	.11	.1	1
66	Rich (approx. 16% fat).	½ gal.	1,188	63	2,635	31	191	105	63	6	214	927	.2	7,840	.24	1.31	1.2	12
67		1 cup	148	63	330	4	24	13	8	1	27	115	Trace	980	.03	.16	.1	1
	Ice milk:																	
68	Hardened	½ gal.	1,048	67	1,595	50	53	29	17	2	235	1,635	1.0	2,200	.52	2.31	1.0	10
69		1 cup	131	67	200	6	7	4	2	Trace	29	204	.1	280	.07	.29	.1	1
70	Soft-serve	1 cup	175	67	265	8	9	5	3	Trace	39	273	.2	370	.09	.39	.2	2

	Yoghurt:																	
71	Made from partially skimmed milk.	1 cup	245	89	125	8	4	2	1	Trace	13	294	.1	170	.10	.44	.2	2
72	Made from whole milk	1 cup	245	88	150	7	8	5	3	Trace	12	272	.1	340	.07	.39	.2	2
	EGGS																	
	Eggs, large, 24 ounces per dozen:																	
	Raw or cooked in shell or with nothing added:																	
73	Whole, without shell	1 egg	50	74	80	6	6	2	3	Trace	Trace	27	1.1	590	.05	.15	Trace	0
74	White of egg	1 white	33	88	15	4	Trace	---	---	---	Trace	3	Trace	0	Trace	.09	Trace	0
75	Yolk of egg	1 yolk	17	51	60	3	5	2	2	Trace	Trace	24	.9	580	.04	.07	Trace	0
76	Scrambled with milk and fat.	1 egg	64	72	110	7	8	3	3	Trace	1	51	1.1	690	.05	.18	Trace	0
	MEAT, POULTRY, FISH, SHELLFISH; RELATED PRODUCTS																	
77	Bacon, (20 slices per lb. raw), broiled or fried, crisp.	2 slices	15	8	90	5	8	3	4	1	1	2	.5	0	.08	.05	.8	---
	Beef,[3] cooked:																	
	Cuts braised, simmered, or pot-roasted:																	
78	Lean and fat	3 ounces	85	53	245	23	16	8	7	Trace	0	10	2.9	30	.04	.18	3.5	---
79	Lean only	2.5 ounces	72	62	140	22	5	2	2	Trace	0	10	2.7	10	.04	.16	3.3	---
	Hamburger (ground beef), broiled:																	
80	Lean	3 ounces	85	60	185	23	10	5	4	Trace	0	10	3.0	20	.08	.20	5.1	---
81	Regular	3 ounces	85	54	245	21	17	8	8	Trace	0	9	2.7	30	.07	.18	4.6	---
	Roast, oven-cooked, no liquid added:																	
	Relatively fat, such as rib:																	
82	Lean and fat	3 ounces	85	40	375	17	34	16	15	1	0	8	2.2	70	.05	.13	3.1	---
83	Lean only	1.8 ounces	51	57	125	14	7	3	3	Trace	0	6	1.8	10	.04	.11	2.6	---
	Relatively lean, such as heel of round:																	
84	Lean and fat	3 ounces	85	62	165	25	7	3	3	Trace	0	11	3.2	10	.06	.19	4.5	---
85	Lean only	2.7 ounces	78	65	125	24	3	1	1	Trace	0	10	3.0	Trace	.06	.18	4.3	---
	Steak, broiled:																	
	Relatively, fat, such as sirloin:																	
86	Lean and fat	3 ounces	85	44	330	20	27	13	12	1	0	9	2.5	50	.05	.16	4.0	---
87	Lean only	2.0 ounces	56	59	115	18	4	2	2	Trace	0	7	2.2	10	.05	.14	3.6	---
	Relatively, lean, such as round:																	
88	Lean and fat	3 ounces	85	55	220	24	13	6	6	Trace	0	10	3.0	20	.07	.19	4.8	---
89	Lean only	2.4 ounces	68	61	130	21	4	2	2	Trace	0	9	2.5	10	.06	.16	4.1	---
	Beef, canned:																	
90	Corned beef	3 ounces	85	59	185	22	10	5	4	Trace	0	17	3.7	20	.01	.20	2.9	---
91	Corned beef hash	3 ounces	85	67	155	7	10	5	4	Trace	9	11	1.7	---	.01	.08	1.8	---
92	Beef, dried or chipped	2 ounces	57	48	115	19	4	2	2	Trace	0	11	2.9	---	.04	.18	2.2	---
93	Beef and vegetable stew	1 cup	235	82	210	15	10	5	4	Trace	15	28	2.8	2,310	.13	.17	4.4	15

[2] Contributed largely from beta-carotene used for coloring.

[3] Outer layer of fat on the cut was removed to within approximately ½-inch of the lean. Deposits of fat within the cut were not removed.

Table of Food Composition (continued)

[Dashes in the columns for nutrients show that no suitable value could be found although there is reason to believe that a measurable amount of the nutrient may be present]

	Food, approximate measure, and weight (in grams)			Water	Food energy	Protein	Fat	Fatty acids: Saturated (total)	Fatty acids: Unsaturated: Oleic	Fatty acids: Unsaturated: Linoleic	Carbohydrate	Calcium	Iron	Vitamin A value	Thiamin	Riboflavin	Niacin	Ascorbic acid
	MEAT, POULTRY, FISH, SHELLFISH; RELATED PRODUCTS—Continued		*Grams*	*Percent*	*kCalories*	*Grams*	*Grams*	*Grams*	*Grams*	*Grams*	*Grams*	*Milligrams*	*Milligrams*	*International units*	*Milligrams*	*Milligrams*	*Milligrams*	*Milligrams*
94	Beef potpie, baked, 4¼-inch diam., weight before baking about 8 ounces.	1 pie	227	55	560	23	33	9	20	2	43	32	4.1	1,860	0.25	0.27	4.5	7
	Chicken, cooked:																	
95	Flesh only, broiled	3 ounces	85	71	115	20	3	1	1	1	0	8	1.4	80	.05	.16	7.4	----
	Breast, fried, ½ breast:																	
96	With bone	3.3 ounces	94	58	155	25	5	1	2	1	1	9	1.3	70	.04	.17	11.2	----
97	Flesh and skin only	2.7 ounces	76	58	155	25	5	1	2	1	1	9	1.3	70	.04	.17	11.2	----
	Drumstick, fried:																	
98	With bone	2.1 ounces	59	55	90	12	4	1	2	1	Trace	6	.9	50	.03	.15	2.7	----
99	Flesh and skin only	1.3 ounces	38	55	90	12	4	1	2	1	Trace	6	.9	50	.03	.15	2.7	----
100	Chicken, canned, boneless	3 ounces	85	65	170	18	10	3	4	2	0	18	1.3	200	.03	.11	3.7	3
101	Chicken potpie, baked 4¼-inch diam., weight before baking about 8 ounces.	1 pie	227	57	535	23	31	10	15	3	42	68	3.0	3,020	.25	.26	4.1	5
	Chili con carne, canned:																	
102	With beans	1 cup	250	72	335	19	15	7	7	Trace	30	80	4.2	150	.08	.18	3.2	----
103	Without beans	1 cup	255	67	510	26	38	18	17	1	15	97	3.6	380	.05	.31	5.6	----
104	Heart, beef, lean, braised	3 ounces	85	61	160	27	5	----	----	----	1	5	5.0	20	.21	1.04	6.5	1
	Lamb,[3] cooked:																	
105	Chop, thick, with bone, broiled.	1 chop, 4.8 ounces.	137	47	400	25	33	18	12	1	0	10	1.5	----	.14	.25	5.6	----
106	Lean and fat	4.0 ounces	112	47	400	25	33	18	12	1	0	10	1.5	----	.14	.25	5.6	----
107	Lean only	2.6 ounces	74	62	140	21	6	3	2	Trace	0	9	1.5	----	.11	.20	4.5	----
	Leg, roasted:																	
108	Lean and fat	3 ounces	85	54	235	22	16	9	6	Trace	0	9	1.4	----	.13	.23	4.7	----
109	Lean only	2.5 ounces	71	62	130	20	5	3	2	Trace	0	9	1.4	----	.12	.21	4.4	----
	Shoulder, roasted:																	
110	Lean and fat	3 ounces	85	50	285	18	23	13	8	1	0	9	1.0	----	.11	.20	4.0	----
111	Lean only	2.3 ounces	64	61	130	17	6	3	2	Trace	0	8	1.0	----	.10	.18	3.7	----

112	Liver, beef, fried	2 ounces	57	57	130	15	6	—	—	—	3	6	5.0	30,280	.15	2.37	9.4	15
	Pork, cured, cooked:																	
113	Ham, light cure, lean and fat, roasted.	3 ounces	85	54	245	18	19	7	8	2	0	8	2.2	0	.40	.16	3.1	—
	Luncheon meat:																	
114	Boiled ham, sliced	2 ounces	57	59	135	11	10	4	4	1	0	6	1.6	0	.25	.09	1.5	—
115	Canned, spiced or unspiced.	2 ounces	57	55	165	8	14	5	6	1	1	5	1.2	0	.18	.12	1.6	—
	Pork, fresh,[3] cooked:																	
116	Chop, thick, with bone	1 chop, 3.5 ounces.	98	42	260	16	21	8	9	2	0	8	2.2	0	.63	.18	3.8	—
117	Lean and fat	2.3 ounces	66	42	260	16	21	8	9	2	0	8	2.2	0	.63	.18	3.8	—
118	Lean only	1.7 ounces	48	53	130	15	7	2	3	1	0	7	1.9	0	.54	.16	3.3	—
	Roast, oven-cooked, no liquid added:																	
119	Lean and fat	3 ounces	85	46	310	21	24	9	10	2	0	9	2.7	0	.78	.22	4.7	—
120	Lean only	2.4 ounces	68	55	175	20	10	3	4	1	0	9	2.6	0	.73	.21	4.4	—
	Cuts, simmered:																	
121	Lean and fat	3 ounces	85	46	320	20	26	9	11	2	0	8	2.5	0	.46	.21	4.1	—
122	Lean only	2.2 ounces	63	60	135	18	6	2	3	1	0	8	2.3	0	.42	.19	3.7	—
	Sausage:																	
123	Bologna, slice, 3-in. diam. by ⅛ inch.	2 slices	26	56	80	3	7	—	—	—	Trace	2	.5	—	.04	.06	.7	—
124	Braunschweiger, slice 2-in. diam. by ¼ inch.	2 slices	20	53	65	3	5	—	—	—	Trace	2	1.2	1,310	.03	.29	1.6	—
125	Deviled ham, canned	1 tbsp.	13	51	45	2	4	2	2	Trace	0	1	.3	—	.02	.01	.2	—
126	Frankfurter, heated (8 per lb. purchased pkg.).	1 frank	56	57	170	7	15	—	—	—	1	3	.8	—	.08	.11	1.4	—
127	Pork links, cooked (16 links per lb. raw).	2 links	26	35	125	5	11	4	5	1	Trace	2	.6	0	.21	.09	1.0	—
128	Salami, dry type	1 oz.	28	30	130	7	11	—	—	—	Trace	4	1.0	—	.10	.07	1.5	—
129	Salami, cooked	1 oz.	28	51	90	5	7	—	—	—	Trace	3	.7	—	.07	.07	1.2	—
130	Vienna, canned (7 sausages per 5-oz. can).	1 sausage	16	63	40	2	3	—	—	—	Trace	1	.3	—	.01	.02	.4	—
	Veal, medium fat, cooked, bone removed:																	
131	Cutlet	3 oz.	85	60	185	23	9	5	4	Trace	—	9	2.7	—	.06	.21	4.6	—
132	Roast	3 oz.	85	55	230	23	14	7	6	Trace	0	10	2.9	—	.11	.26	6.6	—
	Fish and shellfish:																	
133	Bluefish, baked with table fat.	3 oz.	85	68	135	22	4	—	—	—	0	25	.6	40	.09	.08	1.6	—
	Clams:																	
134	Raw, meat only	3 oz.	85	82	65	11	1	—	—	—	2	59	5.2	90	.08	.15	1.1	8
135	Canned, solids and liquid.	3 oz.	85	86	45	7	1	—	—	—	2	47	3.5	—	.01	.09	.9	—
136	Crabmeat, canned	3 oz.	85	77	85	15	2	—	—	—	1	38	.7	—	.07	.07	1.6	—

[3] Outer layer of fat on the cut was removed to within approximately ½-inch of the lean. Deposits of fat within the cut were not removed.

Table of Food Composition (continued)

[Dashes in the columns for nutrients show that no suitable value could be found although there is reason to believe that a measurable amount of the nutrient may be present]

	Food, approximate measure, and weight (in grams)			Water	Food energy	Protein	Fat	Fatty acids: Saturated (total)	Fatty acids: Unsaturated: Oleic	Fatty acids: Unsaturated: Linoleic	Carbohydrate	Calcium	Iron	Vitamin A value	Thiamin	Riboflavin	Niacin	Ascorbic acid
	MEAT, POULTRY, FISH, SHELLFISH; RELATED PRODUCTS—Continued																	
	Fish and shellfish—Continued		Grams	Per-cent	kCalories	Grams	Grams	Grams	Grams	Grams	Grams	Milli-grams	Milli-grams	Inter-national units	Milli-grams	Milli-grams	Milli-grams	Milli-grams
137	Fish sticks, breaded, cooked, frozen; stick 3¾ by 1 by ½ inch.	10 sticks or 8 oz. pkg.	227	66	400	38	20	5	4	10	15	25	0.9	----	0.09	0.16	3.6	----
138	Haddock, breaded, fried	3 oz.	85	66	140	17	5	1	3	Trace	5	34	1.0	----	.03	.06	2.7	2
139	Ocean perch, breaded, fried.	3 oz.	85	59	195	16	11	----	----	----	6	28	1.1	----	.08	.09	1.5	----
140	Oysters, raw, meat only (13–19 med. selects).	1 cup	240	85	160	20	4	----	----	----	8	226	13.2	740	.33	.43	6.0	----
141	Salmon, pink, canned	3 oz.	85	71	120	17	5	1	1	Trace	0	[4] 167	.7	60	.03	.16	6.8	----
142	Sardines, Atlantic, canned in oil, drained solids.	3 oz.	85	62	175	20	9	----	----	----	0	372	2.5	190	.02	.17	4.6	----
143	Shad, baked with table fat and bacon.	3 oz.	85	64	170	20	10	----	----	----	0	20	.5	20	.11	.22	7.3	----
144	Shrimp, canned, meat	3 oz.	85	70	100	21	1	----	----	----	1	98	2.6	50	.01	.03	1.5	----
145	Swordfish, broiled with butter or margarine.	3 oz.	85	65	150	24	5	----	----	----	0	23	1.1	1,750	.03	.04	9.3	----
146	Tuna, canned in oil, drained solids.	3 oz.	85	61	170	24	7	2	1	1	0	7	1.6	70	.04	.10	10.1	----
	MATURE DRY BEANS AND PEAS, NUTS, PEANUTS; RELATED PRODUCTS																	
147	Almonds, shelled, whole kernels.	1 cup	142	5	850	26	77	6	52	15	28	332	6.7	0	.34	1.31	5.0	Trace
	Beans, dry:																	
	Common varieties as Great Northern, navy, and others:																	
	Cooked, drained:																	
148	Great Northern	1 cup	180	69	210	14	1	----	----	----	38	90	4.9	0	.25	.13	1.3	0

149	Navy (pea)	1 cup	190	69	225	15	1	----	----	----	40	95	5.1	0	.27	.13	1.3	0
	Canned, solids and liquid:																	
	White with—																	
150	Frankfurters (sliced).	1 cup	255	71	365	19	18	----	----	----	32	94	4.8	330	.18	.15	3.3	Trace
151	Pork and tomato sauce.	1 cup	255	71	310	16	7	2	3	1	49	138	4.6	330	.20	.08	1.5	5
152	Pork and sweet sauce.	1 cup	255	66	385	16	12	4	5	1	54	161	5.9	----	.15	.10	1.3	----
153	Red kidney	1 cup	255	76	230	15	1	----	----	----	42	74	4.6	10	.13	.10	1.5	----
154	Lima, cooked, drained.	1 cup	190	64	260	16	1	----	----	----	49	55	5.9	----	.25	.11	1.3	----
155	Cashew nuts, roasted	1 cup	140	5	785	24	64	11	45	4	41	53	5.3	140	.60	.35	2.5	----
	Coconut, fresh, meat only:																	
156	Pieces, approx. 2 by 2 by 1/2 inch.	1 piece	45	51	155	2	16	14	1	Trace	4	6	.8	0	.02	.01	.2	1
157	Shredded or grated, firmly packed.	1 cup	130	51	450	5	46	39	3	Trace	12	17	2.2	0	.07	.03	.7	4
158	Cowpeas or blackeye peas, dry, cooked.	1 cup	248	80	190	13	1	----	----	----	34	42	3.2	20	.41	.11	1.1	Trace
159	Peanuts, roasted, salted, halves.	1 cup	144	2	840	37	72	16	31	21	27	107	3.0	----	.46	.19	24.7	0
160	Peanut butter	1 tbsp.	16	2	95	4	8	2	4	2	3	9	.3	----	.02	.02	2.4	0
161	Peas, split, dry, cooked	1 cup	250	70	290	20	1	----	----	----	52	28	4.2	100	.37	.22	2.2	----
162	Pecans, halves	1 cup	108	3	740	10	77	5	48	15	16	79	2.6	140	.93	.14	1.0	2
163	Walnuts, black or native, chopped.	1 cup	126	3	790	26	75	4	26	36	19	Trace	7.6	380	.28	.14	.9	----
	VEGETABLES AND VEGETABLE PRODUCTS																	
	Asparagus, green:																	
	Cooked, drained:																	
164	Spears, 1/2-in. diam. at base.	4 spears	60	94	10	1	Trace	----	----	----	2	13	.4	540	.10	.11	.8	16
165	Pieces, 1 1/2 to 2-in. lengths.	1 cup	145	94	30	3	Trace	----	----	----	5	30	.9	1,310	.23	.26	2.0	38
166	Canned, solids and liquid	1 cup	244	94	45	5	1	----	----	----	7	44	4.1	1,240	.15	.22	2.0	37
	Beans:																	
167	Lima, immature seeds, cooked, drained.	1 cup	170	71	190	13	1	----	----	----	34	80	4.3	480	.31	.17	2.2	29
	Snap:																	
	Green:																	
168	Cooked, drained	1 cup	125	92	30	2	Trace	----	----	----	7	63	.8	680	.09	.11	.6	15
169	Canned, solids and liquid.	1 cup	239	94	45	2	Trace	----	----	----	10	81	2.9	690	.07	.10	.7	10

[4] If bones are discarded, value will be greatly reduced.

Table of Food Composition (continued)

[Dashes in the columns for nutrients show that no suitable value could be found although there is reason to believe that a measurable amount of the nutrient may be present]

	Food, approximate measure, and weight (in grams)			Water	Food energy	Protein	Fat	Fatty acids: Saturated (total)	Fatty acids: Unsaturated: Oleic	Fatty acids: Unsaturated: Linoleic	Carbohydrate	Calcium	Iron	Vitamin A value	Thiamin	Riboflavin	Niacin	Ascorbic acid
			Grams	*Percent*	*kCalories*	*Grams*	*Grams*	*Grams*	*Grams*	*Grams*	*Grams*	*Milligrams*	*Milligrams*	*International units*	*Milligrams*	*Milligrams*	*Milligrams*	*Milligrams*
	VEGETABLES AND VEGETABLE PRODUCTS—Continued																	
	Beans—Continued																	
	Snap—Continued																	
	Yellow or wax:																	
170	Cooked, drained	1 cup	125	93	30	2	Trace	---	---	---	6	63	0.8	290	0.09	0.11	0.6	16
171	Canned, solids and liquid.	1 cup	239	94	45	2	1	---	---	---	10	81	2.9	140	.07	.10	.7	12
172	Sprouted mung beans, cooked, drained.	1 cup	125	91	35	4	Trace	---	---	---	7	21	1.1	30	.11	.13	.9	8
	Beets:																	
	Cooked, drained, peeled:																	
173	Whole beets, 2-in. diam.	2 beets	100	91	30	1	Trace	---	---	---	7	14	.5	20	.03	.04	.3	6
174	Diced or sliced	1 cup	170	91	55	2	Trace	---	---	---	12	24	.9	30	.05	.07	.5	10
175	Canned, solids and liquid.	1 cup	246	90	85	2	Trace	---	---	---	19	34	1.5	20	.02	.05	.2	7
176	Beet greens, leaves and stems, cooked, drained.	1 cup	145	94	25	3	Trace	---	---	---	5	144	2.8	7,400	.10	.22	.4	22
	Blackeye peas. See Cowpeas.																	
	Broccoli, cooked, drained:																	
177	Whole stalks, medium size.	1 stalk	180	91	45	6	1	---	---	---	8	158	1.4	4,500	.16	.36	1.4	162
178	Stalks cut into ½-in. pieces.	1 cup	155	91	40	5	1	---	---	---	7	136	1.2	3,880	.14	.31	1.2	140
179	Chopped, yield from 10-oz. frozen pkg.	1⅜ cups	250	92	65	7	1	---	---	---	12	135	1.8	6,500	.15	.30	1.3	143
180	Brussels sprouts, 7–8 sprouts (1¼ to 1½ in. diam.) per cup, cooked.	1 cup	155	88	55	7	1	---	---	---	10	50	1.7	810	.12	.22	1.2	135
	Cabbage:																	
	Common varieties:																	

	Raw:																	
181	Coarsely shredded or sliced.	1 cup	70	92	15	1	Trace	...	...	...	4	34	.3	90	.04	.04	.2	33
182	Finely shredded or chopped.	1 cup	90	92	20	1	Trace	...	...	...	5	44	.4	120	.05	.05	.3	42
183	Cooked	1 cup	145	94	30	2	Trace	...	...	...	6	64	.4	190	.06	.06	.4	48
184	Red, raw, coarsely shredded.	1 cup	70	90	20	1	Trace	...	...	...	5	29	.6	30	.06	.04	.3	43
185	Savoy, raw, coarsely shredded.	1 cup	70	92	15	2	Trace	...	...	...	3	47	.6	140	.04	.06	.2	39
186	Cabbage, celery or Chinese, raw, cut in 1-in. pieces.	1 cup	75	95	10	1	Trace	...	...	...	2	32	.5	110	.04	.03	.5	19
187	Cabbage, spoon (or pakchoy), cooked.	1 cup	170	95	25	2	Trace	...	...	...	4	252	1.0	5,270	.07	.14	1.2	26
	Carrots:																	
	Raw:																	
188	Whole, 5½ by 1 inch, (25 thin strips).	1 carrot	50	88	20	1	Trace	...	...	...	5	18	.4	5,500	.03	.03	.3	4
189	Grated	1 cup	110	88	45	1	Trace	...	...	...	11	41	.8	12,100	.06	.06	.7	9
190	Cooked, diced	1 cup	145	91	45	1	Trace	...	...	...	10	48	.9	15,220	.08	.07	.7	9
191	Canned, strained or chopped (baby food).	1 ounce	28	92	10	Trace	Trace	...	...	...	2	7	.1	3,690	.01	.01	.1	1
192	Cauliflower, cooked, flowerbuds.	1 cup	120	93	25	3	Trace	...	...	...	5	25	.8	70	.11	.10	.7	66
	Celery, raw:																	
193	Stalk, large outer, 8 by about 1½ inches, at root end.	1 stalk	40	94	5	Trace	Trace	...	...	...	2	16	.1	100	.01	.01	.1	4
194	Pieces, diced	1 cup	100	94	15	1	Trace	...	...	...	4	39	.3	240	.03	.03	.3	9
195	Collards, cooked	1 cup	190	91	55	5	1	...	...	...	9	289	1.1	10,260	.27	.37	2.4	87
	Corn, sweet:																	
196	Cooked, ear 5 by 1¾ inches.[5]	1 ear	140	74	70	3	1	...	...	...	16	2	.5	[6] 310	.09	.08	1.0	7
197	Canned, solids and liquid.	1 cup	256	81	170	5	2	...	...	...	40	10	1.0	[6] 690	.07	.12	2.3	13
198	Cowpeas, cooked, immature seeds.	1 cup	160	72	175	13	1	...	...	...	29	38	3.4	560	.49	.18	2.3	28
	Cucumbers, 10-ounce; 7½ by about 2 inches:																	
199	Raw, pared	1 cucumber	207	96	30	1	Trace	...	...	...	7	35	.6	Trace	.07	.09	.4	23
200	Raw, pared, center slice ⅛-inch thick.	6 slices	50	96	5	Trace	Trace	...	...	...	2	8	.2	Trace	.02	.02	.1	6
201	Dandelion greens, cooked	1 cup	180	90	60	4	1	...	...	...	12	252	3.2	21,060	.24	.29	...	32

[5] Measure and weight apply to entire vegetable or fruit including parts not usually eaten.

[6] Based on yellow varieties; white varieties contain only a trace of cryptoxanthin and carotenes, the pigments in corn that have biological activity.

Table of Food Composition (continued)

[Dashes in the columns for nutrients show that no suitable value could be found although there is reason to believe that a measurable amount of the nutrient may be present]

	Food, approximate measure, and weight (in grams)			Water	Food energy	Protein	Fat	Fatty acids: Saturated (total)	Fatty acids: Unsaturated: Oleic	Fatty acids: Unsaturated: Linoleic	Carbohydrate	Calcium	Iron	Vitamin A value	Thiamin	Riboflavin	Niacin	Ascorbic acid
	VEGETABLES AND VEGETABLE PRODUCTS—Continued		*Grams*	*Per-cent*	*kCalories*	*Grams*	*Grams*	*Grams*	*Grams*	*Grams*	*Grams*	*Milli-grams*	*Milli-grams*	*Inter-national units*	*Milli-grams*	*Milli-grams*	*Milli-grams*	*Milli-grams*
202	Endive, curly (including escarole).	2 ounces	57	93	10	1	Trace	---	---	---	2	46	1.0	1,870	0.04	0.08	0.3	6
203	Kale, leaves including stems, cooked.	1 cup	110	91	30	4	1	---	---	---	4	147	1.3	8,140	---	---	---	68
	Lettuce, raw:																	
204	Butterhead, as Boston types; head, 4-inch diameter.	1 head	220	95	30	3	Trace	---	---	---	6	77	4.4	2,130	.14	.13	.6	18
205	Crisphead, as Iceberg; head, 4¾-inch diameter.	1 head	454	96	60	4	Trace	---	---	---	13	91	2.3	1,500	.29	.27	1.3	29
206	Looseleaf, or bunching varieties, leaves.	2 large	50	94	10	1	Trace	---	---	---	2	34	.7	950	.03	.04	.2	9
207	Mushrooms, canned, solids and liquid.	1 cup	244	93	40	5	Trace	---	---	---	6	15	1.2	Trace	.04	.60	4.8	4
208	Mustard greens, cooked	1 cup	140	93	35	3	1	---	---	---	6	193	2.5	8,120	.11	.19	.9	68
209	Okra, cooked, pod 3 by ⅝ inch.	8 pods	85	91	25	2	Trace	---	---	---	5	78	.4	420	.11	.15	.8	17
	Onions:																	
	Mature:																	
210	Raw, onion 2½-inch diameter.	1 onion	110	89	40	2	Trace	---	---	---	10	30	.6	40	.04	.04	.2	11
211	Cooked	1 cup	210	92	60	3	Trace	---	---	---	14	50	.8	80	.06	.06	.4	14
212	Young green, small, without tops.	6 onions	50	88	20	1	Trace	---	---	---	5	20	.3	Trace	.02	.02	.2	12
213	Parsley, raw, chopped	1 tablespoon	4	85	Trace	Trace	Trace	---	---	---	Trace	8	.2	340	Trace	.01	Trace	7
214	Parsnips, cooked	1 cup	155	82	100	2	1	---	---	---	23	70	.9	50	.11	.12	.2	16
	Peas, green:																	
215	Cooked	1 cup	160	82	115	9	1	---	---	---	19	37	2.9	860	.44	.17	3.7	33
216	Canned, solids and liquid.	1 cup	249	83	165	9	1	---	---	---	31	50	4.2	1,120	.23	.13	2.2	22

217	Canned, strained (baby food).	1 ounce	28	86	15	1	Trace	-----	-----	-----	3	3	.4	140	.02	.02	.4	3
218	Peppers, hot, red, without seeds, dried (ground chili powder, added seasonings).	1 tablespoon	15	8	50	2	2	-----	-----	-----	8	40	2.3	9,750	.03	.17	1.3	2
	Peppers, sweet:																	
	Raw, about 5 per pound:																	
219	Green pod without stem and seeds.	1 pod	74	93	15	1	Trace	-----	-----	-----	4	7	.5	310	.06	.06	.4	94
220	Cooked, boiled, drained	1 pod	73	95	15	1	Trace	-----	-----	-----	3	7	.4	310	.05	.05	.4	70
	Potatoes, medium (about 3 per pound raw):																	
221	Baked, peeled after baking.	1 potato	99	75	90	3	Trace	-----	-----	-----	21	9	.7	Trace	.10	.04	1.7	20
	Boiled:																	
222	Peeled after boiling	1 potato	136	80	105	3	Trace	-----	-----	-----	23	10	.8	Trace	.13	.05	2.0	22
223	Peeled before boiling	1 potato	122	83	80	2	Trace	-----	-----	-----	18	7	.6	Trace	.11	.04	1.4	20
	French-fried, piece 2 by ½ by ½ inch:																	
224	Cooked in deep fat	10 pieces	57	45	155	2	7	2	2	4	20	9	.7	Trace	.07	.04	1.8	12
225	Frozen, heated	10 pieces	57	53	125	2	5	1	1	2	19	5	1.0	Trace	.08	.01	1.5	12
	Mashed:																	
226	Milk added	1 cup	195	83	125	4	1	-----	-----	-----	25	47	.8	50	.16	.10	2.0	19
227	Milk and butter added.	1 cup	195	80	185	4	8	4	3	Trace	24	47	.8	330	.16	.10	1.9	18
228	Potato chips, medium, 2-inch diameter.	10 chips	20	2	115	1	8	2	2	4	10	8	.4	Trace	.04	.01	1.0	3
229	Pumpkin, canned	1 cup	228	90	75	2	1	-----	-----	-----	18	57	.9	14,590	.07	.12	1.3	12
230	Radishes, raw, small, without tops.	4 radishes	40	94	5	Trace	Trace	-----	-----	-----	1	12	.4	Trace	.01	.01	.1	10
231	Sauerkraut, canned, solids and liquid.	1 cup	235	93	45	2	Trace	-----	-----	-----	9	85	1.2	120	.07	.09	.4	33
	Spinach:																	
232	Cooked	1 cup	180	92	40	5	1	-----	-----	-----	6	167	4.0	14,580	.13	.25	1.0	50
233	Canned, drained solids	1 cup	180	91	45	5	1	-----	-----	-----	6	212	4.7	14,400	.03	.21	.6	24
	Squash:																	
	Cooked:																	
234	Summer, diced	1 cup	210	96	30	2	Trace	-----	-----	-----	7	52	.8	820	.10	.16	1.6	21
235	Winter, baked, mashed.	1 cup	205	81	130	4	1	-----	-----	-----	32	57	1.6	8,610	.10	.27	1.4	27
	Sweetpotatoes:																	
	Cooked, medium, 5 by 2 inches, weight raw about 6 ounces:																	
236	Baked, peeled after baking.	1 sweet-potato.	110	64	155	2	1	-----	-----	-----	36	44	1.0	8,910	.10	.07	.7	24
237	Boiled, peeled after boiling.	1 sweet-potato.	147	71	170	2	1	-----	-----	-----	39	47	1.0	11,610	.13	.09	.9	25

Table of Food Composition (continued)

[Dashes in the columns for nutrients show that no suitable value could be found although there is reason to believe that a measurable amount of the nutrient may be present]

	Food, approximate measure, and weight (in grams)			Water	Food energy	Protein	Fat	Fatty acids: Saturated (total)	Fatty acids: Unsaturated: Oleic	Fatty acids: Unsaturated: Linoleic	Carbohydrate	Calcium	Iron	Vitamin A value	Thiamin	Riboflavin	Niacin	Ascorbic acid
	VEGETABLES AND VEGETABLE PRODUCTS—Continued		Grams	Per-cent	kCalo-ries	Grams	Grams	Grams	Grams	Grams	Grams	Milli-grams	Milli-grams	Inter-national units	Milli-grams	Milli-grams	Milli-grams	Milli-grams
	Sweetpotatoes—Continued																	
238	Candied, 3½ by 2¼ inches.	1 sweet-potato.	175	60	295	2	6	2	3	1	60	65	1.6	11,030	0.10	0.08	0.8	17
239	Canned, vacuum or solid pack.	1 cup	218	72	235	4	Trace	---	---	---	54	54	1.7	17,000	.10	.10	1.4	30
	Tomatoes:																	
240	Raw, approx. 3-in. diam. 2⅛ in. high; wt., 7 oz.	1 tomato	200	94	40	2	Trace	---	---	---	9	24	.9	1,640	.11	.07	1.3	[7] 42
241	Canned, solids and liquid.	1 cup	241	94	50	2	1	---	---	---	10	14	1.2	2,170	.12	.07	1.7	41
	Tomato catsup:																	
242	Cup	1 cup	273	69	290	6	1	---	---	---	69	60	2.2	3,820	.25	.19	4.4	41
243	Tablespoon	1 tbsp.	15	69	15	Trace	Trace	---	---	---	4	3	.1	210	.01	.01	.2	2
	Tomato juice, canned:																	
244	Cup	1 cup	243	94	45	2	Trace	---	---	---	10	17	2.2	1,940	.12	.07	1.9	39
245	Glass (6 fl. oz.)	1 glass	182	94	35	2	Trace	---	---	---	8	13	1.6	1,460	.09	.05	1.5	29
246	Turnips, cooked, diced	1 cup	155	94	35	1	Trace	---	---	---	8	54	.6	Trace	.06	.08	.5	34
247	Turnip greens, cooked	1 cup	145	94	30	3	Trace	---	---	---	5	252	1.5	8,270	.15	.33	.7	68
	FRUITS AND FRUIT PRODUCTS																	
248	Apples, raw (about 3 per lb.).[5]	1 apple	150	85	70	Trace	Trace	---	---	---	18	8	.4	50	.04	.02	.1	3
249	Apple juice, bottled or canned.	1 cup	248	88	120	Trace	Trace	---	---	---	30	15	1.5	---	.02	.05	.2	2
	Applesauce, canned:																	
250	Sweetened	1 cup	255	76	230	1	Trace	---	---	---	61	10	1.3	100	.05	.03	.1	[8] 3
251	Unsweetened or artificially sweetened.	1 cup	244	88	100	1	Trace	---	---	---	26	10	1.2	100	.05	.02	.1	[8] 2

	Apricots:																	
252	Raw (about 12 per lb.)[5]	3 apricots	114	85	55	1	Trace	…	…	…	14	18	.5	2,890	.03	.04	.7	10
253	Canned in heavy sirup	1 cup	259	77	220	2	Trace	…	…	…	57	28	.8	4,510	.05	.06	.9	10
254	Dried, uncooked (40 halves per cup).	1 cup	150	25	390	8	1	…	…	…	100	100	8.2	16,350	.02	.23	4.9	19
255	Cooked, unsweetened, fruit and liquid.	1 cup	285	76	240	5	1	…	…	…	62	63	5.1	8,550	.01	.13	2.8	8
256	Apricot nectar, canned	1 cup	251	85	140	1	Trace	…	…	…	37	23	.5	2,380	.03	.03	.5	[8] 8
	Avocados, whole fruit, raw:[5]																	
257	California (mid- and late-winter; diam. 3⅛ in.).	1 avocado	284	74	370	5	37	7	17	5	13	22	1.3	630	.24	.43	3.5	30
258	Florida (late summer, fall; diam. 3⅝ in.).	1 avocado	454	78	390	4	33	7	15	4	27	30	1.8	880	.33	.61	4.9	43
259	Bananas, raw, medium size.[5]	1 banana	175	76	100	1	Trace	…	…	…	26	10	.8	230	.06	.07	.8	12
260	Banana flakes	1 cup	100	3	340	4	1	…	…	…	89	32	2.8	760	.18	.24	2.8	7
261	Blackberries, raw	1 cup	144	84	85	2	1	…	…	…	19	46	1.3	290	.05	.06	.5	30
262	Blueberries, raw	1 cup	140	83	85	1	1	…	…	…	21	21	1.4	140	.04	.08	.6	20
263	Cantaloups, raw; medium, 5-inch diameter about 1⅔ pounds.[5]	½ melon	385	91	60	1	Trace	…	…	…	14	27	.8	[9] 6,540	.08	.06	1.2	63
264	Cherries, canned, red, sour, pitted, water pack.	1 cup	244	88	105	2	Trace	…	…	…	26	37	.7	1,660	.07	.05	.5	12
265	Cranberry juice cocktail, canned.	1 cup	250	83	165	Trace	Trace	…	…	…	42	13	.8	Trace	.03	.03	.1	[10] 40
266	Cranberry sauce, sweetened, canned, strained.	1 cup	277	62	405	Trace	1	…	…	…	104	17	.6	60	.03	.03	.1	6
267	Dates, pitted, cut	1 cup	178	22	490	4	1	…	…	…	130	105	5.3	90	.16	.17	3.9	0
268	Figs, dried, large, 2 by 1 in.	1 fig	21	23	60	1	Trace	…	…	…	15	26	.6	20	.02	.02	.1	0
269	Fruit cocktail, canned, in heavy sirup.	1 cup	256	80	195	1	Trace	…	…	…	50	23	1.0	360	.05	.03	1.3	5

[5] Measure and weight apply to entire vegetable or fruit including parts not usually eaten.

[7] Year-round average. Samples marketed from November through May, average 20 milligrams per 200-gram tomato; from June through October, around 52 milligrams.

[8] This is the amount from the fruit. Additional ascorbic acid may be added by the manufacturer. Refer to the label for this information.

[9] Value for varieties with orange-colored flesh; value for varieties with green flesh would be about 540 I.U.

[10] Value listed is based on products with label stating 30 milligrams per 6 fl. oz. serving.

Table of Food Composition (continued)

[Dashes in the columns for nutrients show that no suitable value could be found although there is reason to believe that a measurable amount of the nutrient may be present]

	Food, approximate measure, and weight (in grams)			Water	Food energy	Protein	Fat	Fatty acids			Carbohydrate	Calcium	Iron	Vitamin A value	Thiamin	Riboflavin	Niacin	Ascorbic acid
								Saturated (total)	Unsaturated									
									Oleic	Linoleic								
	FRUITS AND FRUIT PRODUCTS—Con.		Grams	Percent	kCalories	Grams	Grams	Grams	Grams	Grams	Grams	Milligrams	Milligrams	International units	Milligrams	Milligrams	Milligrams	Milligrams
	Grapefruit:																	
	Raw, medium, 3¾-in. diam.[5]																	
270	White	½ grapefruit.	241	89	45	1	Trace	-----	-----	-----	12	19	0.5	10	0.05	0.02	0.2	44
271	Pink or red	½ grapefruit.	241	89	50	1	Trace	-----	-----	-----	13	20	0.5	540	0.05	0.02	0.2	44
272	Canned, sirup pack	1 cup	254	81	180	2	Trace	-----	-----	-----	45	33	.8	30	.08	.05	.5	76
	Grapefruit juice:																	
273	Fresh	1 cup	246	90	95	1	Trace	-----	-----	-----	23	22	.5	(11)	.09	.04	.4	92
	Canned, white:																	
274	Unsweetened	1 cup	247	89	100	1	Trace	-----	-----	-----	24	20	1.0	20	.07	.04	.4	84
275	Sweetened	1 cup	250	86	130	1	Trace	-----	-----	-----	32	20	1.0	20	.07	.04	.4	78
	Frozen, concentrate, unsweetened:																	
276	Undiluted, can, 6 fluid ounces.	1 can	207	62	300	4	1	-----	-----	-----	72	70	.8	60	.29	.12	1.4	286
277	Diluted with 3 parts water, by volume.	1 cup	247	89	100	1	Trace	-----	-----	-----	24	25	.2	20	.10	.04	.5	96
278	Dehydrated crystals	4 oz.	113	1	410	6	1	-----	-----	-----	102	100	1.2	80	.40	.20	2.0	396
279	Prepared with water (1 pound yields about 1 gallon).	1 cup	247	90	100	1	Trace	-----	-----	-----	24	22	.2	20	.10	.05	.5	91
	Grapes, raw:[5]																	
280	American type (slip skin).	1 cup	153	82	65	1	1	-----	-----	-----	15	15	.4	100	.05	.03	.2	3
281	European type (adherent skin).	1 cup	160	81	95	1	Trace	-----	-----	-----	25	17	.6	140	.07	.04	.4	6
	Grapejuice:																	
282	Canned or bottled	1 cup	253	83	165	1	Trace	-----	-----	-----	42	28	.8	-----	.10	.05	.5	Trace
	Frozen concentrate, sweetened:																	
283	Undiluted, can, 6 fluid ounces.	1 can	216	53	395	1	Trace	-----	-----	-----	100	22	.9	40	.13	.22	1.5	(12)

284	Diluted with 3 parts water, by volume.	1 cup	250	86	135	1	Trace	...	...	...	33	8	.3	10	.05	.08	.5	(12)
285	Grapejuice drink, canned	1 cup	250	86	135	Trace	Trace	...	...	...	35	8	.3		.03	.03	.3	(12)
286	Lemons, raw, 2⅛-in. diam., size 165.[5] Used for juice.	1 lemon	110	90	20	1	Trace	...	...	...	6	19	.4	10	.03	.01	.1	
287	Lemon juice, raw	1 cup	244	91	60	1	Trace	...	...	...	20	17	.5	50	.07	.02	.2	112
	Lemonade concentrate:																	
288	Frozen, 6 fl. oz. per can	1 can	219	48	430	Trace	Trace	...	...	...	112	9	.4	40	.04	.07	.7	66
289	Diluted with 4⅓ parts water, by volume.	1 cup	248	88	110	Trace	Trace	...	...	...	28	2	Trace	Trace	Trace	.02	.2	17
	Lime juice:																	
290	Fresh	1 cup	246	90	65	1	Trace	...	...	...	22	22	.5	20	.05	.02	.2	79
291	Canned, unsweetened	1 cup	246	90	65	1	Trace	...	...	...	22	22	.5	20	.05	.02	.2	52
	Limeade concentrate, frozen:																	
292	Undiluted, can, 6 fluid ounces.	1 can	218	50	410	Trace	Trace	...	...	...	108	11	.2	Trace	.02	02	.2	26
293	Diluted with 4⅓ parts water, by volume.	1 cup	247	90	100	Trace	Trace	...	...	...	27	2	Trace	Trace	Trace	Trace	Trace	5
294	Oranges, raw, 2⅝-in. diam., all commercial, varieties.[5]	1 orange	180	86	65	1	Trace	...	...	...	16	54	.5	260	.13	.05	.5	66
295	Orange juice, fresh, all varieties.	1 cup	248	88	110	2	1	...	...	...	26	27	.5	500	.22	.07	1.0	124
296	Canned, unsweetened	1 cup	249	87	120	2	Trace	...	...	...	28	25	1.0	500	.17	.05	.7	100
	Frozen concentrate:																	
297	Undiluted, can, 6 fluid ounces.	1 can	213	55	360	5	Trace	...	...	...	87	75	.9	1,620	.68	.11	2.8	360
298	Diluted with 3 parts water, by volume.	1 cup	249	87	120	2	Trace	...	...	...	29	25	.2	550	.22	.02	1.0	120
299	Dehydrated crystals	4 oz.	113	1	430	6	2	...	...	...	100	95	1.9	1,900	.76	.24	3.3	408
300	Prepared with water (1 pound yields about 1 gallon).	1 cup	248	88	115	2	1	...	...	...	27	25	.5	500	.20	.07	1.0	109
301	Orange-apricot juice drink	1 cup	249	87	125	1	Trace	...	...	...	32	12	.2	1,440	.05	.02	.5	[10] 40

[5] Measure and weight apply to entire vegetable or fruit including parts not usually eaten.

[10] Value listed is based on product with label stating 30 milligrams per 6 fl. oz. serving.

[11] For white-fleshed varieties value is about 20 I.U. per cup; for red-fleshed varieties, 1,080 I.U. per cup.

[12] Present only if added by the manufacturer. Refer to the label for this information.

Table of Food Composition (continued)

[Dashes in the columns for nutrients show that no suitable value could be found although there is reason to believe that a measurable amount of the nutrient may be present]

	Food, approximate measure, and weight (in grams)			Water	Food energy	Protein	Fat	Fatty acids: Saturated (total)	Fatty acids: Unsaturated: Oleic	Fatty acids: Unsaturated: Linoleic	Carbohydrate	Calcium	Iron	Vitamin A value	Thiamin	Riboflavin	Niacin	Ascorbic acid
	FRUITS AND FRUIT PRODUCTS—Con.		*Grams*	*Percent*	*kCalories*	*Grams*	*Grams*	*Grams*	*Grams*	*Grams*	*Grams*	*Milligrams*	*Milligrams*	*International units*	*Milligrams*	*Milligrams*	*Milligrams*	*Milligrams*
	Orange and grapefruit juice:																	
	Frozen concentrate:																	
302	Undiluted, can, 6 fluid ounces.	1 can	210	59	330	4	1	----	----	----	78	61	0.8	800	0.48	0.06	2.3	302
303	Diluted with 3 parts water, by volume.	1 cup	248	88	110	1	Trace	----	----	----	26	20	.2	270	.16	.02	.8	102
304	Papayas, raw, ½-inch cubes.	1 cup	182	89	70	1	Trace	----	----	----	18	36	.5	3.190	.07	.08	.5	102
	Peaches:																	
	Raw:																	
305	Whole, medium, 2-inch diameter, about 4 per pound.[5]	1 peach	114	89	35	1	Trace	----	----	----	10	9	.5	[3]1.320	.02	.05	1.0	7
306	Sliced	1 cup	168	89	65	1	Trace	----	----	----	16	15	.8	[13]2,230	.03	.08	1.6	12
	Canned, yellow-fleshed, solids and liquid:																	
	Sirup pack, heavy:																	
307	Halves or slices	1 cup	257	79	200	1	Trace	----	----	----	52	10	.8	1,100	.02	.06	1.4	7
308	Water pack	1 cup	245	91	75	1	Trace	----	----	----	20	10	.7	1,100	.02	.06	1.4	7
309	Dried, uncooked	1 cup	160	25	420	5	1	----	----	----	109	77	9.6	6,240	.02	.31	8.5	28
310	Cooked, unsweetened, 10–12 halves and juice.	1 cup	270	77	220	3	1	----	----	----	58	41	5.1	3,290	.01	.15	4.2	6
	Frozen:																	
311	Carton, 12 ounces, not thawed.	1 carton	340	76	300	1	Trace	----	----	----	77	14	1.7	2,210	.03	.14	2.4	[14]135
	Pears:																	
312	Raw, 3 by 2½-inch diameter.[5]	1 pear	182	83	100	1	1	----	----	----	25	13	.5	30	.04	.07	.2	7
	Canned, solids and liquid:																	
	Sirup pack, heavy:																	
313	Halves or slices	1 cup	255	80	195	1	1	----	----	----	50	13	.5	Trace	.03	.05	.3	4

	Pineapple:																	
314	Raw, diced	1 cup	140	85	75	1	Trace	-----	-----	-----	19	24	.7	100	.12	.04	.3	24
	Canned, heavy sirup pack, solids and liquid:																	
315	Crushed	1 cup	260	80	195	1	Trace	-----	-----	-----	50	29	.8	120	.20	.06	.5	17
316	Sliced, slices and juice.	2 small or 1 large.	122	80	90	Trace	Trace	-----	-----	-----	24	13	.4	50	.09	.03	.2	8
317	Pineapple juice, canned	1 cup	249	86	135	1	Trace	-----	-----	-----	34	37	.7	120	.12	.04	.5	[8] 22
	Plums, all except prunes:																	
318	Raw, 2-inch diameter, about 2 ounces.[5]	1 plum	60	87	25	Trace	Trace	-----	-----	-----	7	7	.3	140	.02	.02	.3	3
	Canned, sirup pack (Italian prunes):																	
319	Plums (with pits) and juice.[5]	1 cup	256	77	205	1	Trace	-----	-----	-----	53	22	2.2	2,970	.05	.05	.9	4
	Prunes, dried, "softenized", medium:																	
320	Uncooked [5]	4 prunes	32	28	70	1	Trace	-----	-----	-----	18	14	1.1	440	.02	.04	.4	1
321	Cooked, unsweetened, 17–18 prunes and 1/3 cup liquid.[5]	1 cup	270	66	295	2	1	-----	-----	-----	78	60	4.5	1,860	.08	.18	1.7	2
322	Prune juice, canned or bottled.	1 cup	256	80	200	1	Trace	-----	-----	-----	49	36	10.5	-----	.03	.03	1.0	[8] 5
	Raisins, seedless:																	
323	Packaged, 1/2 oz. or 1 1/2 tbsp. per pkg.	1 pkg.	14	18	40	Trace	Trace	-----	-----	-----	11	9	.5	Trace	.02	.01	.1	Trace
324	Cup, pressed down	1 cup	165	18	480	4	Trace	-----	-----	-----	128	102	5.8	30	.18	.13	.8	2
	Raspberries, red:																	
325	Raw	1 cup	123	84	70	1	1	-----	-----	-----	17	27	1.1	160	.04	.11	1.1	31
326	Frozen, 10-ounce carton, not thawed.	1 carton	284	74	275	2	1	-----	-----	-----	70	37	1.7	200	.06	.17	1.7	59
327	Rhubarb, cooked, sugar added.	1 cup	272	63	385	1	Trace	-----	-----	-----	98	212	1.6	220	.06	.15	.7	17
	Strawberries:																	
328	Raw, capped	1 cup	149	90	55	1	1	-----	-----	-----	13	31	1.5	90	.04	.10	1.0	88
329	Frozen, 10-ounce carton, not thawed.	1 carton	284	71	310	1	1	-----	-----	-----	79	40	2.0	90	.06	.17	1.5	150
330	Tangerines, raw, medium, 2 3/8-in. diam., size 176.[5]	1 tangerine	116	87	40	1	Trace	-----	-----	-----	10	34	.3	360	.05	.02	.1	27
331	Tangerine juice, canned, sweetened.	1 cup	249	87	125	1	1	-----	-----	-----	30	45	.5	1,050	.15	.05	.2	55
332	Watermelon, raw, wedge, 4 by 8 inches (1/16 of 10 by 16-inch melon, about 2 pounds with rind).[5]	1 wedge	925	93	115	2	1	-----	-----	-----	27	30	2.1	2,510	.13	.13	.7	30

[5] Measure and weight apply to entire vegetable or fruit including parts not usually eaten.

[8] This is the amount from the fruit. Additional ascorbic acid may be added by the manufacturer. Refer to the label for this information.

[13] Based on yellow-fleshed varieties; for white-fleshed varieties value is about 50 I.U. per 114-gram peach and 80 I.U. per cup of sliced peaches.

[14] This value includes ascorbic acid added by manufacturer.

Table of Food Composition (continued)

[Dashes in the columns for nutrients show that no suitable value could be found although there is reason to believe that a measurable amount of the nutrient may be present]

No.	Food, approximate measure, and weight (in grams)			Water	Food energy	Protein	Fat	Fatty acids: Saturated (total)	Fatty acids: Unsaturated: Oleic	Fatty acids: Unsaturated: Linoleic	Carbohydrate	Calcium	Iron	Vitamin A value	Thiamin	Riboflavin	Niacin	Ascorbic acid
	GRAIN PRODUCTS		Grams	Percent	kCalories	Grams	Grams	Grams	Grams	Grams	Grams	Milligrams	Milligrams	International units	Milligrams	Milligrams	Milligrams	Milligrams
	Bagel, 3-in. diam.:																	
333	Egg	1 bagel	55	32	165	6	2	---	---	---	28	9	1.2	30	0.14	0.10	1.2	0
334	Water	1 bagel	55	29	165	6	2	---	---	---	30	8	1.2	0	.15	.11	1.4	0
335	Barley, pearled, light, uncooked.	1 cup	200	11	700	16	2	Trace	1	1	158	32	4.0	0	.24	.10	6.2	0
336	Biscuits, baking powder from home recipe with enriched flour, 2-in. diam.	1 biscuit	28	27	105	2	5	1	2	1	13	34	.4	Trace	.06	.06	.1	Trace
337	Biscuits, baking powder from mix, 2-in. diam.	1 biscuit	28	28	90	2	3	1	1	1	15	19	.6	Trace	.08	.07	.6	Trace
338	Bran flakes (40% bran), added thiamin and iron.	1 cup	35	3	105	4	1	---	---	---	28	25	12.3	0	.14	.06	2.2	0
339	Bran flakes with raisins, added thiamin and iron.	1 cup	50	7	145	4	1	---	---	---	40	28	13.5	Trace	.16	.07	2.7	0
	Breads:																	
340	Boston brown bread, slice 3 by ¾ in.	1 slice	48	45	100	3	1	---	---	---	22	43	.9	0	.05	.03	.6	0
	Cracked-wheat bread:																	
341	Loaf, 1 lb.	1 loaf	454	35	1,190	40	10	2	5	2	236	399	5.0	Trace	.53	.41	5.9	Trace
342	Slice, 18 slices per loaf.	1 slice	25	35	65	2	1	---	---	---	13	22	.3	Trace	.03	.02	.3	Trace
	French or vienna bread:																	
343	Enriched, 1 lb. loaf	1 loaf	454	31	1,315	41	14	3	8	2	251	195	10.0	Trace	1.27	1.00	11.3	Trace
344	Unenriched, 1 lb. loaf.	1 loaf	454	31	1,315	41	14	3	8	2	251	195	3.2	Trace	.36	.36	3.6	Trace
	Italian bread:																	
345	Enriched, 1 lb. loaf	1 loaf	454	32	1,250	41	4	Trace	1	2	256	77	10.0	0	1.32	.91	11.8	0
346	Unenriched, 1 lb. loaf.	1 loaf	454	32	1,250	41	4	Trace	1	2	256	77	3.2	0	.41	.27	3.6	0
	Raisin bread:																	
347	Loaf, 1 lb.	1 loaf	454	35	1,190	30	13	3	8	2	243	322	5.9	Trace	.23	.41	3.2	Trace

348	Slice, 18 slices per loaf.	1 slice	25	35	65	2	1				13	18	.3	Trace	.01	.02	.2	Trace
	Rye bread:																	
	American, light (⅓ rye, ⅔ wheat):																	
349	Loaf, 1 lb.	1 loaf	454	36	1,100	41	5				236	340	7.3	0	.82	.32	6.4	0
350	Slice, 18 slices per loaf.	1 slice	25	36	60	2	Trace				13	19	.4	0	.05	.02	.4	0
351	Pumpernickel, loaf, 1 lb.	1 loaf	454	34	1,115	41	5				241	381	10.9	0	1.04	.64	5.4	0
	White bread, enriched: [15]																	
	Soft-crumb type:																	
352	Loaf, 1 lb.	1 loaf	454	36	1,225	39	15	3	8	2	229	381	11.3	Trace	1.13	.95	10.9	Trace
353	Slice, 18 slices per loaf.	1 slice	25	36	70	2	1				13	21	.6	Trace	.06	.05	.6	Trace
354	Slice, toasted	1 slice	22	25	70	2	1				13	21	.6	Trace	.06	.05	.6	Trace
355	Slice, 22 slices per loaf.	1 slice	20	36	55	2	1				10	17	.5	Trace	.05	.04	.5	Trace
356	Slice, toasted	1 slice	17	25	55	2	1				10	17	.5	Trace	.05	.04	.5	Trace
357	Loaf, 1½ lbs.	1 loaf	680	36	1,835	59	22	5	12	3	343	571	17.0	Trace	1.70	1.43	16.3	Trace
358	Slice, 24 slices per loaf.	1 slice	28	36	75	2	1				14	24	.7	Trace	.07	.06	.7	Trace
359	Slice, toasted	1 slice	24	25	75	2	1				14	24	.7	Trace	.07	.06	.7	Trace
360	Slice, 28 slices per loaf.	1 slice	24	36	65	2	1				12	20	.6	Trace	.06	.05	.6	Trace
361	Slice, toasted	1 slice	21	25	65	2	1				12	20	.6	Trace	.06	.05	.6	Trace
	Firm-crumb type:																	
362	Loaf, 1 lb.	1 loaf	454	35	1,245	41	17	4	10	2	228	435	11.3	Trace	1.22	.91	10.9	Trace
363	Slice, 20 slices per loaf.	1 slice	23	35	65	2	1				12	22	.6	Trace	.06	.05	.6	Trace
364	Slice, toasted	1 slice	20	24	65	2	1				12	22	.6	Trace	.06	.05	.6	Trace
365	Loaf, 2 lbs.	1 loaf	907	35	2,495	82	34	8	20	4	455	871	22.7	Trace	2.45	1.81	21.8	Trace
366	Slice, 34 slices per loaf.	1 slice	27	35	75	2	1				14	26	.7	Trace	.07	.05	.6	Trace
367	Slice, toasted	1 slice	23	35	75	2	1				14	26	.7	Trace	.07	.05	.6	Trace
	Whole-wheat bread, soft-crumb type:																	
368	Loaf, 1 lb.	1 loaf	454	36	1,095	41	12	2	6	2	224	381	13.6	Trace	1.36	.45	12.7	Trace
369	Slice, 16 slices per loaf.	1 slice	28	36	65	3	1				14	24	.8	Trace	.09	.03	.8	Trace
370	Slice, toasted	1 slice	24	24	65	3	1				14	24	.8	Trace	.09	.03	.8	Trace

[15] Values for iron, thiamin, riboflavin, and niacin per pound of unenriched white bread would be as follows:

	Iron *Milligrams*	Thiamin *Milligrams*	Riboflavin *Milligrams*	Niacin *Milligrams*
Soft crumb	3.2	.31	.39	5.0
Firm crumb	3.2	.32	.59	4.1

Table of Food Composition (continued)

[Dashes in the columns for nutrients show that no suitable value could be found although there is reason to believe that a measurable amount of the nutrient may be present]

	Food, approximate measure, and weight (in grams)			Water	Food energy	Protein	Fat	Fatty acids: Saturated (total)	Fatty acids: Unsaturated: Oleic	Fatty acids: Unsaturated: Linoleic	Carbohydrate	Calcium	Iron	Vitamin A value	Thiamin	Riboflavin	Niacin	Ascorbic acid
			Grams	*Percent*	*kCalories*	*Grams*	*Grams*	*Grams*	*Grams*	*Grams*	*Grams*	*Milligrams*	*Milligrams*	*International units*	*Milligrams*	*Milligrams*	*Milligrams*	*Milligrams*
	GRAIN PRODUCTS—Continued																	
	Bread—Continued																	
	Whole-wheat bread, firm-crumb type:																	
371	Loaf, 1 lb.	1 loaf	454	36	1,100	48	14	3	6	3	216	449	13.6	Trace	1.18	0.54	12.7	Trace
372	Slice, 18 slices per loaf.	1 slice	25	36	60	3	1	---	---	---	12	25	.8	Trace	.06	.03	.7	Trace
373	Slice, toasted	1 slice	21	24	60	3	1	---	---	---	12	25	.8	Trace	.06	.03	.7	Trace
374	Breadcrumbs, dry, grated	1 cup	100	6	390	13	5	1	2	1	73	122	3.6	Trace	.22	.30	3.5	Trace
375	Buckwheat flour, light, sifted.	1 cup	98	12	340	6	1	---	---	---	78	11	1.0	0	.08	.04	.4	0
376	Bulgur, canned, seasoned	1 cup	135	56	245	8	4	---	---	---	44	27	1.9	0	.08	.05	4.1	0
	Cakes made from cake mixes:																	
	Angelfood:																	
377	Whole cake	1 cake	635	34	1,645	36	1	---	---	---	377	603	1.9	0	.03	.70	.6	0
378	Piece, 1/12 of 10-in. diam. cake.	1 piece	53	34	135	3	Trace	---	---	---	32	50	.2	0	Trace	.06	.1	0
	Cupcakes, small, 2 1/2 in. diam.:																	
379	Without icing	1 cupcake	25	26	90	1	3	1	1	1	14	40	.1	40	.01	.03	.1	Trace
380	With chocolate icing	1 cupcake	36	22	130	2	5	2	2	1	21	47	.3	60	.01	.04	.1	Trace
	Devil's food, 2-layer, with chocolate icing:																	
381	Whole cake	1 cake	1,107	24	3,755	49	136	54	58	16	645	653	8.9	1,660	.33	.89	3.3	1
382	Piece, 1/16 of 9-in. diam. cake.	1 piece	69	24	235	3	9	3	4	1	40	41	.6	100	.02	.06	.2	Trace
383	Cupcake, small, 2 1/2 in. diam.	1 cupcake	35	24	120	2	4	1	2	Trace	20	21	.3	50	.01	.03	.1	Trace
	Gingerbread:																	
384	Whole cake	1 cake	570	37	1,575	18	39	10	19	9	291	513	9.1	Trace	.17	.51	4.6	2
385	Piece, 1/9 of 8-in. square cake.	1 piece	63	37	175	2	4	1	2	1	32	57	1.0	Trace	.02	.06	.5	Trace
	White, 2-layer, with chocolate icing:																	
386	Whole cake	1 cake	1,140	21	4,000	45	122	45	54	17	716	1,129	5.7	680	.23	.91	2.3	2

387	Piece, 1/16 of 9-in. diam. cake.	1 piece	71	21	250	3	8	3	3	1	45	70	.4	40	.01	.06	.1	Trace
	Cakes made from home recipes:[16]																	
388	Boston cream pie; piece 1/12 of 8-in. diam.	1 piece	69	35	210	4	6	2	3	1	34	46	.3	140	.02	.08	.1	Trace
	Fruitcake, dark, made with enriched flour:																	
389	Loaf, 1-lb.	1 loaf	454	18	1,720	22	69	15	37	13	271	327	11.8	540	.59	.64	3.6	2
390	Slice, 1/30 of 8-in. loaf.	1 slice	15	18	55	1	2	Trace	1	Trace	9	11	.4	20	.02	.02	.1	Trace
	Plain sheet cake:																	
	Without icing:																	
391	Whole cake	1 cake	777	25	2,830	35	108	30	52	21	434	497	3.1	1,320	.16	.70	1.6	2
392	Piece, 1/9 of 9-in. square cake.	1 piece	86	25	315	4	12	3	6	2	48	55	.3	150	.02	.08	.2	Trace
393	With boiled white icing, piece, 1/9 of 9-in. square cake.	1 piece	114	23	400	4	12	3	6	2	71	56	.3	150	.02	.08	.2	Trace
	Pound:																	
394	Loaf, 8½ by 3½ by 3in.	1 loaf	514	17	2,430	29	152	34	68	17	242	108	4.1	1,440	.15	.46	1.0	0
395	Slice, ½-in. thick	1 slice	30	17	140	2	9	2	4	1	14	6	.2	80	.01	.03	.1	0
	Sponge:																	
396	Whole cake	1 cake	790	32	2,345	60	45	14	20	4	427	237	9.5	3,560	.40	1.11	1.6	Trace
397	Piece, 1/12 of 10-in. diam. cake.	1 piece	66	32	195	5	4	1	2	Trace	36	20	.8	300	.03	.09	.1	Trace
	Yellow, 2-layer, without icing:																	
398	Whole cake	1 cake	870	24	3,160	39	111	31	53	22	506	618	3.5	1,310	.17	.70	1.7	2
399	Piece, 1/16 of 9-in. diam. cake.	1 piece	54	24	200	2	7	2	3	1	32	39	.2	80	.01	.04	.1	Trace
	Yellow, 2-layer, with chocolate icing:																	
400	Whole cake	1 cake	1,203	21	4,390	51	156	55	69	23	727	818	7.2	1,920	.24	.96	2.4	Trace
401	Piece, 1/16 of 9-in. diam. cake.	1 piece	75	21	275	3	10	3	4	1	45	51	.5	120	.02	.06	.2	Trace
	Cake icings. See Sugars, Sweets.																	
	Cookies:																	
	Brownies with nuts:																	
402	Made from home recipe with enriched flour.	1 brownie	20	10	95	1	6	1	3	1	10	8	.4	40	.04	.02	.1	Trace
403	Made from mix	1 brownie	20	11	85	1	4	1	2	1	13	9	.4	20	.03	.02	.1	Trace

[16] Unenriched cake flour used unless otherwise specified.

Table of Food Composition (continued)

[Dashes in the columns for nutrients show that no suitable value could be found although there is reason to believe that a measurable amount of the nutrient may be present]

	Food, approximate measure, and weight (in grams)			Water	Food energy	Protein	Fat	Fatty acids: Saturated (total)	Fatty acids: Unsaturated: Oleic	Fatty acids: Unsaturated: Linoleic	Carbohydrate	Calcium	Iron	Vitamin A value	Thiamin	Riboflavin	Niacin	Ascorbic acid
			Grams	*Percent*	*kCalories*	*Grams*	*Grams*	*Grams*	*Grams*	*Grams*	*Grams*	*Milligrams*	*Milligrams*	*International units*	*Milligrams*	*Milligrams*	*Milligrams*	*Milligrams*
	GRAIN PRODUCTS—Continued																	
	Cookies—Continued																	
	Chocolate chip:																	
404	Made from home recipe with enriched flour.	1 cookie	10	3	50	1	3	1	1	1	6	4	0.2	10	0.01	0.01	0.1	Trace
405	Commercial	1 cookie	10	3	50	1	2	1	1	Trace	7	4	.2	10	Trace	Trace	Trace	Trace
406	Fig bars, commercial	1 cookie	14	14	50	1	1	—	—		11	11	.2	20	Trace	.01	.1	Trace
407	Sandwich, chocolate or vanilla, commercial.	1 cookie	10	2	50	1	2	1	1	Trace	7	2	.1	0	Trace	Trace	.1	0
	Corn flakes, added nutrients:																	
408	Plain	1 cup	25	4	100	2	Trace	—	—	—	21	4	.4	0	.11	.02	.5	0
409	Sugar-covered	1 cup	40	2	155	2	Trace	—	—	—	36	5	.4	0	.16	.02	.8	0
	Corn (hominy) grits, degermed, cooked:																	
410	Enriched	1 cup	245	87	125	3	Trace	—	—	—	27	2	.7	[17] 150	.10	.07	1.0	0
411	Unenriched	1 cup	245	87	125	3	Trace	—	—	—	27	2	.2	[17] 150	.05	.02	.5	0
	Cornmeal:																	
412	Whole-ground, unbolted, dry.	1 cup	122	12	435	11	5	1	2	2	90	24	2.9	[17] 620	.46	.13	2.4	0
413	Bolted (nearly whole-grain) dry.	1 cup	122	12	440	11	4	Trace	1	2	91	21	2.2	[17] 590	.37	.10	2.3	0
	Degermed, enriched:																	
414	Dry form	1 cup	138	12	500	11	2	—	—	—	108	8	4.0	[17] 610	.61	.36	4.8	0
415	Cooked	1 cup	240	88	120	3	1	—	—	—	26	2	1.0	[17] 140	.14	.10	1.2	0
	Degermed, unenriched:																	
416	Dry form	1 cup	138	12	500	11	2	—	—	—	108	8	1.5	[17] 610	.19	.07	1.4	0
417	Cooked	1 cup	240	88	120	3	1	—	—	—	26	2	.5	[17] 140	.05	.02	.2	0
418	Corn muffins, made with enriched degermed cornmeal and enriched flour; muffin $2\frac{3}{8}$-in. diam.	1 muffin	40	33	125	3	4	2	2	Trace	19	42	.7	[17] 120	.08	.09	.6	Trace

419	Corn muffins, made with mix, egg, and milk; muffin 2⅜-in. diam.	1 muffin	40	30	130	3	4	1	2	1	20	96	.6	100	.07	.08	.6	Trace
420	Corn, puffed, presweetened, added nutrients.	1 cup	30	2	115	1	Trace				27	3	.5	0	.13	.05	.6	0
421	Corn, shredded, added nutrients.	1 cup	25	3	100	2	Trace				22	1	.6	0	.11	.05	.5	0
	Crackers:																	
422	Graham, 2½-in. square	4 crackers	28	6	110	2	3				21	11	.4	0	.01	.06	.4	0
423	Saltines	4 crackers	11	4	50	1	1		1		8	2	.1	0	Trace	Trace	.1	0
	Danish pastry, plain (without fruit or nuts):																	
424	Packaged ring, 12 ounces.	1 ring	240	22	1,435	25	80	24	37	15	155	170	3.1	1,050	.24	.51	2.7	Trace
425	Round piece, approx. 4¼-in. diam. by 1 in.	1 pastry	65	22	275	5	15	5	7	3	30	33	.6	200	.05	.10	.5	Trace
426	Ounce	1 oz.	28	22	120	2	7	2	3	1	13	14	.3	90	.02	.04	.2	Trace
427	Doughnuts, cake type	1 doughnut	32	24	125	1	6	1	4	Trace	16	13	[18].4	30	[18].05	[18].05	[18].4	Trace
428	Farina, quick-cooking, enriched, cooked.	1 cup	245	89	105	3	Trace				22	147	[19].7	0	[19].12	[19].07	[19]1.0	0
	Macaroni, cooked:																	
	Enriched:																	
429	Cooked, firm stage (undergoes additional cooking in a food mixture).	1 cup	130	64	190	6	1				39	14	[19]1.4	0	[19].23	[19].14	[19]1.8	0
430	Cooked until tender	1 cup	140	72	155	5	1				32	8	[19]1.3	0	[19].20	[19].11	[19]1.5	0
	Unenriched:																	
431	Cooked, firm stage (undergoes additional cooking in a food mixture).	1 cup	130	64	190	6	1				39	14	.7	0	.03	.03	.5	0
432	Cooked until tender	1 cup	140	72	155	5	1				32	11	.6	0	.01	.01	.4	0
433	Macaroni (enriched) and cheese, baked.	1 cup	200	58	430	17	22	10	9	2	40	362	1.8	860	.20	.40	1.8	Trace
434	Canned	1 cup	240	80	230	9	10	4	3	1	26	199	1.0	260	.12	.24	1.0	Trace
435	Muffins, with enriched white flour; muffin, 3-inch diam.	1 muffin	40	38	120	3	4	1	2	1	17	42	.6	40	.07	.09	.6	Trace
	Noodles (egg noodles), cooked:																	
436	Enriched	1 cup	160	70	200	7	2	1	1	Trace	37	16	[19]1.4	110	[19].22	[19].13	[19]1.9	0
437	Unenriched	1 cup	160	70	200	7	2	1	1	Trace	37	16	1.0	110	.05	.03	.6	0

[17] This value is based on product made from yellow varieties of corn; white varieties contain only a trace.

[18] Based on product made with enriched flour. With unenriched flour, approximate values per doughnut are: Iron, 0.2 milligram; thiamin, 0.01 milligram; riboflavin, 0.03 milligram; niacin, 0.2 milligram.

[19] Iron, thiamin, riboflavin, and niacin are based on the minimum levels of enrichment specified in standards of identity promulgated under the Federal Food, Drug, and Cosmetic Act.

Table of Food Composition (continued)

[Dashes in the columns for nutrients show that no suitable value could be found although there is reason to believe that a measurable amount of the nutrient may be present]

No.	Food, approximate measure, and weight (in grams)			Water	Food energy	Protein	Fat	Fatty acids: Saturated (total)	Fatty acids: Unsaturated: Oleic	Fatty acids: Unsaturated: Linoleic	Carbohydrate	Calcium	Iron	Vitamin A value	Thiamin	Riboflavin	Niacin	Ascorbic acid
	GRAIN PRODUCTS—Continued		Grams	Per-cent	kCalo-ries	Grams	Grams	Grams	Grams	Grams	Grams	Milli-grams	Milli-grams	Inter-national units	Milli-grams	Milli-grams	Milli-grams	Milli-grams
438	Oats (with or without corn) puffed, added nutrients.	1 cup	25	3	100	3	1	---	---	---	19	44	1.2	0	0.24	0.04	0.5	0
439	Oatmeal or rolled oats, cooked.	1 cup	240	87	130	5	2	---	---	1	23	22	1.4	0	.19	.05	.2	0
	Pancakes, 4-inch diam.:																	
440	Wheat, enriched flour (home recipe).	1 cake	27	50	60	2	2	Trace	1	Trace	9	27	.4	30	.05	.06	.4	Trace
441	Buckwheat (made from mix with egg and milk).	1 cake	27	58	55	2	2	1	1	Trace	6	59	.4	60	.03	.04	.2	Trace
442	Plain or buttermilk (made from mix with egg and milk).	1 cake	27	51	60	2	2	1	1	Trace	9	58	.3	70	.04	.06	.2	Trace
	Pie (piecrust made with unenriched flour):																	
	Sector, 4-in., 1/7 of 9-in. diam. pie:																	
443	Apple (2-crust)	1 sector	135	48	350	3	15	4	7	3	51	11	.4	40	.03	.03	.5	1
444	Butterscotch (1-crust)	1 sector	130	45	350	6	14	5	6	2	50	98	1.2	340	.04	.13	.3	Trace
445	Cherry (2-crust)	1 sector	135	47	350	4	15	4	7	3	52	19	.4	590	.03	.03	.7	Trace
446	Custard (1-crust)	1 sector	130	58	285	8	14	5	6	2	30	125	.8	300	.07	.21	.4	0
447	Lemon meringue (1-crust).	1 sector	120	47	305	4	12	4	6	2	45	17	.6	200	.04	.10	.2	4
448	Mince (2-crust)	1 sector	135	43	365	3	16	4	8	3	56	38	1.4	Trace	.09	.05	.5	1
449	Pecan (1-crust)	1 sector	118	20	490	6	27	4	16	5	60	55	3.3	190	.19	.08	.4	Trace
450	Pineapple chiffon (1-crust).	1 sector	93	41	265	6	11	3	5	2	36	22	.8	320	.04	.08	.4	1
451	Pumpkin (1-crust)	1 sector	130	59	275	5	15	5	6	2	32	66	.7	3,210	.04	.13	.7	Trace
	Piecrust, baked shell for pie made with:																	
452	Enriched flour	1 shell	180	15	900	11	60	16	28	12	79	25	3.1	0	.36	.25	3.2	0
453	Unenriched flour	1 shell	180	15	900	11	60	16	28	12	79	25	.9	0	.05	.05	.9	0

	Piecrust mix including stick form:																	
454	Package, 10-oz., for double crust.	1 pkg.	284	9	1,480	20	93	23	46	21	141	131	1.4	0	.11	.11	2.0	0
455	Pizza (cheese) 5½-in. sector; ⅛ of 14-in. diam. pie.	1 sector	75	45	185	7	6	2	3	Trace	27	107	.7	290	.04	.12	.7	4
	Popcorn, popped:																	
456	Plain, large kernel	1 cup	6	4	25	1	Trace	-	-	-	5	1	.2	-	-	.01	.1	0
457	With oil and salt	1 cup	9	3	40	1	2	1	Trace	Trace	5	1	.2	-	-	.01	.2	0
458	Sugar coated	1 cup	35	4	135	2	1	-	-	-	30	2	.5	-	-	.02	.4	0
	Pretzels:																	
459	Dutch, twisted	1 pretzel	16	5	60	2	1	-	-	-	12	4	.2	0	Trace	Trace	.1	0
460	Thin, twisted	1 pretzel	6	5	25	1	Trace	-	-	-	5	1	.1	0	Trace	Trace	Trace	0
461	Stick, small, 2¼ inches	10 sticks	3	5	10	Trace	Trace	-	-	-	2	1	Trace	0	Trace	Trace	Trace	0
462	Stick, regular, 3⅛ inches.	5 sticks	3	5	10	Trace	Trace	-	-	-	2	1	Trace	0	Trace	Trace	Trace	0
	Rice, white:																	
	Enriched:																	
463	Raw	1 cup	185	12	670	12	1	-	-	-	149	44	[20]5.4	0	[20].81	[20].06	[20]6.5	0
464	Cooked	1 cup	205	73	225	4	Trace	-	-	-	50	21	[20]1.8	0	[20].23	[20].02	[20]2.1	0
465	Instant, ready-to-serve.	1 cup	165	73	180	4	Trace	-	-	-	40	5	[20]1.3	0	[20].21	[20]-	[20]1.7	0
466	Unenriched, cooked	1 cup	205	73	225	4	Trace	-	-	-	50	21	.4	0	.04	.02	.8	0
467	Parboiled, cooked	1 cup	175	73	185	4	Trace	-	-	-	41	33	[20]1.4	0	[20].19	[20]-	[20]2.1	0
468	Rice, puffed, added nutrients.	1 cup	15	4	60	1	Trace	-	-	-	13	3	.3	0	.07	.01	.7	0
	Rolls, enriched:																	
	Cloverleaf or pan:																	
469	Home recipe	1 roll	35	26	120	3	3	1	1	1	20	16	.7	30	.09	.09	.8	Trace
470	Commercial	1 roll	28	31	85	2	2	Trace	1	Trace	15	21	.5	Trace	.08	.05	.6	Trace
471	Frankfurter or hamburger.	1 roll	40	31	120	3	2	1	1	1	21	30	.8	Trace	.11	.07	.9	Trace
472	Hard, round or rectangular.	1 roll	50	25	155	5	2	Trace	1	Trace	30	24	1.2	Trace	.13	.12	1.4	Trace
473	Rye wafers, whole-grain, 1⅞ by 3½ inches.	2 wafers	13	6	45	2	Trace	-	-	-	10	7	.5	0	.04	.03	.2	0
474	Spaghetti, cooked, tender stage, enriched.	1 cup	140	72	155	5	1	-	-	-	32	11	[19]1.3	0	[19].20	[19].11	[19]1.5	0

[19] Iron, thiamin, riboflavin, and niacin are based on the minimum levels of enrichment specified in standards of identity promulgated under the Federal Food, Drug, and Cosmetic Act.

[20] Iron, thiamin, and niacin are based on the minimum levels of enrichment specified in standards of identity promulgated under the Federal Food, Drug, and Cosmetic Act. Riboflavin is based on unenriched rice. When the minimum level of enrichment for riboflavin specified in the standards of identity becomes effective the value will be 0.12 milligram per cup of parboiled rice and of white rice.

Table of Food Composition (continued)

[Dashes in the columns for nutrients show that no suitable value could be found although there is reason to believe that a measurable amount of the nutrient may be present]

	Food, approximate measure, and weight (in grams)			Water	Food energy	Protein	Fat	Fatty acids: Saturated (total)	Fatty acids: Unsaturated: Oleic	Fatty acids: Unsaturated: Linoleic	Carbohydrate	Calcium	Iron	Vitamin A value	Thiamin	Riboflavin	Niacin	Ascorbic acid
			Grams	Percent	kCalories	Grams	Grams	Grams	Grams	Grams	Grams	Milligrams	Milligrams	International units	Milligrams	Milligrams	Milligrams	Milligrams
	GRAIN PRODUCTS—Continued																	
	Spaghetti with meat balls, and tomato sauce:																	
475	Home recipe	1 cup	248	70	330	19	12	4	6	1	39	124	3.7	1,590	0.25	0.30	4.0	22
476	Canned	1 cup	250	78	260	12	10	2	3	4	28	53	3.3	1,000	.15	.18	2.3	5
	Spaghetti in tomato sauce with cheese:																	
477	Home recipe	1 cup	250	77	260	9	9	2	5	1	37	80	2.3	1,080	.25	.18	2.3	13
478	Canned	1 cup	250	80	190	6	2	1	1	1	38	40	2.8	930	.35	.28	4.5	10
479	Waffles, with enriched flour, 7-in. diam.	1 waffle	75	41	210	7	7	2	4	1	28	85	1.3	250	.13	.19	1.0	Trace
480	Waffles, made from mix, enriched, egg and milk added, 7-in. diam.	1 waffle	75	42	205	7	8	3	3	1	27	179	1.0	170	.11	.17	.7	Trace
481	Wheat, puffed, added nutrients.	1 cup	15	3	55	2	Trace	—	—	—	12	4	.6	0	.08	.03	1.2	0
482	Wheat, shredded, plain	1 biscuit	25	7	90	2	1	—	—	—	20	11	.9	0	.06	.03	1.1	0
483	Wheat flakes, added nutrients.	1 cup	30	4	105	3	Trace	—	—	—	24	12	1.3	0	.19	.04	1.5	0
	Wheat flours:																	
484	Whole-wheat, from hard wheats, stirred.	1 cup	120	12	400	16	2	Trace	1	1	85	49	4.0	0	.66	.14	5.2	0
	All-purpose or family flour, enriched:																	
485	Sifted	1 cup	115	12	420	12	1	—	—	—	88	18	[19]3.3	0	[19].51	[19].30	[19]4.0	0
486	Unsifted	1 cup	125	12	455	13	1	—	—	—	95	20	[19]3.6	0	[19].55	[19].33	[19]4.4	0
487	Self-rising, enriched	1 cup	125	12	440	12	1	—	—	—	93	331	[19]3.6	0	[19].55	[19].33	[19]4.4	0
488	Cake or pastry flour, sifted.	1 cup	96	12	350	7	1	—	—	—	76	16	.5	0	.03	.03	.7	0
	FATS, OILS																	
	Butter:																	
	Regular, 4 sticks per pound:																	
489	Stick	½ cup	113	16	810	1	92	51	30	3	1	23	0	[21]3,750	—	—	—	0

490	Tablespoon (approx. 1/8 stick).	1 tbsp.	14	16	100	Trace	12	6	4	Trace	Trace	3	0	[21]470	-----	-----	-----	0
491	Pat (1-in. sq. 1/3-in. high; 90 per lb.).	1 pat	5	16	35	Trace	4	2	1	Trace	Trace	1	0	[21]170	-----	-----	-----	0
	Whipped, 6 sticks or 2, 8-oz. containers per pound:																	
492	Stick	1/2 cup	76	16	540	1	61	34	20	2	Trace	15	0	[21]2,500	-----	-----	-----	0
493	Tablespoon (approx. 1/8 stick).	1 tbsp.	9	16	65	Trace	8	4	3	Trace	Trace	2	0	[21]310	-----	-----	-----	0
494	Pat (1 1/4-in. sq. 1/3-in. high; 120 per lb.).	1 pat	4	16	25	Trace	3	2	1	Trace	Trace	1	0	[21]130	-----	-----	-----	0
	Fats, cooking:																	
495	Lard	1 cup	205	0	1,850	0	205	78	94	20	0	0	0	0	0	0	0	0
496		1 tbsp.	13	0	115	0	13	5	6	1	0	0	0	0	0	0	0	0
497	Vegetable fats	1 cup	200	0	1,770	0	200	50	100	44	0	0	0	-----	0	0	0	0
498		1 tbsp.	13	0	110	0	13	3	6	3	0	0	0	-----	0	0	0	0
	Margarine:																	
	Regular, 4 sticks per pound:																	
499	Stick	1/2 cup	113	16	815	1	92	17	46	25	1	23	0	[22]3,750	-----	-----	-----	0
500	Tablespoon (approx. 1/8 stick).	1 tbsp.	14	16	100	Trace	12	2	6	3	Trace	3	0	[22]470	-----	-----	-----	0
501	Pat (1-in. sq. 1/3-in. high; 90 per lb.).	1 pat	5	16	35	Trace	4	1	2	1	Trace	1	0	[22]170	-----	-----	-----	0
	Whipped, 6 sticks per pound:																	
502	Stick	1/2 cup	76	16	545	1	61	11	31	17	Trace	15	0	[22]2,500	-----	-----	-----	0
	Soft, 2 8-oz. tubs per pound:																	
503	Tub	1 tub	227	16	1,635	1	184	34	68	68	1	45	0	[22]7,500	-----	-----	-----	0
504	Tablespoon	1 tbsp.	14	16	100	Trace	11	2	4	4	Trace	3	0	[22]470	-----	-----	-----	0
	Oils, salad or cooking:																	
505	Corn	1 cup	220	0	1,945	0	220	22	62	117	0	0	0	-----	0	0	0	0
506		1 tbsp.	14	0	125	0	14	1	4	7	0	0	0	-----	0	0	0	0
507	Cottonseed	1 cup	220	0	1,945	0	220	55	46	110	0	0	0	-----	0	0	0	0
508		1 tbsp.	14	0	125	0	14	4	3	7	0	0	0	-----	0	0	0	0
509	Olive	1 cup	220	0	1,945	0	220	24	167	15	0	0	0	-----	0	0	0	0
510		1 tbsp.	14	0	125	0	14	2	11	1	0	0	0	-----	0	0	0	0
511	Peanut	1 cup	220	0	1,945	0	220	40	103	64	0	0	0	-----	0	0	0	0
512		1 tbsp.	14	0	125	0	14	3	7	4	0	0	0	-----	0	0	0	0
513	Safflower	1 cup	220	0	1,945	0	220	18	37	165	0	0	0	-----	0	0	0	0
514		1 tbsp.	14	0	125	0	14	1	2	10	0	0	0	-----	0	0	0	0
515	Soybean	1 cup	220	0	1,945	0	220	33	44	114	0	0	0	-----	0	0	0	0
516		1 tbsp.	14	0	125	0	14	2	3	7	0	0	0	-----	0	0	0	0

[19] Iron, thiamin, riboflavin, and niacin are based on the minimum levels of enrichment specified in standards of identity promulgated under the Federal Food, Drug, and Cosmetic Act.

[21] Year-round average.

[22] Based on the average vitamin A content of fortified margarine. Federal specifications for fortified margarine require a minimum of 15,000 I.U. of vitamin A per pound.

Table of Food Composition (continued)

[Dashes in the columns for nutrients show that no suitable value could be found although there is reason to believe that a measurable amount of the nutrient may be present]

	Food, approximate measure, and weight (in grams)			Water	Food energy	Protein	Fat	Fatty acids: Saturated (total)	Fatty acids: Unsaturated: Oleic	Fatty acids: Unsaturated: Linoleic	Carbohydrate	Calcium	Iron	Vitamin A value	Thiamin	Riboflavin	Niacin	Ascorbic acid
	FATS, OILS—Continued		*Grams*	*Percent*	*kCalories*	*Grams*	*Grams*	*Grams*	*Grams*	*Grams*	*Grams*	*Milligrams*	*Milligrams*	*International units*	*Milligrams*	*Milligrams*	*Milligrams*	*Milligrams*
	Salad dressings:																	
517	Blue cheese	1 tbsp.	15	32	75	1	8	2	2	4	1	12	Trace	30	Trace	0.02	Trace	Trace
	Commercial, mayonnaise type:																	
518	Regular	1 tbsp.	15	41	65	Trace	6	1	1	3	2	2	Trace	30	Trace	Trace	Trace	------
519	Special dietary, low-calorie.	1 tbsp.	16	81	20	Trace	2	Trace	Trace	1	1	3	Trace	40	Trace	Trace	Trace	------
	French:																	
520	Regular	1 tbsp.	16	39	65	Trace	6	1	1	3	3	2	.1	------	------	------	------	------
521	Special dietary, low-fat with artificial sweeteners.	1 tbsp.	15	95	Trace	Trace	Trace	------	------	------	Trace	2	.1	------	------	------	------	------
522	Home cooked, boiled	1 tbsp.	16	68	25	1	2	1	1	Trace	2	14	.1	80	.01	.03	Trace	Trace
523	Mayonnaise	1 tbsp.	14	15	100	Trace	11	2	2	6	Trace	3	.1	40	Trace	.01	Trace	------
524	Thousand island	1 tbsp.	16	32	80	Trace	8	1	2	4	3	2	.1	50	Trace	Trace	Trace	Trace
	SUGARS, SWEETS																	
	Cake icings:																	
525	Chocolate made with milk and table fat.	1 cup	275	14	1,035	9	38	21	14	1	185	165	3.3	580	.06	.28	.6	1
526	Coconut (with boiled icing).	1 cup	166	15	605	3	13	11	1	Trace	124	10	.8	0	.02	.07	.3	0
527	Creamy fudge from mix with water only.	1 cup	245	15	830	7	16	5	8	3	183	96	2.7	Trace	.05	.20	.7	Trace
528	White, boiled	1 cup	94	18	300	1	0	------	------	------	76	2	Trace	0	Trace	.03	Trace	0
	Candy:																	
529	Caramels, plain or chocolate.	1 oz.	28	8	115	1	3	2	1	Trace	22	42	.4	Trace	.01	.05	.1	Trace
530	Chocolate, milk, plain	1 oz.	28	1	145	2	9	5	3	Trace	16	65	.3	80	.02	.10	.1	Trace
531	Chocolate-coated peanuts.	1 oz.	28	1	160	5	12	3	6	2	11	33	.4	Trace	.10	.05	2.1	Trace

532	Fondant; mints, uncoated; candy corn.	1 oz.	28	8	105	Trace	1	...	...	...	25	4	.3	0	Trace	Trace	Trace	0
533	Fudge, plain	1 oz.	28	8	115	1	4	2	1	Trace	21	22	.3	Trace	.01	.03	.1	Trace
534	Gum drops	1 oz.	28	12	100	Trace	Trace	...	...	...	25	2	.1	0	0	Trace	Trace	0
535	Hard	1 oz.	28	1	110	0	Trace	...	...	...	28	6	.5	0	0	0	0	0
536	Marshmallows	1 oz.	28	17	90	1	Trace	...	...	...	23	5	.5	0	0	Trace	Trace	0
	Chocolate-flavored sirup or topping:																	
537	Thin type	1 fl. oz.	38	32	90	1	1	Trace	Trace	Trace	24	6	.6	Trace	.01	.03	.2	0
538	Fudge type	1 fl. oz.	38	25	125	2	5	3	2	Trace	20	48	.5	60	.02	.08	.2	Trace
	Chocolate-flavored beverage powder (approx. 4 heaping teaspoons per oz.):																	
539	With nonfat dry milk	1 oz.	28	2	100	5	1	Trace	Trace	Trace	20	167	.5	10	.04	.21	.2	1
540	Without nonfat dry milk.	1 oz.	28	1	100	1	1	Trace	Trace	Trace	25	9	.6	...	.01	.03	.1	0
541	Honey, strained or extracted.	1 tbsp.	21	17	65	Trace	0	...	...	...	17	1	.1	0	Trace	.01	.1	Trace
542	Jams and preserves	1 tbsp.	20	29	55	Trace	Trace	...	...	...	14	4	.2	Trace	Trace	.01	Trace	Trace
543	Jellies	1 tbsp.	18	29	50	Trace	Trace	...	...	...	13	4	.3	Trace	Trace	.01	Trace	1
	Molasses, cane:																	
544	Light (first extraction)	1 tbsp.	20	24	50	...	...	...	...	...	13	33	.9	...	.01	.01	Trace	...
545	Blackstrap (third extraction).	1 tbsp.	20	24	45	...	...	...	...	...	11	137	3.2	...	.02	.04	.4	...
	Sirups:																	
546	Sorghum	1 tbsp.	21	23	55	...	...	...	...	...	14	35	2.6	...	...	.02	Trace	...
547	Table blends, chiefly corn, light and dark.	1 tbsp.	21	24	60	0	0	...	...	...	15	9	.8	0	0	0	0	0
	Sugars:																	
548	Brown, firm packed	1 cup	220	2	820	0	0	...	...	...	212	187	7.5	0	.02	.07	.4	0
	White:																	
549	Granulated	1 cup	200	Trace	770	0	0	...	...	...	199	0	.2	0	0	0	0	0
550		1 tbsp.	11	Trace	40	0	0	...	...	...	11	0	Trace	0	0	0	0	0
551	Powdered, stirred before measuring.	1 cup	120	Trace	460	0	0	...	...	...	119	0	.1	0	0	0	0	0
	MISCELLANEOUS ITEMS																	
552	Barbecue sauce	1 cup	250	81	230	4	17	2	5	9	20	53	2.0	900	.03	.03	.8	13
	Beverages, alcoholic:																	
553	Beer	12 fl. oz.	360	92	150	1	0	...	...	...	14	18	Trace	...	.01	.11	2.2	...
	Gin, rum, vodka, whiskey:																	
554	80-proof	1½ fl. oz. jigger.	42	67	100	...	...	...	...	...	Trace	...	...	...	...	...	...	...
555	86-proof	1½ fl. oz. jigger.	42	64	105	...	...	...	...	...	Trace	...	...	...	...	...	...	...
556	90-proof	1½ fl. oz. jigger.	42	62	110	...	...	...	...	...	Trace	...	...	...	...	...	...	...

Table of Food Composition (continued)

[Dashes in the columns for nutrients show that no suitable value could be found although there is reason to believe that a measurable amount of the nutrient may be present]

	Food, approximate measure, and weight (in grams)			Water	Food energy	Protein	Fat	Fatty acids: Saturated (total)	Fatty acids: Unsaturated: Oleic	Fatty acids: Unsaturated: Linoleic	Carbohydrate	Calcium	Iron	Vitamin A value	Thiamin	Riboflavin	Niacin	Ascorbic acid
	MISCELLANEOUS ITEMS—Continued																	
	Beverages, alcoholic—Continued																	
	Gin, rum, vodka, whiskey—Con.		*Grams*	*Percent*	*kCalories*	*Grams*	*Grams*	*Grams*	*Grams*	*Grams*	*Grams*	*Milligrams*	*Milligrams*	*International units*	*Milligrams*	*Milligrams*	*Milligrams*	*Milligrams*
557	94-proof	1½ fl. oz. jigger.	42	60	115	---	---	---	---	---	Trace	---	---	---	---	---	---	---
558	100-proof	1½ fl. oz.	42	58	125	---	---	---	---	---	Trace	---	---	---	---	---	---	---
	Wines:																	
559	Dessert	3½ fl. oz. glass.	103	77	140	Trace	0	---	---	---	8	8	---	---	.01	.02	.2	---
560	Table	3½ fl. oz. glass.	102	86	85	Trace	0	---	---	---	4	9	.4	---	Trace	.01	.1	---
	Beverages, carbonated, sweetened, nonalcoholic:																	
561	Carbonated water	12 fl. oz.	366	92	115	0	0	---	---	---	29	---	---	0	0	0	0	0
562	Cola type	12 fl. oz.	369	90	145	0	0	---	---	---	37	---	---	0	0	0	0	0
563	Fruit-flavored sodas and Tom Collins mixes.	12 fl. oz.	372	88	170	0	0	---	---	---	45	---	---	0	0	0	0	0
564	Ginger ale	12 fl. oz.	366	92	115	0	0	---	---	---	29	---	---	0	0	0	0	0
565	Root beer	12 fl. oz.	370	90	150	0	0	---	---	---	39	---	---	0	0	0	0	0
566	Bouillon cubes, approx. ½ in.	1 cube	4	4	5	1	Trace	---	---	---	Trace	---	---	---	---	---	---	---
	Chocolate:																	
567	Bitter or baking	1 oz.	28	2	145	3	15	8	6	Trace	8	22	1.9	20	.01	.07	.4	0
568	Semi-sweet, small pieces.	1 cup	170	1	860	7	61	34	22	1	97	51	4.4	30	.02	.14	.9	0
	Gelatin:																	
569	Plain, dry powder in envelope.	1 envelope	7	13	25	6	Trace	---	---	---	0	---	---	---	---	---	---	---
570	Dessert powder, 3-oz. package.	1 pkg.	85	2	315	8	0	---	---	---	75	---	---	---	---	---	---	---
571	Gelatin dessert, prepared with water.	1 cup	240	84	140	4	0	---	---	---	34	---	---	---	---	---	---	---

	Olives, pickled:																	
572	Green	4 medium or 3 extra large or 2 giant.	16	78	15	Trace	2	Trace	2	Trace	Trace	8	.2	40	-----			-----
573	Ripe: Mission	3 small or 2 large.	10	73	15	Trace	2	Trace	2	Trace	Trace	9	.1	10	Trace	Trace		-----
	Pickles, cucumber:																	
574	Dill, medium, whole, 3¾ in. long, 1¼ in. diam.	1 pickle	65	93	10	1	Trace	-----	-----	-----	1	17	.7	70	Trace	.01	Trace	4
575	Fresh, sliced, 1½ in. diam., ¼ in. thick.	2 slices	15	79	10	Trace	Trace	-----	-----	-----	3	5	.3	20	Trace	Trace	Trace	1
576	Sweet, gherkin, small, whole, approx. 2½ in. long, ¾ in. diam.	1 pickle	15	61	20	Trace	Trace	-----	-----	-----	6	2	.2	10	Trace	Trace	Trace	1
577	Relish, finely chopped, sweet.	1 tbsp.	15	63	20	Trace	Trace	-----	-----	-----	5	3	.1	-----	-----	-----	-----	-----
	Popcorn. See Grain Products.																	
578	Popsicle, 3 fl. oz. size	1 popsicle	95	80	70	0	0	0	0	0	18	0	Trace	0	0	0	0	0
	Pudding, home recipe with starch base:																	
579	Chocolate	1 cup	260	66	385	8	12	7	4	Trace	67	250	1.3	390	.05	.36	.3	1
580	Vanilla (blanc mange)	1 cup	255	76	285	9	10	5	3	Trace	41	298	Trace	410	.08	.41	.3	2
581	Pudding mix, dry form, 4-oz. package.	1 pkg.	113	2	410	3	2	1	1	Trace	103	23	1.8	Trace	.02	.08	.5	0
582	Sherbet	1 cup	193	67	260	2	2	-----	-----	-----	59	31	Trace	120	.02	.06	Trace	4
	Soups:																	
	Canned, condensed, ready-to-serve:																	
	Prepared with an equal volume of milk:																	
583	Cream of chicken	1 cup	245	85	180	7	10	3	3	3	15	172	.5	610	.05	.27	.7	2
584	Cream of mushroom.	1 cup	245	83	215	7	14	4	4	5	16	191	.5	250	.05	.34	.7	1
585	Tomato	1 cup	250	84	175	7	7	3	2	1	23	168	.8	1,200	.10	.25	1.3	15
	Prepared with an equal volume of water:																	
586	Bean with pork	1 cup	250	84	170	8	6	1	2	2	22	63	2.3	650	.13	.08	1.0	3
587	Beef broth, bouillon consomme.	1 cup	240	96	30	5	0	-----	-----	-----	3	Trace	.5	Trace	Trace	.02	1.2	-----
588	Beef noodle	1 cup	240	93	70	4	3	1	1	1	7	7	1.0	50	.05	.07	1.0	Trace
589	Clam chowder, Manhattan type (with tomatoes, without milk).	1 cup	245	92	80	2	3	-----	-----	-----	12	34	1.0	880	.02	.02	1.0	-----
590	Cream of chicken	1 cup	240	92	95	3	6	1	2	3	8	24	.5	410	.02	.05	.5	Trace
591	Cream of mushroom.	1 cup	240	90	135	2	10	1	3	5	10	41	.5	70	.02	.12	.7	Trace
592	Minestrone	1 cup	245	90	105	5	3	-----	-----	-----	14	37	1.0	2,350	.07	.05	1.0	-----

Table of Food Composition (continued)

[Dashes in the columns for nutrients show that no suitable value could be found although there is reason to believe that a measurable amount of the nutrient may be present]

	Food, approximate measure, and weight (in grams)			Water	Food energy	Protein	Fat	Fatty acids: Saturated (total)	Fatty acids: Unsaturated: Oleic	Fatty acids: Unsaturated: Linoleic	Carbohydrate	Calcium	Iron	Vitamin A value	Thiamin	Riboflavin	Niacin	Ascorbic acid
	MISCELLANEOUS ITEMS—Continued																	
	Soups—Continued																	
	Canned, condensed, ready-to-serve—Con.																	
	Prepared with an equal volume of water—Con.		Grams	Percent	kCalories	Grams	Grams	Grams	Grams	Grams	Grams	Milligrams	Milligrams	International units	Milligrams	Milligrams	Milligrams	Milligrams
593	Split pea	1 cup	245	85	145	9	3	1	2	Trace	21	29	1.5	440	0.25	0.15	1.5	1
594	Tomato	1 cup	245	90	90	2	3	Trace	1	1	16	15	.7	1,000	.05	.05	1.2	12
595	Vegetable beef	1 cup	245	92	80	5	2	---	---	---	10	12	.7	2,700	.05	.05	1.0	-----
596	Vegetarian	1 cup	245	92	80	2	2	---	---	---	13	20	1.0	2,940	.05	.05	1.0	-----
	Dehydrated, dry form:																	
597	Chicken noodle (2-oz. package).	1 pkg.	57	6	220	8	6	2	3	1	33	34	1.4	190	.30	.15	2.4	3
598	Onion mix (1½-oz. package).	1 pkg.	43	3	150	6	5	1	2	1	23	42	.6	30	.05	.03	.3	6
599	Tomato vegetable with noodles (2½-oz. pkg.).	1 pkg.	71	4	245	6	6	2	3	1	45	33	1.4	1,700	.21	.13	1.8	18
	Frozen, condensed:																	
	Clam chowder, New England type (with milk, without tomatoes):																	
600	Prepared with equal volume of milk.	1 cup	245	83	210	9	12	---	---	---	16	240	1.0	250	.07	.29	.5	Trace
601	Prepared with equal volume of water.	1 cup	240	89	130	4	8	---	---	---	11	91	1.0	50	.05	.10	.5	-----
	Cream of potato:																	
602	Prepared with equal volume of milk.	1 cup	245	83	185	8	10	5	3	Trace	18	208	1.0	590	.10	.27	.5	Trace
603	Prepared with equal volume of water.	1 cup	240	90	105	3	5	3	2	Trace	12	58	1.0	410	.05	.05	.5	-----

	Cream of shrimp:																	
604	Prepared with equal volume of milk.	1 cup	245	82	245	9	16	—	—	—	15	189	.5	290	.07	.27	.5	Trace
605	Prepared with equal volume of water.	1 cup	240	88	160	5	12	—	—	—	8	38	.5	120	.05	.05	.5	—
	Oyster stew:																	
606	Prepared with equal volume of milk.	1 cup	240	83	200	10	12	—	—	—	14	305	1.4	410	.12	.41	.5	Trace
607	Prepared with equal volume of water.	1 cup	240	90	120	6	8	—	—	—	8	158	1.4	240	.07	.19	.5	—
608	Tapioca, dry, quick-cooking.	1 cup	152	13	535	1	Trace	—	—	—	131	15	.6	0	0	0	0	0
	Tapioca desserts:																	
609	Apple	1 cup	250	70	295	1	Trace	—	—	—	74	8	.5	30	Trace	Trace	Trace	Trace
610	Cream pudding	1 cup	165	72	220	8	8	4	3	Trace	28	173	.7	480	.07	.30	.2	2
611	Tartar sauce	1 tbsp.	14	34	75	Trace	8	1	1	4	1	3	.1	30	Trace	Trace	Trace	Trace
612	Vinegar	1 tbsp.	15	94	Trace	Trace	0	—	—	—	1	1	.1	—	—	—	—	—
613	White sauce, medium	1 cup	250	73	405	10	31	16	10	1	22	288	.5	1,150	.10	.43	.5	2
	Yeast:																	
614	Baker's, dry, active	1 pkg.	7	5	20	3	Trace	—	—	—	3	3	1.1	Trace	.16	.38	2.6	Trace
615	Brewer's, dry	1 tbsp.	8	5	25	3	Trace	—	—	—	3	17	1.4	Trace	1.25	.34	3.0	Trace
	Yoghurt. See Milk, Cheese, Cream, Imitation Cream.																	

APPENDIX I: Recommended Dietary Allowances (U.S.)

The main RDA table appears on the inside front cover, and the 1968 U.S. RDA table used for food labeling is on the inside back. Two additional tables go with the RDA. Table 1 shows the estimated safe and adequate intakes of twelve nutrients in addition to those on the main RDA table. Table 2 is the energy table; it shows energy allowances for people of average height and weight for various age and sex groups.

Table 1. Estimated Safe and Adequate Daily Dietary Intakes of Additional Selected Nutrients*

	Vitamins			Trace elements†						Electrolytes		
Age (years)	Vitamin K (μg)	Biotin (μg)	Pantothenic acid (mg)	Copper (mg)	Manganese (mg)	Fluoride (mg)	Chromium (mg)	Selenium (mg)	Molybdenum (mg)	Sodium (mg)	Potassium (mg)	Chloride (mg)
0-0.5	12	35	2	0.5-0.7	0.5-0.7	0.1-0.5	0.01-0.04	0.01-0.04	0.03-0.06	115 - 350	350 - 925	275 - 700
0.5-1	10-20	50	3	0.7-1.0	0.7-1.0	0.2-1.0	0.02-0.06	0.02-0.06	0.04-0.08	250 - 750	425-1,275	400-1,200
1-3	15-30	65	3	1.0-1.5	1.0-1.5	0.5-1.5	0.02-0.08	0.02-0.08	0.05-0.1	325 - 975	550-1,650	500-1,500
4-6	20-40	85	3-4	1.5-2.0	1.5-2.0	1.0-2.5	0.03-0.12	0.03-0.12	0.06-0.15	450-1,350	775-2,325	700-2,100
7-10	30-60	120	4-5	2.0-2.5	2.0-3.0	1.5-2.5	0.05-0.2	0.05-0.2	0.1 -0.3	600-1,800	1,000-3,000	925-2,775
11+	50-100	100-200	4-7	2.0-3.0	2.5-5.0	1.5-2.5	0.05-0.2	0.05-0.2	0.15-0.5	900-2,700	1,525-4,575	1,400-4,200
Adults	70-140	100-200	4-7	2.0-3.0	2.5-5.0	1.5-4.0	0.05-0.2	0.05-0.2	0.15-0.5	1,100-3,300	1,875-5,625	1,700-5,100

*Because there is less information on which to base allowances, these figures are not given in the main table of the RDA and are provided here in the form of ranges of recommended intakes.

†Since the toxic levels for many trace elements may be only several times usual intakes, the upper levels for the trace elements given in this table should not habitually be exceeded.

Table 2. Mean Heights and Weights and Recommended Energy Intakes

Age (years)	Weight (kg)	Weight (lb)	Height (cm)	Height (in)	Energy needs* (cal)	Energy needs* (MJ)†
Infants						
0.0-0.5	6	13	60	24	kg × 115 (95-145)	kg × 0.48
0.5-1.0	9	20	71	28	kg × 105 (80-135)	kg × 0.44
Children						
1-3	13	29	90	35	1,300 (900-1,800)	5.5
4-6	20	44	112	44	1,700 (1,300-2,300)	7.1
7-10	28	62	132	52	2,400 (1,650-3,300)	10.1
Males						
11-14	45	99	157	62	2,700 (2,000-3,700)	11.3
15-18	66	145	176	69	2,800 (2,100-3,900)	11.8
19-22	70	154	177	70	2,900 (2,500-3,300)	12.2
23-50	70	154	178	70	2,700 (2,300-3,100)	11.3
51-75	70	154	178	70	2,400 (2,000-2,800)	10.1
76+	70	154	178	70	2,050 (1,650-2,450)	8.6
Females						
11-14	46	101	157	62	2,200 (1,500-3,000)	9.2
15-18	55	120	163	64	2,100 (1,200-3,000)	8.8
19-22	55	120	163	64	2,100 (1,700-2,500)	8.8
23-50	55	120	163	64	2,000 (1,600-2,400)	8.4
51-75	55	120	163	64	1,800 (1,400-2,200)	7.6
76+	55	120	163	64	1,600 (1,200-2,000)	6.7
Pregnant					+300	
Lactating					+500	

*The energy allowances for the young adults are for men and women doing light work. The allowances for the two older age groups represent mean energy needs over these age spans, allowing for a 2 percent decrease in basal (resting) metabolic rate per decade and a reduction in activity of 200 cal per day for men and women between 51 and 75 years, 500 cal for men over 75 years, and 400 cal for women over 75. The customary range of daily energy output, shown in parentheses, is based on a variation in energy needs of ± 400 cal at any one age, emphasizing the wide range of energy intakes appropriate for any group of people. Energy allowances for children through age 18 are based on median energy intakes of children these ages followed in longitudinal growth studies. The values in parentheses are tenth and ninetieth percentiles of energy intake, to indicate the range of energy consumption among children of these ages.

†MJ stands for megajoules (1 MJ = 1,000 kJ).

APPENDIX J: Recommended Nutrition References

People interested in nutrition often want to know where, in their own town or county, they can find reliable nutrition information. One place you are not likely to find it is the local library, where fad diet books sit side by side on the shelf with books of facts. However, wherever you live, there are several sources you can turn to:

The Department of Health may have a nutrition expert.

The local extension agent is often an expert.

The food editor of your local paper may be well informed.

The dietitian at the local hospital had to fulfill a set of qualifications before he or she became an R.D. (registered dietitian).

There may be professors of nutrition or biochemistry at a nearby college or university who are knowledgeable.

In addition, you might want to begin to accumulate a small library of your own. The references suggested below are of a general nature, related to many topics covered in this book. The prices and addresses are subject to change.

Books

Nutrition Reviews' Present Knowledge in Nutrition, 4th ed. (Washington, D.C.: Nutrition Foundation, 1976), 605 pages (paperback $12) will bring you up to date on fifty-three topics, including energy, obesity, twenty-nine nutrients, diabetes, coronary heart disease, fiber, renal disease, parenteral nutrition, malnutrition, growth and its assessment, brain development, immunity, alcohol, fiber, milk intolerances, dental health, drugs, and toxins. The only major omissions seem to be nutrition and food intake and national nutrition status surveys. Watch for an update; these come out about every five or six years.

A tidy paperback volume containing thirteen thought-provoking articles from the *New England Journal of Medicine*, each about ten pages long, is *Current Concepts in Nutrition* (Massachusetts Medical Society, 1979). A scholarly volume from the *Journal of Nutrition*, five times larger than *Current Concepts*, is *Nutritional Requirements of Man, a Conspectus of Research* (New York and Washington, D.C.: Nutrition Foundation, 1980). The *Conspectus* has a major review article on human requirements for each of the following: protein, amino acids, vitamin A, calcium, zinc, vitamin C, iron, folacin, and copper.

R. S. Goodhart and M. E. Shils, eds., *Modern Nutrition in Health and Disease*, 6th ed. (Philadelphia: Lea and Febiger, 1980), 1153 pages (about $50) is a major technical reference book on nutrition topics, containing forty encyclopedic articles on the nutrients, foods, the diet, metabolism, malnutrition, age-related needs, and nutrition in disease, with twenty-eight appendixes.

Lagua, Claudio, and Thiele's *Reference Dictionary*, 2d ed. (St. Louis: Mosby, 1974), 330 pages ($9.75) is a dictionary of nutrition terminology with thirty-eight appendixes, including dietary standards of other countries, food grouping systems, biochemical pathways, U.S. agencies, research methods, weights and measures, and others.

Many students also like to have a separate copy of the Table of Food Composition (Appendix H in this book), which is available in softcover from the Government Printing Office (address below). Another more comprehensive book of food composition, which also gives foods in household measures, is *Bowes and Church's Food Values of Portions Commonly Used*. The twelfth edition is available from J. B. Lippincott Company, Philadelphia, as of 1975.

Many excellent publications are available on the important subject of food faddism and misinformation. A whole issue of *Nutrition Reviews* was devoted to this topic and includes a list of suggested readings to help the reader identify faddists, quacks, and promoters: *Nutrition Reviews/Supplement: Nutrition Misinformation and Food Faddism*, July 1974. R. Deutsch has recently revised his entertaining and revealing book on food faddism under the title *The New Nuts among the Berries: How Nutrition Nonsense Captured America* (Palo Alto, Calif.: Bull Publishing, 1977).

The syndicated column on nutrition by J. Mayer and J. Dwyer, which appears in many newspapers, presents well-researched, reliable answers to current questions, as does the column by R. Alfin-Slater and Jelliffe. Mayer's book, *A Diet for Living* (New York: Pocket Books, 1977), is also a useful reference. For the athlete, N. J. Smith's *Food for Sport* (Palo Alto, Calif.: Bull Publishing, 1977) is recommended; and for the vegetarian, F. M. Lappe's *Diet for a Small Planet*, rev. ed. (New York: Ballantine Books, 1975) makes excellent reading. Another good general reference is B. Burton, *Human Nutrition: Formerly Heinz Handbook of Nutrition*, 3d ed. (New York: McGraw-Hill, 1976).

One of the most readable, entertaining, and relevant books of readings in nutrition to come out in recent years is L. Hofmann, ed., *The Great American Nutrition Hassle* (Palo Alto, Calif.: Mayfield, 1978). This book would make an excellent discussion-topic source for a course in which *Nutrition: Concepts and Controversies* is assigned. *Hassle* includes articles by recognized authorities on the RDA, fast foods, additives, infant nutrition, fad diets, sugar, alcohol, and most of the other topics treated in this book's Controversies.

Another book that readers may wish to add to their libraries is the latest edition of *Recommended Dietary Allowances*, available from the National Academy of Sciences (address below).

We also recommend our own book, E. N. Whitney and E. M. N. Hamilton, *Understanding Nutrition*, 2d ed. (St. Paul, Minn.: West, 1981), which explains the biochemistry of nutrition to the beginning student, defining each new chemical term as it appears.

Journals

Nutrition Today, the publication of the Nutrition Today Society, is an excellent journal for the interested layperson. It makes a point of raising controversial issues and providing a forum for conflicting opinions. Articles are seldom referenced but are written by recognized authorities and are entertaining and thought-provoking. Six issues per year, $12.50 ($6.25 for dietetics students), from Director of Membership Services, Nutrition Today Society, PO Box 773, Annapolis, MD 21404.

The *Journal of the American Dietetic Association*, the official publication of the ADA, contains articles of interest to dietitians and nutritionists, news of legislative action on food and nutrition, and a very useful section of abstracts of articles from many other journals of nutrition and related areas. Twelve issues per year, $24 ($12 for dietetics students), from the American Dietetic Association (address below).

Nutrition Reviews, a publication of The Nutrition Foundation, Inc., does much of the work for the library researcher, compiling recent evidence on current topics and presenting extensive bibliographies. Twelve issues per year, $12 ($6 for students), from the Nutrition Foundation, Inc., 489 Fifth Avenue, New York, NY 10017.

Other journals that deserve mention here are the *Journal of Nutrition*, *Food Technology*, the *American Journal of Clinical Nutrition*, and the *Journal of Nutrition Education*. *FDA Consumer*, a government publication with many articles of interest to the consumer, is available from the Food and Drug Administration (address below). Many other journals of value are referred to throughout this book.

Catalogs, Publication Lists, Free and Inexpensive Materials

Lists of publications can be obtained from the following organizations.

ADA catalog (free) from:

The American Dietetic Association
430 North Michigan Avenue
Chicago, IL 60611

Publications list (free) from:

The American Medical Association
535 North Dearborn Street
Chicago, IL 60610

Nutrition references and book reviews (54 pages, $2) from:

The Chicago Nutrition Association
8158 Kedzie Avenue
Chicago, IL 60652

A guide to free health materials, listing over 2000 items, can be obtained for $15 from:

Educators Progress Service, Inc.
214 Center Street
Randolph, WIS 53956

Other free and inexpensive materials can be obtained from the following addresses:

U.S. government:

Consumer and Food Economics Research Division
Federal Center Building
Hyattsville, MD 20782

Human Nutrition Research Division
Agricultural Research Center
Beltsville, MD 20705

Extension Service, USDA
Room 5038, South Building
Washington, DC 20250

Food and Nutrition Service, USDA
Washington, DC 20250

Food and Drug Administration (FDA)
5600 Fishers Lane
Rockville, MD 20852

The Food and Nutrition Information Education Resources Center (FNIERC)
National Agriculture Library
10301 Baltimore Boulevard, Room 304
Beltsville, MD 20705
Tel: (301) 344-3719

Information Division
Agricultural Marketing Service, USDA
Washington, DC 20250

National Academy of Sciences/National Research Council (NAS/NRC)
2101 Constitution Avenue NW
Washington, DC 20418

Office of Child Development
Office of Education
Public Health Service
Washington, DC 20204

U.S. Government Printing Office
The Superintendent of Documents
Washington, DC 20402

Professional and service organizations:

American Academy of Pediatrics
PO Box 1034
Evanston, IL 60204

American College of Nutrition
100 Manhattan Avenue #1606
Union City, NJ 07087

American Dental Association
211 East Chicago Avenue
Chicago, IL 60611

American Dietetic Association
620 North Michigan Avenue
Chicago, IL 60611

American Heart Association
7320 Greenville Avenue
Dallas, TX 75231

American Home Economics Association
2010 Massachusetts Avenue NW
Washington, DC 20036

American Institute of Nutrition
9650 Rockville Pike
Bethesda, MD 20014

American Medical Association
Section of Nutrition Information
535 North Dearborn Street
Chicago, IL 60610

The American National Red Cross
Food and Nutrition Consultant
National Headquarters
Washington, DC 20006

American Public Health Association
1015 Fifteenth Street NW
Washington, DC 20005

American Society for Clinical Nutrition, Inc.
9650 Rockville Pike
Bethesda, MD 20014

The Canadian Diabetes Association
1491 Yonge Street
Toronto, Ontario M4T 1Z5 Canada

The Canadian Dietetic Association
123 Edward Street, Suite 601
Toronto, Ontario M5G 1E2 Canada

Food Protein Council
1800 M Street NW
Washington, DC 20036

Institute of Food Technologists
221 North La Salle Street
Chicago, IL 60601

LaLeche League International, Inc.
9616 Minneapolis Avenue
Franklin Park, IL 60131

March of Dimes Birth Defects Foundation
173 West Madison Street
Chicago, IL 60602

Meals for Millions/Freedom
from Hunger Foundation
1800 Olympic Boulevard
PO Drawer 680
Santa Monica, CA 90406

National Nutrition Consortium, Inc.
1635 P Street NW, Suite 1
Washington, DC 20036

Nutrition Foundation
888 Seventeenth Street NW
Washington, DC 20036

Nutrition Today Society
101 Ridgely Avenue
PO Box 465
Annapolis, MD 21404

Society for Nutrition Education
2140 Shattuck Avenue, Suite 1110
Berkeley, CA 94704

Trade organizations produce many excellent free materials that promote nutritional health. Naturally, they also promote their own products. The student must learn to differentiate between "slanted" and valid information. We find the brief reviews in *Contemporary Nutrition* (put out by General Mills), the *Dairy Council Digest*, Ross Laboratories' *Dietetic Currents*, and R. A. Seelig's reviews from the United Fresh Fruit and Vegetable Association to be generally reliable and very useful.

Campbell Soup Company
Food Service Products Division
375 Memorial Avenue
Camden, NJ 08101

Del Monte Kitchens
Del Monte Corporation
215 Fremont Street
San Francisco, CA 94119

General Foods Consumer Center
250 North Street
White Plains, NY 10625

General Mills
PO Box 113
Minneapolis, MN 55440

Gerber Products Company
445 State Street
Fremont, MI 49412

H. J. Heinz
Consumer Relations
PO Box 57
Pittsburg, PA 15230

Hunt-Wesson Foods
Educational Services
1645 West Valencia Drive
Fullerton, CA 92634

Kellogg Company
Department of Home Economics Services
Battle Creek, MI 49016

Mead Johnson Nutritionals
2404 Pennsylvania Avenue
Evansville, IN 47721

National Dairy Council
111 North Canal Street
Chicago, IL 60606

The Nestle Company, Inc.
Home Economics Division
100 Bloomingdale Road
White Plains, NY 10605

Oscar Mayer Company
Consumer Service
PO Box 1409
Madison, WI 53701

Ross Laboratories
Director of Professional Services
Columbus, OH 43216

United Fresh Fruit and Vegetable Association
1019 Nineteenth Street NW
Washington, DC 20036

International organizations (United Nations):

Food and Agriculture Organization of the United Nations (FAO)
North American Regional Office
1325 C Street SW
Washington, DC 20025

Food and Agriculture Organization (FAO)
Via delle Terma di Caracella
0100 Rome, Italy

World Health Organization (WHO)
1211 Geneva 27
Switzerland

APPENDIX K: Canadian and FAO/WHO Recommendations

A variety of organizations have developed guidelines for how much of each nutrient different age and sex groups should consume daily. Table 1 shows nutritional guidelines established by the Canadian government.[1] The Food and Agriculture Organization of the World Health Organization has set its own standards for nutrient intakes.[2]

Protein quality varies greatly from country to country, and the human requirement for protein depends on its quality, so the FAO/WHO standard (see Table 2) is stated in terms of high-quality milk or egg protein to avoid misinterpretation. Other tables published by FAO/WHO assume lower-quality protein, and still others are stated in terms of amino acid needs.

The FAO/WHO iron recommendations (see Table 7) were based on the assumption that the upper limit of iron absorption by normal individuals would be 10 percent if they consumed less than 10 percent of their calories from foods of animal origin; 15 percent, if 10 to 25 percent; and 20 percent, if more than 25 percent.

Table 1. Dietary Standards for Canada, 1975

						Water-Soluble Vitamins							Fat-Soluble Vitamins			Minerals					
Age	Sex	Weight (kg)	Height (cm)	Energy (cal)	Protein (g)	Thiamin (mg)	Niacin (mg equiv)	Riboflavin (mg)	Vitamin B_6[a] (mg)	Folate (μg)	Vitamin B_{12} (μg)	Vitamin C (mg)	Vitamin A (RE)	Vitamin D (μg cholecalciferol)[b]	Vitamin E (mg d-α-tocopherol)	Calcium (mg)	Phosphorus (mg)	Magnesium (mg)	Iodine (μg)	Iron (mg)	Zinc (mg)
0–6 mo	Both	6	—	kg x 117	kg x 2.2(2.0)[c]	0.3	5	0.4	0.3	40	0.3	20[d]	400	10	3	500[f]	250[f]	50[f]	35[f]	7[f]	4[f]
7–11 mo	Both	9	—	kg x 108	kg x 1.4	0.5	6	0.6	0.4	60	0.3	20	400	10	3	500	400	50	50	7	5
1–3 yr	Both	13	90	1400	22	0.7	9	0.8	0.8	100	0.9	20	400	10	4	500	500	75	70	8	5
4–6 yr	Both	19	110	1800	27	0.9	12	1.1	1.3	100	1.5	20	500	5	5	500	500	100	90	9	6
7–9 yr	M	27	129	2200	33	1.1	14	1.3	1.6	100	1.5	30	700	2.5[g]	6	700	700	150	110	10	7
	F	27	128	2000	33	1.0	13	1.2	1.4	100	1.5	30	700	2.5[g]	6	700	700	150	100	10	7
10–12 yr	M	36	144	2500	41	1.2	17	1.5	1.8	100	3.0	30	800	2.5[g]	7	900	900	175	130	11	8
	F	38	145	2300	40	1.1	15	1.4	1.5	100	3.0	30	800	2.5[g]	7	1000	1000	200	120	11	9
13–15 yr	M	51	162	2800	52	1.4	19	1.7	2.0	200	3.0	30	1000	2.5[g]	9	1200	1200	250	140	13	10
	F	49	159	2200	43	1.1	15	1.4	1.5	200	3.0	30	800	2.5[g]	7	800	800	250	110	14	10
16–18 yr	M	64	172	3200	54	1.6	21	2.0	2.0	200	3.0	30	1000	2.5[g]	10	1000	1000	300	160	14	12
	F	54	161	2100	43	1.1	14	1.3	1.5	200	3.0	30	800	2.5[g]	6	700	700	250	110	14	11
19–35 yr	M	70	176	3000	56	1.5	20	1.8	2.0	200	3.0	30	1000	2.5[g]	9	800	800	300	150	10	10
	F	56	161	2100	41	1.1	14	1.3	1.5	200	3.0	30	800	2.5[g]	6	700	700	250	110	14	9
36–50 yr	M	70	176	2700	56	1.4	18	1.7	2.0	200	3.0	30	1000	2.5[g]	8	800	800	300	140	10	10
	F	56	161	1900	41	1.0	13	1.2	1.5	200	3.0	30	800	2.5[g]	6	700	700	250	100	14	9
51 + yr	M	70	176	2300[e]	56	1.4	18	1.7	2.0	200	3.0	30	1000	2.5[g]	8	800	800	300	140	10	10
	F	56	161	1800[e]	41	1.0	13	1.2	1.5	200	3.0	30	800	2.5[g]	6	700	700	250	100	9	9
Pregnancy				+300[h]	+20	+0.2	+2	+0.3	+0.5	+50	+1.0	+20	+100	+2.5[g]	+1	+500	+500	+25	+15	+1[i]	+3
Lactation				+500	+24	+0.4	+7	+0.6	+0.6	+50	+0.5	+30	+400	+2.5[g]	+2	+500	+500	+75	+25	+1[i]	+7

[a] Recommendations are based on estimated average daily protein intake of Canadians.

[b] A μg cholecalciferol equals 1 μg ergocalciferol (40 IU vitamin D activity).

[c] Recommended protein intake of 2.2 grams per kilogram body weight for infants age 0 to 2 months and 2.0 grams per kilogram body weight for those age 3 to 5 months. Protein recommendation for infants 0 to 11 months assumes consumption of breast milk or protein of equivalent quality.

[d] Considerably higher levels may be prudent for infants during the first week of life.

[e] Recommended energy intake for 66 years and over reduce to 2000 calories for men and 1500 calories for women.

[f] The intake of breast-fed infants may be less than the recommendation but is considered adequate.

[g] Most older children and adults receive vitamin D from the sun, but 2.5 μg daily is recommended. This intake should be increased to 5.0 μg daily during pregnancy and lactation and for those confined indoors or otherwise deprived of sunlight for extended periods.

[h] Increased energy intake recommended during second and third trimesters. An increase of 100 calories per day is recommended during the first trimester.

[i] A recommended total intake of 15 mg daily during pregnancy and lactation assumes the presence of adequate stores of iron. If stores are suspected of being inadequate, additional iron as a supplement is recommended.

Table 2. Safe Levels of Protein, FAO/WHO

Age	Body Weight (kg)	Safe Level of Protein Intake: Protein per kg per Day (g)	Safe Level of Protein Intake: Protein per Person per Day (g)	Adjusted Level for Proteins of Different Quality[a] (g per person per day): Score 80	Score 70	Score 60
Infants						
6–11 mo	9.0	1.53	14	17	20	23
Children						
1–3 yr	13.4	1.19	16	20	23	27
4–6 yr	20.2	1.01	20	26	29	34
7–9 yr	28.1	0.88	25	31	35	41
Male adolescents						
10–12 yr	36.9	0.81	30	37	43	50
13–15 yr	51.3	0.72	37	46	53	62
16–19 yr	62.9	0.60	38	47	54	63
Female adolescents						
10–12 yr	38.0	0.76	29	36	41	48
13–15 yr	49.9	0.63	31	39	45	52
16–19 yr	54.4	0.55	30	37	43	50
Adult man	65.0	0.57	37	46[b]	53[b]	62[b]
Adult woman	55.0	0.52	29	36[b]	41[b]	48[b]
Pregnant woman, latter half of pregnancy			add 9	add 11	add 13	add 15
Lactating woman, first 6 months			add 17	add 21	add 24	add 28

[a] Scores are estimates of the quality of the protein usually consumed relative to that of egg or milk. The safe level of protein intake is adjusted by multiplying it by 100 divided by the score of the food protein. For example, 100/60 = 1.67, and for a child of 1 to 4 years, the safe level of protein intake would be 16 x 1.67, or 27 g of protein having a relative quality of 60.

[b] The correction may overestimate adult protein requirements.

Table 3. Energy Requirements of Children and Adolescents, FAO/WHO

Age (years)	Body Weight (kg)	Energy per kg per Day (cal)	Energy per Person per Day (cal)
Children			
1	7.3	112	820
1-3	13.4	101	1360
4-6	20.2	91	1830
7-9	28.1	78	2190
Male adolescents			
10-12	36.9	71	2600
13-15	51.3	57	2900
16-19	62.9	49	3070
Female adolescents			
10-12	38.0	62	2350
13-15	49.9	50	2490
16-19	54.4	43	2310

Table 4a. Energy Requirements of Men, FAO/WHO

Body Weight (kg)	Lightly Active (cal)	Moderately Active (cal)	Very Active (cal)	Exceptionally Active (cal)
50	2100	2300	2700	3100
55	2310	2530	2970	3410
60	2520	2760	3240	3720
65	2700	3000	3500	4000
70	2940	3220	3780	4340
75	3150	3450	4050	4650
80	3360	3680	4320	4960

Table 4b. Energy Requirements of Women, FAO/WHO

Body Weight (kg)	Lightly Active (cal)	Moderately Active (cal)	Very Active (cal)	Exceptionally Active (cal)
40	1440	1600	1880	2200
45	1620	1800	2120	2480
50	1800	2000	2350	2750
55	2000	2200	2600	3000
60	2160	2400	2820	3300
65	2340	2600	3055	3575
70	2520	2800	3290	3850

Activity levels, as defined by FAO/WHO:

Lightly active:

Men: most professional men (lawyers, doctors, accountants, teachers, architects, etc.), office workers, shop workers, unemployed men.

Women: housewives in houses with mechanical household appliances, office workers, teachers, most professional women.

Moderately active:

Men: most men in light industry, students, building workers (excluding heavy laborers), many farm workers, soldiers not in active service, fishermen.

Women: most women in light industry, housewives without mechanical household appliances, students, department store workers.

Very active:

Men: some agricultural workers, unskilled laborers, forestry workers, army recruits and soldiers in active service, mine workers, steel workers.

Women: some farm workers (especially peasant agriculture), dancers, athletes.

Exceptionally active:

Men: lumberjacks, blacksmiths, rickshaw-pullers.

Women: construction workers.

Table 5. Recommended Vitamin Intakes, FAO/WHO

Age	Vitamin A (μg retinol)	Thiamin (mg)	Riboflavin (mg)	Niacin (mg equiv)	Ascorbic Acid (mg)
0–6 mo	a	a	a	a	a
7–12 mo	300	0.4	0.6	6.6	20
1–3 yr	250	0.5–0.6	0.6–0.8	7.6–9.6	20
4–6 yr	300	0.7	0.9	11.2	20
7–9 yr	400	0.8	1.2	13.9	20
10–12 yr	575	1.0	1.4	16.5	20
13–15 yr (boys)	725	1.2	1.7	20.4	30
13–15 yr (girls)	725	1.0	1.4	17.2	30
16–19 yr (boys)	750	1.4	2.0	23.8	30
16–19 yr (girls)	750	1.0	1.3	15.8	30
Adults (men)	750	1.3	1.8	21.1	30
Adults (women)	750	0.9	1.3	15.2	30

[a] It is assumed that the infant will be breast fed by a well-nourished mother. The mother should have 450 additional retinol μg per day during this period.

Table 6. Recommended Intake of Calcium, FAO/WHO

Age	Practical Allowance (mg/day)
0–12 mo[a]	500–600
1–9 yr	400–500
10–15 yr	600–700
16–19 yr	500–600
Adult	400–500

[a] Artificially fed only.

Table 7. Recommended Daily Intake of Iron, FAO/WHO

Age	Absorbed Iron Required (mg)	Recommended Intake According to Type of Diet, Proportion of Animal Foods		
		Below 10% of Calories	10–25% of Calories	Over 25% of Calories
0–4 mo	0.5	[a]	[a]	[a]
5–12 mo	1.0	10	7	5
1–12 yr	1.0	10	7	5
13–16 yr (boys)	1.8	18	12	9
13–16 yr (girls)	2.4	24	18	12
Menstruating women	2.8	28	19	14
Men and non-menstruating women	0.9	9	6	5

[a] It is assumed that breastfeeding will provide adequate iron.

Notes

1. Canada, Department of National Health and Welfare, *Dietary Standards for Canada* (Ottawa, Ontario: Department of Public Printing and Stationery, 1975), pp. 70-71.

2. FAO/WHO, *Energy and Protein Requirements,* WHO Technical Report Series no. 522, 1973, pp. 25, 31, 35, 74. Tables 2 through 7 are presented as examples for comparison with the Canadian and U.S. standards and should not be used as a basis for diet planning without reading the WHO report. Vitamin A recommendations are from FAO/WHO *Requirements of Vitamin A, Thiamine, Riboflavine, and Niacin, 1967,* as cited by R. L. Pike and M. L. Brown, *Nutrition: An Integrated Approach,* 2d ed. (New York: Wiley, 1975), p. 929. The recommendations for the three B vitamins are from *Requirements of Vitamin A, Thiamine, Riboflavine, and Niacin,* report of a joint FAO/WHO expert group (Rome, September 6-17, 1965), part 8, table 6. Ascorbic acid recommendations are from FAO/WHO *Requirements of Ascorbic Acid, Vitamin D, Vitamin B_{12}, Folate, and Iron, 1970* as cited in Pike and Brown, 1975, p. 929. FAO/WHO has published additional recommendations for vitamins D, B_{12}, and folate. Calcium recommendations are from FAO/WHO, *Calcium Requirements,* WHO Technical Report Series no. 230, 1962, as adapted and cited in Pike and Brown, 1975, p. 926. Iron recommendations are from FAO/WHO, *Requirements of Ascorbic Acid, Vitamin D, Vitamin B_{12}, Folate, and Iron,* FAO Nutrition Meeting Report Series no. 47, 1970, p. 54, as adapted and cited by Pike and Brown, 1975, p. 928.

APPENDIX L: Exchange Systems

For an introduction to the use of exchange systems, see Chapter 2. Two exchange systems are presented here, for the use of U.S. and Canadian readers.

The United States system divides foods into six lists—the milk, vegetable, fruit, bread, meat, and fat lists.[1] The items listed first in each group are from the standard exchange lists used in the United States. We have also listed some Chinese foods and some fast foods to show that the exchange system can be adapted to other uses. At the end of the section is a list of "unlimited" foods, which have negligible calories.

The exchange system can be used to plan diets at many different calorie levels. Six such diets, from 1200 to 3000 calories per day, are shown in the Chapter 2 Food Feature.

Milk List (12 g carbohydrate, 8 g protein, 80 cal)*

Amount	Food
Nonfat fortified milk	
1 c	Skim or nonfat milk
1 c	Buttermilk made from skim milk
1 c	Yogurt made from skim milk (plain, unflavored)
1/3 c	Powdered, nonfat dry milk, before adding liquid
1/2 c	Canned evaporated skim milk, before adding liquid
Low-fat fortified milk	
1 c	1% fat fortified milk (add 1/2 fat exchange)†
1 c	2% fat fortified milk (add 1 fat exchange)‡
1 c	Yogurt made from 2% fortified milk (plain, unflavored) (add 1 fat exchange)†
Whole milk (add 2 fat exchanges)	
1 c	Whole milk
1 c	Buttermilk made from whole milk
1 c	Yogurt made from whole milk (plain, unflavored)
1/2 c	Canned evaporated whole milk, before adding liquid
Chinese foods	
1 c	Soybean milk, unsweetened
2 blocks	Soybean curd (21/2 x 21/2 x 11/2 in)
2/3 c	Soybean, cooked
Fast foods§	

*A milk exchange is a serving of food equivalent to 1 c of skim milk in its energy nutrient content. One milk exchange contains substantial amounts of carbohydrate and protein and about 80 cal.

†These milk exchanges contain more fat than skim milk. Add 1/2 fat exchange.

‡These milk exchanges contain more fat than skim milk. Add 1 fat exchange.

§These fast foods contain 1/2 milk exchange and added bread and fat: chocolate shake (31/2 bread, 2 fat, 365 cal); vanilla shake (3 bread, 11/2 fat, 325 cal); strawberry shake (31/2 bread, 11/2 fat, 345 cal).

Vegetable List (5 g carbohydrate, 2 g protein, 25 cal)*

Amount	Food
1/2 c	Asparagus
1/2 c	Bean sprouts
1/2 c	Beets
1/2 c	Broccoli
1/2 c	Brussels sprouts
1/2 c	Cabbage
1/2 c	Carrots
1/2 c	Cauliflower
1/2 c	Celery
1/2 c	Cucumbers
1/2 c	Eggplant
1/2 c	Green pepper
	Greens
1/2 c	Beet greens
1/2 c	Chards
1/2 c	Collard greens
1/2 c	Dandelion greens
1/2 c	Kale
1/2 c	Mustard greens
1/2 c	Spinach
1/2 c	Turnip greens
1/2 c	Mushrooms
1/2 c	Okra
1/2 c	Onions
1/2 c	Rhubarb
1/2 c	Rutabaga
1/2 c	Sauerkraut
1/2 c	String beans, green or yellow
1/2 c	Summer squash
1/2 c	Tomatoes
1/2 c	Tomato juice
1/2 c	Turnips
1/2 c	Vegetable juice cocktail
1/2 c	Zucchini
Chinese foods	
1/2 c	Beansprouts, soy
1/2 c	Lotus root (1/3 segment)
1/2 c	Waterchestnut
1/2 c	Yam bean root

*A vegetable exchange is a serving of any vegetable that contains a moderate amount of carbohydrate, a small but significant amount of protein, and about 25 cal.

Fruit List (10 g carbohydrate, 40 cal)*

Amount	Food
1 small	Apple
1/3 c	Apple juice
1/2 c	Applesauce (unsweetened)
2 medium	Apricots, fresh
4 halves	Apricots, dried
1/2 small	Banana
1/2 c	Blackberries
1/2 c	Blueberries
1/4 small	Cantaloupe melon
10 large	Cherries
1/3 c	Cider
2	Dates
1	Fig, fresh
1	Fig, dried
1 half	Grapefruit
1/2 c	Grapefruit juice
12	Grapes
1/4 c	Grape juice
1/8 medium	Honeydew melon
1/2 small	Mango
1 small	Nectarine
1 small	Orange
1/2 c	Orange juice
3/4 c	Papaya
1 medium	Peach
1 small	Pear
1 medium	Persimmon (native)
1/2 c	Pineapple
1/3 c	Pineapple juice
2 medium	Plums
2 medium	Prunes
1/4 c	Prune juice
1/2 c	Raspberries
2 tbsp	Raisins
3/4 c	Strawberries
1 medium	Tangerine
1 c	Watermelon
Chinese foods	
1 medium	Guava, fresh
3 medium	Kumquats, fresh
4 medium	Lychee, fresh
1/2 small or 1/3 c	Mango
1/2 small or 1/3 c	Papaya
1/2 medium	Persimmon
1/3 medium	Pomelo
Fast foods†	

*A fruit exchange is a serving of fruit that contains about 10 g of carbohydrate and 40 cal. The protein and fat content of fruit is negligible.

†Apple and cherry pies contain 1 1/2 exchanges of fruit but also 1 bread and 3 1/2 fat exchanges.

Bread List (15 g carbohydrate, 2 g protein, 70 cal)*

Amount	Food
Bread	
1 slice	White (including French and Italian)
1 slice	Whole-wheat
1 slice	Rye or pumpernickel
1 slice	Raisin
1 half	Small bagel
1 half	Small English muffin
1	Plain roll, bread
1 half	Frankfurter roll
1 half	Hamburger bun
3 tbsp	Dried bread crumbs
1 6-in	Tortilla
Cereal	
1/2 c	Bran flakes
3/4 c	Other ready-to-eat cereal, unsweetened
1 c	Puffed cereal, unfrosted
1/2 c	Cereal, cooked
1/2 c	Grits, cooked
1/2 c	Rice or barley, cooked
1/2 c	Pasta, cooked (spaghetti, noodles, or macaroni)
3 c	Popcorn, popped, no fat added
2 tbsp	Cornmeal, dry
2 1/2 tbsp	Flour
1/4 c	Wheat germ

*A bread exchange is a serving of bread, cereal, or starchy vegetable that contains appreciable carbohydrate (15 g) and a small but significant amount of protein (2 g), totaling about 70 cal.

Bread List (15 g carbohydrate, 2 g protein, 70 cal) (cont'd)

Amount	Food
Crackers	
3	Arrowroot
2	Graham, 21/2-in square
1 half	Matzoth, 4 × 6 in
20	Oyster
25	Pretzels, 31/8 in long × 1/8 in diameter
3	Rye wafers, 2 × 31/2 in
6	Saltines
4	Soda, 21/2-in sq
Dried beans, peas, and lentils	
1/2 c	Beans, peas, lentils, dried and cooked
1/4 c	Baked beans, no pork, canned
Starchy vegetables	
1/3 c	Corn
1 small	Corn on cob
1/2 c	Lima beans
2/3 c	Parsnips
1/2 c	Peas, green, canned, or frozen
1 small	Potato, white
1/2 c	Potato, mashed
3/4 c	Pumpkin
1/2 c	Squash (winter, acorn, or butternut)
1/4 c	Yam or sweet potato
Prepared foods†	
1	Biscuit, 2-in diameter (add 1 fat exchange)
1	Corn bread, 2 × 2 × 1 in (add 1 fat exchange)
1	Corn muffin, 2-in diameter (add 1 fat exchange)
5	Crackers, round butter type (add 1 fat exchange)
1	Muffin, plain, small (add 1 fat exchange)
8	Potatoes, french fried, 2× 31/2 in (add 1 fat exchange)
15	Potato chips or corn chips (add 2 fat exchanges)
1	Pancake, 5 × 1/2 in (add 1 fat exchange)
1	Waffle, 5 × 1/2 in (add 1 fat exchange)
Chinese foods	
1 small or 2/3 medium	Bow (Chinese steamed dough)
6	Chestnuts
1 c	Congee
1/4 c	Glutinous rice, cooked
2/3 c	Gruel rice, cooked
1/2 c	Noodles, cooked (shrimp, thin rice, flat rice, cellophane)
2 tbsp	Rice flour or glutinous rice flour
3 small or 1/3 c	Taro
4	Wonton wrapper (5 × 5 in)

†These foods contain more fat than bread. When calculating fat values, add fat exchanges as indicated (1 fat exchange = 5 g fat).

Meat List (7 g protein, 3 g fat + variable added fat; 55 cal + calories for added fat)*

Amount	Food
Low-fat meat	
1 oz	Beef—baby beef (very lean), chipped beef, chuck, flank steak, tenderloin, plate ribs, plate skirt steak, round (bottom, top), all cuts rump, spareribs, tripe
1 oz	Lamb—leg, rib, sirloin, loin (roast and chops), shank, shoulder
1 oz	Pork—leg (whole rump, center shank), ham, smoked (center slices)
1 oz	Veal—leg, loin, rib, shank, shoulder, cutlets
1 oz	Poultry—meat-without-skin of chicken, turkey, cornish hen, guinea hen, pheasant

*A meat exchange is a serving of protein-rich food that contains negligible carbohydrate but a significant amount of protein (7 g) and fat (3 g), roughly equivalent to the amounts in 1 oz of lean meat; contains about 55 cal.

Meat List (7 g protein, 3 g fat + variable added fat; 55 cal + calories for added fat) (cont'd)

Amount	Food
1 oz	Fish—any fresh or frozen
1/4 c	Canned salmon, tuna, mackerel, crab, lobster
5 (or 1 oz)	Clams, oysters, scallops, shrimp
3	Sardines, drained
1 oz	Cheese, containing less than 5% butterfat
1/4 c	Cottage cheese, dry and 2% butterfat
1/2 c	Dried beans and peas (add 1 bread exchange)†
Medium-fat meat (add 1/2 fat exchange)†	
1 oz	Beef—ground (15% fat), corned beef (canned), rib eye, round (ground commercial)
1 oz	Pork—loin (all cuts tenderloin), shoulder arm (picnic), shoulder blade, Boston butt, Canadian bacon, boiled ham
1 oz	Liver, heart, kidney, sweetbreads (high in cholesterol)
1/4 c	Cottage cheese, creamed
1 oz	Cheese—mozzarella, ricotta, farmer's cheese, Neufchatel
3 tbsp	Parmesan cheese
1	Egg (high in cholesterol)
High-fat meat (add 1 fat exchange)†	
1 oz	Beef—brisket, corned beef (brisket), ground beef (more than 20% fat), hamburger (commercial), chuck (ground commercial), roasts (rib), steaks (club and rib)
1 oz	Lamb—breast
1 oz	Pork—spare ribs, loin (back ribs), pork (ground), country-style ham, deviled ham
1 oz	Veal—breast
1 oz	Poultry—capon, duck (domestic), goose
1 oz	Cheddar-type cheese
1 slice	Cold cuts, 4 1/2 × 1/8 in
1 small	Frankfurter
Peanut butter	
2 tbsp	Peanut butter (add 2 1/2 fat exchanges)†
Chinese foods‡	
1/4 c	Canned or cooked abalone, crabmeat, eel, lobster, conch, cuttlefish, squid, octopus, fish maw, sea cucumbers, jellyfish, etc.
10 medium	River snails
2 medium	Frog legs
3 medium	Duck feet
1 medium or 1/2 large	Duck egg, salted
1 medium	Egg, preserved or limed
1/2 block	Soybean curd, fresh, 2 1/2 × 1 1/4 × 1 1/2 in
2 pieces	Soybean curd, fried, 3 × 6 × 1/2 inches
Fast foods§	

†These foods contain more carbohydrate or fat than lean meat. When calculating carbohydrate or fat values, add bread or fat exchanges as indicated.

‡These exchanges are not separated into high-, medium-, and low-fat exchanges.

§Most fast-food meats are for variable numbers of exchanges and have other exchanges added: hamburger (1 high-fat meat, 2 bread, 260 cal); cheeseburger (1 1/2 high-fat meat, 2 bread, 306 cal); Quarter Pounder® (3 high-fat meat, 2 bread, 420 cal); Big Mac® (3 high-fat meat, 2 1/2 bread, 1 1/2 fat, 540 cal); Quarter Pounder® with cheese (4 high-fat meat, 2 bread, 520 cal); Egg McMuffin® (2 high-fat meat, 1 1/2 bread, 1 fat, 350 cal); pork sausage (1 high-fat meat, 1 1/2 fat, 185 cal).

Fat List (5 g fat, 45 cal)*

Amount	Food
Polyunsaturated fat	
1 tsp	Margarine (soft, tub, or stick)†
1/8	Avocado (4-in diameter)‡
1 tsp	Oil—corn, cottonseed, safflower, soy, sunflower
1 tsp	Oil, olive‡
1 tsp	Oil, peanut‡
5 small	Olives‡
10 whole	Almonds‡
2 large whole	Pecans‡
20 whole	Peanuts, Spanish‡
10 whole	Peanuts, Virginia‡
6 small	Walnuts
6 small	Nuts, other‡
Saturated fat	
1 tsp	Margarine, regular stick
1 tsp	Butter
1 tsp	Bacon fat
1 strip	Bacon, crisp
2 tbsp	Cream, light
2 tbsp	Cream, sour
1 tbsp	Cream, heavy
1 tbsp	Cream cheese
1 tbsp	French dressing§
1 tbsp	Italian dressing§
1 tsp	Lard
1 tsp	Mayonnaise§
2 tsp	Salad dressing, mayonnaise type§
3/4-in cube	Salt pork
Chinese foods	
1 tsp	Sesame or chili oil
1 piece	Coconut meat, 1 × 1 × 1.2 in
21/2 tsp	Coconut, grated
2 tsp	Coconut cream (no water)
1 tbsp	Sesame seeds
1-in cube	Fatty cured Chinese pork

*A fat exchange is a serving of any food that contains negligible carbohydrate and protein but appreciable fat (5 g), totaling about 45 cal.

†Made with corn, cottonseed, safflower, soy, or sunflower oil only.

‡Fat content is primarily monounsaturated.

§If made with corn, cottonseed, safflower, soy, or sunflower oil, can be assumed to contain polyunsaturated fat.

Unlimited Foods (negligible cal)*

Amount	Food
	Diet calorie-free beverage
	Coffee
	Tea
	Bouillon without fat
	Unsweetened gelatin
	Unsweetened pickles
	Salt and pepper
	Red pepper
	Paprika
	Garlic
	Celery salt
	Parsley
	Nutmeg
	Lemon
	Mustard
	Chili powder
	Onion salt or powder
	Horseradish
	Vinegar
	Mint
	Cinnamon
	Lime
	Raw vegetables—chicory, Chinese cabbage, endive, escarole, lettuce, parsley, radishes, watercress
Chinese foods	
	Plain agar-agar
	Seasonings, spices, herbs† such as soy sauce, monosodium glutamate, star anise, five-spices powder
	Chinese parsley, kelp, sea girdle, laver, and seaweed hair
1 tsp	Shrimp sauce or dried shrimp
1 tsp or 2 nuts	Gingko nuts
1/2 block	White bean curd cheese, 11/2 × 3/4 × 1 in
1/4 block	Red bean curd cheese, 1 × 1/4 × 1/2 in
1 c or less	Watery vegetables, including bamboo shoots, bitter melon, bottle gourd, cabbage (celery, mustard, or spoon; fresh, pickled, spiced, salted, or salted and dried), Chinese broccoli, Chinese eggplant, fungi (black, brown, or white), snow peas, turnips (Chinese or green), watercress, winter melon, wolfberry leaves

*These are "free foods" that contain negligible carbohydrate, protein, and fat and therefore negligible calories.

†Does not include some starchy and sugar-preserved Chinese herbs.

The Canadian system works the same way as the U.S. system, but the serving sizes and some of the foods listed are different.[2] Notable among the differences are:

The standard serving size for milk is ½ cup (not 1 cup), and whole milk rather than skim is the basis for calculation.

Vegetables are listed in two groups, the A group (7 grams carbohydrate, 2 grams protein) and the B group (about half as much carbohydrate and protein). Serving sizes vary. Two group B vegetable servings may be traded for one group A vegetable serving.

Meats are not divided into low-, medium-, and high-fat categories. An ounce of any meat is considered to provide 7 grams protein, 5 grams fat.

Milk List (6 g carbohydrate, 4 g protein, 4 g fat)*

Amount	Food
Whole milk	
1/2 c	Whole milk
1/4 c	Evaporated whole milk
Low-fat milk	
1/2 c	2% milk†
1/2 c	2% buttermilk†
1/2 c	Skim milk‡
2 tbsp	Powdered skim milk (instant)‡
1/2 c	Skim buttermilk‡
1/3 c	Yogurt (plain)‡

*A milk exchange is a serving of food equivalent to 1/2 c of whole milk in its energy-nutrient content.

†These milk exchanges contain less fat than whole milk. Subtract 1/2 fat exchange.

‡These milk exchanges contain less fat than whole milk. Subtract 1 fat exchange.

Vegetable List—Group A (7 g carbohydrate, 2 g protein)

Amount	Food
1/4 c	Beans—dried navy, lima (canned or cooked)
1/4 c	Beans, green lima
1/2 c	Beets, canned or cooked
2/3 c	Beet greens, cooked
4 stalks	Broccoli, cooked
1/2 c	Brussels sprouts, cooked
3 level tbsp	Canned condensed soup (undiluted)†
1/2 c	Carrots, raw, diced, cooked
21/2 tbsp	Corn, canned cream style or niblet†
1/2 c	Dandelion greens, cooked
2 slices 4 × 4 × 1 in	Eggplant, raw

Vegetable List—Group A (7 g carbohydrate, 2 g protein)* *(continued)*

Amount	Food
2/3 c	Kohlrabi, cooked
4 or 1/3 c chopped	Onions, green
1 medium or 1/3 c chopped	Onions, mature, raw
1/3 c	Parsnips, cooked†
1/3 c	Peas, green, frozen†
1/3 c	Peas, fresh, green, cooked
1/4 c	Peas, green, canned (drained)
2 level tbsp	Potatoes, mashed†
1/2 small	Potato, boiled or baked
1/2 c	Pumpkin, canned
3 level tbsp	Rice, cooked†
3/4 c	Sauerkraut, canned
1/2 c	Squash, hubbard or pepper, baked or mashed
3/4 c	Tomatoes, canned
2/3 c	Tomato juice, no sugar added
1/2 c	Turnip, yellow or white cooked
2/3 c	Vegetable juice, mixed
1/2 c	Vegetables, mixed carrots and peas
1/3 c	Vegetables, mixed carrots, peas, green lima beans, corn

*A vegetable exchange is a serving of any vegetable that contains a moderate amount of carbohydrate and a small but significant amount of protein.

†These vegetables also appear on the bread list in larger servings. They are included in group A for those people whose diet is low in calories and to add variety in making up casserole dishes, soups, and the like for any diet.

Vegetable List—Group B*

Amount	Food
5 stalks	Asparagus
1/2 c	Beans, yellow or green, canned or cooked
1 c	Bean sprouts, raw
1/2 c	Cabbage, raw or cooked
1/2 c	Cauliflower, cooked
4 stalks or 1/2 c chopped	Celery, raw
1/2 c	Celery, cooked
1/2 c	Chard, cooked
1/2 medium or 8 slices	Cucumber
1 6-in stalk	Endive
1/2 c	Fiddleheads
1/2 c	Kale
1/8 head 4 large leaves	Lettuce
2	Onions, green
1 medium	Pepper, green, raw, or cooked
3 tbsp	Pimento, canned
6	Radish
1/2 c	Spinach, cooked or canned
1/3 c	Tomato juice (no sugar added)
1 medium (21/4-in diameter)	Tomato, raw
1/2 c	Vegetable marrow, cooked
1/2 c	Zucchini

*Two servings of group B vegetables equal one serving of group A vegetables. One serving from group B may be taken "free" at any meal.

Fruit List (10 g carbohydrate)*

Amount	Food
1/2 medium	Apple, raw
1/3 c	Apple juice
1/2 c	Applesauce
2	Apricots, raw with stone
5 halves + 2 tbsp juice	Apricots, canned, cooked, or dried
1/2 6-in	Banana
1/3 c	Blackberries, raw
1/2 c	Blueberries, raw
1/2 5-in diameter	Cantaloupe with rind
1 c	Cantaloupe cubes or balls
10 large	Cherries, raw
1/3 c + 2 tbsp juice	Cherries, canned, red, pitted, cooked
1 average	Crabapple
2	Dates
2/3 c	Fruit cocktail, canned
1 + 1 tbsp juice	Fig, cooked
1	Fig, dried
3/4 c	Gooseberries, raw
1/2 small (31/2-in diameter)	Grapefruit, raw
1/2 c with juice	Grapefruit sections, raw
1/2 c	Grapefruit juice
14 medium	Grapes, slipskin
14 medium	Grapes, Malaga and seedless
1/4 c	Grape juice
1/2 melon 5-in diameter	Honeydew melon with rind
3/4 c	Honeydew cubes or balls
1/2 c	Huckleberries
1/2 c	Loganberries
1 medium	Nectarine
1 medium (21/2 in diameter)	Orange, raw
1/2 c + juice	Orange sections
1/2 c	Orange juice
3/4 c + juice (14 sections)	Orange, mandarin sections (canned dietetic)
1 medium	Peach, raw with stone
2 large halves + 2 tbsp juice	Peaches, canned or cooked

*One fruit exchange is a serving of fruit that contains about 10 g of carbohydrate. The protein and fat content of fruit is negligible.

Fruit List (10 g carbohydrate) (cont'd)

Amount	Food
1 small	Pear, raw
2 halves + 2 tbsp juice	Pears, canned or cooked
1/2 c	Pineapple, raw, cubed
1/2 c cubes or 2 slices + 2 tbsp juice	Pineapple, canned
1/2 c	Pineapple, crushed
1/3 c	Pineapple juice
2 medium	Plums, raw with stone
2 medium + 2 tbsp juice	Plums, canned or cooked
1/2	Pomegranate
2	Prunes, cooked
1/4 c	Prune juice
2 level tbsp	Raisins
1/2 c	Raspberries, raw
1/2 c	Raspberries, canned or cooked
2 c	Rhubarb, raw
1 c	Rhubarb, cooked
1/2 c	Saskatoons
1 c	Strawberries, raw
3/4 c	Strawberries, canned or cooked
1 (21/2-in diameter)	Tangerines
1 c	Tomato juice (no sugar added)
1 slice 1 in thick and 5 in triangle	Watermelon, with skin
1 c	Watermelon cubes
1/6-pt brick	Ice cream—plain vanilla, strawberry, chocolate (add 5 g butter or 1 fat exchange)

Bread List (15 g carbohydrate, 2 g protein)*

Amount	Food
1 slice	Bread
4 (41/2 in each)	Bread sticks
6 (6 in each)	Bread sticks, thin
1/2	Bagel
1/4 c	Brewis, cooked (Newfoundland)
1/2 bun	Hamburger bun (31/2-in)
1/2 bun	Wiener bun (6-in)
4 rectangular slices or 8 round slices	Melba toast (commercial)
1	Matzo (6-in square)
3	Arrowroots
4	Graham wafers (2-in)
11/2 biscuits	Holland rusks
6	Soda biscuits (2-in)
2 tbsp	Cereals, uncooked (dry weight)
1/2 c	Cereals, cooked
3/4 c	Cereals, cold, flaked
1 c	Cereals, puffed
2/3 biscuit	Cereals, Shredded Wheat
2 tbsp	Cornstarch
21/2 tbsp	Flour
1/3 c	Beans and peas, dried, cooked
1/2 c	Corn, canned
1 cob	Corn on the cob (41/2 × 11/2 × 2 in)
11/4 c	Popcorn
2/3 c	Parsnips
1/2 c	Peas, canned
2/3 c	Peas, frozen
1 small or 1/3 c mashed	Potatoes
1/2 c	Macaroni, cooked
1/3 c	Rice, spaghetti, noodles (cooked)
6 tbsp	Canned condensed soup (undiluted)

*A bread exchange is a serving of bread, cereal, or starchy vegetable equivalent in energy-nutrient content to one slice of cracked or whole-wheat, white, brown, or rye bread weighing 30 g. A bread exchange contains appreciable carbohydrate and a small but significant amount of protein.

Meat List (7 g protein, 5 g fat)*

Amount	Food
1 medium	Egg
Meat and poultry	
1 slice 4 × 2 × 1/4 in	Sliced medium-fat beef, corned beef, lamb, pork, veal, ham, liver, poultry
1 piece 4 × 2 × 1/4 in	Steak
3 11/2-in cubes	Diced beef for stewing
2 tbsp or small patty (3 tbsp raw)	Minced beef
2/3 oz	Salt beef (dried)
1 small	Lamb loin chop
1/2 medium	Pork, veal chop
3 slices	Bacon, back or side (crisp)
1 slice, 1/8 in thick	Luncheon-type meats
1 slice, 1/4 in thick (11/2-2-in diameter)	Liverwurst, salami, summer sausage
11/2 (12 per lb)	Sausages†
1 piece 4 × 2 × 1/4 in	Seal
1 (12 per lb)	Wieners†
Fish	
1 piece 2 × 1 × 1 in	Fillets of haddock, halibut, cod, sole, whitefish‡
1 piece 2 × 1 × 1 in	Fillet of salmon
1 piece 2 × 1 × 1 in	Salmon steak
1/4 c	Canned chicken haddie, crabmeat, lobster, salmon, tuna
3 fish 3-in each	Sardines (drained)
3 medium	Clams, fresh
3 medium	Oysters
2 medium	Scallops
4 medium	Shrimps, prawns
Cheese	
1 cube 11/2 × 1 × 1 in or 1 slice (presliced, packaged) 31/2 × 31/2 × 1/8 in	Cheddar or processed
11/2 sections	Gruyere
4 level tbsp	Dried, grated (Parmesan)
3 tbsp	Cottage, creamed
3 tbsp	Cottage, dry (skim)‡
1 piece 21/2-in diameter and 1/4-in thick or 1 slice presliced, packaged 31/2 × 31/2 × 1/8-in	Skim milk, processed‡

*A meat exchange is a serving of protein-rich food that contains negligible carbohydrate but a significant amount of protein and fat, roughly equivalent to the amounts in 1 oz (30 g) of meat.

†For special sizes of sausages and wieners, check weight and number per package.

‡These items contain less fat than most meats. Subtract 1 fat exchange.

Fat List (5 g fat)*

Amount	Food
1/8 of 4-in avocado	Avocado pear†
1 strip	Bacon (side)
1 tsp or 1 pat (1 × 1 × 1/4 in)	Butter or margarine
1 tsp	Cooking fat or oil
3 tbsp	Cream, cereal (10%)†
2 tbsp	Cream, coffee (18%)
2 tbsp	Cream, commercial sour
1 tbsp	Cream, whipping
1 rounded tbsp	Cream, whipped
1 tbsp	Cream cheese (white)
1 tbsp	French dressing
1 tsp	Mayonnaise
10	Peanuts†
4	Cashews†
6	Almonds, filberts†
4-5 halves	Pecans, walnuts†
2	Brazil nuts†
5 small	Olives, green
3 medium	Olives, ripe with pit
1/2 tbsp	Peanut butter†

*A fat exchange is a serving of food equivalent to 1 tsp butter in its fat content. Most fat exchanges have negligible carbohydrate.

†It is advisable to limit these items to two servings per day because of the carbohydrate content.

Calorie-Free Foods*

Food	
Artificial sweetener	Watercress
Non-caloric carbonated beverages (dietetic)	Food coloring
Clear tea or coffee	Gelatin, plain
Bouillon	Artificially sweetened jelly powders
Clear broth	Horseradish
Consomme	Mushrooms
Flavouring (vanilla, lemon extract)	Parsley
Vinegar	Rennet tablets
Seasoning, spices, and herbs	
Cinnamon	Sage
Curry powder	Poultry seasoning
Ginger	Mixed whole spices
Nutmeg	Salt and pepper
Mint	Onion salt
Marjoram	Garlic salt

*No significant food value. These foods may be used on calorie-restricted diets without restriction.

Calorie-Poor Foods*

Amount	Food
1 tsp	Cream substitute, powdered (nondairy)
1 tsp	Cocoa (plain)
1 tbsp	Cranberries, cooked without sugar
1 medium serving	Dulse
1 tsp	Fruit spread and jelly, dietetic
1 tbsp	Lemon juice
1 medium	Lemon wedge or slice
1 tsp	Catsup
1 tsp	Chili sauce
1 tsp	Steak sauce
1 tbsp	Partridge berries (Newfoundland)
1 medium	Pickle, dill, unsweetened
4	Pickles, sour, mixed
4	Pickles, sweet, mixed (dietetic)
1 tbsp	Pimento or chopped green pepper
1 tsp	Prepared mustard
1 tbsp	Whipped topping, commercial, powder

*Low in calories. These foods may be used in amounts up to two servings a day in calorie-restricted diets.

Notes

1. The U.S. exchange system presented here is based on material in *Exchange Lists for Meal Planning*, prepared by committees of the American Diabetes Association and the American Dietetic Association in cooperation with the National Institute of Arthritis, Metabolic, and Digestive Diseases and the National Heart and Lung Institute, National Institutes of Health, Public Health Service, U.S. Department of Health, Education, and Welfare.

The Chinese foods listed in these tables are reprinted from *Diabetes and Chinese Food*, © 1978, with the written permission of the Canadian Dietetic Association. We have adjusted the Canadian exchanges used in these examples so that they correspond approximately in food value to the U.S. exchanges. *Diabetes and Chinese Food* is available for a nominal charge from the Canadian Diabetes Association (address in Appendix J).

The fast food data are reprinted by permission from "Nutritional Analysis of Foods Served at McDonald's" (© McDonald's, 1976).

2. The Canadian exchange system is taken from *Exchange Lists for Meal Planning for Diabetics in Canada* (Toronto, Ontario: Canadian Diabetes Association, 1977), and is used with permission.

APPENDIX M: Canada's Food Guide

The U.S. Four Food Group Plan was presented in Chapter 2. Canada's Food Guide is similar and was developed with the same intent. The handbook explaining it presents the pattern of nutrient intakes shown in Table 1.[1] As shown in Table 2, the Food Guide recommends, for adults, a pattern slightly different from that presented in the Four Food Group Plan.

Table 1. Interlocking Pattern of Key Nutrients in the Food Groups (Canada)

Nutrient	Milk and milk products	Bread and cereals	Fruits and vegetables	Meat and alternates
Vitamin A	Vitamin A		Vitamin A	Vitamin A
Thiamin		Thiamin		Thiamin
Riboflavin	Riboflavin	Riboflavin		Riboflavin
Niacin		Niacin		Niacin
Folic acid			Folic acid	Folic acid
Vitamin C			Vitamin C	
Vitamin D	Vitamin D			
Calcium	Calcium			
Iron		Iron	Iron	Iron
Protein	Protein	Protein		Protein
Fat	Fat			Fat
Carbohydrate		Carbohydrate	Carbohydrate	

Table 2. Servings in Canada's Food Guide

Food group	Recommended number of servings (adult)	Serving size
Meat and alternates	2	60-90 g (2-3 oz) cooked lean meat, poultry, liver, or fish
		60 ml (4 tbsp) peanut butter
		250 ml (1 c) cooked dried peas, beans, or lentils
		80-250 ml (1/3-1 c) nuts or seeds
		60 g (2 oz) cheddar, processed, or cottage cheese
		2 eggs
Milk and milk products	2*	250 ml (1 c) milk, yogurt, or cottage cheese
		45 g (11/2 oz) cheddar or processed cheese
Fruits and vegetables	4-5†	125 ml (1/2 c) vegetables or fruits
		125 ml (1/2 c) juice
		1 medium potato, carrot, tomato, peach, apple, orange, or banana
Bread and cereals	3-5‡	1 slice bread
		125-250 ml (1/2-1 c) cooked or ready-to-eat cereal
		1 roll or muffin
		125-200 ml (1/2-3/4 c) cooked rice, macaroni, or spaghetti

*Children up to 11 years, 2-3 servings; adolescents, 3-4 servings; pregnant and nursing women, 3-4 servings. Skim, 2%, whole, buttermilk, reconstituted dry, or evaporated milk may be used as a beverage or as the main ingredient in other foods. Cheese may also be chosen. In addition, a supplement of vitamin D is recommended when the milk that is consumed does not contain added vitamin D.

†Include at least two vegetables. Choose a variety of both vegetables and fruits—cooked, raw, or their juices. Include yellow or green or green, leafy vegetables.

‡Whole-grain or enriched. Whole-grain products are recommended.

Notes

1. Canadian Ministry of Health and Welfare, *Canada's Food Guide: Handbook*, cat. no. H21-74/1977 (Ottawa, Ontario, 1977).

Chapter Notes

Chapter 1—The Problem of Food Choices

1. This belief is overly simple. For a more accurate description, see V. G. Dethier, Other tastes, other worlds, *Science* 201 (1978): 224-228.

Chapter 2—First Facts: Foods

1. J. C. King, S. H. Cohenour, C. G. Corrucini, and P. Schneeman, Evaluation and modification of the basic four food guide, *Journal of Nutrition Education* 10 (1978): 27-29.
2. These figures were taken from Items 86 and 142 in Appendix H.

Chapter 3—First Facts: Nutrient Needs and Nutritional Surveys

1. This is a committee of the Food and Nutrition Board (FNB) of the NAS/NRC (National Academy of Sciences/National Research Council).

2. Food and Nutrition Board, Committee on Recommended Allowances, *Recommended Dietary Allowances*, 9th ed. (Washington, D.C.: National Academy of Sciences, 1980).

3. U.S. Department of Agriculture, Agricultural Research Service, *Food and Nutrient Intake of Individuals in the United States, Spring 1965, USDA Household Food Consumption Survey 1965-1966* (Washington, D.C.: Government Printing Office, 1972).

4. FAO Nutrition Meetings, *Requirements of Vitamin A, Thiamine, Riboflavin, and Niacin*, report series 41 (Rome: Food and Agriculture Organization, 1967).

5. U.S. Department of Health, Education, and Welfare, *Ten-State Nutrition Survey 1968-1970*, publication no. (HSM) 72-8130 (Atlanta, Ga.: Center for Disease Control, 1972).

6. Z. I. Sabry, J. A. Campbell, M. E. Campbell, and A. L. Forbes, Nutrition Canada, *Nutrition Today*, January/February 1974, pp. 5-13.

7. Sabry et al, 1974.

8. C. F. Enloe, Jr., How to do a nutrition survey (editorial), *Nutrition Today*, January/February 1974, p. 14.

9. S. Abraham, M. D. Carroll, C. M. Dresser, and C. L. Johnson, Dietary intake of persons 1-74 years of age in the United States, *Advancedata from Vital and Health Statistics of the National Center for Health Statistics*, vol. 6, publication no. (HRA) 77-1250 (Rockville, Md.: U.S. Department of Health, Education, and Welfare, Public Health Service, Health Resources Administration, March 30, 1977).

10. P. Gunby, Federal agencies view food habit surveys (Medical News), *Journal of the American Medical Association* 244 (1980): 1536.

11. Abraham et a, 1977.

12. D. M. Hegsted, Priorities in nutrition in the United States, *Journal of the American Dietetic Association* 71 (1977): 9-13.

13. H. A. Guthrie and C. M. Guthrie, Factor analysis of nutritional status data from Ten State Nutrition Survey, *American Journal of Clinical Nutrition* 29 (1976): 1238-1241.

14. D. M. Hegsted, Energy needs and energy utilization, in *Nutrition Reviews' Present Knowledge in Nutrition*, 4th ed. (Washington, D.C.: Nutrition Foundation, 1976), pp. 1-9.

15. C. L. Krumdieck, Folic acid, in *Nutrition Reviews' Present Knowledge in Nutrition*, 4th ed. (Washington, D.C.: Nutrition Foundation, 1976), pp. 175-190.

16. Implications from a recent Nationwide Food Consumption Survey, *Journal of The American Dietetic Association* 77 (1980): 473.

17. L. M. Henderson, Nutritional problems growing out of new patterns of food consumption, *American Journal of Public Health* 62 (1972): 1194-1198.

Chapter 4—The Carbohydrates

1. U.S. Senate, Select Committee on Nutrition and Human Needs, *Dietary Goals for the United States*, 2d ed. (Washington, D.C.: Government Printing Office, 1977).

2. U. S. Senate, *Dietary Goals*, 1977.

3. K. M. West, Prevention and therapy of diabetes mellitus, in *Nutrition Reviews' Present Knowledge in Nutrition*, 4th ed. (Washington, D.C.: Nutrition Foundation, 1976), pp. 356-364.

4. Food and Nutrition Board, Committee on Recommended Allowances, *Recommended Dietary Allowances*, 9th ed. (Washington, D.C.: National Academy of Sciences, 1980).

5. Y. Jung, R. C. Khurana, D. G. Corredor, A. Hastillo, R. F. Lain, D. Patrick, P. Turkeltaub, and T. S. Danowski, Reactive hypoglycemia in women—results of a health survey, *Diabetes* 20 (June 1971): 428-434.

6. Most adult diabetics secrete insulin, but it is ineffective or delayed. This kind of diabetes is the common type and because of this characteristic has recently been renamed "non-insulin-dependent diabetes." Often the diet can be adjusted to enable the insulin to do its work so that no insulin shots or drugs need be taken. The rarer type of diabetes—juvenile or "insulin-dependent diabetes"—occurs in fewer than 20 percent of all cases and requires insulin shots.

7. Two papers that have demonstrated this effect are: M. J. Albrink, T. Newman, and P. C. Davidson, Effect of high- and low-fiber diets on plasma lipids and insulin, *American Journal of Clinical Nutrition* 32 (1979): 1486-1491; and J. W. Anderson and W.-J. T. Chu, Plant fiber: Carbohydrate and lipid metabolism, *American Journal of Clinical Nutrition* 32 (1979): 346-363.

8. N. V. Bohannon, J. H. Karam, and P. H. Forsham, Endocrine responses to sugar ingestion in man, *Journal of the American Dietetic Association* 76 (1980): 555-560.

9. C. Lecos, Fructose: Questionable diet aid, *FDA Consumer* 14 (March 1980): 20-23.

10. L. R. Brown and G. W. Finsterbusch, *Man and His Environment: Food* (New York: Harper & Row, 1972), p. 34.

11. Brown and Finsterbusch, 1972, p. 37.

12. U. S. Senate, *Dietary Goals,* 1977.

13. They add, "Legumes are important because a one-cup (approximately 200 g) serving provides more vitamin B_6, folate, iron, zinc, and magnesium than a 2 oz serving of animal protein." Improving on the basic four, *Nutrition and the MD,* October 1977.

Chapter 5—The Lipids: Fats and Oils

1. High blood lipid levels can be good or bad—depending on the lipid (Medical news), *Journal of the American Medical Association* 237 (1977): 1066-1070.

2. A brief, interesting, and accurate discussion of the lipoproteins is available from Ross Laboratories: A. K. Khachadurian, ed., Hyperlipoproteinemia, *Dietetic Currents, Ross Timesaver* 4 (July/August 1977).

3. D. C. Fletcher, Lecithin for hyperlipemia: Harmless but useless (questions and answers), *Journal of the American Medical Association* 238 (1977): 64.

4. Choline and lecithin in the treatment of neurologic disorders, *Nutrition and the MD,* April 1980.

5. C. A. Chandler and R. M. Marston, Fat in the U.S. diet, *Nutrition Program News* (a USDA periodical), May/August 1976.

6. Chandler and Marston, 1976.

7. U.S. Senate, Select Committee on Nutrition and Human Needs, *Dietary Goals for the United States,* 2d ed. (Washington, D.C.: Government Printing Office, 1977), p. 4.

Chapter 6—The Proteins: Amino Acids

1. L. R. Brown and G. W. Finsterbusch, *Man and His Environment: Food* (New York: Harper & Row, 1972), p. 37.

2. The body is not literally wise, although we often write as if cells could act purposively. They can't, but they sometimes seem to, as the physiologist W. B. Cannon first observed in his book, *The Wisdom of the Body* (New York: Norton, 1932).

3. D. M. Matthews and S. A. Adibi, Peptide absorption, *Gastroenterology* 71 (1976): 151-161.

4. A. A. Albanese and L. A. Orto, The proteins and amino acids, in *Modern Nutrition in Health and Disease*, ed. R. S. Goodhart and M. E. Shils, 5th ed. (Philadelphia: Lea and Febiger, 1973), p. 59.

5. U. D. Register and L. M. Sonnenberg, The vegetarian diet, *Journal of the American Dietetic Association* 62 (1973): 253-261.

6. M. C. Crim and H. N. Munro, Protein, in *Nutrition Reviews' Present Knowledge in Nutrition*, 4th ed. (Washington, D.C.: Nutrition Foundation, 1976), pp. 43-54.

7. J. T. Dwyer and J. Mayer, Beyond economics and nutrition: The complex basis of food policy, *Science* 188 (1975): 566-570.

8. Albanese and Orto, 1973, p. 56.

9. About 12 million children under five years of age died of hunger in 1978—a UNICEF statistic. D. R. Gwatkin, How many die? A set of demographic estimates of the annual number of infant and child deaths in the world (commentary), *American Journal of Public Health* 70 (1980): 1286-1289.

10. D. B. Jelliffe and E. F. P. Jelliffe, "Breast is best": Modern meanings, *New England Journal of Medicine* 297 (1977): 912-915. See also the several references suggested at the end of Controversy 12.

11. Albanese and Orto, 1973, pp. 28-88; and L. E. Holt, Jr., Protein economy in the growing child, *Postgraduate Medicine* 27 (1960): 783-798.

12. J. G. Chopra, A. L. Forbes, and J. P. Habicht, Protein in the U.S. diet, *Journal of the American Dietetic Association* 72 (1978): 253-258.

Chapter 7—Energy Balance: Feasting, Fasting, Loafing, Exercise

1. G. A. Bray and L. A. Campfield, Metabolic factors in the control of energy stores, *Metabolism* 24 (1975): 99-117.

2. R. A. Hawkins and J. E. Biebuyck, Ketone bodies are selectively used by individual brain regions, *Science* 205 (1979): 325-327.

3. American Medical Association, A critique of low-carbohydrate ketogenic weight reduction regimens (a review of Dr. Atkins' diet revolution), reprinted in *Nutrition Reviews/Supplement: Nutrition Misinformation and Food Faddism*, July 1974, pp. 15-23.

4. *Obesity '73: A Report from the Geigy Symposium on Obesity, Its Problems and Prognosis* (Ardsley, N.Y.: Geigy Pharmaceuticals, 1973).

5. H. T. Randall, Water, electrolytes and acid-base balance, in *Modern Nutrition in Health and Disease*, ed. R. S. Goodhart and M. E. Shils, 5th ed. (Philadelphia: Lea and Febiger, 1973), pp. 324-361.

6. American Medical Association, 1974.

7. American Medical Association, 1974; W. E. Connor and S. L. Connor, Sucrose and carbohydrate, in *Nutrition Reviews' Present Knowledge in Nutrition*, 4th ed. (Washington, D.C.: Nutrition Foundation, 1976), pp. 33-42.

8. American Medical Association, 1974; F. Rickman, N. Mitchell, J. Dingman, and J. E. Dalen, Changes in serum cholesterol during the Stillman Diet, *Journal of the American Medical Association* 228 (1974): 54-58.

9. R. M. Deutsch, *The New Nuts among the Berries: How Nutrition Nonsense Captured America* (Palo Alto, Calif.: Bull Publishing, 1977), p. 229.

10. A. A. Albanese and L. A. Orto, The proteins and amino acids, in *Modern Nutrition in Health and Disease*, ed. R. S. Goodhart and M. E. Shils, 5th ed. (Philadelphia: Lea and Febiger, 1973), p. 56.

11. Morbid obesity: Long-term results of therapeutic fasting, *Nutrition Reviews* 36 (January 1978): 6-7.

12. Food and Nutrition Board, Committee on Recommended Allowances, *Recommended Dietary Allowances*, 8th ed. (Washington, D.C.: National Academy of Sciences, 1974).

13. R. L. Pike and M. L. Brown, *Nutrition: An Integrated Approach*, 2d ed. (New York: Wiley, 1975), p. 835.

Chapter 8—Energy Balance: Overweight and Underweight

1. B. B. Blouin, Diet and obesity (News Digest), *Journal of the American Dietetic Association* 70 (1977): 535.

2. Lab techniques for estimating body composition do exist. The body's density (weight/volume) provides an estimate, because the densities of fat and lean tissue are known. This is the basis of the lab test in which the whole body is submerged in water to discover its volume. The weight is then divided by the volume to derive the density. The extent to which radioactive potassium or heavy water (deuterium oxide) is diluted in the body fluids also provides an estimate, because these will distribute into lean, and not into fat, tissues.

3. F. Grande and A. Keys, Body weight, body composition and calorie status, in *Modern Nutrition in Health and Disease*, ed. R. S. Goodhart and M. E. Shils, 6th ed. (Philadelphia: Lea and Febiger, 1980), pp. 3-34.

4. Grande and Keys, 1980.

5. C. F. Gastineau, Obesity: Risks, causes, and treatment, *Medical Clinics of North America* 56 (July 1972): 1021-1028.

6. J. V. G. A. Durnin, Sex differences in energy intake and expenditure, *Proceedings of the Nutrition Society* 35 (September 1976): 145-154.

7. E. M. Widdowson, The response of the sexes to nutritional stress, *Proceedings of the Nutrition Society* 35 (September 1976): 175-180.

8. J. Mayer, Obesity, in Goodhart and Shils, 1980, pp. 721-740.

9. Juvenile-onset and adult-onset obesity are sometimes called developmental and reactive obesity, respectively.

10. M. Winick, Childhood obesity, *Nutrition Today*, May/June 1974, pp. 6-12.

11. O. Bosello, R. Ostuzzi, F. A. Rossi, F. Armellini, M. Cigolini, R. Micciolo, and L. A. Scuro, Adipose tissue cellularity and weight reduction forecasting, *American Journal of Clinical Nutrition* 33 (1980): 776-782.

12. Food and obesity in the rat, *Nutrition Reviews* 37 (1979): 52-54.

13. The fat-cell theory has been skeptically reviewed by E. M. Widdowson and M. J. Dauncey, Obesity, in *Nutrition Reviews' Present Knowledge in Nutrition*, 4th ed. (Washington, D.C.: Nutrition Foundation, 1976), pp. 17-23. Similar conclusions were reached by J. Kirtland and M. I. Gurr, Adipose tissue cellularity: A review; 2. The relationship between cellularity and obesity, *International Journal of Obesity* 3 (1979): 15-55. These authors have suggested a better way of counting fat cells—by counting their nuclei.

14. Current concepts of obesity (reviewed by M. R. C. Greenwood and J. Hirsch), *Dairy Council Digest* 46 (1975).

15. K. M. West, Prevention and therapy of diabetes mellitus, in *Nutrition Reviews' Present Knowledge*, 1976, pp. 356-364. An article that contradicts this generalization is F. Davidoff, Medical therapies for diabetes: Do they work? *Journal of the American Dietetic Association* 71 (1977): 495-500.

16. Blouin, 1977.

17. R. A. Seelig, *Obesity: A review* (Washington, D.C.: United Fresh Fruit and Vegetable Association, 1976).

18. Gastineau, 1972.

19. Gastineau, 1972.

20. Winick, 1974.

21. The Nutrition Gazette, *Nutrition Today,* July/August 1979, p. 5.

22. E. Eckholm and F. Record, *Worldwatch Paper* 9: *The Two Faces of Malnutrition* (Washington, D.C.: Worldwatch Institute, 1976).

23. Gastineau, 1972.

24. M. Rezek, The role of insulin in the glucostatic control of food intake, *Canadian Journal of Physiology and Pharmacology* 54 (1976): 650-665.

25. *Appetite,* a quarterly journal "for research on intake, its control, and its consequences," from Academic Press Inc., London, starting in March 1980, announcement in the *Journal of the American Dietetic Association* 77 (1980): 226.

26. Among these hormones are cholecystokinin and calcitonin. Both are secreted after food has been eaten and both act on the brain to produce satiety, at least in experimental animals. E. Straus and R. S. Yalow, Cholecystokinin in the brains of obese and nonobese mice, *Science* 203 (1979): 68-69; W. J. Freed, M. J. Perlow, and R. J. Wyatt, Calcitonin: Inhibitory effect on eating in rats, *Science* 206 (1979): 850-852. Other hormones involved in food intake regulation are the pituitary, the adrenal, the thyroid, and the sex hormones (Mayer, 1980).

27. S. P. Dalvit, The effect of the menstrual cycle on patterns of food intake, *American Journal of Clinical Nutrition* 34 (1981): 1811-1815.

28. S. V. Parameswaran, A. B. Steffens, G. R. Hervey, and L. de Ruiter, Involvement of a humoral factor in regulation of body weight in parabiotic rats, *American Journal of Physiology* 232 (1977): R150-R157.

29. J. E. Morley and A. S. Levine, Stress-induced eating is mediated through endogenous opiates, *Science* 209 (1980): 1259-1261.

30. J. Slochower and S. P. Kaplan, Anxiety, perceived control, and eating in obese and normal weight persons, *Appetite* 1 (1980): 75. Abstract cited in *Journal of the American Dietetic Association* 77 (1980): 376.

31. J. A. Deutsch, W. G. Young, and T. J. Kalogeris, The stomach signals satiety, *Science* 201 (1978): 165-167.

32. Influence of intrauterine nutritional status on the development of obesity in later life, *Nutrition Reviews* 35 (1977): 100-102 (and errata on p. 189); Committee on Nutrition of the Mother and Preschool Child, Food and Nutrition Board, National Research Council, National Academy of Sciences, Fetal and infant nutrition and susceptibility to obesity, *Nutrition Reviews* 36 (1978): 122-126.

33. T. B. Van Itallie and R. G. Campbell, Multidisciplinary approach to the problem of obesity, *Journal of the American Dietetic Association* 61 (1972): 385-390.

34. H. Bruch, Role of the emotions in hunger and appetite, *Annals of the New York Academy of Sciences* 63, Part 1 (1955): 68-75.

35. R. I. Simon, Obesity as a depressive equivalent, *Journal of the American Medical Association* 183 (1963): 208-210.

36. S. P. Yang, L. J. Martin, and G. Schneider, Weight reduction utilizing a protein-sparing modified fast, *Journal of the American Dietetic Association* 76 (1980): 343-346.

37. This response to stress has been studied in animals. An example of such a study is C. D. Berdanier, R. Wurdeman, and R. B. Tobin, Further studies on the role of the adrenal hormones in the responses of rats to meal-feeding, *Journal of Nutrition* 106 (1976): 1791-1800.

38. A. J. Stunkard, Eating patterns and obesity, *Psychiatric Quarterly* 33 (1959): 284-295.

39. W. H. Griffith, Food as a regulator of metabolism, *American Journal of Clinical Nutrition* 17 (1965): 391-398.

40. *Obesity '73: A Report from the Geigy Symposium on Obesity, Its Problems and Prognosis* (New York: Ardsley, 1973).

41. Mayer, 1980.

42. R. S. Drabman, D. Hammer, and G. J. Jarvie, Eating rates of elementary school children, *Journal of Nutrition Education* 9 (1977): 80-82.

43. P. Fabry, Metabolic consequences of the pattern of food intake, in *Handbook of Physiology*, ed. C. F. Code (Washington, D.C.: American Physiological Society, 1967), Section 6, pp. 31-49; G. A. Leveille and D. R. Romsos, Meal eating and obesity, *Nutrition Today*, November/December 1974, pp. 4-9.

44. J. Yudkin, Prevention of obesity, *Royal Society of Health Journal*, July 1961, pp. 221-224.

45. J. V. G. A. Durnin, O. G. Edholm, D. S. Miller, and J. C. Waterlow, How much food does man require? *Nutrition Today*, January/February 1974, p. 28.

46. J. Mayer, as quoted by M. Kernan, Inactivity places burden of obesity on America's youth, *St. Petersburg Times*, August 12, 1973; B. Bullen, as quoted in Seelig, 1976.

47. A. Keys and F. Grande, Body weight, body composition and calorie status, in *Modern Nutrition in Health and Disease*, ed. R. S. Goodhart and M. E. Shils, 5th ed. (Philadelphia: Lea and Febiger, 1973), pp. 1-27.

48. Questions doctors ask . . . , *Nutrition and the MD*, October 1977.

49. H. T. Randall, Water, electrolytes and acid-base balance, in Goodhart and Shils, 1973, pp. 324-361.

50. L. Eisenberg, The clinical use of stimulant drugs in children, *Pediatrics* 49 (1972): 709-715.

51. G. R. Edison, Amphetamines: A dangerous illusion, *Annals of Internal Medicine* 74 (1971): 605-610.

52. B. Lucas and C. J. Sells, Nutrient intake and stimulant drugs in hyperactive children, *Journal of the American Dietetic Association* 70 (1970): 373-377. The FDA now proposes warning labels and restrictions on the sale of amphetamine-type drugs: Experts weigh reducing potions, *FDA Consumer* 13 (October 1979): 10-11.

53. Diet-drug interactions (reviewed by D. A. Roe), *Dairy Council Digest* 48 (March/April 1977).

54. *Obesity '73*, 1973.

55. Cellulite is also not in the dictionary and not likely to appear there. L. Fenner, Cellulite: Hard to budge pudge, *FDA Consumer*, May 1980, pp. 5-9.

56. Greenwood and Hirsch, 1975.

57. U.S. Department of Health, Education, and Welfare, Food and Drug Administration, *FDA Consumer Memo*, HEW publication no. (FDA) 77-3035, 1977.

58. G. A. Bray, A. L. Mendeloff, F. L. Iber, H. P. Roth, and W. W. Faloon, Surgical treatment of obesity: Current status, *American Family Physician* 15 (March 1977): 111-113.

59. Nutritional complications of the surgical treatment of morbid obesity, *Nutrition Reviews* 38 (1980): 238-240.

60. *American Journal of Clinical Nutrition* 30, January 1977. This entire issue was devoted to surgery for the obese.

61. *Obesity '73*, 1973.

62. A. E. Kark, Jaw wiring, *American Journal of Clinical Nutrition* 33, supplement no. 2 (February 1980): 420-424.

63. Many of the margin quotes are from this article: L. Haimes, E. Harrison, H. A. Jordan, P. G. Lindner, and J. Rodin, Applying behavioral techniques in a bariatric practice, part 1, *Obesity and Bariatric Medicine* 6 (January/February 1977): 10-16.

64. A. J. Vergroesen, Physiological effects of dietary linoleic acid, *Nutrition Reviews* 35 (January 1977): 1-5.

65. Vergroesen, 1977.

66. Water weight accumulates during fat oxidation because one fatty acid weighing 284 units leaves behind water weighing 324 units, 14 percent more.

67. M. McDowell, Appetite control: An addiction-like component in overeating and its cure, *Obesity and Bariatric Medicine* 9 (September-October 1980): 138-143.

68. An example is described in A. R. Marston, M. R. Marston, and J. Ross, A correspondence course behavioral program for weight reduction, *Obesity and Bariatric Medicine* 6 (July/August 1977): 140. Abstract cited in *Journal of the American Dietetic Association* 71 (1977): 462.

69. L. S. Levitz, Behavior therapy in treating obesity, *Journal of the American Dietetic Association* 62 (1973): 22-26.

70. Questions doctors ask . . . , *Nutrition and the MD*, June 1978.

71. Keys and Grande, 1973.

Chapter 9—The Vitamins

1. A. Kamil, How natural are those "natural" vitamins? *Co-op News* 25 (March 13, 1972): 3. Reprinted in *Nutrition Reviews/Supplement: Nutrition Misinformation and Food Faddism*, July 1974, p. 34.

2. O. Pelletier and M. O. Keith, Bioavailability of synthetic and natural ascorbic acid, *Journal of the American Dietetic Association* 64 (1974): 271-275.

3. T. K. Basu, Vitamin A and cancer of epithelial origin, *Journal of Human Nutrition* 33 (February 1979): 24-31; M. B. Sporn, N. M. Dunlop, D. L. Newton, and J. M. Smith, Prevention of chemical carcinogenesis by vitamin A and its synthetic analogs (retinoids), *Federation Proceedings* 35 (1976): 1332-1338; Vitamin A, tumor initiation and tumor promotion, *Nutrition Reviews* 37 (1979): 153-156.

4. D. P. DePaola and M. C. Alfano, Diet and oral health, *Nutrition Today*, May/June 1977, pp. 6-11, 29-32.

5. WHO/USAID Joint Meeting, *Vitamin A Deficiency and Xerophthalmia*, Technical Report Series 590 (Albany, N.Y.: Q Corporation, 1976).

6. J. C. Gallagher and B. L Riggs, Nutrition and bone disease, in *Current Concepts in Nutrition*, a paperback book containing reprints from the *New England Journal of Medicine* 1977-1978 (Massachusetts Medical Society, 1979), pp. 61-67.

7. L. M. Henderson, Nutritional problems growing out of new patterns of food consumption, in *The Nutrition Crisis: A Reader*, ed. T. P. Labuza (St. Paul, West: 1975), pp. 106-115.

8. C. A. Thomson and I. S. Sheremate, Current issues in infant feeding, *Journal of the Canadian Dietetic Association* 39 (July 1978): 189-194.

9. M. Rudolf, K. Arulanantham, and R. M. Greenstein, Unsuspected nutritional rickets, *Pediatrics* 66 (1980): 72-76; Vitamin D deficiency rickets, revisited, *Nutrition Reviews* 38 (1980): 116-118.

10. F. Konishi and S. L. Harrison, Vitamin D for adults, *Journal of Nutrition Education* 11 (1979): 120-122.

11. J. N. Hathcock, Nutrition: Toxicology and pharmacology, in *Nutrition Reviews' Present Knowledge in Nutrition*, 4th ed. (Washington, D.C.: Nutrition Foundation, 1976), pp. 504-515.

12. Occult vitamin D intoxication . . . , *Nutrition and the MD*, October 1979.

13. Vitamin E, *Nutrition and the MD*, February 1980; D. B. Menzel, Pulmonary medicine, in *Nutritional Support of Medical Practice*, ed. H. A. Schneider, C. E. Anderson, and D. B. Coursin (Hagerstown, Md.: Harper & Row, 1977), Chap. 31, pp. 477-484.

14. Expert Panel on Food Safety and Nutrition, Committee on Public Information, Institute of Food Technologists, Vitamin E, *Contemporary Nutrition* 2 (November 1977).

15. A. L. Tappel, Vitamin E, *Nutrition Today*, July/August 1973, pp. 4-12.

16. H. H. Draper, J. G. Bergan, M. Chiu, A. S. Csallany, and A. V. Boaro. A further study of the specificity of the vitamin E requirement for reproduction, *Journal of Nutrition* 84 (1964): 395-400.

17. J. G. Bieri, Vitamin E, in *Nutrition Reviews' Present Knowledge*, 1976, pp. 98-110.

18. A detailed 194-page bulletin by M. Dicks on vitamin E in foods has been published by the University of Wyoming, according to *Nutrition Today*, July/August 1973, p. 10; and there was an update on the vitamin E contents of various foods in P. J. McLaughlin and J. L. Weihrauch, Vitamin E content of foods, *Journal of the American Dietetic Association* 75 (1979): 647-665.

19. Vitamin K, *Nutrition and the MD*, February 1980.

20. Role of thiamine in regulation of fatty acid and cholesterol biosynthesis in cultured brain cells, *Nutrition Reviews* 37 (1979): 24-25.

21. D. Lonsdale and R. J. Shamberger, Red cell transketolase as an indicator of nutritional deficiency, *American Journal of Clinical Nutrition* 33 (1980): 205-211.

22. M. Brin and J. C. Bauernfeind, Vitamin needs of the elderly, *Postgraduate Medicine* 63 (1978): 155-163.

23. J. C. Hoskin and P. S. Dimick, Evaluation of [the effects of] fluorescent light on flavor and riboflavin content of milk held in gallon returnable containers, *Journal of Food Protection* 42 (1979): 105-109.

24. R. J. Wyatt, Comment, *American Journal of Psychiatry* 131 (November 11, 1974): 1258-1262. The two hormones whose ratio is altered according to this theory are norepinephrine and epinephrine. The theory that "the" biochemical problem in schizophrenia is increased epinephrine production is but one of many that are being actively investigated by researchers. People with mental disorders of many kinds, including depression, have been observed to have altered levels of certain substances in their brains, blood, and urine. It is not known whether the disorder comes first and causes the changed biochemistry or whether a change in the biochemistry causes the disorder. Very possibly, a number of different hormonal systems are involved, including the adrenal and thyroid glands. J. M. Davis, Theories of biological etiology of affective disorders, *International Review of Neurobiology* 12 (1970): 145-175; A. Coppen, The biochemistry of affective disorders, *British Journal of Psychiatry* 113 (1967): 1237-1263.

25. Task Force on Vitamin Therapy in Psychiatry, American Psychiatric Association, Megavitamin and orthomolecular therapy in psychiatry, pp. 44-47. Excerpts reprinted in *Nutrition Reviews/Supplement: Nutrition Misinformation and Food Faddism*, July 1974, 67-70.

26. Task Force, 1974.

27. V. D. Herbert, Megavitamin therapy, *Contemporary Nutrition* 2 (October 1977).

28. For this and other reasons the World Health Organization excludes vitamin B_6 from multivitamin preparations. L. B. Greentree, Dangers of vitamin B_6 in nursing mothers (letter to the editor), *New England Journal of Medicine* 300 (1979): 141-142.

29. Contribution of the microflora of the small intestine to the vitamin B_{12} nutriture of man, *Nutrition Reviews* 38 (1980): 274-275.

30. D. A. Roe, *Drug-Induced Nutritional Deficiencies* (Westport, Conn.: Avi, 1976), pp. 3, 16-17.

31. D. B. McCormick, Biotin, in *Nutrition Reviews' Present Knowledge*, 1976, pp. 217-225; and L. D. Wright, Pantothenic acid, in the same book, pp. 226-231.

32. R. J. Wurtman, as quoted by H. M. Schmeck, Jr., Memory loss curbed by chemical in foods, *The New York Times*, January 9, 1979.

33. Schmeck, 1979.

34. J. Weininger and G. M. Briggs, Bioflavonoids, in *Modern Nutrition in Health and Disease*, ed. R. S. Goodhart and M. E. Shils, 6th ed. (Philadelphia: Lea and Febiger, 1980), pp. 279-281.

35. A. Kallner, D. Hartmann, and D. Hornig, Steady-state turnover and body pool of ascorbic acid in man, *American Journal of Clinical Nutrition* 32 (1979): 530-539.

36. L. C. Pauling, *Vitamin C and the Common Cold* (San Francisco: W. H. Freeman, 1970).

37. T. C. Chalmers, Effects of ascorbic acid on the common cold, *American Journal of Medicine* 58 (1975): 532-536.

38. Chalmers, 1975.

39. E. T. Creagan, C. G. Moertel, J. R. O'Fallon, A. J. Schutt, M. J. O'Connell, J. Rubin, and S. Frytak, Failure of high-dose vitamin C (ascorbic acid) therapy to benefit patients with advanced cancer, *New England Journal of Medicine* 301 (1979): 687-690.
40. Vitamin C toxicity, *Nutrition Reviews* 34 (August 1976): 236-237.
41. T. Udomratn, M. H. Steinberg, G. D. Campbell, Jr., and F. J. Oelshlegel, Jr., Effects of ascorbic acid on glucose-6-phosphate dehydrogenase-deficient erythrocytes: Studies in an animal model, *Blood* 49 (March 1977): 471-475.
42. Herbert, 1977.
43. P. G. Shilotri and K. S. Bhat, Effect of mega doses of vitamin C on bactericidal activity of leukocytes, *American Journal of Clinical Nutrition* 30 (1977): 1077-1081.
44. L. H. Smith, Risk of oxalate stones from large doses of vitamin C (letter to the editor), *New England Journal of Medicine* 298 (1978): 856; S. Lewin, Evaluation of potential effects of high intakes of ascorbic acid, *Comparative Biochemistry and Physiology* 37B (1973): 681-695.
45. Chalmers, 1975.
46. Herbert, 1977.
47. Z. Sabry, Take a sensible stand on vitamin pills, *Nutrition and the MD*, November 1977.
48. According to *Nutrition and the MD*, chicken soup helps more than hot water to speed the flow of mucus during a cold. Tidbits and morsels, *Nutrition and the MD*, January 1979.

Chapter 10—Minerals and Water

1. Calcitonin, made in the thyroid gland, is secreted whenever the calcium concentration rises too high and acts to stop withdrawal from bone and to slow absorption from the intestine. Parathormone, from the parathyroid glands, has the opposite effect when needed.
2. A. Davis, *Let's Eat Right to Keep Fit* (New York: Harcourt Brace Jovanovich). The book has been through many editions since 1946, when it was first published.
3. D. Rosenfield, Nutritional optimization of new foods (commentary), *Journal of the American Dietetic Association* 72 (1978): 475-477.
4. Postmenopausal estrogen therapy, a pamphlet from the American Council on Science and Health, November 1979.
5. J. C. Gallagher and B. L. Riggs, Nutrition and bone disease, in *Current Concepts in Nutrition*, a paperback book containing reprints from the *New England Journal of Medicine* 1977-1978 (Massachusetts Medical Society, 1979), pp. 61-67.
6. R. P. Heaney, R. R. Recker, and P. D. Saville, Calcium balance and calcium requirements in middle-aged women, *American Journal of Clinical Nutrition* 30 (1977): 1603-1611.
7. To the chemist, a salt results from neutralization of an acid and a base. Sodium chloride—table salt—results from the reaction between hydrochloric acid and the base sodium hydroxide. The positive sodium ion unites with the negative chloride ion to form the salt, and the positive hydrogen ion unites with the negative hydroxide ion to form water. Acid + Base = Salt + Water Hydrochloric acid + Sodium hydroxide = Sodium chloride + Water.
8. U.S. Senate, Select Committee on Nutrition and Human Needs, *Dietary Goals for the United States*, 2d ed. (Washington, D.C.: Government Printing Office, 1977), p. 49.

9. The amount of sodium to be returned by the kidneys to the blood is under the control of an adrenal gland hormone, aldosterone.

10. A. M. Altschul and J. K. Grommet, Sodium intake and sodium sensitivity, *Nutrition Reviews* 38 (1980): 393-402.

11. M. Jacobson and B. F. Liebman, Dietary sodium and the risk of hypertension (correspondence), *New England Journal of Medicine* 303 (1980): 817-818.

12. L. Fenner, Salt shakes up some of us, *FDA Consumer*, March 1980, reprint.

13. Salt and high blood pressure, *Consumer Reports*, March 1979, reprint.

14. E. J. Calabrese and R. W. Tuthill, A review of literature to support a sodium drinking water standard, *Journal of Environmental Health* 40 (September/October 1977): 80-83.

15. A. P. Simopoulos and F. C. Bartter, The metabolic consequences of chloride deficiency, *Nutrition Reviews* 38 (1980): 201-205.

16. H. W. Lane and J. J. Cerda, Potassium requirements and exercise, *Journal of the American Dietetic Association* 73 (1978): 64-65.

17. Clinical signs of magnesium deficiency, *Nutrition and the MD*, January 1980.

18. M. S. Seelig and H. A. Heggtreit, Magnesium interrelationships in ischemic heart disease: A review, *American Journal of Clinical Nutrition* 17 (1974): 59-79.

19. P. D. M. V. Turlapaty and B. M. Altura, Magnesium deficiency produces spasms of coronary arteries: Relationship to etiology of sudden death ischemic heart disease, *Science* 208 (1980): 198-200.

20. For example, E. J. Underwood, *Trace Elements in Human and Animal Nutrition*, 4th ed. (New York: Academic Press, 1977).

21. The thyroid gland may also enlarge because of overactivity resulting from some pathological condition; this type of enlargement is known as toxic goiter.

22. The medical name for this anemia is microcytic (small cell) hypochromic (less color) anemia.

23. R. L. Leibel, Behavioral and biochemical correlates of iron deficiency: A review, *Journal of the American Dietetic Association* 71 (1977): 399-404; and E. Pollitt and R. L. Leibel, Iron deficiency and behavior, *Journal of Pediatrics* 88 (1976): 372-381.

24. Leibel, 1977.

25. M. Winick, Nutritional disorders of American women, *Nutrition Today*, September/October-November/December 1975, pp. 26-28.

26. D. M. Czajka-Narins, T. B. Haddy, and D. J. Kallen, Nutrition and social correlates in iron deficiency anemia, *American Journal of Clinical Nutrition* 31 (1978): 955-960.

27. Z. I. Sabry, J. A. Campbell, M. E. Campbell, and A. L. Forbes, Nutrition Canada, *Nutrition Today*, January/February 1974, pp. 5-13.

28. W. H. Crosby, Who needs iron? in *Current Concepts in Nutrition*, a paperback book containing reprints from the *New England Journal of Medicine* 1977-1978 (Massachusetts Medical Society, 1979), pp. 43-50.

29. J. D. Cook and E. R. Monsen, Vitamin C, the common cold, and iron absorption, *American Journal of Clinical Nutrition* 30 (1977): 235-241.

30. D. Rosenfield, Nutritional optimization of new foods (commentary), *Journal of the American Dietetic Association* 72 (1978): 475-477.

31. G. Michaëlsson, L. Juhlin, A. Vahlquist, Effects of oral zinc and vitamin A on acne, *Archives of Dermatology* 113 (1977): 31-36.

32. Questions doctors ask . . . , *Nutrition and the MD*, October 1978.

33. Copper, *Nutrition and the MD*, August 1980.

34. Chromium and CHO metabolism, *Nutrition and the MD*, September 1980.

35. K. M. Hambidge, Zinc and chromium in human nutrition, *Journal of Human Nutrition* 32 (April 1978): 99-110.

Chapter 11—Foods, Food Labels, and Additives

1. A. M. Schmidt, Food and drug law: A 200-year perspective, *Nutrition Today* 10 (4) (1975): 29-32.
2. L. M. Henderson, Nutritional problems growing out of new patterns of food consumption, *American Journal of Public Health* 62 (1972): 1194-1198.
3. F. M. Clydesdale, In defense of technology, *Journal of Food Protection* 40 (1977): 200-205.
4. M. F. Jacobson, quoted by R. A. Seelig, How FDA nutrient labeling rules favor junk foods, *Nutrition Notes* 71 (1977). Dr. Jacobson was speaking as co-director of the Center for Science in the Public Interest.
5. M. Stephenson, Making food labels more informative, *FDA Consumer* 9 (8) (1975): 13-17.
6. Vitamin A RDA for women is 4000 IU; for men, 5000 IU. Food composition tables show vitamin A contents in IU, but 1980 RDAs for vitamin A are expressed in RE: 800 for women, 1000 for men. As of 1980, then, you have to use the factor 1 RE = 5 IU to compare vitamin A amounts derived from food composition tables with the RDA. But the 1968 U.S. RDA are still in IU.
7. M. Burros, Food editors ask: Fact or flack? *Washington Post*, October 11, 1979.
8. H. Appledorf, Nutritional analysis of foods from fast-food chains, *Food Technology* 28 (1974): 50-55.
9. D. Rosenfield, Nutritional optimization of new foods (commentary), *Journal of the American Dietetic Association* 72 (1978): 475-477.
10. M. K. Head and R. J. Weeks, Conventional vs. formulated foods in school lunches: 2. Cost of food served, eaten, and wasted, *Journal of the American Dietetic Association* 71 (1977): 629-632.
11. C. P. Greecher and B. Shannon, Impact of fast food meals on nutrient intake of two groups, *Journal of the American Dietetic Association* 70 (1977): 368-372; Fast food expansion predicted (news item), *Journal of the American Dietetic Association* 70 (1977): 372.
12. L. Schwartzberg, C. George, and M. C. Phillips, Issues in food advertising: The nutrition educator's viewpoint, *Journal of Nutrition Education* 9 (1977): 60-63.
13. 1. True but misleading, because milk is recognized as a poor source of iron. 2. True but misleading, because orange juice contains so many other nutrients by virtue of being a natural food. 3. True and responsible.
14. Schmidt, 1975.
15. H. A. Guthrie, Concept of a nutritious food, *Journal of the American Dietetic Association* 71 (1977): 14-19.
16. A. J. Wittwer, A. W. Sorenson, B. W. Wyse, and R. G. Hansen, Nutrient density—evaluation of nutritional attributes of foods, *Journal of Nutrition Education* 9 (January-March 1977): 26-30.
17. Guthrie, 1977.
18. P. Isom, Nutritive value and cost of "fast food" meals, *USDA Family Economics Review*, Fall 1976. Abstract in *Journal of the American Dietetic Association* 70 (1977): 497.
19. Henderson, 1972.
20. Roslyn B. Alfin-Slater, Nutrition and work performance, *Nutrition and the MD*, August 1979.
21. O. C. Johnson, The Food and Drug Administration and labeling, *Journal of the American Dietetic Association* 64 (1974): 471-475.
22. FDA clears some food items, bans others, *Chemical and Engineering News* 52 (October 7, 1974): 12.
23. R. D. Middlekauf, Legalities concerning food additives, *Food Technology* 28 (May 1974): 42-49.

24. F. J. Ingelfinger, A matter of opinion, *Nutrition Today* 10 (4) (1975): 11, 28.

25. Ingelfinger, 1975. Another lively, accurate, and interesting article on this subject is R. L. Hall, Safe at the plate, *Nutrition Today*, November/December 1977, pp. 6-9, 28-31. Still another thought-provoking piece is C. F. Enloe, Jr., Leslie and Betty and the hobgoblins (editorial), *Nutrition Today*, January/February 1976, pp. 16-17.

26. F. M. Strong, Toxicants occurring naturally in foods, in *Nutrition Reviews' Present Knowledge in Nutrition*, 4th ed. (Washington, D.C.: Nutrition Foundation, 1976), pp. 516-527.

27. Schmidt, 1975.

28. Schmidt, 1975.

29. The deadliest poison, *Nutrition Today*, September/October-November/December 1975, pp. 4-9; J. Huey, When vichyssoise sells slowly, people can get in the soup, *Nutrition Today*, September/October-November/December 1975, pp. 10-11.

30. A. Schmidt, The benefit-risk equation, *FDA Consumer* 7 (8) (1974): 27-31.

31. Schmidt, 1975.

32. Schmidt, 1975.

33. J. M. Coon, Natural food toxicants: A perspective, in *Nutrition Reviews' Present Knowledge*, 1976, pp. 528-546.

34. Strong, 1976.

35. Coon, 1976.

36. R. Levine, Carbohydrates, in *Modern Nutrition in Health and Disease*, ed. R. S. Goodhart and M. E. Shils, 5th ed. (Philadelphia: Lea and Febiger, 1973), p. 108.

37. The importance of trace minerals, especially, has been coming to light, as shown in O. A. Levander, Nutritional factors in relation to heavy metal toxicants, *Federation Proceedings* 36 (April 1977): 1683-1687. Fiber has a mixed effect, as discussed in D. Kritchevsky, Modification by fiber of toxic dietary effects, *Federation Proceedings* 36 (April 1977): 1692-1695.

38. Coon, 1976.

39. Coon, 1976.

40. Coon, 1976.

41. Coon, 1976.

Chapter 12—Mother, Infant, and Growth

1. D. P. DePaola and M. C. Alfano, Diet and oral health, *Nutrition Today*, May/June 1977, pp. 6-11, 29-32.

2. N. M. Lien, K. K. Meyer, and M. Winick, Early malnutrition and "late" adoption: A study of the effects on the development of Korean orphans adopted into American families, *American Journal of Clinical Nutrition* 30 (1977): 1734-1739.

3. S. P. Bessman, The justification theory: The essential nature of the non-essential amino acids, *Nutrition Reviews* 37 (July 1979): 209-220.

4. We are indebted to S. R. Williams, who showed how Erikson's scheme could be integrated with nutrition principles in her book *Nutrition and Diet Therapy* (St. Louis: Mosby, 1973).

5. D. B. Coursin, Maternal nutrition and the offspring's development, *Nutrition Today*, March/April 1973, pp. 12-18.

6. L. B. Bailey, C. S. Mahan, and D. Dimperio, Folacin and iron status in low-income pregnant adolescents and mature women, *American Journal of Clinical Nutrition* 33 (1980): 1997-2001; V. Herbert, The vitamin craze, *Archives of Internal Medicine* 140 (1980): 173-176.

7. The blood protein responsible for iron absorption is transferrin.

8. California Department of Health, as cited in Nutrition and the pregnant obese woman, *Nutrition and the MD*, January 1978.

9. R. L. Huenemann, Environmental factors associated with preschool obesity, 1: Obesity in six-month-old children, *Journal of the American Dietetic Association* 64 (1974): 480-487.

10. National Institute of Child Health and Human Development, Little babies: Born too soon—born too small, DHEW publication no. (NIH) 77-1079 (Washington, D.C: Government Printing Office, 1977).

11. A. Petros-Barvazian and M. Béhar, Low birth weight: What should be done to deal with this global problem? *WHO Chronicle* 32 (June 1978): 231-232; *New Trends and Approaches in the Delivery of Maternal and Child Care in Health Services* (Sixth Report of the WHO Expert Committee on Maternal and Child Health), as cited in *Journal of the American Dietetic Association* 71 (1977): 357.

12. A. C. Higgins, Nutritional status and the outcome of pregnancy, *Journal of the Canadian Dietetic Association* 37 (1976): 17-35.

13. J. Martin, The fetal alcohol syndrome: Recent findings, *Alcohol Health and Research World*, Spring 1977, pp. 8-12.

14. Fetal alcohol syndrome, *Nutrition and the MD*, July 1978.

15. S. R. Williams, Nutritional guidance in prenatal care, in *Nutrition in Pregnancy and Lactation*, ed. B. S. Worthington, J. Vermeersch, and S. R. Williams (St. Louis: Mosby, 1977), pp. 55-92.

16. R. M. Pitkin, ed., Nutrition in pregnancy, *Dietetic Currents, Ross Timesaver* 4 (January/February 1977).

17. D. Erhard, The new vegetarians, 1: Vegetarianism and its consequences, *Nutrition Today*, November/December 1974, pp. 4-12.

18. R. L. Leibel, Behavioral and biochemical correlations of iron deficiency: A review, *Journal of the American Dietetic Association* 71 (1977): 399-404.

19. Coffee: Downs and ups, *Nutrition and the MD*, April 1978.

20. Coursin, 1973.

21. C. Borberg, M. D. G. Gillmer, E. J. Brunner, P. J. Gunn, N. W. Oakley, and R. W. Beard, Obesity in pregnancy: The effect of dietary advice, *Diabetes Care* 3, May/June 1980, pp. 476-481; Guidelines for management of the pregnant diabetic woman are given in D. M. Jouganatos and S. G. Gabbe, Diabetes in pregnancy: Metabolic changes and current management, *Journal of the American Dietetic Association* 73 (1978): 168-171.

22. R. M. Pitkin, H. A. Kaminetsky, M. Newton, and J. A. Pritchard, Maternal nutrition: A selective review of clinical topics, *Journal of Obstetrics and Gynecology* 40 (1972): 773-785.

23. Simple test helps to identify women at risk for toxemia of pregnancy (Medical News), *Journal of the American Medical Association* 237 (1977): 1541-1542.

24. The hormone that controls the breast milk supply is oxytocin (ox-ee-TOCE-in).

25. D. W. Spady, Infant nutrition, *Journal of the Canadian Dietetic Association* 38 (1977): 34-41.

26. L. S. Sims, Dietary status of lactating women, I: Nutrient intake from food and from supplements, *Journal of the American Dietetic Association* 73 (1978): 139-146.

27. M. J. Mellies, K. Burton, R. Larsen, D. Fixler, and C. J. Glueck, Cholesterol, phytosterols, and polyunsaturated/saturated fatty acid ratios during the first 12 months of lactation, *American Journal of Clinical Nutrition* 32 (1979): 2383-2389.

28. For example, it seems that the folacin in breast milk is constant according to T. Tamura, Y. Yoshimura, and T. Arakawa, Human milk folate and folate status in lactating mothers and their infants, *American Journal of Clinical Nutrition* 33 (1980): 193-197. So is thiamin, at least with above-adequate intakes; riboflavin may change a little; and copper, iron, and zinc do not seem to vary except that the concentrations change over the course of lactation; P. A. Nail, M. R. Thomas, and R. Eakin, The effect of thiamin and riboflavin supplementation on the level of those vitamins in human breast milk and urine, *American Journal of Clinical Nutrition* 33 (1980): 198-204; E. Vuori, S. M. Mäkinen, R. Kara, and P. Kuitunen, The effects of the dietary

intakes of copper, iron, manganese, and zinc on the trace element content of human milk, *American Journal of Clinical Nutrition* 33 (1980): 227-231. Even fluoride in breast milk appears not to depend on the woman's water supply; O. B. Dirks, J. M. P. A. Jongeling-Eijndhoven, T. D. Flissebaalje, and I. Gedalia, Total free and ionic fluoride in human and cow's milk as determined by gas-liquid chromatography and the fluoride electrode, *Caries Research* 8 (1974): 181-186.

29. M. R. Thomas, S. M. Sneed, C. Wer, P. A. Nail, M. Wilson, and E. E. Sprinkle, III, The effects of vitamin C, vitamin B_6, vitamin B_{12}, folic acid, riboflavin, and thiamin on the breast milk and maternal status of well-nourished women at 6 months postpartum, *American Journal of Clinical Nutrition* 33 (1980): 2151-2156.

30. L. B. Greentree, Dangers of vitamin B_6 in nursing mothers (letter to the editor), *New England Journal of Medicine* 300 (1979): 141-142.

31. M. J. Whichelow, Success and failure of breast-feeding in relation to energy intake, *Proceedings of the Nutrition Society* 35 (September 1976): 62A-63A.

32. J. C. King and S. Charlet, Current concepts in nutrition—pregnant women and premature infants, *Journal of Nutrition Education*, October-December 1978, pp. 158-159.

33. J. A. McMillan, S. A. Landaw, and F. A. Oski, Iron sufficiency in breast-fed infants and the availability of iron from human milk, *Pediatrics* 58 (1976): 686-691.

34. Acrodermatitis enteropathica, zinc, and human milk, *Nutrition Reviews* 36 (1978): 241-242.

35. R. R. Arnold, M. F. Cole, and J. R. McGhee, A bactericidal effect for human lactoferrin, *Science* 197 (1977): 263-265.

36. S. J. Fomon and S. J. Filer, Milks and formulas, in *Infant Nutrition*, ed. S. J. Fomon, 2d ed. (Philadelphia: Saunders, 1974), pp. 359-407.

37. M. Winick, Infant nutrition: Formula or breast feeding? *Professional Nutritionist*, Spring 1980, pp. 1-3.

38. J. Mayer, A new look at old formulas, *Family Health/Today's Health*, October 1976, pp. 38, 40, 78.

39. M. W. Choi, Breast milk for infants who can't breast feed, *American Journal of Nursing* 78 (1978): 852-855.

40. R. E. Brown, Breast feeding in modern times, *American Journal of Clinical Nutrition* 26 (1973): 556-562.

41. Fomon and Filer, 1974.

42. Committee on Environmental Hazards of the American Academy of Pediatrics, PCBs in breast milk, *Pediatrics* 62 (1978): 407.

43. J. C. Gallagher and B. L. Riggs, Nutrition and bone disease, in *Current Concepts in Nutrition*, a paperback book containing reprints from the *The New England Journal of Medicine 1977-1978* (Massachusetts Medical Society, 1979), pp. 61-67; D. V. Edidin, L. L. Levitsky, W. Schey, N. Dumbovie, and A. Campos, Resurgence of nutritional rickets associated with breast-feeding and special dietary practices, *Pediatrics* 65 (1980): 232-235.

44. Winick, 1980.

45. Questions doctors ask . . ., *Nutrition and the MD*, October 1977.

46. J. C. Breneman, Food allergy, *Contemporary Nutrition* 4 (March 1979).

47. Gerber Products Company, Why we put what we put in Gerber baby foods (advertisement), *Nutrition Today*, September/October 1973, p. 24; J. C. Suerth (chairman of the board, Gerber Products Company), Letter to the editor, *Nutrition Today*, May/June 1977, pp. 34-35. According to *Nutrition and the MD*, January 1980, there was no more sugar in Beechnut foods and much less in Heinz than formerly.

48. C. M. Kerr, Jr., K. S. Reisinger, and F. W. Plankey, Sodium concentration of homemade baby foods, *Pediatrics* 62 (1978): 331-335; Questions readers ask, *Nutrition and the MD*, May 1980.

49. E. Grunwaldt, T. Bates, and D. Guthrie, Jr., The onset of sleeping through the night in infancy, *Pediatrics* 26 (1960): 667-668.

50. Mayer, 1976.

51. G. Friedman and S. J. Goldberg, An evaluation of the safety of a low-saturated-fat, low-cholesterol diet beginning in infancy, *Pediatrics* 58 (1976): 655-657.

52. The prudent diet in pediatric practice, *Nutrition and the MD*, November 1979.

53. L. E. Holt, Jr., Protein economy in the growing child, *Postgraduate Medicine* 27 (1960): 783-798.

Chapter 13—The Early Years

1. R. B. Choate, Selling cavities—U.S. style, address presented at the American Dental Association annual meeting, October 11, 1977. According to the speaker, the taste for sweetness already exists in the fetus, peaks at fourteen years, and is more marked in blacks than in whites.

2. White House Conference on Nutrition, April 13, 1975, reported as: A Tuesday in the White House, *Nutrition Today*, September/October-November/December 1975, pp. 20-25, 53-54.

3. J. Martin, Child nutrition programs: 1946 to 1980, *School Food Service Journal* 34 (1980): 68, 70-71.

4. A. L. Galbraith, ADA's views on school lunch presented to Congress, *Journal of the American Dietetic Association* 70 (1977): 630-632.

5. Breakfast: A second look, *School Foodservice Journal* 31 (March 1977): 36-37.

6. Type A served fast food style, *School Foodservice Journal* 31 (September 1977): 19.

7. San Jose: Moving more nutritious lunches, *Institutions/Volume Feeding Magazine* 81 (August 1, 1977): 42-43.

8. Fulton County school director plays a hunch on health food—and wins, *Institutions/Volume Feeding Magazine* 81 (September 15, 1977): 33-34.

9. Choate, 1977.

10. P. Charren, Advertising of sugar-rich foods: What can the dental profession do? address presented at the American Dental Association annual meeting, October 11, 1977.

11. Choate, 1977.

12. J. T. Dwyer and J. Mayer, Beyond economics and nutrition: The complex basis of food policy, *Science* 188 (1975): 566-570.

13. L. P. DiOrio, Improving nutrition: What should we eat? A dentist's perspective, address presented at the American Dental Association annual meeting, October 11, 1977.

14. N. L. Shory, School confection sale bans: What can the dental profession do? address presented at the American Dental Association annual meeting, October 11, 1977.

15. Shory, 1977.

16. L. Crawford, Junk food in our schools? A look at student spending in school vending machines and concessions, *Journal of the Canadian Dietetic Association* 38 (July 1977): 193. Abstract cited in *Journal of the American Dietetic Association* 71 (1977): 572.

17. San Jose, 1977.

18. E. Ott, Quieting our detractors' voices, *Food Management* 14 (1979): 25-26.

19. DiOrio, 1977; P. E. Stephenson, Physiological and psychotropic effects of caffeine on man, *Journal of the American Dietetic Association* 71 (1977): 240-247.

20. Some constructive ways to improve your diet, *Consumers' Research Magazine*, October 1976, p. 62.

21. J. L. Knittle, Obesity in childhood: A problem in adipose tissue development, *Journal of Pediatrics* 81 (December 1972): 1048-1059.

22. S. J. Fomon, T. A. Anderson, H. Y. W. Stephen, and E. E. Ziegler, *Nutritional Disorders of Children: Prevention, Screening, and Followup*, DHEW publication no. (HSA) 76-5612 (Washington, D.C.: Government Printing Office, 1976), p. 100.

23. Fomon et al., 1976, p. 116.

24. Fomon et al., 1976, p. 118.

25. W. H. Crosby, Current concepts in nutrition: Who needs iron? *New England Journal of Medicine* 297 (1977): 543-545.

26. Crosby, 1977; Committee on Nutrition of the Mother and Preschool Child, Food and Nutrition Board, National Academy of Sciences, *Iron Nutriture in Adolescence*, DHEW publication no. (HSA) 77-5100 (Washington, D.C.: Government Printing Office, 1977).

27. P. C. Elwood, The enrichment debate, *Nutrition Today*, July/August 1977, pp. 18-24.

28. Council on Foods and Nutrition, American Medical Association, Iron in enriched wheat flour, farina, bread, buns, and rolls (a council statement), *Journal of the American Medical Association* 220 (1972): 13-17.

29. Council on Foods and Nutrition, 1972; J. Mayer, ed., *U.S. Nutrition Policies in the Seventies* (San Francisco: W. H. Freeman, 1973).

30. G. C. Frank, A. W. Voors, P. E. Schilling, and G. S. Berenson, Dietary studies of rural school children in a cardiovascular survey, *Journal of the American Dietetic Association* 71 (1977): 31-35.

31. K. M. West, Prevention and therapy of diabetes mellitus, in *Nutrition Reviews' Present Knowledge in Nutrition*, 4th ed. (Washington, D.C.: Nutrition Foundation 1976), pp. 356-364.

32. E. L. Wynder, The dietary environment and cancer, *Journal of the American Dietetic Association* 71 (1977): 385-392.

33. Fomon et al., 1976, inside front cover.

34. Fomon et al., 1976.

35. L. Goldman, Acne prevention in the family, *American Family Physician* 16 (August 1977): 68-71.

36. We are indebted to Dr. Joyce Williams for many of these suggestions.

Chapter 14—The Young Adult and Adult

1. J. A. Thomas and D. L. Call, Eating between meals: A nutrition problem among teenagers? *Nutrition Reviews* 31 (May 1973): 137-139.

2. Committee on Nutrition of the Mother and Preschool Child, Food and Nutrition Board, National Academy of Sciences, *Iron Nutriture in Adolescence*, DHEW publication no. (HSA) 77-5100 (Washington, D.C.: Government Printing Office, 1977).

3. H. Bruch, Anorexia nervosa, *Nutrition Today*, September/October 1978, pp. 14-18.

4. Bruch, 1978.

5. B. S. Worthington, Nutritional needs of the pregnant adolescent, in *Nutrition in Pregnancy and Lactation*, B. S. Worthington, J. Vermeersch, and S. R. Williams (St. Louis: Mosby, 1977), pp. 119-132.

6. Worthington, 1977.

7. B. Lucas, Nutrition and the adolescent, in *Nutrition in Infancy and Childhood*, ed. P. L. Pipes (St. Louis: Mosby, 1977), pp. 132-144.

8. Young people and alcohol, *Alcohol Health and Research World*, Summer 1975, DHEW publication no. (ADM) 75-157, pp. 2-10.

9. Drinking motivations: Habits of youth illuminated by national survey results, *NIAAA Information and Feature Service* 18 (November 26, 1975), DHEW publication no. (ADM) 75-151.

10. D. P. Kraft, College students and alcohol: The 50 + 12 project, *Alcohol Health and Research World*, Summer 1976, DHEW publication no. (ADM) 76-157, pp. 10-14.

11. G. Globetti, as quoted in Young People and Alcohol, 1975.

12. F. Iber, In alcoholism, the liver sets the pace, *Nutrition Today*, January/February 1971, pp. 2-9.

13. The formation of scar tissue in the liver is known as fibrosis (fye-BROH-sis).

14. C. S. Lieber, Liver adaptation and injury in alcoholism, *New England Journal of Medicine* 288 (1973): 356-362.

15. L. Lifton and R. Scheig, Ethanol-induced hypertriglyceridemia: Prevalence and contributing factors, *American Journal of Clinical Nutrition* 31 (1978): 614-618.

16. A. J. Tuyns, Alcohol and cancer, *Alcohol Health and Research World*, Summer 1978, DHEW publication no. (ADM) 78-157, pp. 20-31.

17. E. Mezey, *Practice of Medicine VII* (Hagerstown, Md.: Harper & Row, Medical Department, 1970), Chap. 36, Effects of alcohol on the gastrointestinal system.

18. Mezey, 1970.

19. R. M. Myerson and J. S. Lafair, Alcoholic muscle disease, *Medical Clinics of North America* 54 (May 1977): 723-730.

20. J. H. Mitchell and L. S. Cohen, Alcohol and the heart, *Modern Concepts of Cardiovascular Disease* 39 (July 1970): 7.

21. N. K. Mello, Some aspects of the behavioral pharmacology of alcohol, in *Psychopharmacology: A Review of Progress, 1957-1967*, ed. D. H. Efron et al., PHS publication no. 1836 (Washington, D.C.: Government Printing Office, 1968).

22. Iber, 1971.

23. The hormone that causes the kidney to return water to the bloodstream is the antidiuretic hormone (ADH).

24. This statement is based on the assumption that 80 percent are drinkers and 10 percent of these are problem drinkers or alcoholics.

25. Only about 5 to 8 percent of all the alcoholics in the United States could be classified as skid row bums. The overwhelming majority are employed, have a high degree of work skills, still live with their families, and have an IQ slightly above average, according to the pamphlet "Shattering Myths about Drinking," available from the Bureau of Alcoholic Rehabilitation, Box 1147, Avon Park, FL 33825.

26. A. K. Sim, Ascorbic acid: A survey, past and present, *Chemistry and Industry*, February 19, 1972, pp. 160-165.

27. N. J. Greenberger, Effects of antibiotics and other agents on the intestinal absorption of iron, *American Journal of Clinical Nutrition* 26 (1973): 104-112.

28. H. Spencer, C. Norris, F. Coffey, and E. Wiatrowski, *Gastroenterology* 68 (1975): 990; abstract cited in Diet-drug interactions (reviewed by D. A. Roe), *Dairy Council Digest* 48 (March/April 1977).

29. D. A. Roe, Drugs, diet and nutrition, *Contemporary Nutrition* 3 (June 1978).

30. J. A. Visconti, ed., Drug-food interaction, in *Nutrition in Disease* (Ross Laboratories, May 1977).

31. Roe, 1978.

32. Diet-drug interactions (reviewed by D. A. Roe), *Dairy Council Digest* 48 (March/April 1977).

33. L. J. King, J. D. Teale, and V. Marks, Biochemical aspects of cannabis, in *Cannabis and Health*, ed. J. D. Graham (New York : Academic Press, 1976).

34. L. E. Hollister, Marihuana in man: Three years later, *Science* 172 (1971): 21-29.

35. King et al., 1976; Hollister, 1971.

36. E. L. Abel, Effects of marihuana on the solution of anagrams, memory and appetite, *Nature* 231 (1971): 260-261; C. T. Tart, Marijuana intoxication: Common experiences, *Nature* 226 (1970): 701-704.

37. L. E. Hollister, Hunger and appetite after single doses of marihuana, alcohol, and dextroamphetamine, *Clinical Pharmacology and Therapeutics* 12 (1971): 44-49; J. D.

P. Graham and D. M. F. Li, The pharmacology of cannabis and cannabinoids, in *Cannabis and Health*, 1976.

38. Hollister, 1971.
39. Marijuana: Truth on health problems, *Science News* 107/108 (February 22, 1975): 117.
40. T. H. Maugh II, Marihuana: New support for immune and reproductive hazards, *Science* 190 (1975): 865-867.
41. Graham and Li, 1976; Pot update: Possible motor effects, *Science News* 113 (February 4, 1978): 71.
42. Graham and Li, 1976.
43. Infrequent use might be defined as three cigarettes a week or less. Maugh, 1975.
44. Maugh, 1975.
45. R. T. Frankle and G. Christakis, eds., Some nutritional aspects of "hard" drug addiction, *Dietetic Currents, Ross Timesaver* 2 (July/August 1975).
46. D. Robertson, J. C. Frolich, R. K. Carr, J. T. Watson, J. W. Hollifield, D. G. Shand, and J. A. Oates, Effects of caffeine on plasma renin activity, catecholamines, and blood pressure, *New England Journal of Medicine* 298 (1978): 181-186.
47. Food allergy, *Nutrition and the MD*, July 1978.
48. Coffee: Downs and ups, *Nutrition and the MD*, April 1978.
49. K. Yano, G. G. Rhoads, and A. Kagan, Coffee, alcohol, and risk of coronary heart disease in Japanese-Americans, *New England Journal of Medicine* 297 (1977): 405-409.
50. Coffee, 1978.
51. P. E. Stephenson, Physiologic and psychotropic effects of caffeine on man, *Journal of the American Dietetic Association* 71 (1977): 240-247.
52. Stephenson, 1977.
53. R. M. Leverton, The paradox of teen-age nutrition, *Journal of the American Dietetic Association* 53 (1968): 13-16.
54. Leverton, 1968.
55. Lucas, 1977.
56. Lucas, 1977.
57. Lucas, 1977.

Chapter 15—The Later Years

1. Bureau of the Census, U.S. Department of Commerce, *Money, Income and Poverty Status of Families and Persons in the United States, 1974-1975* (Washington, D.C.: Government Printing Office).
2. Bureau of the Census, 1974-1975.
3. J. Mayer, Aging and nutrition, *Geriatrics* 29 (5) (1974): 57-59.
4. B. L. Strehler, *Time, Cells, and Aging*, 2d ed. (New York: Academic Press, 1977).
5. Strehler, 1977.
6. A. Comfort, *A Good Age* (New York: Crown, 1976).
7. Strehler, 1977.
8. M. Puner, *To the Good Long Life* (New York: Universe Books, 1974).
9. The "aging pigment" is known as lipofuscin (lip-oh-FEW-sin).
10. Strehler, 1977.
11. Puner, 1974.

12. Strehler, 1977.

13. U.S. Department of Health, Education, and Welfare, *Ten-State Nutrition Survey, 1968-1970*, DHEW publication no. (HSM) 72-8130-8133 (Atlanta: Center for Disease Control, 1972).

14. Mayer, 1974.

15. Strehler, 1977.

16. Strehler, 1977.

17. L. Lutwak, Symposium on osteoporosis: Nutritional aspects of osteoporosis, *Journal of the American Geriatrics Society* 17 (2) (1969): 115-119.

18. Lutwak, 1969.

19. I. Dallas and B. E. C. Nordin, The relation between calcium intake and roentgenologic osteoporosis, *American Journal of Clinical Nutrition* 11 (1962): 263-269.

20. Lutwak, 1969.

21. Mayer, 1974.

22. A. F. Morgan, Nutrition of the aging, *The Gerontologist* 2 (1962): 77-84.

23. Lutwak 1969; Dallas and Nordin, 1962.

24. K. H. Sidney, R. J. Shephard, and J. E. Harrison, Endurance training and body composition of the elderly, *American Journal of Clinical Nutrition* 30 (1977): 326-333.

25. J. S. Lyons and M. F. Trulson, Food practices of older people living at home, *Journal of Gerontology* 11 (1956): 66-72.

26. S. R. Gambert and A. R. Guansing, Protein-calorie malnutrition in the elderly, *Journal of the American Geriatrics Society* 28 (1980): 272-275.

27. D. B. Rao, Problems of nutrition in the aged, *Journal of the American Geriatrics Society* 21(8) (1973): 362-367.

28. H. A. DeVries, Physiological effects of an exercise training regimen upon men aged 52 to 88, *Journal of Gerontology* 25 (1970): 325-336.

29. Lutwak, 1969.

30. Mayer, 1974.

31. Lyons and Trulson, 1956.

32. P. Swanson, Adequacy in old age, part II: Nutrition programs for the aging, *Journal of Home Economics* 56 (1964): 728-734.

33. C. S. Davidson, J. Livermore, P. Anderson, and S. Kaufman, The nutrition of a group of apparently healthy aging persons, *American Journal of Clinical Nutrition* 10 (1962): 181-199.

34. Morgan, 1962.

35. Rao, 1973.

36. J. Pelcovits, Nutrition to meet the human needs of older Americans, *Journal of the American Dietetic Association* 60 (1972): 297-300.

37. Lyons and Trulson, 1956.

38. Pelcovits, 1972.

39. Mayer, 1974.

40. Morgan, 1962.

41. H. H. Koehler, H. C. Lee, and M. Jacobson, Tocopherols in canned entrees and vended sandwiches, *Journal of the American Dietetic Association* 70 (1977): 616-620.

42. M. Jordan, M. Kepes, R. B. Hayes, and W. Hammond, Dietary habits of persons living alone, *Geriatrics* 9 (1954): 230-232.

43. M. Balsley, M. F. Brink, and E. W. Speckman, Nutrition in disease and stress, *Geriatrics* 26 (1971): 87-93.

44. Lutwak, 1969; Morgan, 1962.

45. Ratios to look for in B-vitamin supplements are: thiamin, 1.0 mg; riboflavin, 1.1; pyridoxine, 0.8; niacin, 9.0, pantothenic acid, 5.3. Morgan, 1962.

46. Mayer, 1974.

47. Mayer, 1974.

48. Rao, 1973.

49. B. R. Bradshaw, W. P. Vonderhaar, V. T. Keeney, L. S. Tyler, and S. Harris, Community-based residential care for the minimally impaired elderly: A survival analysis, *Journal of the American Geriatrics Society* 24 (1976): 423-429.

50. Balsley, Brink, and Speckman, 1971.

51. Mayer, 1974; Rao, 1973; Pelcovits, 1972; J. Weinberg, Psychologic implications of the nutritional needs of the elderly, *Journal of the American Dietetic Association* 60 (1972): 293-296; L. M. Williams, A concept of loneliness in the elderly, *Journal of the American Geriatrics Society* 26 (1978): 182-187; J. Pelcovits, Nutrition for older Americans, *Journal of the American Dietetic Association* 58 (1971): 17-21.

52. Weinberg, 1972.

53. Mayer, 1974

54. Rao, 1973.

55. Rao, 1973.

56. Pelcovits, 1972.

57. Pelcovits, 1972.

58. Pelcovits, 1971.

59. Bradshaw et al., 1976.

60. R. L. Kane and R. A. Kane, Care of the aged: Old problems in need of new solutions, *Science* 200 (1978): 913-919.

61. E. C. Cole, An alternative to institutional care, *The Interpreter*, March 1975.

62. Cole, 1975; D. Boss, Reaching out: Diet and senior Americans, *Food Management* 12 (November 1977): 70-73, 89, 91-93.

Controversy Notes and For Further Information

Controversy 1—Natural Foods

1. D. M. Hegsted and L. M. Ausman, Sole foods and some not so scientific experiments, *Nutrition Today*, November/December 1973, pp. 22-25.

2. Hegsted and Ausman, 1973.

3. *The Miami Herald*, January 9, 1979.

4. More precisely still, an organic compound contains carbon-carbon or carbon-hydrogen bonds or both: Methane (CH_4) and ethanol (CH_3-CH_2OH) are organic compounds while carbon dioxide (CO_2) and carbon tetrachloride (CCl_4) are not.

5. Position paper on food and nutrition misinformation on selected topics, *Journal of the American Dietetic Association* 66 (1975): 277-279.

6. L. A. Barnes, Nutritional aspects of vegetarianism, health foods, and fad diets, *Nutrition Reviews* 35 (1977): 153-157.

7. R. T. Frankle and F. K. Heussenstamm, Food zealotry and youth: New dimensions for professionals, *American Journal of Public Health* 64 (January 1974): 11-18.

8. B. McPherrin, Mail order health fraud, *ACSH News and Views* 1 (5) (September/October 1980): 10.

9. McPherrin, 1980.

10. McPherrin, 1980.

11. Ginseng abuse syndrome, *Nutrition and the MD*, September 1979.

12. W. H. Lewis, Reporting adverse reactions to herbal ingestants (letter to the editor), *Journal of the American Medical Association* 240 (1978): 109-110.

13. Lewis, 1978.

14. A. Brynjolfsson, Food irradiation and nutrition, *The Professional Nutritionist*, Fall 1979, pp. 7-10.

15. M. W. Pariza, Food safety from the eye of a hurricane, *The Professional Nutritionist*, Fall 1979, pp. 11-14.

16. S. S. Aron, T. F. Midura, K. Damus, B. Thompson, R. M. Wood, and J. Chin, Honey and other environmental risk factors for infant botulism, *Journal of Pediatrics* 94 (February 1979): 331, as quoted in I. B. Vyhmeister, What about honey? *Life and Health*, August 1980, pp. 5-7.

17. Vyhmeister, 1980; R. W. Miller, Honey: Making sure it's pure, *FDA Consumer* 13 (September 1979): 12-13.

18. M. Stephenson, The confusing world of health foods, *FDA Consumer* 12 (July/August 1978): 18-22.

19. Stephenson, 1978.

20. Singing the health food blues, an interview with B. Cavanough, former owner of a health food store, *ACSH News and Views* 1 (2) (February 1980): 10-11.

21. W. H. Allaway, *The Effect of Soils and Fertilizer on Human and Animal Nutrition*, Agriculture Information Bulletin no. 378 (Washington, D.C.: Government Printing Office, March 1975).

22. R. B. Alfin-Slater, Vitamin supplementation: an appraisal of values—and dangers, *The Professional Nutritionist*, Winter 1980, pp. 8-11.

23. J. D. Gussow, The organic alternative, *Nutrition Today*, March/April 1974, pp. 31-32.

For Further Information

An excellent cookbook for families wishing to prepare healthful meals is:

- White, A., and the Society for Nutrition Education. *The Family Health Cookbook*. New York: David McKay Company, 1980.

Among the references cited in this controversy's notes is *ACSH News and Views*, a newsletter from the American Council on Science and Health. This council, composed of reputable, credentialed scientists in several disciplines related to nutrition, makes it its business to provide a balanced view of the controversies raging about consumer issues like the "denutrification" and "embalming" of foods. The council is neither pro-health foods nor pro-industry on principle, but rather looks at the evidence and reports on each case on its merits. A thirty-minute lecture on cassette tape by its president is available:

- Whelan, E. The organic food rip-off. $9.50. Spenco Medical Corporation, P.O. Box 8113, Waco, TX 76710.

Whelan's message is that the real health threats are smoking, overeating fat, overeating generally, and lack of exercise, not food additives.

The council's newsletter is also highly recommended reading for the consumer who wants a balanced picture. The interview with a former health food store owner (Note 20) is especially relevant to this controversy. Refer to Appendix J for the council's address.

Many people believe that health frauds are easy to spot. They are not, and quackery is thriving in this age of enlightenment. A book that proves this point over and over again and shows why people spend fortunes on fraudulent products is:

- Barrett, H. S. and Knight, G., eds. *The Health Robbers* (Philadelphia: Stickley, 1976).

A collection of readings illustrating the many kinds of nutrition misinformation abounding today is:

- *Nutrition Reviews/Supplement: Nutrition Misinformation and Food Faddism* (July 1974).

Several references are available on the toxic effects of plant products. The lead article in a 1979 issue of *Nutrition Reviews*, for example, is:

- Wilson, B. J. Naturally occurring toxicants of foods. *Nutrition Reviews* 37 (1979): 305-312.

Controversy 2—Vitamin Supplements

1. C. Norman, New food regulations make strange bedfellows, *Nutrition Today*, September/October 1973, pp. 20-21.
2. R. J. Williams, J. D. Heffley, M. L. Yew, and C. W. Bode, A renaissance of nutritional science is imminent, in *The Nutrition Crisis, a Reader*, ed. T. P. Labuza (St. Paul: West, 1975), pp. 27-41.
3. One person may even need seven times as much of a nutrient as another—but to say this is to display the full range of needs from the lowest to the highest. That is, the comparison is between someone with extraordinarily small needs and someone with extraordinarily high ones. (R. Dubos, The intellectual basis of nutrition science and practice, an article presented at the NIH conference on the biomedical and behavioral basis of clinical nutrition, June 19, 1978, in Bethesda, Maryland, and reprinted in *Nutrition Today*, July/August 1979, pp. 31-34.) Such a comparison can't be used as the basis for recommending that any normal person take doses of nutrients seven or so times higher than the *average*.
4. P. L. White, Food faddism, *Contemporary Nutrition* 4 (February 1979).
5. White, 1979.
6. V. Herbert, The health hustlers, in *The Health Robbers*, ed. S. Barrett and G. Knight (Philadelphia: George F. Stickley, 1976).
7. This was not because the vitamin C in the pills was different, of course, but because the pills were different. Some other ingredient in the "natural" pills may have interfered with the absorption of the vitamin, for example. O. Pelletier, and M. O. Keith, Bioavailability of synthetic and natural ascorbic acid, in Labuza, 1975, pp. 192-200.
8. A. Kamil, How natural are those "natural" vitamins? *Co-op News* 25 (March 13, 1972): 3, reprinted in *Nutrition Reviews/Supplement: Nutrition Misinformation and Food Faddism*, July 1974, p. 34.
9. Position paper on food and nutrition misinformation on selected topics, *Journal of the American Dietetic Association* 66 (1975): 277-279.
10. B. McPherrin, Mail order health fraud, *ACSH News and Views* 1(5) (September/October 1980): 10.
11. White, 1979.
12. A. E. Harper, Science and the consumer, *Journal of Nutrition Education* 11 (October-December 1979): 171.
13. M. Stephenson, The confusing world of health foods, *FDA Consumer* 12 (July/August 1978): 18-22.
14. Questions doctors ask, *Nutrition and the MD*, December 1978.
15. Stephenson, 1978.
16. Stephenson, 1978.

For Further Information

Three good papers on nutritional individuality are available. The first two are written in easy-to-read style for the layperson, the third is more technical and is for the professional:

• Williams, R. J. Nutritional individuality. *Human Nature*, June 1978, pp. 46-53.

• Dubos, R. The intellectual basis of nutrition science and practice. Article presented at the NIH conference on the biomedical and behavioral basis of clinical nutrition, June 19, 1978, in Bethesda, Maryland. Reprinted in *Nutrition Today*, July/August 1979, pp. 31-34.

• Young, V. R., and Scrimshaw, N. S. Genetic and biological variability in human nutrient requirements. *American Journal of Clinical Nutrition* 32 (1979): 486-500.

The American Association of Pediatrics Committee on Nutrition is concerned about nutrition practices that are potentially harmful to the health of children and has published a special report addressing some of these. It reads in part:

> Most individuals who adhere to unusual nutritional practices, except for balanced vegetarianism, are aware that their ideas run counter to the mainstream of medical and nutritional opinion. Physicians and other health professionals should be prepared to encounter strong resistance. . . it is best to focus on those features of the diet that are of greatest potential harm. . . even with the more extreme dietary practices, it is usually possible to prevent serious harm by striving for dietary variety and balance and working within the value system or philosophy of the group or individual.

The report—Nutritional aspects of vegetarianism, health foods, and fad diets—has been published in two places: *Pediatrics* 59 (March 1977) and *Nutrition Reviews* 35 (June 1977): 153-157.

The Chicago Nutrition Association puts out a list of "books not recommended" as one of its many services to consumers; the list is also available from the American Medical Association. The addresses of both associations are in Appendix J.

The American Dietetic Association has an ongoing committee on food and nutrition misinformation which can be contacted for answers to questions you may have about nutrition facts and rumors. The ADA's address is in Appendix J.

The Nutrition Foundation devoted a whole issue of its *Nutrition Reviews* to problems like those dealt with here:

• *Nutrition Reviews/Supplement: Nutrition Misinformation and Food Faddism* (July 1974).

Especially relevant to nutrition quackery is Darby's article on pages 57-61 in that issue, "The Unicorn and Other Lessons from History," and the references it lists.

Controversy 3—Dietary Guidelines

1. U.S. Senate, Select Committee on Nutrition and Human Needs, *Dietary Goals for the United States* (Washington, D.C.: Government Printing Office, February 1977). The *Goals* were revised and reprinted in a second edition in December 1977.
2. C. F. Enloe, Jr., Takin' away me dyin' (editorial), *Nutrition Today*, November/December 1977, pp. 14-15.
3. E. N. Whitney and E. M. N. Hamilton discuss this problem and present many references relating to it, in the section entitled "Dietary fat and cancer," in *Understanding Nutrition*, 2d ed. (St. Paul: West, 1981), pp. 84-93. See also Controversy 5B in this book.
4. R. Reinhold, A panel that gave thoughts for food, *New York Times*, January 8, 1978.
5. U.S. Senate, *Dietary Goals*, 1977, 1st ed., p. 3 and 2d ed., p. xv.

6. E. L. Wynder, The dietary environment and cancer, *Journal of the American Dietetic Association* 71 (1977): 385-392.
7. E. Eckholm and F. Record, *Worldwatch Paper 9: The Two Faces of Malnutrition* (Washington, D.C.: Worldwatch Institute, 1976).
8. Proper diet saves lives, land, oil . . ., *Science News*, January 17, 1981, pp. 39-40.
9. Reinhold, 1978.
10. Enloe, 1977.
11. C. F. Enloe, Jr., It ain't necessarily so! (editorial), *Nutrition Today*, September/October 1974, p. 16.

For Further Information

A history of the setting of guidelines in the U.S. from the 1957 Four Food Group Plan to the present is:

- McNutt, K. Dietary advice to the public: 1957 to 1980. *Nutrition Reviews* 38 (1980): 353-360.

A. E. Harper has published a thoughtful article on the problems of setting guidelines for the public:

- Dear Secretary—. *Nutrition Today*, March/April 1979, pp. 19-20.

His article is followed by a humorous "behind-the-scenes peak" at the government departments involved in the controversies surrounding these issues:

- Greenberg, D. S. A long wait for a little advice. *Nutrition Today*, March/April 1979, pp. 20-22.

C. F. Enloe's editorial ("The mouse that snored"), and the major article detailing the Dietary Guidelines for Americans on pages 13-18 of that same issue also make lively reading.

The National Nutrition Consortium (a nonprofit organization composed of several professional societies) recommends that in the future, guidelines be stated in quantitative fashion and that they cover more areas, including exercise, immunization programs, smoking, and drug abuse. The consortium also makes suggestions regarding future research to establish policy:

- National Nutrition Consortium. Guidelines for a national nutrition policy. *Nutrition Reviews* 38 (1980): 96-98.

Controversy 4A—Sugar

1. Reprinted from C. W. Lecos, Sugar: How sweet it is—and isn't, *FDA Consumer*, February 1980: 21-23.
2. D. F. Hollingsworth, Translating nutrition into diet, *Food Technology* 31 (February 1977): 38-41, 78.
3. K. M. West, Prevention and therapy of diabetes mellitus, in *Nutrition Reviews' Present Knowledge in Nutrition*, 4th ed. (Washington, D.C.: Nutrition Foundation, 1976), pp. 356-364.
4. W. E. Connor and S. L. Connor, Sucrose and carbohydrate, in *Nutrition Reviews' Present Knowledge*, 1976, pp. 33-42.
5. Connor and Connor, 1976.

6. Connor and Connor, 1976.

7. N. Wightman, Saccharin—are there alternatives? *Journal of Nutrition Education* 9 (1977): 106-108.

8. Wightman, 1977.

9. U. D. Register and L. M. Sonnenberg, The vegetarian diet, *Journal of the American Dietetic Association* 62 (1973): 253-261.

10. Lecos, 1980.

11. Institute of Food Technologists' Expert Panel on Food Safety and Nutrition, Sugars and nutritive sweeteners in processed foods, *Food Technology* 33 (May 1979): 101-105.

12. M. Berger, Dietary management of children with uremia, *Journal of the American Dietetic Association* 70 (1977): 498-505.

13. West, 1976.

14. West, 1976.

15. West, 1976.

16. A. M. Cohen, High sucrose intake as a factor in the development of diabetes and its vascular complications, in U.S. Senate, Select Committee on Nutrition and Human Needs, *Dietary Sugar and Disease* (hearings) (Washington, D.C.: Government Printing Office, 1973), pp. 167-198.

17. West, 1976.

18. T. H. Maugh II, Diet: Drug-free therapy for diabetics, *The Sciences*, January/February 1977, pp. 16-19.

19. Maugh, 1977.

20. L. Lederman, The acid in the sweetness, *The Sciences*, July/August 1974, pp. 6-11.

21. A. T. Brown, The role of dietary carbohydrates in plaque formation and oral disease, in *Nutrition Reviews' Present Knowledge*, 1976, pp. 488-503.

22. R. A. Seelig, Nutrition, diet and the teeth: A review, reprinted by United Fresh Fruit and Vegetable Association, Washington, D.C., 1968.

23. R. L. Glass and S. Fleisch, Diet and dental caries, *Journal of the American Dental Association* 88 (1974): 807-813.

24. S. M. Garn, M. A. Solomon, and A. Schaefer, Internal validation of sugar-food intakes in obese adolescents (letter to the editor), *American Journal of Clinical Nutrition* 33 (1980): 1890.

25. B. L. Cohen, Relative risks of saccharin and calorie ingestion, *Science* 199 (1978): 983.

26. A. R. P. Walter, The relative risks of saccharin and sucrose ingestions (letter to the editor), *American Journal of Clinical Nutrition* 32 (1979): 727-728.

27. J. Ostrander and M. Koch, Sugarless confections, *Journal of the American Dietetic Association* 70 (1977): 156.

28. Wightman, 1977.

29. J. A. Hruban, Selection of snack foods from vending machines by high school students, *Journal of School Health* 47 (1977): 33-37.

30. For example, *The Snacking Mouse*©, 1977, available from The Polished Apple, Malibu, CA 90265

31. L. Warschoff, What Betty Crocker doesn't tell you about sugar! Baltimore: American Friends Service Committee, 1976.

For Further Information, Controversy 4A

Among the books that state the case against sugar emotionally and unfairly is:

- Duffy, W. *Sugar Blues*. New York: Warner Books, 1981.

References that give sugar a fair hearing include those listed in Appendix J and in this chapter's and Controversy's notes.

Controversy 4B—Fiber

1. J. Scala, Fiber, the forgotten nutrient, *Food Technology* 28 (January 1974): 34-36.
2. Scala, 1974.
3. R. D. Smith, Checking out the fiber fad, *The Sciences*, March/April 1976, pp. 25-29.
4. D. P. Burkitt, Relationships between diseases and their etiological significance, *American Journal of Clinical Nutrition* 30 (1977): 262-267.
5. M. A. Howell, Diet as an etiological factor in the development of cancers of the colon and rectum, *Journal of Chronic Diseases* 28 (1975): 67-80.
6. Smith, 1976.
7. H. Trowell, Definition of dietary fiber and hypothesis that it is a protective factor in certain diseases, *American Journal of Clinical Nutrition* 29 (1976): 417-427.
8. Burkitt, 1977.
9. A. I. Mendeloff, Dietary fiber, in *Nutrition Reviews' Present Knowledge in Nutrition*, 4th ed. (Washington, D.C.: Nutrition Foundation, 1976), pp. 393-401.
10. Smith, 1976.
11. The role of fiber in the diet (reviewed by D. P. Burkitt, G. A. Leveille, and A. I. Mendeloff), *Dairy Council Digest* 46 (January/February 1975).
12. C. K. Johnson, K. Kolasa, W. Chenowith, and M. Bennink, Health, laxation, and food habit influences on fiber intake of older women, *Journal of the American Dietetic Association* 77 (1980): 551-557.
13. Scala, 1974.
14. G. A. Spiller, M. C. Chernoff, R. A. Hill, J. E. Gates, J. J. Nassar, and E. A. Shipley, Effect of purified cellulose, pectin, and a low-residue diet on fecal volatile fatty acids, transit time, and fecal weight in humans, *American Journal of Clinical Nutrition* 33 (1980): 754-759.
15. M. S. Mathur, H. Ram, and V. S. Chadda, Effect of bran on intestinal transit time in normal Indians and intestinal amoebiasis, *American Journal of Proctology, Gastroenterology, and Colon and Rectal Surgery*, November-December 1978, pp. 30-32, 34.
16. High-fiber diets and colonic disease, *American Journal of Nursing* 77 (1977): 255.
17. M. A. Eastwood, Fibre and enterohepatic circulation, *Nutrition Reviews* 35 (January 1977): 42-44.
18. A. M. Connell, C. L. Smith, and M. Somsell, Absence of effect of bran on blood-lipids, *Lancet*, March 1, 1975, pp. 496-497; A. S. Truswell and R. M. Kay, Bran and blood-lipids, *Lancet*, February 14, 1976, p. 367.
19. Trowell, 1976.
20. Scala, 1974.
21. K. W. McNutt, Perspective—fiber, *Journal of Nutrition Education* 8 (1976): 150-152.
22. McNutt, 1976.
23. High-fiber diets, 1977.
24. Questions doctors ask. . ., *Nutrition and the MD*, April 1978.
25. D. P. Burkitt, Economic development—not all bonus, *Nutrition Today*, January/February 1976, pp. 6-13.
26. S. Vaisrub, Fiber feeding—Fad or finger of fate? (editorial), *Journal of the American Medical Association* 235 (1976): 182.
27. M. V. Krause and M. A. Hunscher, *Food, Nutrition and Diet Therapy*, 5th ed. (Philadelphia: Saunders, 1972), p. 352.
28. Role of fiber, 1975.
29. M. A. Eastwood, W. D. Mitchell, and J. L. Pritchard, The effect of bran on the excretion of faecal cations, *Proceedings of the Nutrition Society* 35 (September 1976): 78A-79A.
30. A. S. Prasad, Zinc deficiency, *Nutrition and the MD*, January 1979.

31. W. D. Holloway, C. Tasman-Jones, and S. P. Lee, Digestion of certain fractions of dietary fiber in humans, *American Journal of Clinical Nutrition* 31 (1978): 927-930.

32. J. Mayer, and J. Dwyer, Basic research into dietary fiber yields facts about what fiber can and can't do, *Tallahassee Democrat*, March 29, 1979.

33. B. S. Drasar and D. J. A. Jenkins, Bacteria, diet, and large bowel cancer, *American Journal of Clinical Nutrition* 29 (1976): 1410-1416.

34. Smith, 1976.

35. D. Kritchevsky, Modification by fiber of toxic dietary effect, *Federation Proceedings* 36 (1977): 1692-1695.

36. U. D. Register and L. M. Sonnenberg, The vegetarian diet, *Journal of the American Dietetic Association* 62 (1973): 253-261.

For Further Information, Controversy 4B

No reliable popular reference on fiber is available, but for the more technically inclined, we recommend:

- G. E. Inglett and S. I.Falkehag, eds. *Dietary Fibers: Chemistry and Nutrition*, New York: Academic Press, 1979.

Issues 1 and 2 of the *Journal of Plant Foods and Human Nutrition*, 1978, were devoted entirely to fiber.

A book exploring some fascinating possibilities for future research into uses of fiber in the treatment of obesity and other conditions is:

- K. W. Heaton, ed. *Dietary Fibre: Current Developments of Importance to Health.* Westport, Conn.: Food & Nutrition Press, 1979.

Controversy 5A—Atherosclerosis

1. R. B. Alfin-Slater and L. Aftergood, Fats and other lipids, in *Modern Nutrition in Health and Disease*, ed. R. S. Goodhart and M. E. Shils, 5th ed. (Philadelphia: Lea and Febiger, 1973), pp. 117-141.

2. H. C. McGill and G. E. Mott, Diet and coronary heart disease, in *Nutrition Reviews' Present Knowledge in Nutrition*, 4th ed. (Washington, D.C.: Nutrition Foundation, 1976), pp. 376-391.

3. R. I. Levy and N. Ernst, Diet, hyperlipidemia and atherosclerosis, in Goodhart and Shils, 1973, pp. 895-918.

4. J. Gorman, A running argument: Does physical activity help prevent heart attacks? *The Sciences*, January/February 1977, pp. 10-15.

5. R. L. Holman, H. C. McGill, J. P. Strong, and J. C. Greer, The natural history of atherosclerosis: The early aortic lesions as seen in New Orleans in the middle of the 20th century, *American Journal of Pathology* 34 (1958): 209-234.

6. Gorman, 1977.

7. D. C. Glass, Stress, behavior patterns, and coronary disease, *American Scientist* 65 (1977): 177-188.

8. There are in-between types, of course; Type A is at one extreme. Glass, 1977.

9. R. H. Rosenman, R. H. Rahe, N. O. Borhanie, and M. Feinleib, Heritability of personality and behavior pattern, *Proceedings of the First International Congress on Twins*, Rome, 1975, as cited by Glass, 1977.

10. R. Levy, Introduction, in *Proceedings of the Conference on the Decline in Coronary Heart Disease Mortality*, ed. R. J. Havlik and M. Feinleib, U.S. Department of Health, Education, and Welfare, Public Health Service, National Institutes of Health, NIH Publication No. 79-1610, May 1979, p. 1.

11. J. C. Kleinman, J. J. Feldman, and M. A. Monk, Trends in smoking and ischemic heart disease mortality, in *Havlik and Feinleib*, 1979, pp. 195-211.

12. N. O. Borhanie, Mortality trend in hypertension, United States, 1950-1976, in *Havlik and Feinleib*, 1979, pp. 218-235.

13. R. Beaglehole, J. C. LaRosa, G. E. Heiss, C. E. Davis, B. M. Rifkind, R. M. Muesing, and O. D. Williams, Secular changes in blood cholesterol and their contribution to the decline in coronary mortality, in *Havlik and Feinleib*, 1979, pp. 282-297.

14. R. S. Paffenbarger, Jr., Countercurrents of physical activity and heart attack trends, in *Havlik and Feinleib*, 1979, pp. 298-311.

15. J. Stamler, reporting for R. Byington, A. R. Dyer, D. Garside, K. Liu, D. Moss, J. Stamler, and Y. Tsong, Recent trends of major coronary risk factors and CHD mortality in the United States and other industrialized countries, in *Havlik and Feinleib*, 1979, pp. 340-380.

16. Remember this refers to the reduced risk from CVD only. If "risk of death from all causes" is measured, serum cholesterol becomes relatively less important—4 percent—and cigarette smoking considerably more important—65 percent. And exercise is not included because it isn't one of the "big three" in the heart disease picture. Stamler, 1979.

17. Food and Nutrition Board, National Research Council, National Academy of Sciences, *Towards Healthful Diets*, reprinted in *Nutrition Today*, May/June 1980, pp. 7-11.

18. For a more complete description of these factors see Controversy 4: Cholesterol, in the first edition of this book.

19. Food and Nutrition Board, 1980.

20. Food and Nutrition Board, 1980.

21. Food and Nutrition Board, 1980.

22. N. Ernst and R. I. Levy, Diet, hyperlipidemia and atherosclerosis, in *Modern Nutrition in Health and Disease*, ed. R. S. Goodhart and M. E. Shils, 6th ed. (Philadelphia: Lea and Febiger, 1980), pp. 1045-1070.

23. G. J. Miller and N. E. Miller, Plasma high-density-lipoprotein concentration and development of ischaemic heart disease, *Lancet* 1 (1975): 16-19; W. P. Castelli, J. T. Doyle, T. Gordon, C. G. Hames, M. C. Hjortland, S. B. Hulley, A. Kagan, and W. J. Zukel, HDL cholesterol and other lipids in coronary heart disease, *Circulation* 55 (1977): 767-772; T. Gordon, W. P. Castelli, M. C. Hjortland, W. B. Kannel, and T. R. Dawber, High density lipoprotein as a protective factor against coronary heart disease, *The American Journal of Medicine* 62 (1977): 707-714; N. E. Miller, D. S. Thelle, O. H. Førde, and O. D. Mjos, The Tromso Heart Study: High density lipoprotein and coronary heart disease: A prospective case-control study, *Lancet* 5 (1977): 965-967; High blood lipid levels can be good or bad—depending on the lipid (Medical News), *Journal of the American Medical Association* 237 (1977): 1066-1067, 1069-1070.

24. T. O. Von Lossonczy, A. Ruiter, H. C. Bronsgeest-Schoute, C. M. van Gent, and R. J. J. Hermus, The effect of a fish diet on lipids in healthy human subjects, *American Journal of Clinical Nutrition* 31 (1978): 1340-1346.

25. J. W. Anderson and W. L. Chen, Plant fiber: Carbohydrate and lipid metabolism, *American Journal of Clinical Nutrition* 32 (1979): 346-363; Dietary fiber, exercise and selected blood lipid constituents, *Nutrition Reviews* 38 (1980): 207-209.

26. J. L. Marx, The HDL: The good cholesterol carriers? (Research News), *Science* 205 (1979): 677-679.

27. P. D. Wood, W. Haskell, H. Klein, S. Lewis, M. P. Stern, and J. W. Farquhar, The distribution of plasma lipoproteins in middle-aged male runners, *Metabolism* 25 (1976): 1249-1257.

28. A. Weltman, S. Matter, and B. A. Stamford, Caloric restriction and/or mild exercise: Effects on serum lipids and body composition, *American Journal of Clinical Nutrition* 33 (1980): 1002-1009.

29. D. W. Erkelens, J. J. Albers, W. R. Hazzard, R. C. Frederick, and E. L Bierman, High-density lipoprotein-cholesterol in survivors of myocardial infarction, *Journal of the American Medical Association* 242 (1979): 2185-2189; D. Streja and D. Mymin, Moderate exercise and high-density lipoprotein-cholesterol, *Journal of the American Medical Association* 242 (1979): 2190-2192; W. P. Castelli, Exercise and high-density lipoproteins (editorial), *Journal of the American Medical Association* 242 (1979): 2217.

30. Streja and Mymin, 1979.

For Further Information, Controversy 5A

The most useful references on heart disease for the general reader are available from the American Heart Association (see Chapter 5 references).

The controversy over whether dietary fat and cholesterol affect heart disease deaths has been so noisy and lasted so long that it has a name of its own: the diet-heart controversy. Both sides are summed up in a pair of short articles, one by the editor of the *Journal of the American Medical Association* (he says diet has no effect) and the other by the American Heart Association (they say it does):

- Mann, G. V. Diet-heart: End of an era. *New England Journal of Medicine* 297 (1977): 644-650.
- Nutrition Committee, American Heart Association. Diet and coronary heart disease: Another view. *New England Journal of Medicine* 298 (1978).

Both were reprinted in *Current Concepts in Nutrition* (see Appendix J).

Most of the May-June, 1980, issue of *Nutrition Today* was also devoted to this controversy. The cover bore a picture of the eruption of Mount St. Helens and suggested that the diet-heart debate was as violent as that famous volcano.

Controversy 5B— Nutrition and Cancer

1. E. L. Wynder and G. B. Gori, Contribution of the environment to cancer incidence: An epidemiologic exercise, *Journal of the National Cancer Institute* 58 (1977): 825-832.
2. E. L. Wynder, The dietary environment and cancer, *Journal of the American Dietetic Association* 71 (1977): 385-392.
3. R. Weltman, Fat and forty is no joke for colorectal cancer victims, *Journal of the American Medical Association* 238 (1977): 843-844.
4. K. K. Carroll and H. T. Khor, Effects of level and type of dietary fat on incidence of mammary tumors induced in female Sprague-Dawley rats by 7,12-dimethylbenz-α-anthracene, *Lipids* 6 (1971): 415-420.
5. F. J. C. Roe, Food and cancer, *Journal of Human Nutrition* 33 (1979): 405-415.
6. For a more complete description of *trans*-fatty acids, see E. N. Whitney and E. M. N. Hamilton, *Understanding Nutrition*, 2d ed. (St. Paul: West, 1981), pp. 84-93.
7. A. Keys, Alpha lipoprotein (HDL) cholesterol in the serum and the risk of coronary heart disease and death, *Lancet* 20 (September 1980): 603-606.
8. Nutrition and diet in carcinogenesis, *Nutrition and the MD*, April 1976.
9. S. M. Oace, Diet and cancer, *Journal of Nutrition Education* 10 (1978): 106-108; J. L. Lyon and A. I. Mendeloff, Diet fiber and colonic cancer (letter to the editor), *New England Journal of Medicine* 298 (1978): 110-111.

10. News item, *Nutrition Today,* March/April 1978, p. 5; Mutagen formation in beef during cooking, *Nutrition and the MD,* January 1979.

11. National Cancer Institute, as cited in Morsels and tidbits, *Nutrition and the MD,* May 1980.

12. Carroll and Khor, 1975; M. G. Enig, R. J. Munn, and M. Keeney, Dietary fat and cancer trends—a critique, *Federation Proceedings* 37 (1978): 2215-2220.

13. Nutrition and diet in carcinogenesis, *Nutrition and the MD,* April 1976.

14. E. L. Wynder, 1977.

15. M. B. Sporn and D. L. Newton, Chemoprevention of cancer with retinoids, *Federation Proceedings* 38 (1979): 2528-2534; C. Kahn, Inside the cancer labs, *Family Health,* October 1980, pp. 22-25, 58.

16. The Nutrition Gazette, *Nutrition Today,* September/October 1978, p. 5.

17. M. E. Shils, Nutritional problems in cancer patients, in *Nutrition in Disease* (Columbus, Ohio: Ross Laboratories, August, 1976).

18. M. A. Mishkel and D. J. Nazir, The linoleic acid and *trans* fatty acids of margarines (letter to the editor), *American Journal of Clinical Nutrition* 33 (1980): 2055-2056.

19. Food and Nutrition Board, National Research Council, National Academy of Sciences, *Towards Healthful Diets,* as reprinted in *Nutrition Today,* May/June 1980, pp. 7-11.

For Further Information, Controversy 5B

A new research finding not discussed here is the relation between coffee drinking and cancer of the pancreas. The reader will want to keep an eye out for further developments, but the pioneering work was:

- MacMahon, B., Yen, S., Trichopoulos, D., Warren, K., and Nardi, G. Coffee and cancer of the pancreas. *New England Journal of Medicine* 304 (1981): 630-633.

Another topic not treated has to do with the effects of substances in combination, such as sugar and fat, or alcohol and smoking:

- Hunter, K.; Linn, M. W.; and Harris, R. Dietary patterns and cancer of the digestive tract in older patients. *Journal of the American Geriatrics Society* 28 (1980): 405-409.

A major conference was held in the summer of 1978. The highlights of that conference, which included discussions of nutrition both as a cause of cancer and as a part of cancer therapy, are summed up in:

- Hartley, H. L. National conference on nutrition in cancer. *Nutrition Today,* September/October 1978, pp. 6-13, 24-29.

For additional references on the relations between fat and cancer, and specifically on the roles of the *trans*-fatty acids and fiber, see:

- Whitney, E. N., and Hamilton, E. M. N. Highlight 2: Fat and cancer. In *Understanding Nutrition,* 2d ed. St. Paul: West, 1981.

The relationships between nutrition and cancer are so many, and so much is being learned about them, that a new journal has been started to publish the findings: *Nutrition and Cancer,* available from 6503 Pyle Road, Bethesda MD 20034. There are also two good reference books on the subject:

- Winick, M., ed. *Nutrition and Cancer.* Somerset, NJ: Wiley, 1977.
- Whelan, E. *Preventing Cancer.* New York: Norton, 1978.

For the general reader who wants to supply the best nutritional care possible for a cancer patient, the American Cancer Society has many helpful booklets. Examples:

- *Nutrition for Patients Receiving Chemotherapy and Radiation Treatment* (for the patient).
- *Nutrition and Cancer* (for the professional).

Look up the society in your phone book.

The National Cancer Institute also makes available many useful publications. One of the best is:

- *Diet and Nutrition: A Resource for Parents of Children with Cancer.* NIH publication no. 80-2038, December 1979

This booklet can be obtained from USDHHS (address in Appendix J).

Another excellent resource is a recent issue of *Nutrition Today*, which was entitled "Cancer Patient Nourishment":

- *Nutrition Today*, May/June, 1981.

Controversy 6—Liquid Protein

1. W. H. Griffith, Food as a regulator of metabolism, *American Journal of Clinical Nutrition* 17 (1965): 391-398.
2. Griffith, 1965.
3. D. M. Matthews and S. A. Adibi, Peptide absorption, *Gastroenterology* 71 (1976): 151-161.
4. R. Chernoff and A. S. Block, Liquid feedings: Considerations and alternatives, *Journal of the American Dietetic Association* 70 (1977): 389-391.
5. Interdisciplinary Cluster on Nutrition of the President's Biomedical Research Panel, Assessment of the state of nutrition science, Part 2, *Nutrition Today*, January/February 1977, pp. 24-27.
6. L. B. Bailey and H. E. Clark, Plasma amino acids and nitrogen retention of human subjects who consumed isonitrogenous diets containing rice and wheat or their constituent amino acids with and without additional lysine, *American Journal of Clinical Nutrition* 29 (1976): 1353-1358.
7. A. A. Albanese and L. A. Orto, The proteins and amino acids, in *Modern Nutrition in Health and Disease*, ed. R. S. Goodhart and M. E. Shils, 5th ed. (Philadelphia: Lea and Febiger, 1973), p. 37.
8. S. R. Williams, *Nutrition and Diet Therapy*, 3d ed. (St. Louis: Mosby, 1973), p. 464.
9. G. L. Blackburn and J. Flatt, Preservation of lean body mass during acute weight reduction, *Federation Proceedings* 32 (1973): 916. This was was cited in R. Linn and S. L. Stuart, *The Last Chance Diet* (New York: Bantam Books, 1977), bibliography.
10. Linn and Stuart, 1977.
11. P. Girard, Liquid protein new diet weapon, *Atlanta Journal*, October 21, 1977.
12. C. K. Cyborski, Deaths associated with the protein-sparing diet (Questions and Answers), *Journal of the American Medical Association* 239 (1978): 971.
13. FDA Field Services Division, Deaths associated with liquid protein diets, *Morbidity Mortality Weekly Report* 26 (1977): 383.
14. FDA Field Services Division, 1977; P. Felig, Four questions about protein diets, *New England Journal of Medicine* 298 (1978): 1025-1026.

15. G. L. Blackburn, The "liquid protein" controversy—a closer look at the facts, *Obesity and Bariatric Medicine* 7 (January-February 1978): 25-28.

16. R. W. Barclay, Low-calorie protein supplements (Legislative Highlights), *Journal of the American Dietetic Association* 72 (1978): 422.

17. R. A. Fouty, Liquid protein diet magnesium deficiency and cardiac arrest (letter to the editor), *Journal of the American Medical Association* 240 (1978): 2632-2633; M. J. Moore, Liquid protein diets and electrolyte deficiency (letter to the editor), *Journal of the American Medical Association* 241 (1979): 1464.

18. W. E. Jarvis, Myocardial tissue concentrations of magnesium and potassium in men dying suddenly from ischemic heart disease (letter to the editor); and C. J. Johnson, Reply to letter by Jarvis, *American Journal of Clinical Nutrition* 33 (1980): 176.

19. M. A. Hilton, Nutritional need for sulfur amino acids in the "liquid protein" diet—a hypothesis, *Obesity and Bariatric Medicine* 8 (March-April 1979): 49-52.

20. L. M. Klevay, Copper deficiency with liquid protein diet? (letter to the editor), *New England Journal of Medicine* 300 (1979): 241.

21. M. Arenberg, S. E. Warren, W. V. R. Vieweg, G. L. Blackburn, D. H. Hastings, R. R. Michiel, A. Frank, B. R. Bistrian, and P. Felig, "Liquid protein diets" and "protein-sparing modified fast" (correspondence), *New England Journal of Medicine* 299 (1978): 419-421.

22. Liquid protein warning (update), *FDA Consumer* 14 (June 1980): 2.

23. L. M. Henderson, Programs to combat nutritional quackery, *Nutrition Reviews/Supplement: Nutrition Misinformation and Food Faddism*, July 1974, pp. 67-70.

Controversy 7—Athletes

1. American Dietetic Association, Nutrition and physical fitness (a statement), *Journal of the American Dietetic Association* 76 (1980): 437-443.

2. M. E. Shils, Food and nutrition relating to work and environmental stress, in *Modern Nutrition in Health and Disease*, R. S. Goodhart and M. E. Shils, 5th ed. (Philadelphia: Lea and Febiger, 1973), pp. 711-729; O. Mickelson, Nutrition and athletics, *Food and Nutrition News* 41 (April 1970), reprinted in *The Nutrition Crisis: A Reader*, ed. T. P. Labuza (St. Paul: West, 1975), pp. 228-231; M. H. Williams, *Nutritional Aspects of Human Physical and Athletic Performance* (Springfield, Ill.: Charles C. Thomas, 1976).

3. D. R. Lamb, Androgens and exercise, *Medicine and Science in Sports* 7 (1975): 1-5.

4. Lamb, 1975; N. J. Smith, Gaining and losing weight in athletics, *Journal of the American Medical Association* 236 (1976): 149-151.

5. Smith, 1976.

6. Nutrition and athletic performance, *Dairy Council Digest* 46 (1976).

7. T. J. Bassler, Body build and mortality (letter to the editor), *Journal of the American Medical Association* 244 (1980): 1437.

8. ATP is adenosine triphosphate and CP is creatine phosphate. For more about the way these compounds work, look them up in E. N. Whitney and E. M. N. Hamilton, *Understanding Nutrition*, 2d ed. (St. Paul: West, 1981), or in a beginning biology book.

9. Nutrition and athletic performance, 1976.

10. F. I. Katch, W. D. McArdle, and B. R. Boylan, *Getting in Shape* (Boston: Houghton Mifflin, 1979), p. 109.

11. P. Slovic, What helps the long distance runner run? *Nutrition Today* 10 (3) (1975): 18-21.

12. Nutrition and athletic performance, 1976.

13. I am indebted to Dr. Sam Smith for suggesting this summary.
14. Nutrition and athletic performance, 1976.
15. Mickelson, 1970.
16. J. Bergstrom and E. Hultman, Nutrition for maximal sports performance, *Journal of the American Medical Association* 221 (1972): 999.
17. S. Wintsch, Beading the heat, *Science '81* 2 (1981): 80-82.
18. Wintsch, 1981.
19. Wintsch, 1981.
20. Wintsch, 1981.
21. T. W. Bunch, Blood test abnormalities in runners, *Mayo Clinic Proceedings* 55 (1980): 113-117; S. H. Vitousek, Is more better? *Nutrition Today*, November/December 1979, pp. 10-17.
22. D. L. Costill, A scientific approach to distance running, *Track and Field News* (Los Altos, Calif.: 1979), p. 22.
23. Mickelson, 1970.

For Further Information

Recommended references on all aspects of nutrition are listed in Appendix J. In addition, books of special interest to the athlete are:

- Katch, F. I.; McArdle, W. D.; and Boylan, B. R. *Getting in Shape, an Optimum Approach to Fitness and Weight Control.* Boston: Houghton Mifflin, 1979.
- Smith, N. J. *Food for Sport.* Palo Alto, Calif.: Bull Publishing, 1976.
- Williams, M. H. *Nutritional Aspects of Human Physical and Athletic Performance.* Springfield, Ill.: Charles C. Thomas, 1976.

Two important articles are:

- Bergstrom, J., and Hultman, E. Nutrition for maximal sports performance. *Journal of the American Medical Association* 221 (1972): 999-1006.
- Gunby, P. Increasing numbers of physical changes found in nation's runners (Medical News). *Journal of the American Medical Association* 245 (1981): 547-548.

The view was presented here that "athlete's anemia" is an adaptation to training and not a true anemia. An alternative view, that athletes absorb less and excrete more iron than nonathletes, is presented in:

- Ehn, L.; Carlmark, B.; and Hoglund, S. Iron status in athletes involved in intense physical activity. *Medicine and Science in Sports and Exercise* 12 (1980): 61-64.

The entire issue of *Nutrition Today*, November/December 1979, was devoted to food and sports and makes very interesting reading, although many statements are of questionable accuracy.

Controversy 8—Ideal Body Weight

1. A. Keys, Overweight, obesity, coronary heart disease and mortality, *Nutrition Reviews* 38 (1980): 297-307. This lecture was also published in *Nutrition Today*, July/August 1980, pp. 16-22.

2. E. J. Drenick, G. S. Bale, F. Seltzer, and D. G. Johnson, Excessive mortality and causes of death in morbidly obese men, *Journal of the American Medical Association* 243 (1980): 443-445.

3. P. Gunby, A little (body) fat may not hasten death (Medical News), *Journal of the American Medical Association* 244 (1980): 1660. For men, the corresponding figure was 125 to 139 percent of "ideal."

4. J. V. G. A. Durnin, Sex differences in energy intake and expenditure. *Proceedings of the Nutrition Society* 35 (September 1976): 145-154.

5. W. A. Check and J. Elliott, Obesity may reduce survival, increase risk, in breast cancer (Medical News), *Journal of the American Medical Association* 244 (1980): 419-420.

6. L. G. Alonso and T. H. Maren, Effect of food restriction on body composition of hereditary obese mice, *American Journal of Physiology* 183 (1955): 284-290; reprinted as a "Nutrition Classic" in *Nutrition Reviews* 38 (1980): 317-320.

7. G. A. Bray and L. A. Campfield, Metabolic factors in the control of energy stores, *Metabolism* 24 (1975): 99-117.

8. J. V. G. A. Durnin, O. G. Edholm, D. S. Miller, and J. C. Waterlow, How much food does man require? *Nutrition Today*, January/February 1974, p. 28.

9. C. Abraira, M. de Bartolo, and J. W. Myscofski, Comparison of unmeasured versus exchange diabetic diets in lean adults: Body weight and feeding patterns in a 2-year prospective pilot study, *American Journal of Clinical Nutrition* 33 (1980): 1064-1070.

10. Human obesity and adipocyte function, *Nutrition Reviews* 36 (1978): 140-141.

11. The First Ross Conference on Medical Research included a number of papers touching on this problem. For example: J. S. Garrow, Energy balance in obesity, in *Report of the First Ross Conference*, ed. J. Kinney (Columbus, Ohio: Ross Laboratories, 1980), pp. 134-138.

12. E. A. Newsholme, A possible metabolic basis for the control of body weight (Sounding Board), *New England Journal of Medicine* 302 (1980): 400-405.

13. Role of brown fat in obesity, *Nutrition and the MD*, October 1980; J. Elliott, Blame it all on brown fat now (medical news), *Journal of the American Medical Association* 243 (1980): 1983-1985.

14. Food and Nutrition Board, National Research Council, National Academy of Sciences, *Towards Healthful Diets*, as reprinted in *Nutrition Today*, May/June 1980, pp. 7-11.

15. D. M. Hegsted, Energy needs and energy utilization, in *Nutrition Reviews' Present Knowledge in Nutrition*, 4th ed. (Washington, D.C.: Nutrition Foundation, 1976), pp. 1-9.

16. B. B. Alford and M. L. Bogle, *Nutrition and the Life Cycle* (Englewood Cliffs, N.J.: Prentice-Hall, forthcoming).

17. F. Davidoff, Medical therapies for diabetes: Do they work? *Journal of American Dietetic Association* 71 (1977): 495-500.

For Further Information

The major paper from which the information in this Controversy was taken is:

- Keys, A. Overweight, obesity, coronary heart disease and mortality. *Nutrition Reviews* 38 (1980): 297-307. This lecture was also published in *Nutrition Today*, July/August 1980, pp. 16-22.

Among the many references showing the anomalies and discrepancies in people's energy balances and body weights are two excellent reviews:

- Hegsted, D. M. Energy needs and energy utilization.
- Barnes, R. H. Energy.

These appear as Chapters 1 and 2 (pp. 1-9 and 10-16) in *Nutrition Reviews' Present Knowledge in Nutrition*, 4th ed. (Washington, D.C.: Nutrition Foundation, 1976).

Controversy 9—Vitamin B_{15}

1. Most of this story follows closely the excellent review of the history of pangamate: V. Herbert, Pangamic acid ("vitamin B_{15}"), *American Journal of Clinical Nutrition* 32 (1979): 1534-1540.
2. Herbert, 1979.
3. Herbert, 1979.
4. V. Herbert, as quoted in: B_{15} blarney, *ACSH News and Views*, April 1980, pp. 4-5.
5. B_{15} blarney, 1980.
6. American Council of Science and Health, as quoted by ABC World News Tonight, April 1980.
7. Herbert, 1979.
8. Other names you may have read on labels or in literature making exaggerated claims are p-aminobenzoic acid (PABA), hesperidin, lipoic acid, and ubiquinone. These are not vitamins and are not needed by humans. V. Herbert, The vitamin craze, *Archives of Internal Medicine* 140 (1980): 173-176.
9. M. Fisk, ed., *Encyclopedia of Associations*, 11th ed. (Detroit: Gale Research Company, Book Tower, 1977) Look for the latest edition of this reference book.
10. L. M. Henderson, Programs to combat nutritional quackery, *Nutrition Reviews/Supplement: Nutrition Misinformation and Food Faddism*, July 1974, pp. 67-70.
11. The American Medical Association supported such a committee for many years, and the American Dietetic Association also formed such a committee to clear up major misunderstandings about nutrition.

For Further Information

Some fascinating and very readable stories of the kind recounted in this Controversy are told in many of the references listed in Appendix J and at the ends of Controversies 1 and 2. With reference to B vitamins in particular we especially recommend the articles by Herbert referred to in this Controversy's notes.

Controversy 10A—Iron Superenrichment

1. Council on Foods and Nutrition, Iron in enriched wheat flour, farina, bread, buns, and rolls, *Journal of the American Medical Association* 220 (1972): 13-17.
2. Food and Nutrition Board, National Academy of Sciences/National Research Council, Recommendation for increased iron levels in the American diet, 1969 (reprint).
3. Council on Foods, 1972.
4. Iron overload conditions, known as hemochromatosis and hemosiderosis, are described in C. V. Moore, Major minerals, in *Modern Nutrition in Health and Disease*, ed. R. S. Goodhart and M. E. Shils, 5th ed. (Philadelphia: Lea and Febiger, 1973), pp. 297-323.
5. W. H. Crosby, Current concepts in nutrition: Who needs iron? *New England Journal of Medicine* 297 (1977): 543-545. There is an exception to this generalization; see the discussion of athletes' anemia in Controversy 7.

6. P. C. Elwood, The enrichment debate, *Nutrition Today*, July/August 1977, pp. 18-24.
7. This accusation really isn't quite fair. Enrichment is directed at considerably more than 2 percent of the population, and very few would be at risk for iron overload.
8. Elwood, 1977.
9. S. M. Garn, N. J. Smith, and D. C. Clark, The magnitude and the implications of apparent race differences in hemoglobin values, *American Journal of Clinical Nutrition* 28 (1975): 563-568.
10. H. A. Dymsza, Supplementation of foods vs nutrition education: Nutritional improvement debate, in *The Nutrition Crisis: A Reader*, ed. T. P. Labuza (St. Paul: West, 1975), pp. 129-133.
11. M. M. Wintrobe, The proposed increase in the iron fortification of wheat products, *Nutrition Today*, November/December 1973, pp. 18-20.
12. B. Borenstein, Supplementation of foods vs nutrition education: Nutritional improvement debate, in Labuza, 1975, pp. 134-137; and P. A. Lachance and H. Kiesel, Supplementation of foods vs nutrition education: Nutritional improvement debate, in Labuza, 1975, pp. 141-145.
13. E. W. Speckmann and D. McAfee, Supplementation of foods vs nutrition education: Nutritional improvement debate, in Labuza, 1975, pp. 138-141.
14. P. C. Elwood and D. Hughes, Clinical trial of iron therapy on psychomotor function in anaemic women, *British Medical Journal* 3 (1970): 254-255.
15. Crosby, 1977.
16. Elwood, l977.
17. Elwood, 1977.
18. G. W. Gardner, V. R. Edgerton, B. Senewiratne, R. J. Bernard and H. Ohira, Physical work capacity and metabolic stress in subjects with iron deficiency anemia, *American Journal of Clinical Nutrition* 30 (1977): 910-917.
19. E. Pollitt and R. L. Leibel, Iron deficiency and behavior, *Journal of Pediatrics* 88 (1978): 372-381.
20. R. L. Leibel, Behavioral and biochemical correlates of iron deficiency: A review, *Journal of the American Dietetic Association* 71 (1977): 398-404.
21. Interdisciplinary Cluster on Nutrition of the President's Biomedical Research Panel, Assessment of the state of nutrition science, part 2, *Nutrition Today*, January/February 1977, pp. 24-27.
22. Crosby, 1977.
23. Council on Foods, 1972.
24. Anatomy of a decision, *Nutrition Today*, January/February 1978, pp. 6-10, 28-29.
25. Council on Foods, 1972.

For Further Information, Controversy 10A

The superenrichment debate was covered in a lively issue of *Nutrition Today*:

- *Nutrition Today*, July/August 1977.

A more general debate over the question whether to fortify foods or to educate consumers about diet appears on pages 129-145 of:

- LaBuza, T. P. *The Nutrition Crisis: A Reader* St. Paul: West, 1975.

For an insight into the subtle effects of early iron deficiency, read Leibel's 1977 article cited in this Controversy's notes. The other items in the notes are also recommended.

Controversy 10B—Fluoridation

1. E. R. Schlesinger, D. E. Overton, H. C. Chase, and K. T. Cantwell, Newburgh-Kingston caries-fluorine study, 12: Pediatric findings after 10 years, *Journal of the American Dental Association* 52 (1956): 296-306.
2. D. S. Bernstein, N. Sadowsky, D. M. Hegsted, C. D. Guri and F. J. Stare, Prevalence of osteoporosis in high- and low-fluoride areas in North Dakota, *Journal of the American Medical Association* 198 (1966): 499-504. The water in the low-fluoride area contained 0.3 ppm, and the water in the high-fluoride area contained 4 to 5.8 ppm.
3. F. H. Nielsen, Are nickle, vanadium, silicon, fluoride, and tin essential for man? A review, *American Journal of Clinical Nutrition* 27 (1974): 515-520.
4. Food and Nutrition Board, Committee on Recommended Allowances, *Recommended Dietary Allowances*, 9th ed. (Washington, D.C.: National Academy of Sciences, 1980), pp. 156-159.
5. National Nutrition Consortium endorses fluoridation, *Journal of the American Dietetic Association* 70 (1977): 354.
6. National Nutrition Consortium—progress notes, *Journal of the American Dietetic Association* 71 (1977): 59, 63.
7. Letters to the editor, *Journal of Nutrition Education* 11 (October-December 1979): 162-168.

For Further Information, Controversy 10B

A well-researched review of the health benefits of fluoridation is:

- Richmond, V. L. Health effects associated with water fluoridation. *Journal of Nutrition Education* 11 (April-June 1979): 62-64.

This and the letters to the editor, together with the author's response, which appeared in the October-December issue of the *Journal* (pp. 162-168), are highly recommended reading.

Controversy 11A—Freedom of Choice

1. R. S. Goodhart and M. E. Shils, eds., *Modern Nutrition in Health and Disease*, 6th ed. (Philadelphia: Lea and Febiger, 1980).
2. A. E. Harper, Nutritional regulations and legislation: Past developments, future implications, *Journal of the American Dietetic Association* 71 (1977): 601-609.
3. H. S. White, Freedom of choice (Viewpoint), *Journal of Nutrition Education* 10, October-December 1978: 150-151.
4. Harper, 1977.
5. White, 1978.
6. R. C. Atkins and S. Linde, Nutrition medicine: A vitamin and mineral program, in *Dr. Atkins' Superenergy Diet*, reprinted in L. Hofmann, ed., *The Great American Nutrition Hassle* (Palo Alto, Calif.: Mayfield Publishing, 1978), pp. 185-204.
7. National Nutrition Consortium, Laetrile (vitamin B_{17})—a statement, *Journal of the American Dietetic Association* 70 (1977): 354.

8. Toxicity of laetrile, *FDA Drug Bulletin*, November/December 1977, pp. 26, 31-32.
9. Harper, 1977.
10. Laetrile: The political success of a scientific failure (editorial), *Consumer Reports* 42 (August 1977): 444-447.
11. Harper, 1977.
12. C. G. Moertel, A trial of laetrile now, *New England Journal of Medicine* 298 (1978): 218.
13. Laetrile fails, study finds, *Tallahassee Democrat*, May 1, 1981.
14. E. S. Parham, Comparison of responses to bans on cyclamate (1969) and saccharin (1977), *Journal of the American Dietetic Association* 72 (1978): 59-62.
15. D. Kennedy, What animal research says about cancer, *Human Nature*, May 1978, pp. 84-89.
16. *Nutrition Today*, July/August 1977, p. 4.
17. J. Verrett and J. Carper, *Eating May Be Hazardous to Your Health* (New York: Simon and Schuster, 1974), p. 96, as cited by Hofmann, 1978, p. 333.
18. R. D. Lyons, FDA may be ultimate challenge to Carter's pledge on reorganization and consumer aid, *New York Times*, March 15, 1977.

For Further Information, Controversy 11A

To help you keep track of consumer issues the FDA deals with, including foods, drugs, and cosmetics, we highly recommend the lively and colorful magazine:

- *FDA Consumer.*

To get an independent consumer view of the same issues, try the following, available in almost every library:

- *Consumer Reports.*

Controversy 11B—Saccharin and Nitrites

1. G. R. Howe, J. D. Burch, and A. B. Miller, Artificial sweeteners and human bladder cancer, *Lancet*, September 17, 1977, pp. 578-581.
2. Nitrite will not be banned say government agencies, *The Nation's Health*, October 1980. This newspaper is a publication of the American Public Health Association.
3. National Research Council, as quoted in *Science News*112 (July 2, 1977): 12-13.
4. T. H. Jukes, Fact and fancy in nutrition and food science, *Journal of the American Dietetic Association* 59 (1971): 203-211.
5. Jukes, 1971.
6. The final National Academy of Sciences report concluded that it was saccharin alone, and not any associated impurities, that was most likely responsible for the carcinogenic effect. P. B. Hutt and E. Sloan, NAS issues saccharin report, *Nutrition Policy Issues*, March 1979. This publication is a newsletter from General Mills, Inc.
7. B. L. Cohen, Relative risks of saccharin and calorie ingestion, *Science* 199 (1978): 983.
8. R. N. La Du, Analysis of the National Academy of Sciences Food Safety Report, *Food Technology* 33 (November 1979): 53-56.
9. Nitrite research studies evaluated, *School Foodservice Journal* 32 (November-December 1978): 20-24.

10. C. A. Thomson and I. S. Sheremate, Current issues in infant feeding, *Journal of the Canadian Dietetic Association* 39 (July 1978): 189-194.
11. C. Lecos, Fructose: questionable diet aid, *FDA Consumer*, March 1980, 20-23.
12. Update on nitrites, *Nutrition and the MD*, June 1979.
13. E. Whelan, quoted in the following headline: Stop banning things at the drop of a rat, *New World*, November 24, 1979.
14. S. A. Miller, Achieving food safety through regulation, *Food Technology* 33 (November 1979): 57-60.
15. M. Hollands and J. Goeller, A guideline to the use of saccharin, *Journal of the Canadian Dietetic Association* 38 (July 1977): 198. Abstract cited in *Journal of the American Dietetic Association* 71 (1977): 572.
16. There is a greater likelihood of nitrites forming from the nitrates in these vegetables than there is of finding nitrites in the commercial baby-food equivalents. Thomson and Sheremate, 1978.

For Further Information, Controversy 11B

A very readable, thought-provoking series of four articles on food safety regulation appeared in the November 1979 issue of *Food Technology*.

- Zeckhauser, R. Social and economic factors in food safety decision-making. Pp. 47-52, 60.
- La Du, R. N. Analysis of the National Academy of Sciences Food Safety Report. Pp. 53-56.
- Miller, S. A. Achieving food safety through regulation. Pp. 57-60.
- Brown, C. J. Revising the U.S. food safety policy: Government viewpoint. Pp. 61-64.

The saccharin debate is far from over. Some of the newer issues about human risks are raised in an argument in the pages of the:

- *New England Journal of Medicine* 303 (1980): 341-342.

A perspective on additives with two pages of interesting information about nitrates, nitrites, and nitrosamines is:

- Jukes, T. H. Food additives, in *Current Concepts in Nutrition*, a paperback book containing reprints from the *New England Journal of Medicine* 1977-1978 (Massachusetts Medical Society, 1979), pp. 13-22.

Controversy 12—Baby Killers

1. This testimony is as reported in: Infant formulas: Threat to Third World? *Science News*, June 3, 1978, p. 357.
2. Both Dr. Fomon and Dr. Latham are quoted in "Morality vs. Profits—Infant Formula Promotion in the Third World," a leaflet distributed by INFACT in 1978.
3. Dr. Jelliffe, as quoted by L. Edson, Babies in poverty, the real victims of the breast/bottle controversy, *The Lactation Review* IV: 1 (1979): 21-38. (The *Review* is available from 666 Sturges Highway, Westport, CT 06880.)
4. Infant formulas, 1978.

5. Morality vs. profits, 1978.

6. Nestle letter, 1978.

7. Morality vs. profits, 1978.

8. Morality vs. profits, 1978.

9. International Advisory Group on Infant and Child Feeding, The feeding of the very young: An approach to determination of policies, a report to the Nutrition Foundation, October 1978.

10. H. R. Muller, Infant nutrition today: A new rationale in infant feeding? in *Nestle Research News 197* (Lausanne, Switzerland: Nestle Products Technical Assistance Co. Ltd., 1976), pp. 12-23.

11. WHO/UNICEF meeting on infant and young child feeding, *WHO Chronicle* 33 (1979): 435-443. The other issues were: promotion and support of appropriate weaning practices; promotion of information, education, and training of health workers concerning breastfeeding; the health and social status of women in relation to infant and young child feeding; and suggested actions for governments and other groups.

12. Muller, 1976.

13. WHO/UNICEF meeting, 1979.

14. Edson, 1979.

15. The code was the subject of the WHO meeting in Geneva, May 4, 1981.

16. Breast-feeding code gets "no" vote from U.S., *Tallahassee Democrat*, May 21, 1981.

For Further Information

A history of the introduction of formula feeding with a background to the present controversy is presented in

- Schwab, M. G. The rise and fall of the baby's bottle. *Journal of Human Nutrition* 33 (1979): 276-282.

Highly recommended is the report of the WHO meeting with its closing resolutions:

- WHO/UNICEF meeting on infant and young child feeding. *WHO Chronicle* 33 (1979): 435-443.

Nutrition Today provided continuing coverage of the controversy over the WHO code and the United States vote during the summer of 1981. Especially recommended is the guest editorial by N. S. Scrimshaw. Dr. Scrimshaw is institute professor, Department of Nutrition and Food Science at Massachusetts Institute of Technology, and one of the United States' most highly respected authorities in nutrition and health problems in underdeveloped countries. He sees the controversy as oversimplified and the United States vote as "a disgrace to our nation":

- Scrimshaw, N. S. Code not cure. *Nutrition Today*, July/August 1981, pp. 11, 15.

An issue not dealt with here is whether breastfeeding inhibits ovulation so that the next birth is postponed. There are many research articles now published showing that it does, if frequent enough. Typical are:

- Konnwe, M., and Worthman, C. Nursing frequency, gonadal function, and birth spacing among !Kung hunter-gatherers, *Science* 207 (1980): 788-791.
- Knodel, J. Breast-feeding and population growth, *Science* 198 (1977): 1111-1115.
- Prema, K.; Naidu, A. N.; and Kumari, S. N. Lactation and fertility. *American Journal of Clinical Nutrition* 32 (1979): 1298-1303.
- Jelliffe, D. B., and Jelliffe, E. F. P. Postpartum amenorrhea: Hormones versus nutrition (letter to the editor). *American Journal of Clinical Nutrition* 31 (1978): 1977-1978.

• Delgado, H., Lechtig, A., Martorell, R., Brineman, E., and Klein, R. E. Nutrition, lactation, and postpartum amenorrhea. *American Journal of Clinical Nutrition* 31 (1978): 322-327.

A review that includes many additional references to the same effect is:

• Jackson, R. L. Maternal and infant nutrition and health in later life. *Nutrition Reviews* 37 (1979): 33-37.

If you want more information about the current state of affairs with respect to the conflict between INFACT and the Nestle Company, you can get the two sides from:

INFACT	The Nestle Company, Inc.
1701 University Avenue, S.E.	100 Bloomingdale Road
Minneapolis, MN 55414	White Plains, NY 10605

It is really Nestle/Europe, not the U.S.-based company, that INFACT has been fighting, but INFACT has felt that the only way to put pressure on the company effectively was to boycott its domestic branch.

Controversy 13—Hyperactivity

1. L. Eisenberg, The clinical use of stimulant drugs in children, *Pediatrics* 49 (1972): 709-715.
2. Institute of Food Technologists' Expert Panel on Food Safety and Nutrition and the Committee on Public Information, Diet and hyperactivity: Any connection? *Food Technology* 30 (April 1976): 29-34; B. F. Feingold, Hyperkinesis and learning disabilities linked to artificial food flavors and colors, *American Journal of Nursing* 75 (1975): 797-803.
3. M. Morrison, The Feingold diet (letter to the editor), *Science* 199 (1978): 840.
4. M. Nagy, Monosodium glutamate and the "Chinese restaurant syndrome," *Journal of the American Medical Association* 225 (1973): 1665.
5. L. Reif-Lehrer and M. G. Stemmerman, Monosodium glutamate intolerance in children (letter to the editor), *New England Journal of Medicine* 293 (1975): 1204-1205.
6. L. A. Barness, Pediatrics, in *Nutritional Support of Medical Practice*, ed. H. A. Schneider, C. E. Anderson, and D. B. Coursin (Hagerstown, Md.: Harper & Row Medical Department, 1977), pp. 441-462, especially pp. 452-454.
7. V. J. Fontana and F. Moreno-Pagan, Allergy and diet, in *Modern Nutrition in Health and Disease*, ed. R. S. Goodhart and M. E. Shils, 6th ed. (Philadelphia: Lea and Febiger, 1980): pp. 1071-1081.
8. Barness, 1977.
9. W. G. Crook, An alternative method of managing the hyperactive child (letter to the editor), *Pediatrics* 54 (1974): 656.
10. Barness, 1977.
11. Barness, 1977.
12. Update, *Journal of the American Dietetic Association* 70 (1977): 540.
13. National Advisory Committee on Hyperkinesis and Food Additives, *Final Report to the Nutrition Foundation*, October 1980.
14. National Advisory Committee, 1980.
15. Barness, 1977.
16. Eisenberg, 1972.
17. Health watch, *ACSH News and Views*, September/October 1980, p. 8.

18. R. L. Leibel, Behavioral and biochemical correlates of iron deficiency: A review, *Journal of the American Dietetic Association* 71 (1977): 399-404.

19. C. D. May, Food allergy—material and ethereal, *New England Journal of Medicine* 302 (1980): 1142-1143.

For Further Information

A thoughtful editorial by an allergist makes the necessary distinctions and lays down the methodology for the study of food allergy:

- May, C. D. Food allergy—material and ethereal. *New England Journal of Medicine* 302 (1980): 1142-1143.

The connections among malnutrition, learning, and behavior in children are clearly explained in a thirty-three-page pamphlet from the National Institutes of Health:

- National Institute of Child Health and Human Development, Center for Research for Mothers and Children. *Malnutrition, Learning, and Behavior.* DHEW publication no. (NIH) 76-1036. Washington, D.C.: Government Printing Office, 1976.

A review of the recent research on malnutrition and behavior, including 173 references, is:

- Brocek, J. Malnutrition and behavior: A decade of conferences. *Journal of the American Dietetic Association* 72 (1978): 17-23.

A cookbook that helps the parent prepare additive-free, "sugar"-free, milk-free, or grain-free meals for hyperactive/allergic children is the paperback:

- Robb, P. *Cooking for Hyperactive and Allergic Children.* Fort Wayne, Ind.: Cedar Creek Publishers, 1980.

Controversy 14A—Acne

1. Office of Research Reporting and Public Response, National Institute of Allergy and Infectious Diseases, National Institutes of Health, *Acne*, NIH Publication No. 80-188, USDHHS, May 1980.

2. Terminology: The oily secretion is *sebum*, the glands are the *sebaceous glands*, and the ducts through which the oil flows are those of the *hair follicles*.

3. O. A. Roels, Vitamin A physiology, *Journal of the American Medical Association* 214 (1970): 1097-1102; S. J. Yaffe and L. J. Filer, Jr., The use and abuse of vitamin A (American Academy of Pediatrics, joint committee statement on drugs and nutrition), *Pediatrics* 48 (1971): 655-656.

4. Acne, 1980.

5. G. Michaëlsson, L. Juhlin, and A. Vahlquist, Effects of oral zinc and vitamin A in acne, *Archives of Dermatology* 113 (1977): 31-36.

6. T. Cornbleet and I. Gigli, Should we limit sugar in acne? *Archives of Dermatology* 83 (1961): 968-969; J. E. Fulton, G. Plewig, and A. M. Kligman, Effect of chocolate on acne vulgaris, *Journal of the American Medical Association* 210 (1969): 2071-2074; R. M. Reisner, Acne vulgaris, *Pediatric Clinics of North America* 20 (1973): 851-864.

7. L. Goldman, Acne prevention in the family, *American Family Physician* 16 (August 1977): 68-71.

8. Dr. Benjamin L. Bivins, dermatologist, of Tallahassee, Florida, kindly supplied this and other information used in this report.

9. Goldman, 1977.

For Further Information, Controversy 14A

For general information about skin conditions in relation to nutrition, see the term *skin* in the index to this and other nutrition books listed in Appendix J. In reference to acne in particular, the pamphlet referred to in note 1, and the article by Goldman (note 7) are especially informative.

Controversy 14B— Doctors

1. J. B. Schorr, as quoted by L. Hofmann, ed., *The Great American Nutrition Hassle* (Palo Alto, Calif.: Mayfield, 1978), p. 399.
2. P. R. Lee, as quoted by Hofmann, 1978, p. 321.
3. M. Winick, as quoted by R. Kotulak, Many doctors ignorant of nutrition, *Chicago Tribune*, May 1977.
4. Tidbits and morsels, *Nutrition and the MD*, January 1978.
5. S. R. Williams, Nutritional guidance in prenatal care, in *Nutrition in Pregnancy and Lactation*, ed. B. S. Worthington, J. Vermeersch, and S. R. Williams (St. Louis: Mosby, 1977), p. 55.
6. Aside from these contributions, Adelle Davis's writings may have done more harm than good. She publicized many mistaken notions about nutrition, promoting health food fads and other unnecessary, dangerous, and expensive practices. Her book *Let's Eat Right to Keep Fit* (New York: Harcourt Brace Jovanovich), first published in 1946, is listed among the "Books Not Recommended" of the Chicago Nutrition Society, available from the American Medical Association (addresses in Appendix J).
7. E. S. Nelson, Nutrition instruction in medical schools—1976, *Journal of the American Medical Association* 236 (1976): 2534.
8. C. K. Cyborski, Nutrition content in medical curricula, *Journal of Nutrition Education* 9 (1977): 17-18.
9. W. J. Darby, The renaissance of nutrition education, *Nutrition Reviews* 35 (February 1977): 33-38.
10. Nelson, 1976.
11. C. F. Enloe, Jr., For whom the bell tolls (editorial), *Nutrition Today*, July/August 1973, p. 14.
12. J. Gutman, Physicians' exposure to health topics through mass media: An avenue for improving the dietitian's image, *Journal of the American Dietetic Association* 71 (1977): 505-509.
13. L. J. Filer and E. F. Calesa, Multi-media education about infant nutrition for physicians, *Journal of the American Dietetic Association* 72 (1978): 404-406.
14. Nutrition: No longer a stepchild in medicine (Medical News), *Journal of the American Medical Association* 238 (1977): 2245.
15. C. A. Hall, L. J. Howard, and J. A. Halsted, The clinical nutrition program at Albany Medical College, *Nutrition Today*, September/October-November/December 1975, pp. 31-33. Albany was not the first to inaugurate such a program, but this brief description provides a model for others to follow.
16. C. E. Butterworth, The skeleton in the hospital closet, *Nutrition Today*, March/April 1974, pp. 4-8. Dr. Butterworth is professor of medicine and pediatrics and director of the Nutrition Program at the University of Alabama in Birmingham and chairman of the Council on Foods and Nutrition of the American Medical Association.

17. Butterworth, 1974.

18. G. L. Blackburn and B. R. Bistrian, A report from Boston, *Nutrition Today*, May/June 1974, p. 30. Dr. Blackburn is assistant professor of surgery, Harvard University; research associate, Department of Nutrition and Food Science, Massachusetts Institute of Technology; and director of the Intensive Care Unit and Nutritional Services, Boston City and New England Deaconess Hospitals. Dr. Bistrian is research associate, Department of Nutrition and Food Science, Massachusetts Institute of Technology; visiting physician, Department of Medicine, Boston City Hospital; and research assistant, New England Deaconess Hospital.

19. A. Fonaroff, Undernutrition (letter to the editor), *Journal of the American Medical Association* 237 (1977): 1825-1826.

20. An example of such a hospital survey is reported by H. N. Jacobson, Dietary practices, services and trends in the teaching hospitals in New Jersey, *Nutrition Today*, September/October-November/December 1975, pp. 14-18.

21. Veterans Administration Hospital, New York City, Height and weight data in the patient's medical record, *Journal of the American Dietetic Association* 72 (1978): 409-410.

22. C. E. Butterworth and G. L. Blackburn, Hospital malnutrition, *Nutrition Today*, March/April 1975, pp. 8-18. *Nutrition Today* has since made available a teaching aid on this subject (lecture and slide presentation); see address in Appendix J.

23. J. E. Wade, Role of a clinical dietitian specialist on a nutrition support service, *Journal of the American Dietetic Association* 70 (1977): 185-189.

24. This view was expressed in a letter to the editor of the *Journal of the American Medical Association* suggesting that the recognition of the importance of nutrition in surgery was the fourth major advance in the field: J. C. Stevens, Surgical nutrition: The fourth coming, *Journal of the American Medical Association* 239 (1978): 192.

25. G. L. Blackburn and B. R. Bistrian, Curative nutrition: Protein-calorie management, in H. A. Schneider, C. E. Anderson, and D. B. Coursin, eds., *Nutritional Support of Medical Practice* (Hagerstown, Md.: Harper & Row Medical Department, 1977), pp. 80-100.

26. N. E. Schwartz and S. I. Barr, Mothers: Their attitudes and practices in perinatal nutrition, *Journal of Nutrition Education* 9 (1977): 169-172.

27. B. K. Hollen, Attitudes and practices of physicians concerning breast-feeding and its management, *Journal of Tropical Pediatrics and Environmental Child Health* 22 (December 1976): 288-293.

28. J. T. Dwyer and J. Mayer, Beyond economics and nutrition: The complex basis of food policy, *Science* 188 (1975): 566-570. Dr. Dwyer is director of the Frances Stern Nutrition Center, New England Medical Center Hospital; associate professor, Tufts University School of Medicine; and lecturer in maternal and child nutrition, Harvard School of Public Health. Dr. Mayer, professor of nutrition at Harvard University from 1950 to 1976, is now president of Tufts University.

29. Task force, John E. Fogarty International Center for Advanced Study in the Health Sciences, National Institutes of Health, and American College of Preventive Medicine, *Preventive Medicine, USA: Health Promotion and Consumer Health Education* (New York: Prodist, Neale Watson Academic Publications, 1976), pp. 48-49.

30. Task Force, 1976.

For Further Information, Controversy 14B

A high-quality textbook in nutrition for medical students is:

- Schneider, H. A.; Anderson, C. E.; and Coursin, D. B., eds. *Nutritional Support of Medical Practice*. Hagerstown, Md.: Harper & Row Medical Department, 1977.

But even medical students would do well to start first with a good introductory college text with an emphasis on foods.

Reading lists in nutrition for physicians are available from The Nutrition Foundation, Inc. (address in Appendix J). Also, free to physicians is Ross Labs' series of eleven papers on nutrition topics:

- *Nutrition Education for Physicians—Problems and Opportunities.* Ross Labs, 625 Cleveland Avenue, Columbus, OH 43215.

A newsletter is available that is a must for the busy doctor who wants to catch up and keep up:

- *Nutrition and the MD.*

Four to six pages of reading each month, this little newsletter features nutritional strategies in patient care, alerts the physician to new findings in the clinical literature (and cites its sources), notes important new publications, and provides authoritative answers to questions patients commonly ask. It is available from P.M., Inc., P.O. Box 2160, Van Nuys, CA 91405.

Controversy 15—Vitamin E

1. D. B. Menzel, Pulmonary medicine, in *Nutritional Support of Medical Practice*, ed. H. A. Schneider, C. E. Anderson and D. B. Coursin (Hagerstown, Md.: Harper & Row Medical Department, 1977), pp. 477-484.
2. Vitamin E and bronchopulmonary dysplasia, *Nutrition and the MD*, July 1979.
3. C. L. Natta, L. J. Machlin, and M. Brin, A decrease in irreversibly sickled erythrocytes in sickle cell anemia patients given vitamin E, *American Journal of Clinical Nutrition* 33 (1980): 968-971.
4. L. Corash, S. Spielberg, C. Bartsocas, L. Boxer, R. Steinherz, M. Sheetz, M. Egan, J. Schlessleman, and J. D. Schulman, Reduced chronic hemolysis during high-dose vitamin E administration in Mediterranean-type glucose-6-phosphate dehydrogenase deficiency, *New England Journal of Medicine* 303 (1980): 416-420.
5. C. F. Nockels, Protective effects of supplemental vitamin E against infection, *Federation Proceedings* 38 (1979): 2134-2138; B. E. Sheffy and R. D. Schultz, Influence of vitamin E and selenium on immune response mechanisms, *Federation Proceedings* 38 (1979): 2139-2143; M. K. Horwitt, Therapeutic uses of vitamin E in medicine, *Nutrition Reviews* 38 (1980): 105-113.
6. Horwitt, 1980.
7. Another use for vitamin E? (Medical News), *Journal of the American Medical Association* 243 (1980): 1025.
8. Vitamin E relieves most cystic breast disease; may alter lipids, hormones (Medical News), *Journal of the American Medical Association* 244 (1980): 1077-1078.
9. I. Machtey and L. Ouaknine, Tocopherol in osteoarthritis: A controlled pilot study, *Journal of the American Geriatrics Society* 26 (1978): 328-330.
10. Horwitt, 1980.
11. Expert Panel on Food Safety and Nutrition, Committee on Public Information, Institute of Food Technologists, Vitamin E, *Contemporary Nutrition* 2 (November 1977); A. L. Tappel, Vitamin E, *Nutrition Today*, July/August 1973, pp. 4-12; H. H. Draper, J. G. Bergan, M. Chiu, A. S. Csallany, and A. V. Boaro, A further study of the specificity of the vitamin E requirement for reproduction, *Journal of Nutrition* 84 (1964): 395-400.
12. R. E. Gillilan, B. Mondell, and J. R. Warbasse, Quantitative evaluation of vitamin E in the treatment of angina pectoris, *American Heart Journal* 93 (April 1977): 444-449; Vitamin E: A scientific status summary by the Institute of Food Technologists' Expert

Panel on Food Safety and Nutrition and the Committee on Public Information, *Food Technology* 31 (1977): 77-80.

13. E. T. G. Leonhardt, Effects of vitamin E on serum cholesterol and triglycerides in hyperlipidemic patients treated with diet and clofibrate, *American Journal of Clinical Nutrition* 31 (1978): 100-105.

14. Questions readers ask, *Nutrition and the MD*, May 1980.

15. Questions, 1980.

16. J. G. Bieri, Vitamin E, in *Nutrition Reviews' Present Knowledge in Nutrition*, 4th ed. (Washington, D.C.: Nutrition Foundation, 1976), pp. 98-110; Menzel, 1977; Committee on Safety, Toxicity, and Misuse of Vitamins and Trace Minerals, National Nutrition Consortium, Inc., *Vitamin-Mineral Safety, Toxicity, and Misuse* (Chicago: The American Dietetic Association, 1978).

17. J. S. Prasad, Effect of vitamin E supplementation on leukocyte function, *American Journal of Clinical Nutrition* 33 (1980): 606-608.

18. L. A. Barness, Nutritional aspects of vegetarianism, health foods, and fad diets, *Nutrition Reviews* 35 (1977): 153-157.

19. N. Y. J. Yang and I. D. Desai, Effect of high levels of dietary vitamin E on hematological indices and biochemical parameters in rats, *Journal of Nutrition* 107 (1977): 1410-1417.

20. V. Herbert, Vitamin E report (letter to the editor), *Nutrition Reviews* 35 (1977): 158.

21. N. B. Belloc and L. Breslow, Relationship of physical health status and health practices, *Preventive Medicine* 1 (1972):409-421.

For Further Information

The references listed in Appendix J provide abundant additional information about vitamin E. As for the aging process and its relation to nutrition, the information to be found in the following journals is generally reliable:

- *Geriatrics.*
- *The Gerontologist.*
- *Journal of the American Geriatrics Society.*
- *Journal of Gerontology.*

See also the references for Chapter 15.

Index

Numbers in bold face refer to pages where definitions are given.
Numbers followed by "t" refer to pages where a table appears.
Numbers in italics refer to pages where a figure appears.

A

B

C

D

E

F

G

H

I

J

K

M

N

O

P

T

U

X

Y

Z

†